THE PHYSICIAN MANAGER'S HANDBOOK

Essential Business Skills for Succeeding in Health Care

Robert J. Solomon, PhD
The College of William and Mary
Williamsburg, Virginia

AN ASPEN PUBLICATION®
Aspen Publishers, Inc.
Gaithersburg, Maryland
1997

Library of Congress Cataloging-in-Publication Data

Solomon, Robert J., 1947–
The physician manager's handbook: essential business skills for succeeding in health care/Robert J. Solomon.
p. cm.
Includes bibliographical references and index.
ISBN 0-8342-0768-0
1. Health services administration—United States—Handbooks, manuals, etc. 2. Health facilities—United States—Business management—Handbooks, manuals, etc. 3. Physician executives—United States—Handbooks, manuals, etc. I. Title.
[DNLM: 1. Practice management, Medical—organization & administration—United States. 2. Financial Management—organization & administration—United States. 3. Personnel Management—methods—United States. W 80 S689p 1997]
RA971.S677 1997
'.68—dc21
DNLM/DLC
for Library of Congress
96–24308
CIP

Orders: (800) 638-8437
Customer Service: (800) 234-1660

About Aspen Publishers • For more than 35 years, Aspen has been a leading professional publisher in a variety of disciplines. Aspen's vast information resources are available in both print and electronic formats. We are committed to providing the highest quality information available in the most appropriate format for our customers. Visit Aspen's Internet site for more information resources, directories, articles, and a searchable version of Aspen's full catalog, including the most recent publications: **http://www.aspenpub.com**
Aspen Publishers, Inc. • The hallmark of quality in publishing
Member of the worldwide Wolters Kluwer group

Editorial Resources: Sandra L. Lunsford
Library of Congress Catalog Card Number: 96-24308
ISBN: 0-8342-0768-0

Printed in the United States of America

1 2 3 4 5

Table of Contents

Acknowledgments

Many people made valuable contributions to my thinking about this book, as well as in some instances to its material content. In particular, I thank Jack Bruggeman, Aspen Publishers; Michael Camp, VHA; William Geary, Ph.D.,The College of William and Mary; Kevin Hendricks, Ph.D., The College of William and Mary; Alfred Herzog, M.D., Hartford Hospital; Kevin Hutchinson, VHA; Irving M. Pike, M.D., Gastroenterology Consultants, Ltd.; James Roberts, M.D., VHA; and Alan Snell, M.D., Memorial Health System.

The following individuals reviewed parts of the manuscript. Their comments were very helpful: Henry Mallue, J.D., Ed.D., The College of William and Mary; Garland Tillery; and Godwin T. White, Ph.D., C.P.A., The College of William and Mary.

In addition, I want to thank my wife, Bernadette Jones, L.C.S.W., B.C.D., who deserves credit in two regards. First, she was instrumental in adjusting our lives to all that was necessary in order to complete this project. Second, she first enunciated and then evolved two of the most powerful management themes that are expressed in this book, responsibility and consequence, and had the courage to put them into effect in her own practice.

CHAPTER 1

Succeeding as a Physician Manager: Essential Business Skills

Many physicians think of physician managers as having developed an alternative employment path to traditional clinical practice. Generally, this path is seen as one that emphasizes management responsibility instead of clinical practice, in some cases to the total exclusion of clinical practice. The focus of this book is at odds with this limited view of the physician manager. It is my contention that management skills should now be an essential part of the physician's repertoire and that physicians who don't possess these skills are less able to provide their patients with the highest levels of clinical care as well as personally survive and prosper in the current health care environment.

At the core of the physician manager's job description is the use of medical knowledge, medical technology, physicians, and "medical thinking" to help organizations make better medical and management decisions. Managers who are trained only in administration cannot adequately bring medical considerations into the decision-making process. Physicians who are not knowledgeable about business concepts and language cannot contribute effectively to discussions and decisions that have both medical and business aspects.

Physicians who possess management skills can more effectively consider and balance both the medical and the administrative aspects of an issue. Physicians who can communicate in the language of business can sit across the table from administrators and effectively represent the medical perspective because they understand the positions of both professional managers and physicians. Finally, physicians with business skills can best represent their own self-interests when working with their own employees, consultants, insurers, and other groups within and outside their organization.

Many physician managers are employed by large health care organizations, including hospitals, health maintenance organizations (HMOs), physician–hospital organizations, and large single-specialty or multispecialty private practices. There is another physician manager, however, who often is overlooked and who needs to be as much the physician manager as his or her colleagues working in large managed care organizations. This physician manager works in and probably owns part of a small group or solo practice. Historically, private practice physicians have always had to manage their practices' business affairs. Often, these responsibilities are undertaken by one physician, perhaps reluctantly, through default, rotation, or self-interest. All too often, important management responsibilities are delegated to a practice business manager, without physicians retaining appropriate control. This can be a formula for disaster because there are many situations in which a business manager's self-interest does not coincide with that of those who own the practice. Other physicians, realizing the importance of their participation in management decision making, actively manage their practices, although many do so without adequate management skills.

All these physicians are in situations that call for physician manager skills. The core of knowledge that physician managers need is the same irrespective of whether they manage in a large HMO, a solo private practice, or any organization in between. What varies as one progresses from a solo practice to a large managed care organization is the complexity of the situation, the amount of data available, and the degree to which and the immediacy with which decisions will directly affect you, the decision maker. All physician managers must become proficient in the *same* body of knowledge. *How* a physician uses this knowledge, and the extent to which it will be the central focus of his or her work, will vary depending upon the specific nature of the physician manager's responsibilities.

Medical practices, hospitals, and health care systems *are* businesses. Health care currently constitutes about 17 percent of the U.S. Gross National Product. Unfortunately, the recognition of this fact by physicians and those who train them is only now beginning to occur. Medicine has been slow to acquire management skills for two reasons. First, for most of the 20th century, medicine was very profitable. When times are good, patients are plentiful, and an industry is growing, many don't feel the need to operate efficiently. A thick salve of cash will cover many business mistakes and inefficiencies! Second, medical school and residency curricula are designed by academicians, who are often unfamiliar with and uninterested in the nonmedical aspects of health care. As a result, they generally

have no appreciation of the need for their students and their profession to acquire business and management skills. As a result, these skills are generally not adequately represented in their curricula.

The business skills that physician managers need are the same as those that top-level managers use in most other types of business. In some ways, health care organizations are like any other business, and thus physician managers can benefit from the methods and concepts that have proven useful in other types of organizations. For example, observing how long it takes to collect fees (aging of accounts) is an accepted business procedure that certainly has application in any health care organization. Similarly, utilizing marketing methods that result in an attractive medical product/service is as important to a practice or hospital as customer-focused products are to Wal-Mart. Understanding and managing how much it costs to provide a product or service are as critical to a managed care organization or a private practice evaluating a capitated contract as they are to an airplane manufacturer who is deciding whether to build a new aircraft. In short, the business skills that managers need are fundamentally the same irrespective of the industry. Therefore, the lessons learned by the IBMs, Wal-Marts, and Microsofts of the world do not have to be rediscovered through trial and error by physician managers.

THE PHYSICIAN MANAGER'S ROLE DEFINITION

In working and consulting with medical practices, I have seen two fundamental errors as physician managers try to determine their appropriate role. Some physician managers make the mistake of being a micro-manager. Micro-managers are looking over everyone's shoulder. They routinely second guess subordinates' daily operational decisions and in general become very intrusive in everyone's lives. This reduces employee discretion and initiative, and in some cases employees become fearful and resentful of not being trusted to do their work. In addition, practice-based micro-managing physician managers are doing less of what arguably is the most critical function in their job description, and what only they can do: generating revenue! Time devoted to micro-managing is time taken away from clinical work.

The other role definition mistake that physician managers may make is to be the absentee manager. These physician managers often say, "I hired a business manager and staff to take care of all that stuff." Going to this other extreme also creates problems. If the physician manager is totally uninvolved in important decisions, then choices will be made without your input, and perhaps without physician input. Subordinate managers and partners will make decisions reflecting their knowledge, self-interest, and professional perspective, which may or may not adequately represent your self-interest.

To help you define the appropriate level of physician manager involvement, I propose the following criteria. Physician managers should be involved enough in decision making to:

- know when they are getting a good job from employees and others. For example, you must know enough about employment methods so that you can lead your business manager or human resources director to move beyond unstructured anecdotal interviews. You personally will not be involved in the selection process. That would be getting too far down in the trenches unless the position was directly reporting to you, such as a surgical assistant. Your role in this case is to make certain that the *employment system* is functioning appropriately.
- ask questions and obtain critical information for decision making. For example, if you are on a hospital committee considering purchasing new ophthalmological surgery equipment, then you need to know enough to ask for the necessary financial information to make a *financially*, as well as medically, informed decision.
- set reasonable standards that meet your needs. For example, your health care system is in the process of selecting an electronic medical record (EMR). You have seen several of the proposed systems, and note that from a physician's perspective they are all deficient in fundamental ways, such as appropriate fields, intrusive data entry, decision support, etc. You need to have a vision of the physician manager's appropriate role in the EMR system selection and design process, so that you can say, "Wait! We are going about this in the wrong way! The process that we are using is wrong and we will invariably select or develop an inadequate EMR!"

PHYSICIAN MANAGER SKILLS

For physician managers to achieve these objectives, they must develop skills and comfort with several technical business skills. The skill areas in which physician managers need to develop proficiency form the chapters of this book. Below is a brief description of some of the major subject areas that are discussed in this book.

Management

Management is the glue that holds all organizations together. It is the process of obtaining, organizing, and directing all the human resources associated with a health care organization. Whether you manage in a solo practice with one secretary, in a group practice with many physicians and diverse job descriptions, or in a large hospital system, the quality of management will determine whether personnel operate as an effective team. In some organizations, employees and groups are constantly fighting border disputes; in others, they work together synergistically to achieve a common vision of what needs to be achieved.

There are many aspects of managing a health care organization's human resources. They include the following:

- *Leadership:* guiding and inspiring physician and nonphysician employees to work toward your vision of what needs to be achieved. This vision may include incorporating others' perspectives and totally delegating a decision to them. Leadership skills can range from being directive, to consulting with others, to delegating tasks to others. It can also involve empowering others, such as giving subordinates decision-making responsibilities that might normally be reserved for more senior managers. Often, in larger health care organizations, physician managers are working with groups of employees where there is no clear manager–subordinate relationship. Physician managers also must learn, therefore, to lead where they don't have line control. Leadership therefore is not only leading through inspiration but knowing how to involve others, when to be directive, and when to hand off a decision to others.

- *Performance appraisal:* evaluating the job performance of employees, and using this information to make personnel decisions, such as training needed, compensation, discipline, termination, and the like. Appraisal of physician performance is becoming increasingly important. Medical outcomes, patient satisfaction, and cost are increasingly being used to evaluate physician performance. The physician manager's role is to ensure that performance appraisal systems are in place that motivate appropriate employee, peer, and partner behavior.

- *Employment methods:* knowing how to hire both professional and clerical employees. Knowledge of this function fits the classic physician manager role definition. You will not do the hiring, but as a physician you clearly have to live with the consequences of good or poor employment decisions. The physician manager should have a vision of what a good employment process looks like, so that he or she knows enough to turn to the business manager or the human resource department and say "Using unstructured anecdotal interviews isn't good enough. We need to consider the following methods. . . . "

- *Motivation:* understanding what drives employees to act in specific ways when given a task to perform or a goal to achieve. By understanding what motivates employees, you can structure the work–reward relationship to best achieve your objectives. Similarly, you can influence your organization to structure rewards to better meet employees' needs.

- *Compensation:* determining equitable pay and benefits for employees, including physicians.

- *Organization structure, design, and integration:* putting the parts of the health care organization together so that they make sense, reporting relationships are logical and contribute to productivity, and jobs are composed of tasks that fit together logically and require an appropriate amount of work. Achievement of these goals is the basis for achieving integration—getting the parts of the health care organization to work together in a synergistic manner.

- *Change:* all organizations are confronted with the need to change. Changing medical procedures, information technology, managed care, and legal issues, to name a few, all result in health care organizations having to change. Often, people will resist change because it threatens their own self-interest. Physician managers must be able to recognize the need to change and be able to prevent or overcome resistance that may hinder them from putting needed changes into effect.

- *Negotiation:* physicians are constantly negotiating with patients, employees, partners, and colleagues. As physicians manage larger organizations, their ability to negotiate with factions within their organization and with other organizations, such as HMOs, insurers, employers, and hospitals, will become more important.

- *Total quality management (TQM):* understanding that a primary component of the physician manager's job description is managing systems as well as people. These systems may include the employment system, collection system, management information system, clinical treatment systems, and others. TQM is a management philosophy that emphasizes fixing processes and creating incentives for employees to look for ways to improve processes. It uses statistical control and charting methods to document and plan for improvement.

Marketing

Most physicians assume that marketing is simply a different word for advertising. This is not the case. Marketing begins with identifying customers' needs and then proceeds to identify internal and external organization factors when determining services offered, location, promotion, and pricing (including, for example, participation in an HMO). Advertising, which is a form of promotion, is one small part of the marketing process.

The marketing concept is distinctly different from that of selling, which is the process of persuading patients, for example, that they need a particular service. Sellers ask "Where and how can I find patients to buy the services that I currently offer?" In contrast, marketers begin with patients, determine what they need, can afford, and so on, and then design, package, price, and provide services so that patients have a natural affinity for them.

A fundamental change that has occurred in health care is the nature of the customer. Health care providers have a very complex definition of a *customer* that generally includes, but is not limited to, the patient. In the 1990s, another customer is often the purchaser of health care, who may be employers, insurers, and governments. Often, the incentives of these different customers are not aligned. For example, patients may want unrestricted access to services, whereas a health care provider who has taken a capitated contract may have more concern about the relationship between benefit and cost. This complicates the picture for the physician manager who

accepts the marketing model because now must carefully determine how to balance these needs.[1]

Some physicians question the ethics of including marketing considerations in medical decision making. The reality at the turn of the century is that marketing considerations *are* very much involved in health care decision making. What you as a physician consider ethical, given the local and national standards of the profession and the actions of competitors, is a personal matter. Certainly, what is generally considered ethically acceptable today is different from what was considered acceptable in the recent past. Chapter 9 is designed to familiarize you with the marketing mind set and to give you the tools to implement marketing methods consistent with your personal ethical standards.

Financial Management

Financial management is the process of using accounting and financial information to make management decisions. Practices, hospitals, and all other organizations create a lot of financial information in the normal course of their daily operation. It is critical for the physician manager to *use* this information to make management decisions. Often, health care organizations use financial information in the autopsy mode; that is, they look at outcomes two years after a decision was made and then use the financial data to describe what went wrong, and how badly it went wrong! A better approach is to use the financial information *proactively*, before you make a decision. By doing this, you can reduce the chance of failure and identify critical success factors that will have to be paid attention to and actively managed to succeed.

Financial management skills will help you answer the following questions:

- If I increase the size of my practice, what effect will this have on my profit?
- If I introduce a new program or procedure, how much volume must I have at a given

price before I break even or achieve a profit target?

- How do I evaluate a capital investment, such as building a new hospital wing, purchasing a second magnetic resonance imager, or acquiring two primary care practices?

Business Law

Physician managers constantly interact with other entities, such as patients, insurance companies, landlords, suppliers, employees, and contractors. Many of these interactions have legal implications. Ideally, the time to address the legal implications of an arrangement is *before* the arrangement goes into effect. Documents must anticipate anything that can go wrong, provide for what you would like to have occur if something does go wrong, and be legally binding. You certainly will want to consult an attorney during this process and have him or her draft all written agreements.

Employment law is another area where physician managers need knowledge. Knowing how to comply with Equal Employment Opportunity legislation, including compliance with provisions against sexual harassment and discrimination against those with disabilities, are critical for avoiding legal confrontations.

There also will be situations when you must make decisions without being able to contact your attorney immediately. By knowing how to recognize the legal implications of such situations, you may be able to avoid a legal blunder in daily decision making. Chapter 14 provides you with basic business law concepts, so that you will be able to respond in more appropriate ways on a daily basis and know when and how to utilize your attorney.

Information Systems

Physician managers are increasingly finding themselves at the center of medical management information systems. Systematically collecting the right kind of information, and getting that in-

formation to those who can make decisions to modify treatment and cost processes, can be a physician manager's most important organizational contributions. For example, a cardiac surgery unit can collect outcome and cost data on coronary artery bypass grafts. The data may be an assemblage of patient demographics, comorbid conditions, treatment provided, perhaps including diagnosis-related group (DRG), *International Classification of Diseases*, or Current Procedural Terminology codes or totally new coding schemes, with additional information being coded by case managers as patients progress through treatment. Potentially, the data may be used to improve case management procedures, reduce excess costs, and improve patient care.

Physician managers need to understand the basics of how information systems work, so that the systems they put in place are the ones that they need and will enhance their ability to manage. These systems can range from practice medical office management software to health care system–wide clinical assessment tools that track and evaluate physician, department, and health system performance.

Strategic Management

Strategic management is the process of developing a plan for business success. It involves thinking about events in a larger context than today's immediate needs. Many practices and larger health care organizations have no strategic plan. Their actions are a response to immediate and sometimes personal goals, or they are a reaction to the transitory demands of the marketplace. Without a strategy, each management decision may be treated as a unique event. There will be no basis for determining whether specific decisions contribute to or work against achieving larger objectives.

Strategic planning is the process of identifying internal organizational strengths and weaknesses as well as external environmental opportunities and threats and then using these data, along with a clear understanding of the organization's mission, to create a plan for the future.

Collection

Revenue is the wealth that medical organizations generate by providing services. An organization's collection methods must be thorough enough to convert a large proportion of this revenue into cash. Many businesses generate enough revenue to survive but nevertheless do not prosper and sometimes fail because they do not efficiently convert the revenue into cash.

Chapter 8, on collection of revenues, emphasizes the physician manager's role in the collection *process*. You will learn how to use management reports to manage the collection administration process and to assist in developing more effective methods. You will learn how to manage the receivable process so that problems are caught early and are prevented from growing into larger, profit-threatening, or even organization-threatening issues.

PROBLEMS FOR THE PHYSICIAN MANAGER

Many physician managers who also have some clinical responsibilities are probably thinking about now "Easy for him to say! When am I supposed to do this? In the 60th through the 65th hour of each week?" This response does point out some difficulties in attending to these management responsibilities.

Many physician managers do have a full-time job as a clinician. They have to be a manager on top of being a physician. To put this in perspective, however, this is the same challenge faced by all professions. Lawyers, accountants, and architects, for example, similarly must either reduce their professional hours or work additional hours to handle the management part of their business.

Another difficulty is that acquiring business skills requires learning a new language and developing new skills, which take time and effort. What you need to learn, however, is not rocket science. The most powerful ideas that are contained in an MBA program can be conveyed in a relatively short period of time and form the basis of this book. In addition, physicians are smart. They quickly grasp ideas, readily apply them, and then acquire additional knowledge of specific subjects when this becomes job relevant.

Another difficulty is that occasionally clinical and business issues come into conflict. For example, several years ago I had the opportunity to work with physicians in an oncology practice, who understood that to bid effectively for managed care contracts they needed to understand what it cost them to provide a service. One particular cost of about $3,500, which was never reimbursed, kept recurring. I asked one of the physicians about this, and he commented that this was an antinausea medication that Blue Cross and many other insurers wouldn't pay for. "Their attitude is that the patient will be sick as a dog for a few days, but 6 months from now they won't remember it," he commented. He then went on to say that he and his practice colleagues felt that, to provide the standard of care with which they were comfortable, they would simply provide the medication.

As a consultant who is not a physician, I couldn't advise these physicians one way or another on whether to provide the medication. I could, however, point out the financial cost, which was in fact substantial. The physicians, who now understood both the medical and the financial implications of their decision, could then appropriately evaluate both aspects of the decision. Ideally, they would also begin to look at their own financial data to identify issues such as this and begin making more informed decisions.

In this case, the medical and financial information did come into conflict. I suggest, however, that the conflict was there all along. Acquiring the financial information simply brought it to the surface and allowed for a conscious, considered decision, as opposed to a decision without knowledge and by default.

Finally, it is important to recognize that providing medical services is not the same as producing computer software or selling soap. There are important qualitative considerations to health care that would be lost by simply transferring accepted business practices to the health care setting. This uniqueness is a result of several factors. The close, personal relationship that often exists between the patient and the physician removes many of the adversarial boundaries normally defining a customer's relationship to a business. If the nature of the physician–patient relationship is not properly addressed, a conflict can arise between the humanitarian and ethical aspects of health care and the financial considerations that are necessary for organizational survival. Physician managers often make decisions that involve the quality and quantity of patient life, and these are interwoven with the cost of services, the history of accepted medical practice, and the welfare of their organization. Few managers in other industries face challenges with this magnitude of professional, ethical, legal, and organizational implications.

APPLICATION TO MANAGED MEDICINE

How do these business skills relate to the current challenges posed by managed medicine, such as managed care, HMOs, preferred provider organizations, capitation contracting, and the like? Let me address this question by posing another question: What would IBM's top-level executives do if they were faced with two challenges: They thought that price competition would force the price of computers down, and consumers were demanding higher-quality products. Specifically, what questions would they ask, and what data would they want to see?

I have presented this scenario to countless groups of physicians. Uniformly, they enthusiastically tackle it with questions that are right on target, such as these:

- Who is our customer?
- What do our customers specifically want regarding computer characteristics?
- What do customers perceive as quality?
- Who is our competition?
- What does it cost us to make our computer?

- What does it cost them to make a computer?
- How many do we have to sell to break even or meet a profit goal?
- How high is our current quality?
- Where in the production process are there opportunities to improve quality, work smarter, and so forth?

The question that I posed for IBM executives is directly analogous to two of the major challenges presented by managed care. How do you survive in a world where revenues will be reduced? If profit is what is left over after you subtract costs from revenues, then getting a handle on costs will be a critical success factor. Understanding what it costs to provide a procedure and how many procedures will be needed to obtain a profit target becomes critical. These are *financial management* skills. Knowing who your customers are and what they want, so that you can satisfy it as well or better than competitors, becomes critical. These are *marketing* and *marketing strategy* skills. Managing physicians to work more effectively with nursing and laboratory staff, and all these to work more effectively with intake and billing, so that on average a hospital discharges its patients three hours sooner for a DRG than a competitor across town, thereby obtaining a cost advantage, is *integration*, a *management* skill.

The most fundamental way of improving quality is to improve employee performance. Performance appraisal is a *management* skills. Similarly, improving employment procedures so that you automatically increase the quality and reduce the training time of new employees by, say, 20 percent improves quality as an input. Finally, adopting a TQM philosophy, in which we encourage and reward employees to think about ways of improving the service process and to create change as opposed to resisting it, is fundamental to improving quality.

The answer to the question of how business skills relate to the challenge of managed care is that *managed care creates business problems, and they are amenable to the same types of analyses and solutions as are other business problems.* Sometimes I think that everyone in health care is hoping for a magic solution, and that it will probably be found in some obscure technical article in *Health Care Forum* on how to create an MSO. I disagree. The answer to managed care is to understand at a fundamental level how to operate a business, a health care business. Once you acquire these necessary skills, then applying a layer of unique information about managed care can be a helpful refinement. Concentrating on managed care strategy without a fundamental understanding of health care business skills is analogous to adding more sail to a ship in a stiff breeze—a ship with an inadequate keel, a warped rudder, and leaking seams. You will roll all over the place, first this way then that; you will try one adjustment, then another, undershoot, overreact; but you won't get where you want to go, and you may in fact sink, *because the underlying structure is faulty*.

CONCLUSION

This book covers the major business skills that physician managers need to acquire. Coinci-

dentally, many of these subjects also form the core of the MBA curriculum. The goal is to provide physician managers with an understanding of how the science (and art) of business administration can be applied to their roles in health care organizations.

Some physician managers are full-time executives and spend all their time managing. They use their physician training for context and background. Other physician managers are primarily clinicians and use their management skills in an ancillary manner. Many private practice physician managers are the chief executive officers of their practices and are ultimately responsible for the survival of their practices. To perform effectively in all these roles, physicians must know enough about how a health care business *should* operate to be able to evaluate the performance of subordinates and consultants, step in at appropriate critical times in the management process, know the crucial questions to ask, and determine overall organization strategy. This book is designed to provide this necessary knowledge.

REFERENCE

1. L. Crane and J. Lynch, Consumer Selection of Physicians and Dentists: An Examination of Choice Criteria and Cue Usage, *Journal of Health Care Marketing* 8, no. 3 (1988): 16–19.

CHAPTER 2

Evaluating Performance

Chapter Objectives

In this chapter, you will learn how to evaluate the job performance of your employees, including physicians, so that you can improve their effectiveness and, as a result, improve organizational effectiveness. One goal will be for you to develop personal performance evaluation skills so that the direct management of your employees improves. In addition, you will learn how to develop performance appraisal systems that ensure the effectiveness of the performance appraisal skills of other physicians and managers. These performance appraisal systems provide internal control, so that management can assess and improve overall organizational productivity.

Finally, effective performance appraisal methods focus on the eventual outcome: improving employee performance. All too often, organizations focus on performance appraisal *methods* and become overly concerned with form over substance. As a result, they create rigid, time-consuming evaluation methods that both managers and subordinates dread. This chapter emphasizes the evaluation of employee *behavior* and *behaviorally* what you need to do to achieve this end. I will not offer, therefore, a set of forms or methods for you to use because they almost certainly would be inappropriate for your specific circumstance. What I will provide, instead, is a philosophy of performance appraisal and a strategy for you to develop methods that will work best in your organization.

Not all employees will do what you want them to do. Reasons for this include:

- limitations in ability that prevent an employee from properly performing the job
- personality characteristics that limit an employee's willingness to follow directions
- the widespread view that institutions and organizations, such as medical practices, hospitals, and health care systems, exist to serve the needs of the employee as opposed to the employer

There are several reasons for developing a performance appraisal system and then using it to evaluate job performance. First, the performance appraisal process is important because it is the organization's formal way of changing and improving job performance. Inadequate employee job performance has the potential to lower the quality of health care provided, to reduce profits, and ultimately to jeopardize an organization's existence. It is essential, therefore, that physician managers routinely and effectively evaluate job performance, change employee performance when it is inadequate, and terminate employees who will not or cannot improve their performance. Performance appraisals also provide employees with direct guidance regarding how you wish them to perform their jobs. If, for example, a business manager is devoting too much time to producing unused financial reports and not enough time to working old accounts, then comment on it *now*. In the absence of your comments, the business manager may assume that you approve of the current apportioning of work. By documenting your dissatisfaction and then evaluating and rewarding the business manager's future performance, you will tie behavior to rewards, thereby motivating the employee to perform in the interest of the organization.

Performance appraisals can also tell you what additional training, supervision, and task changes might be needed by your employees. For example, if you find that your accounting data are not being kept in a timely enough manner, this may indicate that the employee who is responsible needs more direction regarding when you expect the data to be available. It also may indicate that the employee needs some additional training in the use of your accounting software, or that the employee's workload is too heavy and some accounting tasks should be transferred to another employee or to your accountant.

Second, in a positive sense, performance appraisal is a strong motivational tool. Just as most physicians take real satisfaction when they are complimented on a job well done, most other employees will similarly be energized and motivated to perform well when their efforts are recognized. Similarly, absence of recognition when performance meets or exceeds expectations can be demoralizing. Many employees adopt the attitude "Why should I care if management doesn't care enough to notice." Self-actualized, internally motivated employees can be particularly demoralized when they see lower perform-

ers receiving the same compliments, pay raises, and promotions that they receive. Once again, this can be a dysfunctional outcome from an inadequate performance appraisal system.

Finally, performance appraisal should be the basis for personnel actions. By basing pay raises, promotions, access to training, discipline, and termination on performance appraisal, you create equity, so that employees perceive that the organization is treating them fairly. Also, you create a legal defense against any allegations of wrongful discharge and infractions of Equal Employment Opportunity laws.

There are, however, costs to performance appraisal. As you will see, one critical physician manager role is to ensure that performance appraisal systems are in place. It takes time and effort to develop these systems. It also takes time and effort to use the performance appraisal system to evaluate job performance, whether we are talking about evaluating front office clericals, laboratory directors, or physicians. Finally, it can be personally difficult to discuss substandard performance. It can be an intimidating, if not distasteful, process to sit across a table from someone and say "George, there are some real problems with part of your work, and we need to talk about it."

The process of determining how well an employee, peer, or partner is performing is called performance appraisal, and the document that results from this process is called a performance evaluation, although often these two terms are used interchangeably. The performance appraisal process includes:

- identifying the appropriate issues on which to evaluate performance
- evaluating the quality and quantity of work performed
- constructing a performance appraisal document to record the conclusions reached as a result of the performance evaluation
- informing the employee of your observations
- using this information to improve job performance by setting goals and providing,

for example, training, coaching, additional equipment, and so on

All supervisors, physician managers, and even many physicians without formal management responsibilities should be proficient in using performance appraisal methods. Physicians may be involved in the evaluation of hospital nursing and support personnel with whom they work but over whom they have no direct line authority. For example, a physician may provide a nursing supervisor with observations regarding a nurse's job performance, which the supervisor will then take into consideration when writing the nurse's performance evaluation. Physician managers may be responsible for directly evaluating technical, clerical, and medical personnel, including other physicians. A physician manager who is directing a hospital's medical staff office may also supervise several administrative and clerical positions.

PERFORMANCE APPRAISAL: THE SHORT COURSE

The performance appraisal process that evolves in many large organizations can be a bureaucratic, form-laden affair. It doesn't need to be that way. Below are six skills that form the foundation for conducting effective performance appraisals. This is the place to begin in terms of both personally conducting appraisals and designing a performance appraisal system for your practice or health care organization. Subsequent parts of this chapter will elaborate with additional details and refinements, but if you can really instill these six concepts into your own and your organization's evaluations, you will get the first 85 percent of the value to be gained. If your organization currently has a performance appraisal system that does not have these characteristics, consider superimposing them on this current system. Generally, there is nothing incompatible about adding some details that make a difference to your current system. Politically, you may find it advantageous to add elements instead of trying to tear down the old

system. These six rules can take you a long way toward personally conducting effective performance appraisals. They also should form the foundation for your organization's performance appraisal methods.

Immediate Feedback Is the Most Effective Form of Performance Appraisal

The single most effective performance appraisal procedure is to observe and comment on employee performance *as it occurs*. Immediate feedback has a number of benefits. If job performance is good, your comments will provide motivation and encouragement. If job performance is poor, you will immediately begin to modify the substandard behavior. If an employee's performance is inadequate and you don't comment on it, you have implicitly told the employee that the performance is acceptable. For example, if a deadline for getting a radiology report out is missed by a day and you don't remark on this, then you have indicated that deadlines are not really that important. Delaying your comments until a periodic annual or semiannual performance review will probably result in many missed deadlines. In addition, if you don't comment on inadequate performance as it occurs, some employees may conclude that you are afraid of a confrontation. Employees who perceive that their supervisor is afraid of distasteful or confrontational situations may use this knowledge to achieve their own objectives at your expense or your organization's expense.

Some employees will be honestly confused by a failure to comment immediately. For example, you review a report that indicates that there are a number of patients who are not making their copayments at the time of service. You don't inquire or comment on this to the business manager, who is ultimately responsible for all financial matters in your practice. The business manager knows the practice's policy that copayments must be made at the time of service but assumes that, because you have seen the report and haven't commented, you are satisfied with the current level of policy enforcement. In effect, not commenting has resulted in others assuming that you concur with their actions, and that policy has been changed.

Many physician managers have difficulty providing immediate feedback, particularly when it is critical. It can be difficult to sit across a table from an employee and say "John, I have a problem with how you are. . . ." It is much easier to be critical of an employee to your spouse or to your golfing partner because he or she is likely to nod in agreement. All this does, however, is provide a safe outlet and temporarily relieve your frustration. It does not achieve the most important objective: changing the employee's behavior. On the other hand, some physician managers are only too happy to be critical of an employee but are slow to provide deserved compliments. This is a quick way to generate employee dissatisfaction and turnover. Effectively using immediate feedback is a difficult skill to master. It takes both experience and good judgment to distinguish between the occasional inconsequential error or achievement and a failure or triumph of real significance.

The meaning of the word *immediate* should also be understood. This does not mean providing comments in front of other employees, physicians, and peers. This does mean getting the employee aside, perhaps in the ensuing hours or in the next day or so, to provide the needed comments. Remember, the goal is to change behavior, not to embarrass or degrade an employee.

Review Your Direct Subordinates at Least Annually, and Have Your Managers Who Are Subordinate to You Review All Their Employees Annually

Periodic performance appraisals should be conducted regularly. Typically, these are done annually, although new employees should receive a review after two or three months on the job. By telling new employees at the time of employment that they will be formally evaluated in two or three months, you achieve two objectives. First, you give the new employee an extra incentive to learn the new job and to excel. Second, you emphasize that you are very concerned about job performance and will recognize when the employee's performance is inadequate, outstanding, or in between. In effect, this initial periodic review provides an opportunity to shape the development of a new employee.

Periodic reviews of a continuing employee provide an opportunity to evaluate the employee's record and establish a coherent plan for improvement. Without periodic reviews, the feedback provided by daily supervision can simply amount to a series of unconnected comments. The review helps place these comments into a larger perspective and allow plans for improvement to be based on the employee's current strengths, weaknesses, and personal goals.

An important tool to use in conjunction with a periodic review is a critical incident file (Exhibit 2–1). A critical incident file contains brief comments regarding noteworthy events in the working life of an employee. Generally, if an event is significant enough for you to comment on it directly to the employee, then it is appropriate to put a note in the employee's critical incident file. The word *critical* in this instance means "out of the ordinary *and* important," not necessarily "bad." A critical incident file should include comments about praiseworthy as well as blameworthy incidents. The comments should be very brief. If they are not, then the time involved in documenting incidents will become burdensome, and the file will not be maintained.

A critical incident file will be particularly useful at the time of an employee's periodic review because it provides a link between daily observations and summarizing conclusions. It provides the supervisor with behavioral examples from the entire year, thus allowing a more balanced and accurate evaluation. Without a critical incident file, your memory may become selective. You may tend to remember only more recent events or may disproportionately recall positive (or negative) incidents. Critical incident files are maintained by the employee's direct supervisor, so you personally should maintain critical incident files only on those subordinates who report directly to you.

Exhibit 2–1 Critical Incident File Excerpts

2/11/90	VISA bill not paid on time. $36.62 finance charge.
4/29/90	941 tax form not prepared until the last day. Preparation done only after I reminded her.
7/17/90	Ran long computer reports during day instead of overnight, tying up computer during day. When asked, she had no reason for doing this. Poor time management.
11/3/90	Went out of her way to make Frank feel welcome on his first day by taking him to lunch.
12/9/90	Got us a $6,000 advance from CHAMPUS against claims that they are slow paying on.

Each employee should be able to review the contents of his or her own critical incident file. Remember, the object is to improve job performance. You can't do that by keeping your comments, either positive or negative, secret. Correspondingly, any incident worthy of entering in a critical incident file is important enough to be discussed with the employee near the time of the occurrence. By commenting on performance as it occurs, and then documenting important deviations from the norm in a critical incident file, you will make the assessment of performance an integral part of your management technique.

Next, be certain that those below you in the management hierarchy also similarly evaluate their employees on both immediate and periodic bases. Finally, be certain that all managers are evaluated on their ability to conduct performance appraisals. In this way, accountability cascades down the organization.

How do you know if a subordinate manager is doing a good job of performance appraisal? Obviously, you can't sit in on all of his or her evaluation interviews with subordinates, nor can you constantly observe the performance of the subordinates and compare this to his or her evaluations of their job performance! What you can do, however, is to look at the documented evidence. If the manager evaluates all his or her subordinates as "outstanding" but a sampling of critical incident files doesn't support this, then you have reason to believe that the manager isn't being totally accurate. Similarly, use a "reality check."

If the manager's subordinate evaluations seem inconsistent with the work group's performance or with your personal observations of an employee, you may also want to question the accuracy of the evaluation. Ultimately, of course, you can't judge your subordinates' ability to conduct performance appraisals with a micrometer. It's a judgment call. If there are inconsistencies, the goal is to improve the subordinate manager's observation and reporting skills. Additional training and, ultimately, tying raises and promotion opportunities to this factor, just like any other important area of job performance, should result in improved appraisals.

Set Goals for Those Who Report to You, and Have Them Set Goals for Those Who Report to Them

Goal setting is one of the most powerful tools available to managers. The simple act of telling an employee "This is what I want" or "This is where we are headed and how your performance can best help us get there" is a powerful way of directing and improving both employee and organization performance. When employees have specific goals, it gives then something concrete against which to match their daily actions. It also gives them predictability. There is nothing more frustrating to a subordinate than having to guess what a manager wants, especially if a wrong guess can result in criticism. Finally, setting difficult but realistically attainable goals stretches employees beyond where many would normally perform if they had no goals or a generalized goal such as "do the best you can."[1] When a surgeon, for example, truly accepts the goal of reducing operating room costs by standardizing procedures and materials for patients when it is medically acceptable to do so, he or she begins looking at the whole work environment differently. How do you get employees to accept goals that they perceive are not in their self-interest? You can't, but that is another story, and another aspect of managing that we will discuss in Chapter 5. Suffice it to say at this point that the way to motivate employees is to align their goals with the goals of the organization.

Setting goals for your subordinate managers and having them set goals for their subordinates result in coordinated goal setting cascading down through the organization. Those at the top, who are setting policy, will identify goals for their direct subordinates that are consistent with their view of where the organization is heading. These subordinate managers, in turn, will set even more specific goals for their subordinates that are consistent with the goals that they received from the highest levels. As this goal setting-process cascades down through the organization, it creates coordinated, directed behavior that coincides with top management's objectives.

Table 2–1 summarizes how a goal cascade might play out in a hospital adjusting to an increasingly managed care environment. It begins with the chief executive officer (CEO) identifying cost reduction as a critical goal. The implications for each level below the CEO become more specific and operational as we descend the organization's hierarchy, but each ties in with the policy goal set at the top.

You Will Get the Job Performance That You Are Willing To Accept. Don't Be a "Moab Manager"!

A few summers ago I was vacationing in the Moab, Utah area visiting Canyonlands and Arches National Parks. One afternoon around 3:00 P.M. my wife and I returned to town after a hard day of hiking. My wife had burned up her breakfast, with four hours to go to our dinner reservation. Solution: Get a quick burger at a brand new outlet of a national hamburger chain.

We park in the lot. My wife waits in the car, and I go inside. There are two lines being

Table 2–1 Cascading Goals

Position	Goal
Chief Executive Officer	Reduce operating costs
Vice President, Cardiac Services	Train staff physicians on cost issues Develop activity-based costing of selected procedures
Director, Cardiac Surgical Care	Develop standard treatment protocols Develop methods to assess clinical outcomes "Clean up" clinical coding Develop outcome database
Director, Cardiac Care Case Managers	Develop case management software Develop case management procedures Identify sources of invalid coding Specify outcome database variables

worked by two servers. I get into a line with one couple in front of me. The server takes the couple's order: two burgers, two fries, two sodas. The server disappears.

Several additional people enter the restaurant. Some get in the line behind me, and some go to the other line. Eventually those behind me move into the other line. That line is moving; mine is not. I'm feeling relaxed—after all, I'm on vacation, and have just had a great day in a beautiful national park. After about 5 minutes, I realize that nothing is happening. The other line is moving to some degree and is apparently being served by the store manager, who is running around frantically and obviously doing several jobs. I ask her "Is anyone serving this line?" She responds "Yes," drops her head, and continues working on the order in front of her.

Several more minutes go by. Nothing happens. At about this time I notice that to the manager's right there is another worker, who is drying a stack of trays with a towel very, very slowly. A customer whom this worker knows enters the restaurant and begins to talk to her. She puts the trays and towel down and talks casually with her friend. The shop manager is working 5 feet to her left, yet neither seems concerned!

Then the drive-in clerk shouts back to the cook as he picks up a burger: "Last Double Belchfire Burger!" I'm distracted by the towel clerk again. She has picked up a tray now and continues to talk to her friend. Is she a mime doing slowness? Now the cook responds, about 2 minutes after the drive-in clerk's admonition. He mumbles in response to the drive-in clerk's comment "What did ya say?"

Ten minutes now in line. I'm beginning to feel trapped! I comment to the manager working the other line "Is anyone working this line?" She responds, with exasperation, "Yes sir." A few moments go by, and she calls out "Where *is* Sherry?" The slow towel dryer mumbles (very, very slowly) "Dunn-nnoohh." The manager calls out "Sherry, where *are* you?" Sherry now calls out from the back of the restaurant "I'm makin' fries!" Sherry is not making fries. The fry maker is in the front of the restaurant, and she

is somewhere in the back. The manager goes scurrying off to finish some undone task, then rushes back to grab a handful of burgers and keep some movement in her line.

Finally, Sherry shuffles back to her line and completes the order for the couple. She then takes my order—very, very slowly. When I leave to take the food to my wife in the car, total elapsed time is *twenty* minutes. No exaggeration. *Twenty* minutes!

Incredible! I can't take it! My code of ethics as a management professor and consultant requires me to help! Besides, I'm madder than hell! I go back into the restaurant, walk to the front of the line, and state to the manager, in the calmest, quietest most controlled voice that I can muster, "This is the *slowest* fast food restaurant that I've ever been in!" She immediately responds "We're short of help." I stare at her.

"That's not the problem!" I say. "The problem is that everyone, with the exception of you, is moving *SLOWLY*!" We both stare at each other. I turn and leave. I had not completed the consultation. Perhaps the pay was a little too low, and after all, I was on vacation. To complete the consultation, I should have added, " . . . and in addition to moving slowly, they are doing it in front of you, and your response is to do nothing other than compensate by working harder and faster yourself!"

This case is a good example of a basic management principle: You get what you are willing to accept. There are many employees who will give you the lowest level of performance that you will tolerate. This manager's employees worked slowly—*very, very slowly*—and did it right in front of her. Yet she didn't demand anything more of them, so naturally they didn't give it. The message that she gave her subordinates was, "That's O.K." The message that she should have given is "If we're understaffed, we work that much harder and faster, and then some!" Instead, this "manager" stopped managing, and tried to compensate personally for underperforming employees.

Be on the lookout for "Moab Management," both when you are personally supervising subordinates and in your subordinate managers. If you find yourself or your subordinate managers compensating for subordinates who don't meet standards, but you don't directly demand improvement, then you are a "Moab Manager." The inevitable consequence is patient/customer dissatisfaction.

What should the manager have done? I would suggest closing the shop doors for 5 minutes and providing a clear explanation of performance expectations, assurance of training to those who haven't mastered skills yet, and an offer of resignation for those who can't or won't excel. What should you do if you find yourself Moab Managing? The same thing. Let subordinates know what you need, train them if they are not adequately trained, and give them their notice if they choose not to perform.

Finally, if you are in Moab, Utah, go to dinner at the Center Street Cafe and order the chocolate crème brulée for dessert. It may not cure Moab Management, but I guarantee that it will take your mind off of it until tomorrow. It worked for me![2]

People Do What They *Want* To Do: Hold Your Employees Responsible for Their Behavior

This is a corollary to "Moab Management," but nevertheless very important. As a manager, you do not have the luxury of excusing employee behavior as accidental or unintentional. Why did the tray dryer in Moab put the trays and towels down to talk with a friend? Because she *wanted* to! Her need to chat greatly exceeded her work standards or her fear of retribution from her manager, who was working 5 feet to her left. Similarly, Sherry was slogging through the day in a fog because she (pick one):

- was hung over from the previous evening and didn't care enough about her work performance to drink in moderation the evening before
- was an underemployed college graduate and was thoroughly bored with her work

- was lazy and didn't want to give any more effort than was demanded
- had never been asked to perform any better

The reason that she was choosing to give substandard performance is irrelevant. The point is that she was doing it; the customer didn't care why, and the supervisor was responsible for fixing this problem. Similarly, your patients or your organization's patients don't care why the service is inadequate or slow, so as a manager that can't be your first concern either. You don't have the luxury to play psychiatrist. Stick to managing behavior, not intentions, explanations, or unconscious motivations. If you do otherwise, you will find yourself in a swamp of justifications and attempts to pass off responsibility to you and to others.

Have Realistic Expectations of Others. Is Getting That Last 5 Percent Really Worthwhile?

This is a *question*! If it *is* worthwhile, then go for it—if it's *not*, back off! There are two management stereotypes of physician managers. The first is the absentee manager, the physician who doesn't manage. The second is the martinet who overmanages and is always demanding more than what most would perceive as reasonable. This skill applies to the latter stereotype. In a sense, it contradicts some of the earlier skills. The theme underlying the previous skills is "Hold employees strictly accountable, set high standards, and push, push, push!" There is a time, however, to back off.

Effective physician managers set high standards but only ask for 110 percent when this is absolutely essential. Ineffective physician managers continually ask for 110 percent, and generally they never get it. One aspect of the art of management is knowing when to ask for that extra effort. Beyond asking you to be introspective and consider as objectively as possible the level of demands that you place on your employees, this issue is a subjective, judgmental skill.

THE PERFORMANCE APPRAISAL PROCESS

The performance appraisal process, like all personnel processes, begins with the job description. The goal of the appraisal process is to evaluate incumbent performance in each major area of job performance. Without a good job description, there is a chance that you will miss some important aspect of performance. As the time for an employee's annual appraisal approaches, it is a good idea to give the incumbent a copy of his or her job description and ask whether anything of consequence has changed. If the job has changed, revise the description. Exhibit 2-2 contains a job description for a typical business manager position.

Conducting the Periodic Appraisal

The first step in the periodic appraisal process is to schedule a date for the review. Provide enough notice so that you and the employee will have time to prepare. Next, ask the employee to write a self-evaluation. Have the employee

---

Exhibit 2–2 Practice Business Manager Job Description

1. *Collection*. Responsible for the collection of all revenue. This includes using current office procedures and developing new ones to ensure the collection of all copayments and insurance. This will involve working with the other front office staff to develop these procedures, and to make them work. Responsible for making certain that all accounts are paid within a reasonable time, which is normally not to exceed 90 days past current.
2. *Insurance Billing*. Generating accurate insurance bills and mailing them on a regular basis.
3. *Payroll*. Maintain and generate accurate payroll records, including collections for each physician, determine physicians' monthly income based upon collections; calculate and assemble the physician payroll and front office payroll; calculate and pay retirement benefits to appropriate retirements plans.
4. *Taxes*. Calculate all federal (941, 940, etc.) and state taxes; ensure proper withholding for each payroll, make tax deposits in a timely manner; file all tax reports such as 941 quarterly, VEC quarterly, and state monthly in a timely manner.
5. *Accounts Payable*. Pay all practice bills. Manage the practice checkbook and savings account, including keeping an accurate running balance. Forward all appropriate financial information to the practice accountant when necessary, and at the end of each fiscal year.
6. *Posting and Accounting for Payments*. Post all payments received into the *MediMac* medical office management system. Reconcile all payments made the previous day with cash, checks, insurance remits, credit card receipts, etc. to provide accuracy and accountability.
7. *Fee Negotiation*. Negotiate patient fees in a manner that achieves practice financial objectives and protects practice financial integrity, but makes provision for patients with real financial hardships.
8. *Management Reports and Database Management*. Generate or cause to be generated management reports that are necessary for conducting the daily operation of the practice and provide accountability and problem identification. Examples include, but are not limited to, aging analyses, earned receipts by producer, daily receipts, etc. Insure the integrity of these databases including accuracy and backups.
9. *Problem Identification and Resolution*. Identify problems in any area of the practice, immediately bring them to the attention of the managing physician, and propose and implement solutions.
10. *Supervision*. Supervise and evaluate the job performance of all front office employees.
11. *Scheduling*. Ensure the validity of the patient scheduling system. Troubleshoot any problems and redesigning the system as necessary.
12. *Additional*. Additional duties and responsibilities and issues as they are determined to be appropriate by the managing physician.

organize his or her remarks around the major job performance issues noted in the job description. An example of a narrative self-evaluation by a practice business manager is found in Exhibit 2–3. This particular evaluation was written by a new business manager who was being evaluated after 90 days on the job. Generally, it is a good idea to formally evaluate all new employees af-

ter 60 to 90 days using your standard annual review process. Doing this with new employees helps to clarify responsibilities and identify where additional training is needed. This also tells the new employee that job performance is important. Instruct the employee to get the written remarks to you several days prior to when you plan to write your performance evaluation.

Exhibit 2–3 Self Evaluation, December 3, 1996

1. *Collection.* This is probably the area of most improvement from when I took over the job. Collection has gone extremely well. I have begun to tell patients more and more to call their insurance company themselves if there is a problem and then let me know if there is anything that I can do. I have felt overwhelmed by all the accounts that have needed my attention since I took over the position, but things are under better control now.
2. *Insurance Billing.* I am very confident in this area. I have developed procedures that have achieved consistency. Claims are sent out bi-weekly on Wednesdays and Fridays.
3. *Payroll.* Payroll has been a challenge as there is always something different to do, such as different deductions, phone charges, refunds, etc. I feel, overall, that I am mastering the process.
4. *Taxes.* The 941 taxes have gone smoothly. I have needed help coming up with the figures for state taxes. I have made a note on how to calculate state taxes, so this month it should not be a problem. Two concerns: What are the 940 taxes and the VEC taxes? Are these in my job description? Should I do these also or are they the accountant's responsibility? After looking at the job description they appear to be my responsibility but I need some clarification and instruction.
5. *Accounts Payable.* There have been no problems in this area that I am aware of. I have used George's system for keeping track of bill due dates and it is working well.
6. *Posting and Accounting.* I have not had any difficulty with posting payments and making deposits save the MEDWORK EAP checks. I have been clear about making EAP checks a

separate deposit, but it seems to be confusing in the accounting system. We like to keep the check for office space rental on a separate deposit from patient payments, but at times MEDWORK puts both kinds of payments in the same check.
7. *Fee Negotiations.* I have negotiated fees for several patients. I feel comfortable with this area.
8. *Management Reports and Database Management.* I have had some difficulty with the aging analysis reports. Specifically, I am having trouble using the *Excel* spreadsheet to sort each physician's aging in the manner that you want. For the most part, I have mastered the reports that I need for my daily work, such as daily receipts and adjustments, insurance aging, production reports, adjustment reports, etc. I need some clarification on how to use the categories in the referrals database. Specifically, when do I use the "newspaper ad" and "generated by practice" categories. I get confused between these two.
9. *Problem Identification and Resolution.* I am skilled in the area of problem identification. We have constructed several office forms and eliminated others to make the office run more efficiently. "No pay" and "no show" bills are now sent out the next day. I have fixed the problem for getting timely releases signed by the physicians.
10. *Scheduling.* There have been a few errors with scheduling by Amanda for whatever reason. Overall this seems to be going well. Problems have been avoided by confirming patient visits. We have this up to almost 100 percent attempts within two days of scheduled appointments.

The process of writing a self-evaluation causes the employee to think about his or her job performance, to examine it as a supervisor might, and to begin thinking about what needs to be done in the future. The self-evaluation also tells you how the employee has interpreted your feedback, and it gives you an indication of what to expect in the appraisal interview. Schedule the periodic review at a time during normal work hours, and explain to the employee that the purpose of the meeting is to review past performance and to begin planning for the next year.

The appraisal information that you will be discussing in the meeting and will be in your written appraisal should contain no surprises. If you are doing an adequate job of keeping the employee appraised of his or her performance on a daily basis, the periodic review will simply be a reiteration of what has been said over the year. At some point, it will be useful to review the employee's critical incident file. Classify incidents according to the factors noted on the job description. In addition, collect any other pieces of pertinent information, such as objective measures of job performance and comments from peers and other physician managers.

You are now ready to write the employee's performance evaluation report. Your evaluation should always be put in writing. A written report provides documentation that will be useful for tracking an employee's progress over the years. Written documentation also can be useful in defending against legal challenges to personnel decisions (see Chapter 14). Exhibit 2–4 contains excerpts from a business manager's annual evaluation. This evaluation is based on the job description found in Exhibit 2–2, but it is for a different business manager from the one whose comments are found in Exhibit 2–3.

It is important to evaluate the employee separately on each job description factor. Be as specific and behavioral as possible. Notice that the performance appraisal in Exhibit 2–4 directly parallels the job description factor by factor. Notice also that it focuses on job relevant behav-

iors, not on personality characteristics or sweeping generalities. Finally, notice that it makes distinctions across factors. Performance on some factors is very good, while other areas need substantial improvement.

When writing an evaluation, it is important to use clear, concise language. This will save you time and will provide the subordinate with an unambiguous statement regarding strengths and weaknesses. Initially, you may find it difficult to be direct, especially if there are performance problems. It is important to remember, however, that careers can be ruined by supervisors who are kind and softhearted. *Avoiding the difficult issues until performance is so inadequate that you must discipline or fire the employee is not doing anyone a favor.* It is important that your comments remain related to job performance and are not condescending or personally derogatory. In summary, stick to the facts and work with the employee to develop reasonable solutions.

Next, meet with the employee to discuss your evaluation. Begin the performance appraisal interview by giving the employee a copy of your written analysis. Then review the sources of data that you used in developing your evaluation, including critical incidents, observations of others, and objective measures (e.g., aging analyses). This tells the employee that your evaluation is based on fact, not conjecture, and that the appraisal is important enough for you to have taken time to assemble a written document based on data. Use the interview time to elaborate on your written appraisal and to begin planning for the future. Solicit employee comments, and explore any areas in which the employee has suggestions for how job performance might be improved. Although weaknesses and areas needing improvement should certainly be discussed, don't dwell on them. Most employees have strengths, and it is important to discuss these and build upon them.

At this point, you have reached a fork in the road. Less effective organizations essentially tell the employee at this point "Go out there and continue what you are doing" or "Go out there and

Exhibit 2–4 Performance Evaluation (Excerpts) XXXXXXXX July 15, 1996

1. *Collection.* The overall level of collection in the 120- to 180-day category is back into the acceptable range. This winter, however, collection totals exceeded $6,000 in this category, which was not acceptable. In addition, I had to closely supervise you to get the receivables back down. This should be a self-managing function. This pattern, however, of losing control and then having to be closely worked with to regain control has occurred consistently over the years. The fact that you can get the receivables back under control shows that you can do it. However, we want you to take more responsibility for dealing with this yourself, before it becomes a problem, and before it has to be addressed by me.

   You continue not to enforce the 90-day patient payment policy. Patients should be called when their balance reaches the 60-day category, encouraged to contact their insurance company at that point, and told that they will have to pay when the balance reaches 90 days.

   In addition, each day you should review the next day's appointments, so that patients can be called before an appointment and reminded to bring in past due balances.

2. *Insurance Billing.* You get the insurance bills out in a very timely manner. You have really turned the posting and billing operations into a consistent and efficient process. This is a real strength.

3. *Payroll.* The basic payroll processing operates well in that we always pay the payroll on time. There have been some minor problems revolving around infrequent events. For example, you did not account accurately for physicians' Yellow Pages display ads. This was fixed only after I noted the error. It appears that personal long distance telephone charges have been dropped again. This was a problem that was noted last year. It got better for a while, but it is a problem again.

4. *Taxes.* There was one instance when a 941 payment was underpaid, but that was caught before the end of a quarter. With that exception, you did a lot better this past year.

5. *Accounts Payable.* This area has developed into a strength. You have consistently paid the bills on time without reminder. We incurred no interest expenses on our bills last year.

6. *Posting and Accounting for Payments.* This occurs in a timely and consistent manner. In addition, the posting process is highly accurate. There have been no instances of incorrectly posted money. In addition, you routinely handle the adjustments to payroll; bounced checks, insurance retractions, transfers, etc. correctly without the need for supervision.

7. *Fee Negotiation.* The fee agreements that you negotiate with patients show good discretion in getting the best fee from patients who need a fee agreement. Your payment plans are highly structured and convey the message that we expect patients to meet their financial obligations. You have used good judgment in making decisions that protect the practice's revenue, yet are responsive to patients with real hardships. The McKlintock case in particular showed good judgment in setting a reasonable payment plan that respected the family's financial situation, yet still will provide fairness for Dr. Johnson.

8. *Management Reports and Database Management.* I am routinely getting aging analyses now. This is an improvement from last year. Your consistency with write-off and adjustment reports and the aging database report could be improved. These should always be part of the package of reports that you give to me each month.

   Patient records were put into storage, and there was no update to the archived patient files database. In addition, some charts were in the wrong boxes.

   The referral database contains many omissions and errors. It is not a reliable source of information about referrals. Specifically, the categorizations of referrals have no consistency, and I have found eight internal referrals in the last month that were not properly recorded. We have talked about this several

continues

Exhibit 2–4 continued

times over the last year. This is one of our most important databases. This is a major problem.

9. *Problem Identification and Resolution.* Thinking about the future consequences of events is still an area that needs attention. Generally, you react to problems once they occur and have been brought to your attention, but an important part of your job is to be looking for ways to improve things and prevent problems before they occur.

    Most of the physicians feel that we rarely get request sheets back in a timely manner. The request sheet process was developed to help you remember requests, and to provide a process to return information. If you feel that this system is too cumbersome or time consuming, then you need to develop a better one. Responding to physicians' needs in a timely manner (typically on the same day) is important, and providing feedback is critical if we are to operate in a coordinated manner. If you can't get to something on the same day, then tell the physician, and estimate when you will be able to get to it.

10. *Supervision.* Your day-to-day supervision of the other front office employees on routine activities is adequate. The duties and responsibility are logically assigned and the quality of your written appraisals of subordinates is behavioral and specific. Morale appears to be high.

    It took longer than usual to get Janet fully trained. It appeared that the training program that you designed to train her in our medical office management software was not as complete as it could have been.

11. *Scheduling.* Scheduling has been a problem. It is up to you to manage this system. If the scheduling system is not working, it is your job as office manager to make it work. If this means calling a meeting with physicians and other office staff to understand why problems are occurring, and then changing the way the scheduling process works, then that is what you have the responsibility to do.

11. *Additional.* Last year in your performance review we noted that there appeared to be problems with concentration and short-term memory loss. In the last 6 months it appears that your memory impairment has worsened. Last year you forgot things but remembered them once you were reminded of them. In the last few months, even when reminded, you seem to have no memory that some events occurred. This is a change and is a different type of short-term memory impairment. We feel that you need to consult with your physician and perhaps seek a consultation with a specialist. This is, however, only a suggestion, and it is totally at your prerogative. I will provide you with a list of specific examples that you can share with your doctor and may help him or her identify a cause.

Areas of Improvement Since July 12, 1995 Evaluation

1. You now consistently use the financial warnings in MediMac and are filling out day sheets on this basis. This was a major goal and you succeeded in doing this.
2. You are doing a better job of utilizing our standard procedures including consistently verifying insurance and having all patients sign MOP forms.

Summary

Overall, your job performance is good. You have some real strengths where your performance is excellent. Also, there are some areas that are important and need attention. Overall, the front office operates well. We get the patients through, we get the bills out; we get the money in, and the office operates in a generally effective manner.

My biggest concern is your ability to adapt to the changes that occur in the job and to identify and fix problems before they become serious. As managed care continues to change the challenges that we face, this increasingly becomes a critical part of your job. I am concerned about your health as memory problems have persisted and changed in their nature.

fix it!" More effective organizations do what is called goal setting. Goal setting is characterized by the following:

- Goals should be behavioral. This means that the goals should be observable job behavior as opposed to mentalistic impressions of improvement.
- You, perhaps with the employee's help, should identify a *path* for the employee to follow to achieve the goal. Don't leave this up to the employee. Many employees can't figure out how to get from here to there. Help them work through the details of that process. Similarly, there may be occasions where you don't know enough to identify the details of the path. For example, suppose that you conclude that a business manager's collection problems are due to insufficient knowledge of how to use your medical office management software. You can't instruct the manager, but you can say "I want you to come back to me in a week with a *plan* for how you will acquire this knowledge."
- There should be a time frame for completion. Always state deadlines for specific objectives. If you don't, then many employees will always find other things to do rather than deal with difficult learning objectives. Also, this gives you a "freedom date," so that you know that you can take another action as of a specific date.
- Periodically check to monitor the employee's progress. Don't assume that, just because performance has improved, it will remain that way. This, of course, ties in with the admonition to continuously observe and comment on job performance as it happens.

Exhibit 2–5 contains goals set by the manager to follow up on the performance appraisal in Exhibit 2–4. Notice that the discussion is factual and that specific behavioral targets as well as time deadlines are identified.

Evaluation Errors

There are a number of errors that physician managers can make when evaluating job performance. Leniency errors occur when supervisors consistently rate employees either too high or too low. Some supervisors tend to evaluate subordinates consistently too favorably (positive leniency bias) because they think that a more accurate evaluation would have an adverse impact on morale. Some give high evaluations because they have not been paying close enough attention to subordinate performance, and no one ever objected to a high evaluation! Other supervisors feel that a less-than-outstanding evaluation reflects poorly on their own leadership ability. Finally, some supervisors lack assertiveness, and they become overly dependent on acceptance and approval from their subordinates. Giving an accurate appraisal may threaten this approval.

Similarly, there are a number of reasons why some supervisors consistently downgrade subordinate performance. Some supervisors project their own failings onto their subordinates. If it is always a subordinate's fault, the supervisor does not have to accept personal responsibility. Other supervisors have unreasonably high standards. It is important to remember that a medical practice owner or a physician in an executive management position will generally have a far greater degree of commitment to the organization than many other employees. It is important to be realistic about the degree of commitment and performance that can be expected from employees. Consistently giving low evaluations and demanding performance that employees perceive as unreasonable will only result in employee dissatisfaction and turnover.

Another common evaluation mistake is called a halo error. A halo error occurs when a supervisor allows an employee's performance on one job factor to influence the evaluation on another factor. For example, if Dr. Smith is outstanding at diagnosis, you should not allow this to influence your evaluation of her performance on communications with patients and "bedside

Exhibit 2–5 Goals

These are areas to work on. We will meet in late September to see how you are progressing in these areas.

1. Respond to all request sheets on the day that you receive them. Begin doing this immediately.

2. Develop a method to reduce scheduling errors. The goal is zero errors. This will require you to work with physicians and the front office staff; get their ideas and develop as a team a process that works. I suggest that you use the scheduling problems that have already occurred as a point of discussion to talk with physicians and the staff about better ways to handle scheduling. The new procedure should be in place by August 15.

3. Call all patients when they have money in 60 days and inform them that in 3 to 4 weeks they will have to pay unless their insurance company responds. The patient will not be surprised if you thoroughly review the method of payment with them at the time of the initial office visit. It is not sufficient simply to accept the patient's statement that he or she cannot pay. Failure to do this has delayed collecting funds that the office needs. Begin putting this policy into effect immediately.

    This was your number one goal last year. It really is important for you to make this a top priority.

4. The referral database problem needs to be fixed. This needs to be a zero error area. I want you to determine why referrals are occasionally omitted and develop a solution to this problem. Also, it appears to me that we need to clarify the referral categorization guidelines. I want you to develop new written guidelines. Please let me know your findings by August 15. In the interim, please carefully review all new referrals to be certain that they are entered into the database correctly.

5. I strongly encourage you to immediately contact your physician regarding the memory issue. This is, however, totally at your discretion. I am concerned about you and your health.

6. Work accounts aggressively on your own initiative to keep collection statistics at their current favorable levels. Begin doing this immediately.

7. The nature of your job is changing. It is requiring you to look more inquisitively at the front office operation, identify problems, and come up with solutions before the problems become serious. It is important for you to be continuously examining processes to see how they can be improved and to take a more proactive approach to your job. This should be a daily, ongoing part of your job.

    In addition, I want you to develop a list of practice management areas where our current methods could be improved. We will then discuss this list together, refine it, and develop improvement projects if appropriate. I want to see this list by September 15.

manner." Similarly, if Vice President Andersen has developed an outstanding cost accounting system for oncology services, this should not raise his evaluation on supervisory skills if they in fact need improvement. These are separate, distinct issues and should be treated as such in the performance appraisal process. A particularly insidious type of halo error occurs when the supervisor allows a factor that is not job relevant, such as physical attractiveness, to influence some or all of the evaluations of job-relevant factors. Sometimes this halo process can be very subtle, and it may occur at an unconscious or semiconscious level. Systematically conducting evaluations factor by factor based on job descriptions helps eliminate these types of halo errors.

PERFORMANCE EVALUATION DATA

The data that you will use to evaluate an employee can be classified as either objective or subjective. Objective data are produced in the normal course of work activities. Examples include "typing error rate," "reinfection rate," "percentage of insurance dollars collected within 90 days," "number of patients treated per week," "number of referrals generated per month," "average length of stay," and so on. Be very careful when using objective data. Unless you fully understand the numbers, they can be misleading. For example, suppose that you are evaluating a physician based on the number of referrals that he or she has generated over the past year. Can you separate referrals generated by the organization, such as those caused by a Yellow Pages ad that mentions your colleague's name, from referrals generated directly by the physician?

Similarly, mortality rates and other measures of physician performance can be very misleading unless they take into account extenuating circumstances, such as comorbid conditions, sometimes referred to as illness burden or case mix (see Chapter 15, Information Technology). Also, an increase in accounts receivable may be indicative of either a performance problem or organization growth. If the organization is growing, you may have to adjust the accounts receivable numbers to obtain a valid picture of a business manager's performance. You could, for example, take the accounts receivable money that is 90 days old as a percentage of the current accounts receivable. Objective data can be very useful for evaluating an employee's performance if the data truly reflect the performance.

Another problem with using direct measures is that they can be "gamed." For example, a business manager who is evaluated on accounts receivable over 120 days can write off these balances. Unless you are observant and note or anticipate this behavior by being certain to review write-off reports (as you should!), the manager will look good on the performance evaluation *while at the same time producing a counterproductive, unintended outcome.* Similarly, a physician who is evaluated on the basis of clinical outcomes that are not properly adjusted for the illness burden of his or her patients may undertreat or overrefer sicker patients. Once again, the performance appraisal process will have generated counterproductive behavior.

Subjective data include your personal interpretation of events, such as your judgment of an employee's ability to work with patients, diagnostic skills, supervisory skills, knowledge of software, and the like. Subjective data are generally susceptible to the rating errors mentioned above. Most of the data available for evaluating health care employees are subjective. Even those practices and hospitals that maintain databases on productivity and finances find that, in the final analysis, performance appraisals are largely subjective because the objective data usually are relevant to only a part of each job.

As a physician manager, your challenge is to develop a set of evaluation criteria that draw on objective and subjective data and that in total will present a fair, complete picture of the employee's performance. When jobs contain evaluation issues that are both objective and subjective in nature, be especially vigilant for halo errors. It is very easy to let subjective data bask in the halo of objective data. For example, you have good, hard evidence that Dr. Hoskins is an excellent surgeon. His reinfection and rework rates are low compared with those of his peers and national statistics. You may, unconsciously or semiconsciously, tend to allow these facts to bias your evaluations of other, less measurable issues, such as his bedside manner and treatment of staff. Similarly, Mr. Carney does a great job of collecting revenue, but he tends to look the other way when physicians provide incomplete documentation and notes. Once again, you may be inclined to overrate his ability to obtain physician compliance out of gratitude for his success in keeping the money flowing. It is important for supervisors to evaluate factors separately because these independent evaluations are the basis for providing employees with the opportunity to improve in those areas that need development.

PERFORMANCE STANDARDS

Performance standards (Exhibit 2–6) are statements describing what any employee on a particular job must do or achieve to perform adequately. Performance standards relate to the *job*.

Exhibit 2–6 Typical Performance Standards

Checkbook

- Checkbook is reconciled with the bank statement no later than five days after the statement is received.
- Monthly income should always balance against the monthly collection for physicians plus other income.

Accounts Receivable

- Total accounts receivable should never exceed two times current accounts receivable.
- Accounts receivable report should be run each week.
- Cash box should be balanced against receipts printout each day.

Word Processing

- Documents should contain no typing, spelling, or grammatical errors.

- Documents should be completed no later than three days after they are submitted for typing.

Database Maintenance

- Referral database should be revised at least weekly.
- All transactions should be entered into McNeal Office Management software daily.
- All other databases should be revised at least weekly.
- All databases should be backed up daily.

Referrals

- Twenty-five percent of a physician's referrals should be self-generated.
- Two public information seminars should be presented each year.
- Two network primary care physician training programs on new GI pharmaceuticals should be conducted each year.

Irrespective of who occupies the position, the incumbent will be expected to meet the performance standards for that job. Performance standards should not be confused with employee goals. An employee's goal is a personal objective that may equal or exceed a particular performance standard. For example, a performance standard for the position of business manager may be to keep accounts receivable in 180+ days below 5 percent of total accounts receivable. By definition, any business manager who does this is doing at least an adequate job on this factor. A specific goal for Mr. Carney, however, may be to reduce accounts receivable from its current 4.3 percent level to an average 3.3 percent across the last six-month period within one year.

Many large organizations like to have written performance standards for virtually all factors on most jobs. This is a waste of time. It is difficult to write meaningful performance standards for some factors, and others are so obvious that it makes no sense to ponder the issue. For example, the following might be a performance

standard for patient relations: "Employee is always courteous and attentive to patient needs." This statement is so bland that it is virtually meaningless. It states the obvious and provides no guidance to the employee. Don't waste your time or your employees' time writing or trying to apply meaningless performance standards.

On the other hand, if you have a clear standard of acceptable behavior and the job performance issue is important, then it will be helpful to your employees if you share those standards with them. Performance standards should always be discussed with employees at the time of employment. They should also be communicated to employees in written form, either as part of the job description or in a separate document.

RATING FORMS

Many supervisors consider completing a rating form (Exhibit 2–7) equivalent to doing a performance appraisal. As we have seen, performance appraisal is a much more broadly

Exhibit 2–7 Typical Performance Appraisal Rating Scales

1. When unsure about a problem, discusses it with supervisor.
   Almost Always   1   2   3   4   5   Almost Never

2. Has mastered the information provided in technical manuals for the office equipment and software used on the job.
   Almost Always   1   2   3   4   5   Almost Never

3. Has a sense of humor even with difficult patients.
   Almost Always   1   2   3   4   5   Almost Never

4. Accepts and adapts to change.
   Almost Always   1   2   3   4   5   Almost Never

5. Adequately delegates work.
   Almost Always   1   2   3   4   5   Almost Never

6. Gets written reports completed on time.
   Almost Always   1   2   3   4   5   Almost Never

7. Gets all appropriate paperwork signed by patients.
   Almost Always   1   2   3   4   5   Almost Never

8. Communicates appropriately with patients.
   Almost Always   1   2   3   4   5   Almost Never

encompassing process than simply completing a form. Completing a rating form should instead be viewed as just a way to record the evaluation information and conclusions.

Evaluation forms of this type have their own special problems. Standardized rating forms take a lot of time and effort to construct. As a result, some organizations use "one size fits all" appraisal factors across many, if not all, jobs. This approach is worthless. As we have seen, it is essential to identify specific aspects of performance *for each individual job*. Generic factors, such as quality, quantity, and willingness to follow directions, are not going to be appropriate or specific enough for many jobs. In addition, using standard forms allows managers to be lazy. If the factors to be evaluated are not job specific, the manager can complete the form without having to provide a lot of detail about the employee's performance.

Standardized rating forms can be useful, however, in larger organizations. Sometimes it is necessary to make comparisons across many employees, such as when a clerical supervisor

position is being filled internally. It would be time consuming to try to equate the narrative performance appraisal reports across the several dozen applicants to determine who is most worthy of the promotion. Many large organizations, recognizing the critical importance of the performance appraisal process, have invested the time and money to develop performance appraisal forms for groups of jobs, although not necessarily for every single job in the organization. For example, all clerk/typists have a custom-developed performance evaluation form, as do licensed practical nurses, registered nurses, pharmacists, nursing supervisors, and so forth.

To do this effectively, supervisors of these positions, and ideally job incumbents, must be involved in the development of these evaluation forms. In addition, supervisors have as part of their job the responsibility to suggest changes to the standard evaluation form as the duties of the position change.

Because medical practices rarely need to make comparisons among large numbers of employees, rating forms such as the one in Exhibit

2–7 are not necessary. Usually, performance appraisals in medical practices are aimed at assessing a few employees in great depth. The object is to compare the employee against the demands of the job instead of with other employees. A narrative evaluation constructed around the job description factors for the position is the most appropriate type of evaluation to achieve this end. In effect, a blank piece of paper and an accurate job description are the key to conducting a superior performance evaluation, irrespective of the job.

IMPROVING PERFORMANCE

Job performance can be improved by selectively using four techniques: training, incentives, discipline, and job restructuring. The choice of which method or methods to use depends on the employee's current circumstances. The performance appraisal process will help you determine the best strategy. Training is appropriate for increasing an employee's skills if the low performance is due to limited ability *and if you believe that he or she has both the capacity and motivation to improve.* It is also beneficial in the case of an outstanding employee who still has some room to grow.

Incentives will be discussed more fully in Chapters 4 and 5. At this point, it is sufficient to say that providing an incentive, such as a pay raise or a bonus based on production, will only change behavior when the employee sees the incentive as valuable and related to job performance and if he or she has the ability to improve. If the employee lacks any of these elements, then incentives are not an appropriate behavioral change strategy. The same holds true for discipline. Threats and the removal of rewards only change performance when the threats are perceived as credible, the rewards are desired, each is perceived as tied to achievement, and the employee has the skill to improve. If the employee really doesn't want the job or the rewards or is unable to improve, then discipline will have no effect.

Job restructuring involves changing a job to compensate for an employee's strengths and weaknesses. For example, suppose an otherwise valuable secretary has difficulty collecting fees from patients at the time of service. Your business manager tries to improve performance by giving the secretary guidelines and having him or her work closely with another employee who is good at this task; the secretary reads articles on self-esteem, practices collection methods by role-playing with other employees, and so on. Performance, however, does not significantly improve. At this point, you may choose to rethink the tasks performed on this job and the other front office jobs.

If it is possible to restructure some of the jobs so that this employee will spend little if any time collecting fees, you will have solved the performance problem. Obviously, you must use this method carefully. If other employees perceive that they must bear an extra burden because of a coworker's incompetence or reluctance, you will simply be trading one kind of problem for another. Used skillfully, however, this can be an effective way to improve organizational performance while salvaging otherwise valuable employees.

EVALUATING PHYSICIAN PERFORMANCE

As more physicians work in managed care organizations and salaried positions, the need to evaluate physician performance increases. Physicians are arguably in the best position to influence directly the quality and cost of the care delivered. Both are central to the success of health care organizations as we move into an era requiring ever-increasing efficiency. As a result, evaluating physician performance will become increasingly central to organizational success, whether we are talking about a private practice, a hospital, a health maintenance organization, or any other type of health care organization.

Historically, physician evaluation has been handled through a peer review process. For peer review to be effective, there must be a collegial atmosphere that supports an honest and thorough evaluation. All too often, peer review has meant "If you don't give me a hard time, I won't give you one when the roles are reversed."

Traditionally, physicians in fee-for-service arrangements had at least one objective measure on one job performance factor because providing more service resulted in higher revenues. As with any reward system based largely on a single factor, this is a situation ripe for manipulation. Patient overtreatment and a disinterest in the cost of services are predictable outcomes.

Managed care can in many ways reverse the incentives in physician evaluation plans. Because physicians working under managed care are being held accountable for additional factors, such as quality, cost, rule compliance, and the like, evaluation systems must reflect this complexity. If it does not, the physician might "game" the evaluation plan, with disastrous consequences for the health care organization and its patients.

Evaluation of physicians follows the same model as for any other type of job. Begin with the job description, and build the evaluation process around its content. What makes this a more challenging process for the physician manager is that many physicians have never been in positions where they were the subject of regular and thorough evaluations. As a result, personal sensitivities and the skill with which the process is managed become particularly important.

One way to address this problem is to involve physicians in the development of the appraisal system. This achieves two positive results. First, physicians who will be evaluated are in the best position to ensure that the appraisal plan actually captures all the complexity and nuances of their work. Their involvement can ensure that the evaluation plan is complete and realistic. Second, a general principle of management is that ownership increases the probability of acceptance. In this case, physicians who are instrumental in designing a plan that they accept as valid are more likely to use it willingly and to accept evaluations under it.

Some may counter that involving physicians in the evaluation plan's design gives them the power to produce an ineffectual plan. In a climate of distrust and adversarial scheming, that certainly could be the case. If that is the nature of your physician management–labor relations climate, then there are more fundamental issues that must be discussed with physicians before the development of a performance appraisal plan. In a somewhat healthier environment, the inclusion of line physicians in the design of the evaluation plan can help ensure teamwork and acceptance.

Kongstvedt has provided some examples of evaluation factors for typical closed (Table 2–2) and open (Table 2–3) physician panels.[3] As with any job, however, it is important to develop evaluation factors from the *physician job description or descriptions as they exist in your organization*. Remember, identifying appropriate factor content and assessment methods will determine the ultimate success of the plan. Use of objective measures (e.g., audits of patient records for compliance with plan standards), surveys to assess patient satisfaction, and development of cost measures and management reports to quantify utilization are all feasible.

Does this level of monitoring cost something in terms of administrative overhead and physician manager time? Certainly. But what are the costs to an organization whose reason for existence is to use health care resources efficiently when those who are instrumental in providing care while managing cost considerations do not have to live with the consequences of their actions?

PERFORMANCE APPRAISAL SUMMARY

The assessment of performance should be a continuous process. Formal appraisals provide an opportunity for you to review progress, solicit personal goals, and plan for the future. Performance appraisals help you motivate your employees, peers, and partners, and provide you with critical information for making management decisions, including training, job restructuring, compensation, and termination decisions.

Table 2–2 Potential Closed Panel Physician Evaluation Factors

Factor	Description
Productivity	Volume and efficiency of work as measured against plan norms. *Examples:* visits per week, complication rate, rework rate, etc.
Medical charting	Compliance with charting standards, legibility, timeliness, etc.
Dependability	Compliance with plan rules, time constraints, etc.
After hours on-call	Appropriate use of medical emergency services, availability, patient continuity, etc.
Medical knowledge	Level of technical skills and appropriate professional judgment.
Management of patient care	Compliance with treatment protocols and appropriate deviation from them, appropriate follow-up intervals, etc.
Management of outside resources	Appropriate and cost-effective use of consultants for diagnosis and treatment.
Patient relations	Patient perception of treatment quality, patient relations.
Teamwork	Flexibility and responsiveness in working with others, including physicians, nurses, clericals; committee work and attendance; etc.
Leadership	Training and motivating others to work toward plan goals.

Source: Adapted from P.R. Kongstvedt, Formal Physician Performance Evaluations, *The Managed Health Care Handbook*, 2nd Edition, pp. 189–197, © 1993, Aspen Publishers, Inc.

Table 2–3 Potential Open Panel Physician Evaluation Factors

Factor	Description
Productivity	Office visits, per member per year, and other objective standards
Referral utilization	Referrals per member per year, cost per referral, etc.
Hospital utilization	Objective measures of utilization, such as days per physician panel, days per 1,000 patients, etc.
Ancillary utilization	Use of ancillary services, such as radiology, pharmacy, laboratory, etc.
Precertification and authorization compliance	Compliance with plan requirements
Use of plan network	Utilization of plan physicians, hospitals, etc.
Plan policies and procedures	Fees, committee attendance, etc.
Quality management	Compliance with plan standards for preventive care and health maintenance
Patient relations	Patient satisfaction, including patient retention, transferring patients to other providers, waiting time, availability, etc.

Source: Adapted from P.R. Kongstvedt, Formal Physician Performance Evaluations, *The Managed Health Care Handbook*, 2nd Edition, pp. 189–197, © 1993, Aspen Publishers, Inc.

You should personally conduct all performance appraisals of your direct subordinates. It is also desirable for you occasionally to observe the appraisal interviews conducted by subordinate managers of their subordinates. At a minimum, you should read their evaluations and review them with your subordinate managers. This will help prevent subordinate managers from using the performance appraisal process to satisfy their own needs for power and control at the expense of their subordinates. Reading evaluations will also provide you with an efficient way of learning more about your employees and their strengths and weaknesses.

REFERENCES

1. M.E. Tubbs, Goal-Setting: A Meta-Analysis Examination of the Empirical Evidence, *Journal of Applied Psychology* 91 (1986):474–483.

2. R. Solomon, You Can't Win by Doing Employees' Work for Them, *American Medical News*, 19 July 1993, p. 26.

3. P.R. Kongstvedt, "Formal Physician Performance Evaluations," in *The Managed Health Care Handbook*, 2nd ed. (Gaithersburg, Md.: Aspen Publishers, Inc., 1993), 189–197.

CHAPTER 3

Employment Methods

Chapter Objectives

This chapter will tell you how to hire front office and professional employees, including physicians, using scientific selection methods. By using these methods, you will reduce personnel costs due to turnover, absenteeism, poor job performance, and increased training as well as legal costs associated with infractions of the Equal Employment Opportunity laws. You will learn how to:

1. use interviews, tests, references, resumes, and work samples to ensure that the best available personnel are hired
2. organize the employment process, so that it is as inexpensive and time efficient as possible
3. define your appropriate role in the employment process as well as the roles of subordinates and consultants
4. recruit effectively, so that you can apply the selection methods to a well-qualified pool of applicants

Whenever you hire someone, you are placing a bet. You are betting that the new employee *can* perform the job adequately, will *want* to perform the job adequately, and will *remain* with you for a reasonable amount of time. This chapter is about changing the odds on the employment bet so that they become more favorable. Employment methods, including interviews, tests, work samples, references, and the like, when properly used, can improve your chance of making a good hiring decision. Using methods that don't work at all, or using good employment methods inappropriately, is equivalent to making a decision by tossing a coin.

Generally, you will not be personally conducting interviews, administering tests, and scanning resumes, with the exception of those times when you are hiring someone who will work directly with you, such as a physician or surgical assistant. Instead, your business manager or human resources director will perform these tasks. Ultimately, however, you are responsible for the adequacy of the employment process, and you certainly will have to live with its consequences. Your appropriate role as a physician manager, therefore, is to ensure that those who will be doing the hiring know what to do. To do this, you need a vision of what a thorough, competent employment process looks like. Figure 3–1 summarizes the personnel management process. This chapter covers the recruiting, selection, and evaluation process in Figure 3–1.

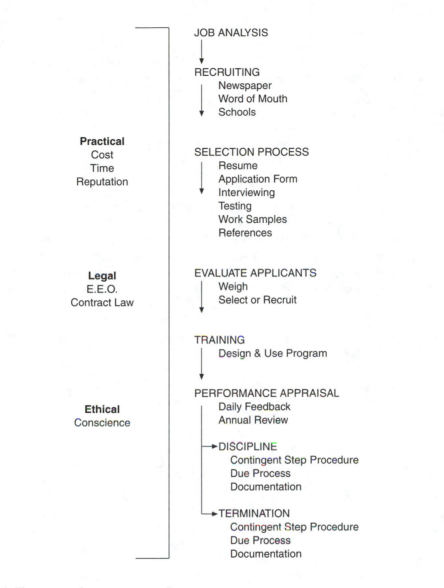

Figure 3–1 The personnel management process.

Let's use some common sense. One obvious way to know whether a person can perform a job is to put him or her on the job for a period of time, observe his or her performance, and determine whether it is both minimally adequate and superior to that of other competing applicants. In an ideal world, this is how we would employ people. Unfortunately, there are problems with this approach, the most obvious of which are that it would take excessive time and would be organizationally disruptive to other staff, patients, and so forth to have new applicants cycling through a position. Perhaps, however, we can take this principle of obtaining a work sample, reduce its size and length, and isolate applicants from the rest of the organization and patients. If we do this effectively, we may still get a good indication of the applicant's skills.

A commonly used example of this strategy is a typing test. This is especially the case if the material to be typed is drawn from existing files and charts, so that it is typical of what the job incumbent will do on a daily basis. This approach to identifying applicant skills is called a work sample. Work samples may not always be appropriate. Some job issues are difficult to simulate. Sometimes, applicants will need extensive training after hiring, such as in the operation of scheduling software, so that a pre-employment work sample doesn't make sense. A work sample, however, is a useful metaphor to introduce the strategy of hiring, and we will revisit this selection method in more detail later.

To use a work sample and the other employment methods that will be discussed, you must first determine which tasks are actually performed on the job. If you don't really understand what an employee does, then you won't know what tasks to put into the work sample or to assess in other ways. This process of discovering what employees really do is called job analysis, and it results in a document called a job description. Just as a job description provides the basis of performance appraisal (Chapter 2), it will provide the basis for determining what job applicant skills to assess.

Once you know the content of the job, you can choose appropriate tools for making the hiring decision. These tools include work samples, interviews, tests, references, and resumes, to name a few. Because each tool has distinct strengths and weaknesses, you will have to learn when to use each one. Many employers limit their choice of employment methods to interviews or, perhaps, to a particular test routinely used for all jobs. This strategy will result in less than ideal employment decisions. It is analogous to having only two tools in your garage and using them for all jobs performed around the house. Try digging a ditch with a rake or cutting the lawn with a hedge trimmer. It *can* be done, but the costs are high in terms of time, effort, and the quality of the final product.

It is also important to generate a large pool of applicants. Even if you develop a perfectly good employment procedure, it will not help you much if competent applicants don't apply for the job. The process of generating an applicant pool is called recruiting. It is important to know how to recruit a good applicant pool as well as how to select from it effectively.

Finally, you will need a selection strategy for sifting through the applicant pool. In addition to identifying the best applicant, you must be able to apply your selection tools efficiently and cost effectively. If you don't have a workable selection strategy, you will get bogged down in a swamp of applicants and waste valuable time evaluating candidates who should have been eliminated at the beginning of the process.

First, we will cover these topics by focusing on the hiring of clerical, administrative, and supervisory personnel, such as office managers, computer operators, and secretaries. A significant proportion of employment by medical practices, hospitals, and managed care organizations is concerned with these types of positions. The strategy for hiring physicians and other professionals, such as nurses and technicians, is generally the same, although the specific tests, questions, and work samples will be different. The selection of physicians and other professionals is discussed in a separate section of this chapter.

Instituting a selection process for a job proceeds in the following manner. First, determine the tasks that are performed on the job. Second, identify appropriate selection tools. Third, develop a recruiting strategy. Fourth, construct a decision-making procedure to identify the best applicant. Finally, do all these things in as simple, timely, effective, and inexpensive a manner as possible.

All the methods discussed in this chapter can be carried out by a hospital human resources administrator or a practice business manager under the initial guidance of a human resources professional. Remember, you personally are not in the business of hiring; you are in the business of practicing medicine or managing medically related affairs, which is where you should devote your time. Because of the value of your time, you will want to involve yourself personally only at selected critical points in the process, and then only for filling certain jobs. Nevertheless, it is essential that you understand what *should* occur, so that you can appropriately assign tasks to subordinates or consultants and determine whether they have properly completed their work. This responsibility strikes to the heart of the physician manager's job responsibilities. The word *you* is used throughout this chapter to indicate the person performing the action being discussed. Often, therefore, this will not refer personally to the physician manager but to the subordinate to whom the physician manager has delegated the task.

JOB ANALYSIS: IDENTIFYING SELECTION FACTORS

To hire the right person for a job, you must first understand the content of the job in detail. If you don't know what skills and abilities are needed to perform the job, then you cannot determine whether an applicant has the appropriate skills or abilities. Employee selection, therefore, always starts with collecting information about the job. The process of collecting this information is called job analysis, and the resulting document describing the job is called a job description. Exhibit 2–2 in Chapter 2 contains a sample job description for a practice business manager position.

Job analysis can be performed in a number of different ways. If you are a physician manager in a large organization, such as a hospital, health maintenance organization (HMO), or large group practice, there may already be job descriptions in existence. If this is the case, these job descriptions are a good place to start. Never assume, however, that an existing job description, especially if it is several years old, is still valid. Job content can change rapidly, especially in a high-technology, rapidly changing environment such as health care. If the job description is wrong or incomplete, you might not assess the right skills. Existing job descriptions can be validated by talking to current incumbents or their supervisors. If you have any doubt about the ac-

curacy of the job description, reanalyze the job.

There are several ways to conduct a job analysis. If there is an employee currently performing the job, you can interview that employee. You want to know exactly what the employee does and how often he or she does it. You might ask the employee to verbally walk you through a typical workday. Also, have the employee describe any tasks that are performed only weekly or monthly. Talk to the employee's supervisor. He or she may have a somewhat different perspective on the position's content.

Another good way to obtain job analysis information is to observe the employee performing the job. Keep in mind that, because of your presence, the employee may change the job content or speed up or slow down the performance of tasks. Although employees may tend to exaggerate the importance or frequency of some tasks, it is rare that they will fabricate or totally eliminate tasks. This is especially true in smaller organizations such as a medical practice, where the employee might well expect that whoever is conducting the job analysis already knows the content of the job.

Finally, sometimes you can obtain important information about a job by briefly performing it yourself. This technique familiarizes you with the small points that might easily be missed in an interview. For example, when analyzing a secretarial position, I sat in for the secretary for a morning. I discovered that it was not unusual for a patient to be at the window making a copayment while another was waiting to schedule an appointment, the telephone was ringing, and someone else was grabbing the appointment book. Performing the work conveyed an intensity that was not readily apparent from interviewing or observing the incumbent.

Any job analysis method can lead to judgments that may be altered when the information is checked using another method. A good example of this was a job analysis I conducted for a bus company. After interviewing several bus drivers, I was very impressed with the complexity of the job, to such a degree that I was inclined to rate the job as only slightly less demanding than that of an astronaut or polar explorer. To check my observations, I bought a ticket and rode the buses for a few hours. This put things back into perspective. The tasks were performed exactly as the drivers had described to me in the interviews. The circumstances under which they were performed, however, were very different. The level of complexity and intensity was not as I had imagined. The drivers had not tried to deceive me. Quite the contrary, they were very aware of what they did on a daily basis and had accurately conveyed this to me. As an outsider, however, the impression that their words created was not as the job appeared when it was actually observed.

Once you have a good sense of what the job entails, write a job description. The job description in Exhibit 2–2 (Chapter 2) is typical. Job descriptions should be written in concise, clear language. There is no point to using excessive, flowery, or imprecise language. The goal is to identify the major job performance issues. It is not necessary for the job description to describe the position down to the last detail. For example, you don't need to know how many times a day the business manager picks up a pen, but it is important not to miss any major job performance issues. The next step involves reducing the job description down to a handful of major performance issues.

The whole job analysis and description process should not take much time. The job analyst should be able to interview a typical clerical incumbent in about 30 to 60 minutes. Perhaps observation of any critical or confusing parts of the job will take another 30 minutes. Writing the job description should take no more than an hour. Once the job description has been assembled, give it to the incumbent for his or her comments. The cost associated with this process is minimal when you consider how difficult it would be to fix the problems that would result from hiring the wrong person. The job description only needs to be changed if the job changes. It is quite possible, therefore, to use the same job description for many years and for the selection of several job holders.

Job descriptions should be written before you need them. When employees give notice or are fired, you must move as quickly as possible. In addition, terminated employees and employees who resign because they are unhappy tend not to be cooperative. It is best, therefore, to write the descriptions in advance, so that they will be available in an emergency. You will also use job descriptions in most other personnel management procedures, including performance evaluation, training, and compensation. Thus having job descriptions on hand also will expedite these procedures.

If you are starting a new medical practice, you obviously can't interview the job incumbent. There are, however, a number of ways to obtain the information you need. Start by mentally visualizing all the tasks that must be performed in the practice, and then separate them into logical clusters. These logical clusters will be jobs. If you couple this "what if" analysis with a healthy dose of adaptability and flexibility, your initial job descriptions will be adequate. Another way of acquiring job analysis information is to obtain access to a colleague's practice and to interview and unobtrusively observe the personnel there.

Once you have constructed a job description for a position, you must distill it down to the major employment issues, which are called selection factors. Using the job description in Exhibit 2–2, the typical selection factors for a practice business manager might reduce down to supervision, collection, taxes, problem identification, and teamwork. Applicants would be evaluated on only these factors. There are two reasons for this reduction process:

1. It would take too much time to evaluate applicants on their ability to perform *all* tasks that make up a job. Concentrate, therefore, on the most important job performance issues. If tasks are not important, then don't waste expensive selection time on them.

2. Many tasks cluster together because they require the same fundamental skills or knowledge. For example, it is not necessary to assess whether an applicant can type letters as opposed to memos or address labels. There is an underlying factor here: typing ability. If the applicant pos-

sesses the basic skill of typing, it is reasonable to assume that this skill can be applied to a number of circumstances that only differ superficially.

Exhibit 3–1 contains a job description for a computer operator/secretary position, and Table 3–1 shows how this description can be reduced down to a set of selection factors. Generally, you can adequately describe a job using between four and seven selection factors. If you draft more than eight selection factors, look at them carefully to see whether some factors can be combined. If you can't, then you should consider whether the job is too broad for any one person to perform adequately. It may be that a broad job can be performed if the workload is relatively light. As your organization grows and the workload increases, however, the employee may become overburdened.

The most appropriate person to perform the job analysis task is the supervisor of the position to be filled. You should only consider becoming personally involved for positions that report directly to you, such as the position of nurse or business manager if you are practice based. In this case, the size of your practice will determine your involvement. If, for example, the open position is a surgical assistant, then your business manager would probably conduct the job analysis and draft the job description, but with substantial input on your part. If you are a physician manager in a hospital or large health care organization, it is likely that the personnel or human resources department will do the job analysis. If this is the case, try to review the job description before applicant selection begins, so that you can add or delete content.

Positions that don't report directly to you should be analyzed by their supervisors. For ex-

---

Exhibit 3–1 Job Description for Position of Computer Operator/Secretary

Primary Duties

The Computer Operator/Secretary is the primary practice expert in the operation of the computer system. Duties include the operation of all computer hardware and software, troubleshooting problems with hardware and software, learning how to use new hardware and software, training new employees in the operation of hardware and software, making recommendations for the acquisition of new hardware and software, and developing procedures for and taking the responsibility for being certain that all databases are backed up on a regular basis.

In addition, it is the responsibility of the Computer Operator/Secretary to identify methods and procedures for the operation of the office in the event that the computer system becomes temporarily inoperative and to train appropriate personnel regarding these procedures.

The Computer Operator/Secretary must be proficient in the operation of *Medic*, word processing programs (Microsoft *Word* 6.0), database pro-

grams (*Filemaker Pro* 3.0), spreadsheet programs (Microsoft *Excel* 5.0), and any other programs necessary for the operation of the practice.

Secretarial duties include patient interaction, answering telephones, scheduling appointments, collecting fees, word processing, and other duties and responsibilities as assigned by the supervisor.

Major Job Performance Factors

- Operate and troubleshoot computer hardware and software
- Proficiency in various programs, including *Medic*, Microsoft *Word* 6.0, Microsoft *Excel* 5.0, *Filemaker Pro* 3.0.
- Patient interaction: personal and telephone
- Office activities: word processing, filing, scheduling appointments, etc.
- Collecting fees

Supervision

Reports to the business manager.

Table 3–1 Selection Factors for the Job of Computer Operator/Secretary

Factor	Description
Word Processing/software	Ability to use *Word* 6.0, *Filemaker Pro* 3.0, *Excel* 5.0, *Medic*, or similar types of programs; ability to learn these programs
Typing skills	Ability to type correctly and with speed
Interpersonal skills	Ability to communicate in socially appropriate ways with others
Anticipatory skills	Ability to anticipate the effects of actions on patients and peers
Language skills	Appropriate use of grammar and syntax

ample, the business manager of a practice should conduct the job analysis and write the job description for secretary, collection, and billing positions.

Assuming that you will delegate these tasks to someone, you should examine the final list of selection factors and compare them with the job description. You should be able to discern a logical relationship between the two documents. Personally performing this check will serve as a control, providing some assurance that the job analysis was properly performed.

In a private practice or smaller health care organization, all this work could easily be contracted out to a consultant. If you choose to use a consultant, it is a good idea to have the consultant simultaneously train one of your employees in job analysis methods because these skills are easily learned. By doing this, you will reduce the likelihood of having to pay future consulting fees. A management consultant should be able to do a job analysis of most office jobs in a few hours and write the job description and identify selection factors in another one to two hours. These time estimates are longer than those for medical practice personnel because consultants will be less familiar with the content of the jobs and will produce more polished documents, thus requiring additional time.

SELECTION METHODS

There are many different selection methods from which to choose. Table 3–2 contains some of the more common ones and the job performance factors for which they are generally appro-

priate. As we have seen previously, one way to think about a selection method is as a sample of applicant behavior. This is a good place to begin, but there will be some situations where other strategies are more appropriate. For example, suppose the new job incumbent will have to use specialized medical office management software, such as *MediMac*, *Medic*, or scheduling software. If you restrict the applicant pool to only those who already have experience using this specific software, you might reject many applicants who otherwise could have performed the job very well. In addition, your search for the right applicant may take much longer because you will be looking for the relatively rare applicant who is already trained *and* who is acceptable on all other employment factors.

Under these circumstances, it would probably make sense to look for an applicant who had the underlying ability to learn how to use your medical office management software. In this situation, it would be best to look for applicants with learning ability, sometimes also called IQ or intelligence, because this is a good predictor of which applicants will be able to benefit the most from a training program. If, during the course of screening applicants, someone appeared who was already trained in the software, he or she clearly would have an advantage in the selection process, but you are no longer counting on being able to find someone such as this.

An alternative strategy to a work sample, therefore, is to look for underlying human abilities that are clearly job relevant, based on the content of the job description. Psychological tests and ability tests can be very helpful to as-

Table 3–2 Employment Methods and Their Uses

Method	Performance Factors
Resume	A work sample Experience Education Work history Practicalities
Application form	Same as resume, and compare across applicants Obtain legal protections
Interview	Interpersonal skills Verbal skills Communication skills Motivation/career goals Sell applicant on job
Testing	Technical job knowledge Technical proficiency Aptitude (ability to learn) Personality Honesty (?)
Work samples and simulations	Technical job knowledge Technical proficiency Decision making Problem solving
In basket	Decision making Problem solving
References	Verification of data (?)

sess applicant abilities. Human abilities such as learning ability, adaptability, accuracy, stress tolerance, receptiveness to being managed, and attention to detail, to mention only a few, can be assessed by various tests.

We will now explore in more detail the available employment method choices and job performance issues that they generally measure best. Then we will discuss how to assemble the various employment methods for a job into an effective, time-efficient, and cost-effective employment process.

THE RESUME

Resumes are valuable sources of information for two reasons. First, resumes are samples of applicants' behaviors. They are statements that applicants prepare themselves at their own pace, stating what they feel is important about themselves and what qualifies them for a job. Look at a resume first, therefore, as a sample of behavior. Second, each resume is a statement of what the applicant has been doing with his or her life.

When examining a resume as a behavior sample, consider its orderliness, neatness, and organization. How clearly and concisely does it convey information? If the applicant takes two pages to express what could be presented in one page, this may indicate that the applicant will not be able to construct concise documents or arguments or "get to the point" on the job. This may be a hypothesis to evaluate during the employment process if you feel the applicant is otherwise qualified for the position. Does it appear that some thought has gone toward organizing information in a logical manner? If the resume is confusing or illogically organized, this is an indication that the applicant may not be able to present information in a logical, understandable manner to you, your employees, patients, and so forth. Are spelling, punctuation, and grammar correct? If you find mistakes, it may mean that the applicant does not have basic language skills, is a lazy or sloppy worker, or tends to be rushed and make mistakes.

After you have evaluated the resume as a work sample, evaluate its content. First, examine the applicant's previous experience and education to determine whether he or she has the skills required for the job. This doesn't mean that the applicant must have performed a job with the same job title or previously worked for a medical organization. For example, bookkeeping in a medical practice is little different from bookkeeping in any other type of professional or service organization. An applicant who has worked for an accounting firm, a lawyer, or an architect should have little difficulty making the transition to a medical practice.

Examine how frequently the applicant has changed jobs. Eliminate applicants who have a history of frequent job changes. They are job hoppers who will be dissatisfied in any situation, and their dissatisfaction will cause disruption and dissension. Look for a logical order or progression to the job changes. Good applicants will show a history of increased skills and responsibilities. A bookkeeper who then became a secretary, and then the receivables administrator for a 15-physician practice, and who now is applying to become the manager of a 4-physician practice is moving in the right direction. A manager of a 4-physician practice who is now willing to take a secretarial position is going the wrong way. The associated pay and status reductions can create all sorts of acting out and displaced anger. Going back to our betting analogy, this latter employee is a bad bet.

Examine the resume for unexplained gaps in employment. If you find any, the applicant must account for them—*all of them*. An employment gap sometimes indicates failure at a job, perhaps even time in jail. Discuss any gaps with the applicant during the interview. You will have to make a judgment concerning the reasonableness of the applicant's explanation.

On many jobs, education and experience are to some degree interchangeable. An applicant for a bookkeeping position who has no previous experience but has received appropriate, documented education might well be able to perform the job. Jobs requiring skills that normally aren't obtained through formal education, such as insurance billing, are best performed by people who have had previous experience. This, of course, creates a problem for the inexperienced applicant: how to obtain experience if the only people who are hired are people with experience. This is a problem, but it is not *your* problem.

Generally, the person screening the resumes for a position should be the one to whom the incumbent will report. Physician managers may be tempted to delegate initial resume screening to others. Your ability to judge with whom you can work, however, can rarely be matched, and never exceeded, by the judgment of others.

THE APPLICATION FORM

Generally, the initial screening of applicants will be based on resumes, followed by short telephone interviews. Survivors will then be invited in for additional interviewing, testing, and so on. It is desirable at this point to have all applicants complete an application form. This will make it easier to compare applicants on education, previous experience, and the like. The alternative is to dig this information out of the resumes, which is a frustrating, time-consuming job. Another important reason for using an application form is that it can provide justification for immediate dismissal of an employee who lied about qualifications, credentials, previous experience, and so on. The application form should state that supplying false information may result in the denial or immediate termination of employment.[1]

Application forms should only request job-relevant information. Do not ask applicants about their race, religion, sex, national origin, or age because these are not relevant to evaluating applicant performance. Exhibit 3–2 contains a sample application form. State laws vary consid-

erably regarding what questions are permissible, and you should contact your attorney before using any application form. For example, federal law allows the use of Ms., Mrs., Miss, and Mr. on application forms, whereas some states, such as New York and Michigan, forbid this prac-

Exhibit 3–2 Application Form

Last Name		First Name			Middle Name			
Present Address (Street, City, State, Zip Code)			Telephone Number			Social Security Number		
Position Applying For			Date Available					

Names and Addresses of Schools Attended	Dates From	To	Degree	Major or Subject Area	G.P.A. Major	Overall

Licenses or Certificates	Granting Agency	Expiration Date

Honor Societies, Professional Societies, Etc.:

List All Previous Work Experiences. Begin With Most Recent Position Held. Use Additional Application Forms if Necessary.

Employer's Name and Address	Supervisor's Name and Title	Job Title & Work Description	Salary	Employed From

Work or Educational References. Name of Reference	Name of Organization	This Reference Was Your:

I acknowledge that I am seeking employment with _____. I further state that all of the information that I have provided is true. By signing this application form I acknowledge that employment may be denied or terminated if I have supplied false or misleading information. I also understand that the position that I am applying for is an at-will position, and that if I am hired my employment can be terminated at the sole discretion of the employer.

Job Applicant's Signature_____ Date _____

tice.[2] Refer to Chapter 14 for a more complete discussion of Equal Employment Opportunity and how to utilize your attorney.

Finally, if the employee is to work without a written contract, the application form should contain a strong at-will employment provision. At-will employment gives you flexibility to terminate an unsatisfactory employee. Once again, refer to Chapter 14 for a discussion of at-will employment and written contract employment arrangements.

THE INTERVIEW

The interview is the most commonly used selection tool. Unfortunately, given the way that it is normally used, it is also one of the least effective.[3] Management research beginning as early as 1915 has consistently indicated that interviews tend to have low reliability. This means that if you interview the same person on two different occasions, your conclusions might not agree. Similarly, if two interviewers interview the same applicant, they might not reach the same conclusion. Research also indicates that the interview has low validity.[4] This means that interviewer predictions of eventual employee job performance tend to be inaccurate. If this is the case, why is the interview the most commonly used selection tool, and why has its use persisted over the years?

The answers to these questions tell us a lot about employers and how they tend to misuse the interview. Many employers view the hiring process as a test of their own personal intuition. They don't view the interview as a distinct tool. Instead, they believe that their personal intuition is the tool and that the interview simply provides a time, a place, and a process in which to utilize their intuition. If in fact the interview is really nothing more than an opportunity to apply intuition and perspicacity, then it requires no prior preparation. In addition, most employers, physicians and their business managers included, don't want to take the time to prepare a proper interview! As a result, the interview is typically a morass of questions that are either "pets"

(posed to all applicants irrespective of the job) or created on the spot with little or no thought regarding what is being measured or how to evaluate the applicant's response.

Irrespective of the research evidence, interviewers are usually convinced that they make good employment decisions. Two factors usually operate to create this fallacious belief in success. First, many tend to remember the past selectively. Good employment decisions tend to be remembered, and bad ones tend to be forgotten or explained away. Second, there will always be a natural incidence of success in choosing from any pool of applicants. Even if you make hiring decisions by tossing a coin, some of those chosen will be successful employees. If a job is minimally demanding or if your recruiting is effective, some proportion of the applicants might well have the appropriate skills because those who are unable or uninterested will tend to self-select out. As a consequence, even poor interviewing will result in some hiring success, and the interviewer will be led to overestimate his or her contribution to this success. The interviewer will then continue to use the interview in ways that contribute little or nothing to obtaining better employees.

Fortunately, all of this does not mean that the interview is useless; rather, it is a testimonial to its routine misuse. Many review studies, such as the one conducted by Weisner and Cronshaw (1988),[5] have consistently pointed to the superiority of structured interviews over the unstructured anecdotal interviews conducted in most health care organizations. A structured interview has the following characteristics:

- The interview is limited to measuring factors that have been identified in a job analysis.
- Questions are written ahead of time.
- Scoring standards are identified for each question. That is, the characteristics of a good answer and a bad answer, at a minimum, are written down. Often interviewers write "great" questions, only to learn later

that they can't determine what constitutes a good or a poor answer!

- All applicants are asked the same questions in the same order, thereby giving everyone a "level playing field."
- Applicant answers are then compared to the scoring standards to evaluate how well an applicant has performed, and to determine how applicants compare to each other.

The effect of standardizing the interview is dramatic. Weisner and Cronshaw reported that the average correlation between interviewers' predictions of job performance and actual job performance was 0.20 when they used unstructured interviews. This is on a scale in which 1.00 means perfect association, 0.00 means random association, and –1.00 means perfect but inverse association between the interviewer's conclusions and subsequent job performance. When interviewers used a structured interview method, the correlation increased to 0.63. Because of the nature of the number scale for these values, the degree of predictability for the structured interview was actually over nine times higher than for the unstructured interview.[6]

Now, let's return to our idea of a work sample that requires applicants to perform as they would on the job and consider what you are asking applicants to do during an interview: *communicate* and *interact* in a social situation. A successful interview strategy, therefore, will utilize the interview to assess those things for which it is a natural work sample and will do this in a structured manner.

You would probably unconsciously abide by the work sample rule for interviewing in extreme cases. Few employers, for example, would ask an applicant whether he or she is a good typist! Obviously, applicants could say whatever they please, whereas a simple typing test would provide much more accurate information. Once we go beyond foolish examples, however, employers are inclined to misuse the interview in other absurd, if less obvious, ways. For example, if you use the interview to assess technical skills, reliability, learning ability, intelligence, work attitudes, honesty, or personality traits, you are misusing it. These factors can be more accurately assessed using other methods.

Exhibit 3–3 contains some examples of structured interview questions and response categories for a factor of supervisory skills. Notice that the scoring categories are not specific answers but instead delineate the *characteristics* of what constitutes a good versus a poor response. People are very creative, and you will never anticipate all the unique answers that applicants will produce. Generally, however, there will be three or four themes that run through answers and characterize their quality. This is what you are trying to build your scoring categories around. *If you can't write good scoring categories, then you probably have a poorly worded or ill-conceived question!*

It is usually sufficient to anticipate three levels of response to a question, such as "outstanding," "acceptable," and "not acceptable." The number of evaluation categories is arbitrary and should depend on what you find to be useful. Some questions could generate five easily separated categories, whereas other questions could be evaluated with only two categories.

When you are conducting the interview, you should concentrate on what the applicant is saying and take notes for later evaluation. After the interview, you can rewrite your notes into a more complete narrative evaluation, so that you can more easily recall the applicant's responses. You can also then classify the responses into scoring categories. If the applicant says something that you want to pursue during the interview, feel free to pursue it. Be certain, however, to come back to the point of departure and proceed from there.

It is very important to understand that your evaluation criteria express a value system. For example, look at question 3 in Exhibit 3–3. Some physicians consider the very poor answer the best answer and would evaluate applicants who would discuss the personal and business implications of a personal problem with a subordinate as having poor supervisory skills. The

Exhibit 3–3 Structured Interview Questions and Response Categories

Supervisory Skills for Business Manager Position: Exhibiting patience and tactfulness when dealing with fellow employees, remaining open to new ideas and suggestions, and listening to and understanding employee needs.

1. How would you handle a situation in which there is a deterioration in a subordinate's performance?

   A. *Good:* Answer refers to attempts to determine the cause and to institute corrective actions.
   B. *Fair:* Answer refers to confrontation with and warning of subordinate.
   C. *Poor:* Answer refers to dismissal of subordinate with no attempt at corrective action or to corrective actions that do not directly address the performance problem.

2. Lori is a secretary who collects patient fees and does typing and other clerical tasks. She comes to you with an idea for improving the negotiation of patient fees. Negotiation of patient fees is your job, not hers. How would you respond?

   A. *Good:* Answer refers to sincere evaluation of the subordinate's suggestion and to attempt to understand the reasons why it was suggested.
   B. *Poor:* Answer refers to superficial acceptance without evaluation or to outright rejection of the idea of a subordinate making such a suggestion.

3. An employee comes to you to discuss a personal problem. How would you respond to this situation?

   A. *Good:* Answer characterized by setting aside time to examine with the employee the problem's possible job-related consequences as well as the personal consequences.
   B. *Fair:* Answer characterized by a discussion of the job-related consequences only.
   C. *Poor:* Answer characterized by discussion of the personal consequences only.
   D. *Very poor:* Answer characterized by refusal to discuss the problem and telling the employee, implicitly or explicitly, to leave personal problems at home.

scoring categories often represent a value system that should reflect *your* preferences. There is nothing wrong with this, as long as you understand your preferences and *consciously* build them into the applicant evaluation process.

Problems arise when you select employees on one basis but then ask them to perform in a contrary manner. To achieve consistency between your preferences and employee characteristics, you may have to engage in some serious introspection. If you feel that the best strategy for running an office is to refuse to discuss personal problems, then don't hire applicants whose natural inclination is to do the contrary.

Keep in mind that the interview will best assess applicants' abilities when they are using their skills as they would use them on the job. For example, if you are trying to assess medical terminology skills, then develop questions around discussions with previous job incumbents that require the understanding and correct utilization of medical language. On the other hand, if you are trying to assess general language skills, including the ability to use good grammar, get the applicant to talk on any familiar topic, such as hobbies, career goals, or previous jobs. Concentrate on *how* applicants communicate as opposed to the *content* of their communication.

If you are familiar with the job and have developed a clear list of selection factors, it should take an hour or two to develop questions and evaluation criteria for all the interview factors. Keep in mind that the questions and evaluation criteria for each factor may be used for other jobs that require that same factor. If you have several clerical jobs that require good verbal skills, for example, you can use the same questions and criteria for all these jobs.

Interviewing is a task within the capacity of most business managers and office managers. In general, it should not be contracted out to a consultant unless none of your staff has the time available. The personal involvement of your staff in selecting their associates will more than compensate for their initial lack of structured interviewing experience. Generally, an employee will be more knowledgeable than a consultant about the position. Finally, using employees to conduct structured interviews will develop their interview skills, thereby giving you the flexibility to respond to unexpected employment needs and keep your consulting costs down.

Whether you get personally involved should depend on the position. If you will be working closely with whomever is selected, you will probably want some involvement. Obviously, you will only want to use your time to interview the best applicants—those who have already cleared several other selection hurdles. Positions more removed from the focus of your activities might not require your personal attention. This is, however, a matter of personal preference. Some practice-based physician managers insist on personally interviewing all their employees. Using the interview to hire physicians is discussed in a later section in this chapter.

TESTING

Testing can assess job-relevant skills and personality characteristics that cannot be accurately assessed using an interview, such as intelligence, personality, work ethic, sense of responsibility, motivation, and supervisory capacity. Have you ever had an employee who was good technically but just couldn't seem to get along with anyone? If your answer is yes, then testing is an alternative you should consider. Similarly, most job proficiency skills and aptitudes can also be best assessed using tests. Unfortunately, many employers who could greatly benefit from testing do not utilize it. There seem to be three general reasons for this. First, it never occurs to some physician managers that they could use testing. Second, some feel uncomfortable using an unfamiliar technology. Third, some believe that federal Equal Employment Opportunity laws have made testing difficult to use, if not illegal.

Should these reasons prevent you from utilizing testing? As to the first, obviously not. You are now informed: Testing is an available alternative that is cost effective and applicable to jobs found in health care organizations of all sizes. As to the second, although you and your staff may currently be unfamiliar with how to use testing, you or they can develop the competence in a relatively short time and at a reasonable cost. In addition, larger health care organizations, such as hospitals and health care systems, should have personnel or human resources staff with testing skills. If they don't, then this department desperately needs to upgrade its capabilities. As to the third, there is nothing in the 1964 Civil Rights Act, the Equal Employment Opportunity Commission's *Uniform Guidelines*, or any other piece of federal civil rights legislation that precludes using employment tests.[7] The *Uniform Guidelines* do raise some issues with which both you and your staff should be familiar, but these relate to any employment method, including unstructured and structured interviewing. These issues are discussed in detail in Chapter 14.

Tests should be selected with the following considerations:

- Select tests based on a logical fit with the job description. If the job description calls for learning ability and stress tolerance, then these should be constructs to look for in a test.
- Use published, validated tests. By this I mean tests that have been developed by a reputable test publisher. Have them show you evidence that the test really measures what it purports to measure.
- Utilize human resources professionals to set up your initial testing and selection pro-

grams. These can then be used as a model for future efforts.

- Construct simple work samples, such as for word processing and collection skills.

Generally, I recommend that smaller health care organizations retain a consultant to create a selection program for a position. This is analogous to retaining an accountant to set up your accounting software, procedures, and bookkeeping methods. After this has been done, the bookkeeping process can be managed by organizational personnel, with occasional consults as technical questions arise. Similarly, a human resources professional can help you with setting up a selection process and selecting tests. Subsequently, the process can be managed by your employed personnel. The goal is to work with the consultant to learn the process of selection and test identification, so that your staff can work the consultant out of a job.

The process that I will now describe for developing a testing program is essentially what a consultant would do for you. Obviously, you can follow the same process, especially once you have seen it applied by a consultant. After conducting a thorough job analysis, identifying selection factors, and then selecting those that can be best measured by a test, the challenge is to find appropriate tests. One source of information about tests is published reference books. They provide descriptions of tests and information about how to obtain them. One of the best is *Tests: A Comprehensive Reference for Assessment in Psychology, Education, and Business*.[8] An alternative, more academic in its orientation, is *The Tenth Mental Measurements Yearbook*, which is generally available in college libraries.[9]

An example of a test review from *Tests* is given in Exhibit 3–4. Test reviews can provide much useful information, including what the test measures, how long it takes to administer, appropriate uses, scoring, cost, and source. Exhibit 3–5 shows the cover page and sample test items from the Wonderlic Personnel Test, which is described in Exhibit 3–4.

Exhibit 3–4 Wonderlic Test Review

THE WONDERLIC PERSONNEL TEST
E.F. Wonderlic

Adult

Purpose: Measures level of mental ability in business and industrial situations. Used for selection and placement of business personnel and for vocational guidance.

Description: 50-item paper-pencil test measuring general learning ability in verbal, spatial, and numerical reasoning. The test is used to predict an individual's ability to adjust to complex and rapidly changing job requirements and complete complex job training. The test also measures potential turnover and dissatisfaction on routinized or simple labor intensive jobs. Test items include analogies, analysis of geometric figures, arithmetic problems, disarranged sentences, sentence parallelism with proverbs, similarities, logic, definitions, judgment, direction following, and others. Examiner required. Suitable for group use. Available in Spanish, French, Mexican, Cuban, and Puerto Rican.

Timed: 12 minutes; may also be administered untimed.

Scoring: Hand key
aptitude and skills screening

Cost: 25 tests $45.00; 100 tests $105.00; complete package (25 or 100 equivalent forms, answer key for scoring, manual)

Publisher: E.F. Wonderlic Personnel Test, Inc.

Source: Reprinted with permission from R.C. Sweetland and D.J. Keyser, *Tests-A Comprehensive Reference for Assessments in Psychology, Education, and Business,* 3rd edition, © 1991, Pro-Ed.

As you examine the sample items from this test, they may look somewhat familiar. You probably encountered questions such as these at some point during schooling, when the school system conducted standardized testing. In other words, the Wonderlic is a simple, fast intelligence test. Intelligence underlies success on many jobs and is directly related to the ability to benefit from training programs. In addition, employees with higher IQs grasp principles and can apply them to new situations. Each new event, in effect, is not totally unique.

Recently, for example, an applicant for a front office position, who was well dressed and had good conversational English skills, scored in the 12th percentile on the Wonderlic. She could not answer an item that was similar to the following:

> An auto dealer bought some cars for $100,000. He sold them for $200,000, making $5,000 on each car. How many cars were involved?

Evaluation of her verbal skills and her motivation to get the job would never lead you to believe that she could not deal with a simple reasoning problem such as the one above. If we use a selection strategy, that we would rather reject 10 qualified applicants who would have succeeded than hire one who would fail, then it is obvious that you would not want to place a bet on this applicant.

Once you find a test that seems appropriate in terms of factor coverage, testing time, and cost, call the publisher. Most of the big publishing houses have toll-free telephone numbers. Describe the job for which you will be using the test, and discuss the appropriateness of the test for your application. If there is enough time, have the publisher mail you literature on the test, or order a specimen set. A specimen set usually includes one copy of the test, the test manual, and other literature describing the test's appropriate application.

Whenever you obtain a test, pay particular attention to its manual. A good test manual should contain easily understood administration and scoring instructions. It should also contain information about the appropriate use of the test and the test's reliability and validity. Reliability is the ability of a test to give consistent results. With a reliable test, applicants would get similar test scores if tested on two separate occasions. Validity concerns the question of whether a test really does measure what it is intended to measure. If a test is called the XYZ Test of Verbal Skills, it possesses validity if it really does measure verbal skills. Test manuals often provide a reference list of published papers and books that comment on the test. Many of these publications discuss using the test for specific jobs. By consulting some of these publications, reviewing information in the test manual, and carefully examining the test itself, you should be able to gain a sense of the test's appropriateness for your application.

DRUG TESTING

Drug testing of applicants may be appropriate under certain circumstances. Because drug testing is a relatively expensive procedure, you should give careful consideration to when and how you use it. There are a number of different drug tests. The least expensive, at a cost of about $10 to $15, is thin-layer chromatography (TLC). It is also the most subjective. Enzyme immunoassay (EIA) and radioimmunoassay (RIA) are slightly more expensive but provide more definitive results. These tests can detect the eight major abused drugs or drug classes: amphetamines, barbiturates, benzodiazepines, cannabinoids, cocaine, methaqualone, opiates, and phencyclidine. EIA and RIA are the most commonly used employment drug tests and cost between $15 and $20. Finally, gas chromatography and mass spectroscopy offer much greater sensitivity than EIA, RIA, and TLC. Because they are significantly more expensive, they must be reserved for situations in which extreme accuracy is essential, such as a follow-up to an initially positive finding.

All the tests discussed are susceptible to various degrees of cross-reaction. A cross-reaction is when a legal substance, such as poppy seeds, falsely indicates the presence of an illegal substance, such as heroin. With these facts in mind,

Exhibit 3–5 Wonderlic Personnel Test

WONDERLIC

PERSONNEL TEST
FORM V

NAME _____   Date_____

Social Security Number_____--____--_____

READ THIS PAGE CAREFULLY. DO EXACTLY AS YOU ARE TOLD.
DO NOT TURN OVER THIS PAGE UNTIL YOU ARE
INSTRUCTED TO DO SO.

PROBLEMS MUST BE WORKED WITHOUT THE AID OF A CALCULATOR
OR OTHER PROBLEM-SOLVING DEVICE.

This is a test of problem-solving ability. It contains various types of questions. Below is a sample question correctly filled in:

PLACE
ANSWERS
HERE

REAP is the opposite of
    1 obtain,   2 cheer,   3 continue,   4 exist,   5 sow .... (_____)
The correct answer is "sow." (It is helpful to underline the correct word.) The correct word is numbered 5. Then write the figure 5 in the brackets at the end of the line.
Answer the next sample question yourself.
Paper sells for 23 cents per pad. What will 4 pads cost? .... (_____)
The correct answer is 92¢. There is nothing to underline so just place "92¢" in the brackets.

Here is another example:
MINER MINOR—Do these words
    1 have similar meanings, 2 have contradictory meanings,
    3 mean neither the same nor opposite? .... (_____)

The correct answer is "mean neither same nor opposite" which is number 3 so all you have to do is place a figure "3" in the brackets at the end of the line.

When the answer to a question is a letter or a number, put the letter or number in the brackets. All letters should be printed.

This test contains 50 questions. It is unlikely that you will finish all of them, but do your best. After the examiner tells you to begin, you will be given exactly 12 minutes to work as many as you can. Do not go so fast that you make mistakes since you must try to get as many right as possible. The questions become increasingly difficult, so do not skip about. Do not spend too much time on any one problem. The examiner will not answer any questions after the test begins.

Now, lay down your pencil and wait for the examiner to tell you to begin!

Do not turn the page until you are told to do so.

Source: Reprinted with permission from Wonderlic Personnel Test, Inc., © 1988, Libertyville, Illinois.

you may want to consider testing an applicant in the following instances:

- The applicant, once hired, would have ready access to prescription drugs or large sums of cash.
- Other information indicates that the applicant may have a history of illicit drug abuse.
- The drug screen is the final employment hurdle.

In such situations, employers will generally use an EIA or RIA. If a positive finding is returned, the possibility of a false positive is evaluated using either gas chromatography or mass spectroscopy. Obviously, it is essential for the testing laboratory to retain all samples so that retesting is feasible.

WORK SAMPLES

As we have seen, a work sample uses a portion of the actual job to assess job applicants. A work sample provides a very effective way to evaluate applicants because it gives each applicant the opportunity actually to perform part of the job. *A work sample is only appropriate when you do not intend to train the new employee in the particular skill.* For example, word processing ability is a good work sample candidate because you certainly wouldn't intend to train a new employee to use Microsoft *Word* or Corel *WordPerfect* when there are many trained applicants looking for jobs. The limiting factor in using work samples is the complexity of the simulation that you will have to devise and the amount of time that it will take to assess an applicant. For example, you may be able to devise a work sample for word processing that would take five hours to administer and would be very indicative of applicants' abilities, but it would take so much time and be so expensive that it would be impractical.

Here is how to construct a work sample, using word processing skills as an example. The same basic procedures can be used to design other work sample measures. First, review the job description to get a good idea of the nature of documents typed and the word processing program used. If you have any doubt, talk to an incumbent, and also review documents from current office files. The work sample should be typical of the kind of word processing normally performed, such as a letters, reports, speeches, and the like. Because your goal is to make the work sample representative of office word processing, the range of skills, such as commands, macros, formatting, printing, merging addresses into form letters, exporting to other programs, and so forth, also should be represented in your work sample. This may be achieved by pulling together parts from several different documents. It may also require you to construct an item or document that is typical in character and gives applicants a good opportunity to exhibit their skills in a particular area, such as developing style sheets.

Generally, it is best to make the work sample long enough that even the very best applicants won't be able to finish. This will ensure that you get plenty of range in the scores. It is very important to standardize the work sample testing conditions, so that everyone is tested under similar conditions. Avoid testing in noisy rooms or where applicants may get interrupted by current employees.

Give the applicants plenty of time to learn the "feel" of your word processing equipment. The test should provide enough time for applicants to exhibit their word processing ability fully, including speed and accuracy. Use your common sense to develop reasonable scoring criteria. Set reasonable minimum standards in obvious knowledge areas, such as speed, errors, and ability to format, use tables, macros, and style sheets. The particular scoring criteria that you adopt are not as crucial as the consistency with which you apply them. As long as the rules are generally reasonable, the scoring criteria relate to actual job performance, and the criteria are consistently applied across applicants, the resulting rank ordering of applicants should reflect their relative skill levels.

There are many other opportunities to develop work samples. For example, telephone skills can be assessed by staging a work sample during an interview. Play the role of a caller, and have the applicant turn away so as not to react to your facial expressions or body language. Then develop a conversation to assess the applicant's abilities to use language, respond appropriately to questions, and so on. Keep the evaluation criteria simple; this will increase reliability. Develop two or three evaluation criteria, such as these:

- *Adequate:* Handled all questions and situations using appropriate language or tact.
- *Minimal:* Had some problems with appropriate language or tact.
- *Inadequate:* Had substantial problems with appropriate language or tact.

It is important not to confuse style preferences with skill. For example, if there is a particular way you like the telephone answered, it is not appropriate to expect your preference to be anticipated by applicants. The new employee can be trained in these matters of style. Instead, you should be looking for fundamental telephone answering skills, such as tact, appropriate language, and cordiality. In addition, keep your notes to support your conclusions. Later, you may want to review your evaluation of an applicant, and your original notes will allow you to reevaluate and weight the test conclusions.

Collection is another candidate for work sampling. You can construct a work sample around an aging analysis. See whether applicants can determine the highest-priority cases to work. Then have simulated case folders available for the worst cases. Have applicants draft letters, set up follow-up dates, recommend actions, and so forth. This process can be much more effective than asking applicants during an interview "How good are you at collection?" Other factors amenable to work sample assessment include writing, filing, checkbook balancing, interacting with patients (using a simulated patient), negotiating patient payment plans or fees (using a simulated patient), problem solving, and completing insurance forms.

CASE APPLICATION

Exhibit 3–6 contains the job description for a radiology practice's scheduling coordinator. Exhibit 3–7 presents the job performance factors that are derived from this job description. Table 3–3 identifies possible selection methods for each factor. This job provides a good example of where traditional assessment methods of interviewing and references would almost certainly be inadequate if used by themselves. Imagine, for example, asking applicants whether they can tolerate stress, whether they are good at problem solving, or whether they can work effectively as part of a team! For most applicants, the hope of getting a high-paying job would result in giving socially desirable answers in an interview: "Yes, I really enjoy solving challenging problems, and Stress Tolerance is my middle name!"

It can be seen in Table 3–3 that work samples are used to assess typing speed and word processing ability, whereas the interview assesses oral communications skills, presence, and motivation. The remaining factors are assessed with various tests. The Testing Time column indicates the time necessary to test one applicant. The Cost column contains the cost for one package of tests, and the Tests column indicates the number of applicants that can be tested for the cost. Twenty-three applicants can be assessed for a materials cost of about $585, with a few tests left over.[10]

Using this job as an example, let's examine some of these tests in more detail. We have previously examined the Wonderlic Personnel Test. In this instance, it will be used to assess learning ability because the job requires learning a complex, proprietary, computer-based scheduling system and physician preferences for times, hospitals, coworkers, and so forth. Those who are smarter, all things else equal, will probably learn the scheduling intricacies and deduce underlying principles of scheduling and physicians'

Exhibit 3–6 Job Description: Scheduling Coordinator

Job Summary

Generates and prepares weekly physician schedule for 21+ physicians in a timely manner, including assignment of physicians to more than 24 hospital and clinic cells. Communicates with physicians regarding scheduling process, and keeps administrator informed of changes and problems. Participates as a team member by performing additional assignments, such as word processing.

Supervision Received

Administrator

Supervision Given

None

Physical Demands

Those associated with an office environment, including use of computer.

Performance Requirements

Knowledge of skills and preferences of each physician and preferences of the various locations and facilities. Operate personal computer. Grammar, spelling, and punctuation appropriate for business communication. Ability to work effectively with demanding physicians. Ability to work under stress. Ability to work as a team member. Must be assertive and confident, but not abrasive.

Position Responsibilities

- Develop weekly schedules for 21+ physicians across 24+ locations/positions, which are forwarded to the Calendar Committee for review
- Adjust proposed schedules based on comments of Calendar Committee members
- Adjust schedules based on requests of physicians
- Maintain calendar of scheduled meetings and conferences
- Maintain master schedule of vacations, days/half days off, weekend work, and on-call
- Maintain log of special physician scheduling requests
- Update changes made to schedule during the week
- Maintain statistical reports for variables identified by Calendar Committee
- Maintain final schedules issued

preferences more easily, quickly, and effectively than those with lower levels of learning ability. The Wonderlic provides a good measure of this ability in 12 minutes for about $2.20 per applicant.[11]

Problem solving is assessed by the Judgment Test. This test measures aptitude for logical thinking and ability to deduce solutions to abstract problems.[12] Attention to detail is assessed with the Name-Finding Test, which measures short-term memory and attention to detail.

The NPF test measures stress tolerance, ability to adjust to challenging situations, and overall adjustment. It comprises 40 questions. Exhibit 3–8 provides descriptions of how people tend to behave when they score at various levels on the test. As you read these descriptions, consider how stress intolerant an applicant would have to be before you could accurately assess this in an interview. Most of us would probably be able to identify applicants in stanine categories 1 and 2. We might easily miss those in stanines 3 and 4 if they were having a good day. Now, examine the descriptions of stanines 7 through 9. Applicants who score in these categories would really excel on this high-stress scheduling job. How well do you think you would be able to identify them using an interview? Do you really think that you could consistently identify applicants from stanine 7 versus those from

Exhibit 3–7 Major Job Performance Selection Factors

Abilities	
Learning ability (intelligence)	Ability to take principles and apply to unique situations.
Problem solving	Constant problems resolving conflicting physician needs and desires with facility needs. Complex schedules.
Attention to detail	
Typing speed	Back-up office support. Probably a low weight factor.
Word processing	*WordPerfect, Excel*
Oral communications skills	Very important. Must be able to communicate reasons for scheduling choices to physicians and negotiate compliance.
Personality-Related Issues	
Ability to work under stress	Managing 24 physicians' work lives. Some will try to coerce what they want. Some don't like working at certain locations or with others.
Goal-oriented work orientation	No time for chit-chat. Needs to concentrate on the task at hand.
Ability to work as part of a team	Essence of job is coordination. Must be able to work with physicians and other personnel to get information necessary to make good scheduling choices.
Assertiveness and self-confidence	Must be strong enough not to be bullied by physicians, yet self-confident so that there is appropriate flexibility.
Additional Selection Factors	
Presence	Appropriate dress and demeanor for a professional office.
Motivation	Life circumstances conducive to remaining on the job. Appropriateness of the position to applicant's career progression and salary history.

stanine 5 or separate a "9" from a "7" using an interview? I don't think so, but this test can do it reliably and accurately. In addition, the test has a scale to measure whether the applicant is trying to "fake good," or provide an overly positive image of him- or herself.

The final two test measures are the Employment Inventory (EI) and the Customer Service Inventory (CSI).[13] The EI assess dependability, responsibility, and conscientiousness. The CSI identifies applicants who can be courteous, persistent, pleasant, helpful, customer-oriented, and tactful when working with difficult customers. High scorers on the CSI show enthusiasm in customer interactions, have a tolerance for rudeness, and are focused on finding solutions to the customer's problems.[14] In this case the customers, of course, are the physicians!

HONESTY/INTEGRITY TESTS

All of us have heard stories about the trusted employee who embezzles funds.[15] Theft of cash, supplies, and inventory is an important business problem, with annual estimates of financial losses running between $40 billion and $50 billion. One attempt to reduce losses due to theft was to use a polygraph or lie detector test to screen applicants. Research has indicated quite strongly that the polygraph is not effective at screening applicants.[16] In addition, the Employee Polygraph Protection Act of 1988 makes

Table 3–3 Scheduling Position Selection Methods Time and Cost Estimates

Job Performance Factors	Assessment Method	Testing Time (min.)	Cost	Number of Tests
Learning ability	Wonderlic Personnel Test	12	$55.00	25
Problem solving	Judgment Test	6	$30.00	23
Attention to detail	Name-Finding Test	4	$40.00	25
Typing speed	Typing/work sample	15	$0.00	
Word processing—*WordPerfect*	Typing/work sample		$0.00	
Oral communications skills	Interview			
Personality-related issues				
Ability to work under stress	NPF test	10	$35.00	23
Goal-oriented work behavior	Employment Inventory (EI)	15	$212.50	25
Ability to work as part of a team	Customer Service Inventory (CSI)			
Assertiveness and self-confidence	CSI	15	$212.50	25
Presence	Interview			
Motivation	Interview			
Tenure	EI			
TOTAL		65	$585.00	

the use of polygraphs for screening applicants illegal for virtually all organizations.[17]

Generally, organizations try to reduce theft through cash control methods, such as separating the collection of cash from the accounting for it, and regular monitoring and reconciling of financial reports, such as revenue, receipts, and write-off reports. Although these tactics are important, they are essentially defensive and passive in nature.

Recent research findings suggest that physician managers can use an additional method to reduce theft and gain other benefits as well. Integrity tests, sometimes called honesty tests, are easily administered and scored paper-and-pencil tests that can be used to screen job applicants for "organizationally delinquent" behaviors, including likelihood to steal or commit sabotage, alcohol and drug abuse, absenteeism, lying, unreliability, immaturity, and insubordination.

Conceptually, integrity tests assess deviance from accepted socialization standards. Socialization appears to be normally distributed, with a few individuals being overly conscientious, most being generally rule compliant, and a few being rule resistant, which in extreme cases results in law violations. Hogan and Hogan, who have conducted extensive research on identifying organizational delinquents, concluded:

> . . . there are people who, although hostile to rules, manage to avoid becoming involved with the legal system, and, therefore, are not identified as delinquent. We believe that they are the people who cause most of the problems in organizations.[18(p.273)]

How well do integrity tests work? Before answering that question, you need to understand four ideas fundamental to employee selection. First, no selection procedure including tests, interviews, references, or your subjective gut intuition, works perfectly. A reasonable objective, therefore, is to shift the odds of making a good hiring decision more in your favor.

Exhibit 3–8 Scoring for the NFP Test

STANINE	PERCENTILE RANGE	DESCRIPTION	STANINE	PERCENTILE RANGE	DESCRIPTION
4	24–40	People who score at this level may approach new situations somewhat cautiously because they are not confident enough of their ability to deal with unknown challenges. They do not handle stress as well as many others who score higher. However, this should not interfere with good performance if job responsibilities and demands are moderate.	9	96–99	The overall level of emotional adjustment of people at this level is excellent. They tend to view issues with great objectivity and realism and appear to be highly dependable. They approach new situations calmly and usually have the inner resources to cope with every challenge they encounter. As employees they are likely to display outstanding emotional stability, responsibility, and resistance to stress.
3	12–23	People who score at this level have relatively low frustration tolerance. They are quite frequently viewed by others as impatient, emotional and overreactive. They are best placed in job situations where unpredictability is low. This way, they can use the talents they have without having to face significant emotional strain.	8	89–95	People who score at this level can be placed in positions in which the need for dependability, loyalty, and stability is great. They aren't easily upset by changing circumstances and generally react well to stress.
			7	77–88	People who score at this level generally appear to be cool-headed and even-tempered. They are able to approach most situations calmly and handle them with practical sense.
2	5–11	People who score at this level describe themselves as tense, high-strung, irritable, and anxious. They may be easily shattered by events and worry unreasonably that things aren't going right. Because they often overreact to situations, others may find them difficult to get along with and work with for any extended period of time.	6	60–76	Scores at this level suggest above average emotional stability and self-confidence. People with such scores can generally be counted on to respond appropriately when they are confronted with new situations.
1	1–4	At this level, overall adjustment is very poor. It is hard for people who score this low to find the strength they need to face each day's challenges. In their answers to the test questions they describe themselves as extremely tense and anxious.	5	41–59	People who score at this level are average in terms of emotional stability and overall adjustment. They can cope successfully when normal demands are placed on them but are not likely to perform well in really high-pressure situations.

Source: Copyright © 1992 by Industrial Psychology International, LTD., Champaign, Il. Used by permission.

Second, you can make two types of selection errors. A false positive is when you decide that an applicant will be successful and he or she fails. A false negative is when you decide that an applicant will fail, but if hired he or she would have actually succeeded.

Third, as you raise the cut-off score on your test, you increase the chance of a false negative but decrease the chance of a false positive. For example, colleges that have very high entrance requirements turn away many applicants who in fact would have succeeded, but at the same time these high standards result in very high success rates for those who are admitted.

Fourth, from the employer's perspective, false negatives are not considered a cost. *In effect, you don't care if you reject 10 applicants who would have succeeded, as long as the one whom you do hire is not a false positive.* These concepts of false positive and false negative, and how they affect selection success, are discussed in more detail in a later part of this chapter.

Now, let's look at the results of one study to illustrate the potential strengths and weaknesses of integrity testing.[19] An integrity test was given to 482 grocery store applicants before employment. Because this was an experiment, the test results were not used, and all 482 applicants were hired. After 8 months, 17 had been identified as thieves, and of these 94 percent (16 of 17) had failed the integrity test. Of the rest, however, 48 percent also had failed the test. Some of these may have been thieves who had not been caught or who hadn't stolen yet, but some were undoubtedly false positives.

From a decision-making perspective, if we had used the test to make hiring decisions and rejected all applicants who failed the test, we would have eliminated 94 percent of the theft, but we also would have had to identify an additional 225 applicants to fill all 482 positions. Recruiting and screening an additional 225 applicants is obviously an expensive and time-consuming process. Scaling this down to selection ratios more typical of a health care organization, this would suggest that if your current employment methods require you to evaluate 10 applicants for a receptionist position, you might have to evaluate on average 15 to find an applicant who both is qualified on your current performance standards and passes the integrity test.

What about legal issues? There is a substantial body of data indicating that professionally developed integrity tests do not discriminate unfairly on the basis of race, gender, or age. Privacy law has generally focused on the invasiveness of the information collection process, such as blood, urine, and polygraph testing. There are virtually no privacy cases that challenge the content of integrity tests. The Employee Polygraph Protection Act of 1988, which essentially outlawed polygraph testing by private employers, specifically excludes oral and written tests. As with most aspects of life these days, however, you may want to consult your attorney for any recent cases or statutes in your state.

Integrity testing is controversial, and there is still some disagreement in the field about whether it really provides a useful indication of counterproductive behavior. There have been some allegations, for example, that the tests can be faked easily and that coaching can affect scores.[20] Few applicants, however, will have access to coaching help, and most integrity tests contain scales that effectively detect faking. In addition, a number of the earlier studies were not methodologically sound, although more recent studies have successfully addressed many of these earlier problems. Finally, there has been controversy over whether the tests provide a useful level of predictability. Recent reviews indicate that validities are equivalent to or higher than those of many other widely used tests.

If integrity testing sounds as if it might be helpful, and if you feel ethically comfortable using this type of instrument, contact several of the publishers listed in Exhibit 3–9. Have your business manager or personnel/human resources department consider the specific delinquency issues tested for, cost, administration time, validation data demonstrating that the test really works, and convenience of scoring when deciding whether to use a particular test. Integrity tests cost between $10 and $25 per applicant, so use them only on finalists who otherwise are fully qualified. This will keep your evaluation costs down.

OBTAINING TESTS

Although most psychological tests are available and usable by anyone, it is desirable to consult with a human resources professional who is knowledgeable about testing before starting a testing program. Exhibit 3–9 contains a limited list of test publishers. Distribution of some psychological tests is restricted to those with appropriate qualifications. If you or your staff don't meet the publisher's qualifications, don't try to circumvent these restrictions because this indicates that the test requires a sophisticated understanding of testing theory or specific training in the test to use it effectively. Remember, if you use a test improperly, you may deceive yourself regarding the quality of applicants whom you hire. Continue looking for another test that assesses the same factor. There are thousands of tests available, and usually any given factor can be assessed using literally dozens of published, unrestricted tests. The difference between restricted and unrestricted tests is often analogous to the difference between the prescription and nonprescription strengths of some medications. The "nonprescription" test may be more than adequate for your purpose as well as easier to score and less expensive.

Most tests come with hand scoring templates that make scoring relatively fast and error free. Many published tests also are supported by scoring services. A scoring service will provide you with an interpretive report at a reasonable cost with turnaround in a week or less. Some services provide scoring over the telephone with faxed reports, thereby providing an immediate evaluation. The quality and quantity of data provided in these reports is generally very high. The cost varies from about $10 to $25 per applicant. A scoring service should be used, therefore, only

Exhibit 3–9 Selected Test Publishers

E.F. Wonderlic, Inc. Test, Inc.
820 Frontage Road
Northfield, IL 60093
(800) 323-3742

Hogan Assessment Systems
P.O. Box 521176
Tulsa, OK 74152
(918) 749-0632
(800) 756-0632

Personnel Decisions, Inc.
2000 Plaza VII Tower
45 South Seventh Street
Minneapolis, MN 55403-1608
(612) 399-0927

London House, Inc.
9701 West Higgins Road
Rosemont, IL 60018
(800) 221-8378

IPI, Ltd.
4106 Fieldstone Road
Champaign, IL 61821
(800) 747-1119

for finalists and for important performance issues.

Many tests can also be scored using personal computer software. This software is sold by the test publisher. It will provide you with scoring and an interpretive report for a stated number of applicants.

WHO SHOULD DESIGN AND CONDUCT YOUR TESTING?

Testing is truly a double-edged sword. It provides considerable power, but considerable knowledge is required if this power is not to be abused. As was pointed out above, it is possible for your staff to identify employment factors, select tests, and put the process into operation without any outside help. This is especially the case if you have a staff person who is interested in the subject and is willing to do a little reading and self-education. Generally, however, physician managers working in private practices and smaller health care organizations that don't employ a human resources specialist should consider using a consultant to help guide the introduction of testing. One cost-effective way to find a knowledgeable consultant is to contact the business or psychology department at a local college or university.

The consultant will help your staff select tests and other employment methods that are appropriate for the job and your staff's skills, will train your staff to administer the employment methods correctly, and will arrange to obtain the testing materials. Remember, once you find a test that satisfactorily measures a job-related factor, it can be used for any other job that requires that same performance factor. Ideally, the employment tests that a consultant recommends should be scorable by your staff or a scoring service. Be suspicious if a consultant recommends tests, other than work samples, that are "self-developed" or only scorable by the consultant. Locking yourself into this kind of arrangement may limit your future flexibility as well as result in inflated consulting fees. Your staff should be able to do a creditable job of constructing work samples, especially if the initial attempts are supervised by a knowledgeable consultant.

Test administration, scoring, and evaluation generally are within the capability of office staff. Once again, you may choose initially to use a consultant to perform these tasks. The trade-off will be between the convenience of using a consultant and the timeliness and cost savings achieved by doing the work in house.

Physician managers in larger health care organizations should expect the personnel/human resources staff to be thoroughly competent in the use of tests, structured interviews, and work samples. If this is not the case, the appropriate role for the physician manager is to set goals for the staff to obtain these skills. This may include hiring someone with the appropriate expertise or having a current staff member obtain formal training in testing and testing theory.

REFERENCES AND RECOMMENDATIONS

References and recommendations are very difficult tools to use because you can never be certain what motivates those who provide them.[21] Employers can have many reasons for giving former employees a good reference, including keeping their own unemployment insurance rates down and fear of legal action on the part of the former employee. It is important to determine the reference's ability to evaluate the applicant and the extent of his or her knowledge of the applicant's job performance. Remember, everyone can find someone who will provide a good reference. Even Al Capone had his friends and beneficiaries.

It is very important to limit references to those people who had an employment relationship with the applicant. A personal reference is generally worthless because the motivation of the person giving the reference is highly suspect. You may be talking to the applicant's brother-in-law. You may be doing this even with an employer reference! It is wise, therefore, to ask whether the employee is related to the person providing the reference.

The best way to use a reference is as a means to verify or validate information that you have obtained elsewhere in the employment process. Personally, I find that it is best to talk on the telephone with whomever is providing a reference. You can often obtain more information than the person is willing to commit to writing, and on occasion the person will inadvertently reveal some unintended information by voice inflection, pauses, and so on.

If you are using the reference for verification, construct a list of questions to ask. For example, if psychological testing indicates that an applicant should have outstanding interpersonal abilities, attempt to verify this by asking "Could you describe some of John's most outstanding qualities?" If the reference doesn't mention the applicant's interpersonal abilities, you might then say "Give me an example of an incident that is typical of John's ability to work with others." Similarly, if an applicant has indicated that a significant part of his or her job involved insurance collection, you could ask the reference "What were some of the major duties that Sally had?" The answer should verify whether insurance collection was a primary or secondary responsibility.

Asking good questions and designing a strategy by which to use the reference to confirm or disconfirm hypotheses generated in previous employment steps take time and thought. As a result, obtaining references should be the *final* step in the selection process. Ideally, it should only be used for the top one or two applicants as determined by your other employment methods.

EVALUATION OF APPLICANT PERFORMANCE

Once you have collected all the applicant data, you will have to interpret it. You are looking for the applicant with the best *overall* performance across all interviews, tests, work samples, qualifications, and the like, without a "failing" score on any single component. Although the data can be combined statistically to form an overall composite score for each applicant, this can be a difficult process that should not be attempted unless you have significant statistical skills. It is all too easy to produce a number that is meaningless. For example, combining numbers from a structured interview with those from skill tests, psychological tests, and work samples can create a meaningless number unless they are all on the same number scale and have similar variances. You will do better to examine narrative reports and testing outcomes and to categorize applicants subjectively into two or three broad outcome groups such as "superior," "OK," and "not acceptable."

Sometimes, it is helpful to construct a table in which the rows are applicants, the columns are selection methods, and the cells contain outcomes. You then can graphically display and simultaneously view all of the applicants' outcomes. Generally, when you examine all of the assembled data, one or two applicants will stand out as having the best set of performance indicators; fully acceptable in all areas, and generally higher than most in most areas. If the performance level of top applicants is very good, small differences between applicants will not be of any real significance, so you probably will not materially change your chance of picking an acceptable applicant if you choose from any of the top contenders.

RECRUITING

Recruiting is the process of getting applicants to apply for a job. The object is to attract those applicants who are likely to have the required skills, will find the job attractive, and will want to work for you.

The most commonly used recruiting tools are word of mouth and published advertisements, such as in general distribution newspapers and professional newspapers and journals. Word-of-mouth recruiting has the advantage of quickly conveying information to people who have indicated to you or your employees that they are in the job market. If your current employees are high performers, word-of-mouth recruiting may help screen out unsuitable applicants. Usually, competent employees will not recommend people who they know are incompetent because they will not want to work with them. Word-of-mouth recruiting can also result in your employees' persuading friends or associates to enter the job market and become applicants. Many people are not dissatisfied enough with their current job to take the risk or expend the effort to search for a new job. If opportunity knocks, however, they may respond. The danger of word-of-mouth recruiting is that the applicant who learns of a position from a friend may feel an allegiance to this friend that competes with the allegiance to the employer.

Classified newspaper advertising is another excellent way of generating an applicant pool for office and technical positions. The advertisement should clearly state the major duties of the job, the compensation level, and the work hours, so that applicants can self-select based on these considerations. Newspaper ads generate a low proportion of useful resumes. Expect between 50 percent and 75 percent of these applicants to be eliminated in the resume screening process. Newspaper ads compensate for this by generating large numbers of applicants.

Generally, employment agencies are not a desirable recruiting source for nonprofessional and nonmanagerial employees. If you hire one of their applicants, you will usually have to pay some form of fee. In addition, their screening methods are often ineffective, and you should *not* delegate a major part of the selection process to the employment agency. Employment agencies can be useful for supplying temporary replacements, thus allowing you enough time to find well-qualified applicants.

Employment agencies may be more helpful for executive and professional positions and positions with salaries exceeding $50,000. Executive recruiters, as they are called, may have access to successful managers who are not currently in the job market. Generally, these recruiters are more sophisticated in their screening methods than employment agencies that concentrate on lower level positions. Here are some guidelines to consider if you plan to use an executive recruiter:[22]

1. Be certain that the agency you are choosing can conduct a thorough search. Does it have the resources and contacts in the health care industry to be successful?
2. Ask to meet the individual who will be handling your assignment. Would you be impressed with this person if he or she was trying to recruit you?

3. Clarify the search firm's fees, and get a signed contract. Be certain that contract termination clauses and payment schedules are clearly stated. Generally, fees range from 25 percent to 35 percent of the income of the position to be filled, plus expenses.
4. Choose a recruiter whom you can trust. This person will become aware of your organization's strengths and weaknesses, so you need to be able to trust this person with privileged information. If, during your conversations, the recruiter is revealing inappropriate information about other clients to you, he or she will probably not respect your confidentiality either.
5. Talk to some of the recruiter's clients. Ask these clients whether the consultant's appraisal of applicants was accurate.

Other potential recruiting sources include local colleges and technical schools. In general, these sources are best used for jobs that require little or no previous experience. Schools have several distinct advantages:

- A school placement office can send you a large number of applicants with little effort on your part.
- Applicants with little or no experience will generally work for lower wages than experienced applicants. If the job doesn't require experience, why pay for it?
- A school may do some preliminary screening, so that you only get the better applicants. One way to increase the chance of this happening is to tell the placement office that you will evaluate a few of their applicants and will discontinue recruiting if the quality of applicants is low.

Finally, job posting is a useful method of recruiting in larger health care organizations. With this method, open positions are posted in a designated place, such as on a specific bulletin board. Initially, positions are only open to current employees. Job posting is good for employee morale because it tells employees that the organization encourages career growth and that the employer has a commitment to working with current employees before searching elsewhere. This, in turn, generates employee commitment.

SELECTION STRATEGY

After reviewing all the selection tools that are available, you may feel that doing a good job of hiring employees is a time-consuming and complicated process. It doesn't have to be. The key to hiring good employees, and doing it in a timely, cost-effective manner, is understanding how to *organize* the employee search process.

The first step in implementing a successful selection strategy is to create a large applicant pool as quickly as possible. The applicant pool is the set of applicants who apply for the job. It is a waste of time and effort to identify and evaluate sequentially a few applicants and then repeat the whole process. First, there is always a time delay between recruiting efforts and the receipt of resumes. Obviously, if you have to repeat the whole process even once, you will waste considerable time simply waiting for the arrival of additional resumes.

A second and perhaps more important consideration is that a sequential recruiting process may not identify the most qualified applicant. For example, suppose you only use a limited recruiting method, such as word of mouth, that generates a selection pool of three or four applicants. One of these applicants may appear to be an adequate, although not outstanding, prospect. As a result, you find yourself in the difficult position of having to decide between offering this applicant the job or resuming your recruiting efforts. There will be a strong temptation to hire the "bird in hand" because this will relieve your anxiety and allow you to move on to other, more pressing matters (such as practicing medicine, managing cardiology services, running the physician services office, etc.). It may be, however, that a far more qualified applicant is out there and that a broader initial search, using a newspa-

per ad or an announcement posted at a local university, for example, would have identified this applicant.

Also necessary for developing a successful selection strategy is understanding how to sequence the events and how to process all the applicant information. The best way of sequencing is to use "multiple hurdles." This means that you order the selection process into sequential stages, so that subsequent employment methods are only applied to the survivors of previous stages. An effective sequencing uses the least expensive and least time-consuming procedures early in the employment process and reserves the more expensive and more time-consuming procedures for those applicants who have survived the initial hurdles. For example, a reasonable order of events for a clerical position might be as follows:

1. resume review
2. telephone interview of applicants
3. face-to-face interview and testing of applicants
4. work sample and role play tests
5. telephone reference check

Ideally, you would only conduct the telephone reference check for your top candidate.

An example of a selection sequence for processing 26 applicants is illustrated in Exhibit 3–10. In step 1, the 26 resumes are classified as good or bad. Only the 14 good applicants pass on to step 2 and are interviewed by telephone. Of these survivors, seven pass the telephone interview and move on to step 3, which involves testing and initial face-to-face interviewing. After testing and interviewing, two applicants, D and A, stand out. These are the only applicants to be rated superior in both the interview and the test. D and A are invited back for step 4, the second interview and personality testing. The object of this interview is to resolve any questions raised by the first interview; the personality testing is an expensive procedure. Applicant D is evaluated as superior and expresses interest in the job, so his or her references are checked. The references' comments are consistent with the previous testing and interviewing, so D is offered the position. If he or she declines the job, A's references will be checked, and A might be offered the job. If A were to decline, then you would have to decide whether to proceed with applicants E and H or obtain a new applicant pool. Exhibit 3–10 indicates that 26 applicants could be evaluated and a job offer realistically made with the expenditure of about 15.75 hours of someone's time.

It is also possible to reduce the time expended if you are willing to risk lengthening the employment process. For example, suppose in Exhibit 3–10, that A and D greatly impressed you during their telephone interviews. You could delay testing and interviewing of E, H, L, M, and Q until after you tested and interviewed A and D. If you then conclude that either A or D is about as good as an applicant can get, you could further delay evaluating the others until you reach a final decision on A and D. If you eventually hire A or D, you will save at least 5 hours. The danger here is that one of the other applicants might be superior.

You will also benefit from providing applicants with detailed, realistic information about the job early in the selection process. This is called a realistic job preview. Realistic job previews enable uninterested applicants to drop out of the process, saving you the trouble of evaluating their qualifications. For example, always indicate the salary range early in the evaluation process, such as in the initial telephone contact or perhaps even in the advertising. Similarly, you should describe the job in some detail in the telephone interview so that uninterested applicants can drop out at that point. During the first face-to-face interview, review the position's duties and responsibilities, and, if possible, show the applicant where he or she would work. Fill in any gaps left by the job description, and provide a fair statement of the work, warts and all. Applicants who have unrealistic job expectations and would be likely to quit after a short time on the job tend to self-select out when told the truth.

Finally, an effective selection strategy is one that is put into practice with *patience*. It is disruptive and perhaps frightening to have an im-

Exhibit 3–10 Sequence of Employment Steps

---

1. Resumes

Day 1
Time: 4 hours
Good applicants: A, B, C, D, E, F, G, H, I, L, M, Q, P, W
Bad applicants: J, K, N, O, R, S, T, U, V, X, Y, Z

2. Telephone interview

Day 1
Time: 3.25 hours
Good applicants: A, D, E, H, L, M, Q
Bad applicants: B, C, F, G, P, W

3. Test

Days 2-4
Time: 1 hour (directions only)
High: A, D, E
Adequate: H, M
Not adequate: Q

Interview

Days 2-4
Time: 3 hours
High: A, D, H, Q
Adequate: E, M

4. Second interview and personality testing

Day 5
Time: 1.5 hours and 3 hours (for top two applicants, respectively)
Ranking: D, A

5. Reference check

Day 5
Time: 0.25 hour
Hire: D

---

portant position vacant. It is far worse, however, to fill the position with the wrong person. Your employment methods may give you answers you don't like. They may indicate that many applicants who initially appeared to be well qualified are not good employment risks. Be persistent, and don't easily take a less than adequate applicant just to fill the position and move on to other issues.

FALSE POSITIVES AND FALSE NEGATIVES

As was pointed out above, employee selection is analogous to betting. The interviews, tests, work samples, and other selection tools and procedures change the odds, but they do not guarantee that you will hire an adequate employee. If you are using valid, job-related employment methods, applicants who perform better on the selection procedures will have higher probabilities of succeeding on the job.

Following is an explanation of the relationship among false positives, false negatives, and successful employment decisions. Figure 3–2 illustrates this relationship. The horizontal (x) axis of each graph represents applicant performance on the selection procedure. This could be an interview, test, or work sample or a composite evaluation based on several employment procedures. The vertical (y) axis represents the job performance.[23] Each dot in the scatter plot indicates how a particular applicant scored on both the selection procedure and job performance.[24] The line encircling the scatter plot provides a visual summary of the selection procedure–job performance relationship. Notice that as selection procedure performance increases, job performance generally increases, although this does not happen in every instance. Nevertheless, higher selection procedure performance correlates with higher job performance. An applicant who performs well on the selection procedure is more likely to perform well on the job than an applicant who performs poorly on the selection procedure.

The y axis of graph A in Figure 3–2 is bisected to distinguish acceptable and unacceptable job performance. The effect of hiring at any given level of selection procedure performance can be observed by drawing a vertical line through the scatter plot. The scatter plot is now divided into four areas: the false-positive area, the false-negative area, the true-positive area, and the true-negative area.

True negatives occur when the selection procedure predicts that the applicant will fail and the applicant does in fact fail. True positives occur when the selection procedure predicts that the applicant will succeed and the applicant does in fact succeed. False positives occur when the selection procedure predicts success but the applicant fails. False negatives occur when the selection procedure predicts failure but the applicant succeeds. Notice the size of the true-positive area relative to the size of the false-positive area. The ratio of these two areas is an index of the employment method's effectiveness.

Now examine graph B in Figure 3–2. The only difference between this graph and graph A is that the acceptable–not acceptable line is moved to the right. This means that the employer is demanding higher performance on the selection procedure, such as a higher test score or more favorable structured interview evaluation, before an applicant will be hired. Notice the effect that this has on the selection procedure's effectiveness. The ratio of the true-positive area to the false-positive area has increased. Notice also that the ratio of the true-positive area to the false-negative area has decreased. *Demanding higher applicant scores increases the probability that those hired will succeed, but at the cost of rejecting more applicants who would have been successful.*

From your perspective as an employer, a false-positive error is far more expensive and dangerous than a false-negative error. It is better not to hire someone who would succeed than to hire someone who fails. Therefore, you want to bias your decision making so that you minimize the probability of making a false-positive error, even though that may increase the chance of making several false-negative errors and continuing the employment process.

It should be apparent that, theoretically, an employer could demand a selection procedure performance score so high that the probability of applicant success would be 100 percent. The limiting factor, however, is that the employer has to fill the position, and it may take a very

A

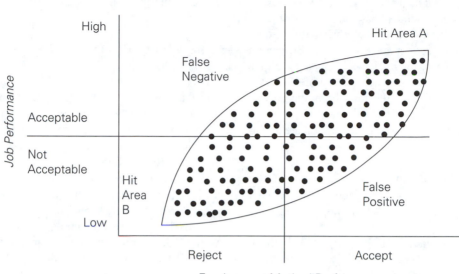

B

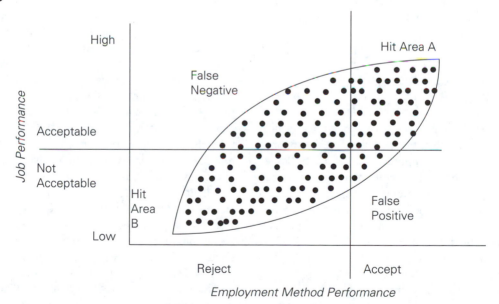

Figure 3–2 False positives, false negatives, and hits.

long time to find an applicant who scores high enough for that degree of certainty. This illustration also demonstrates that you should not jump at the first applicant whose selection procedure performance scores are acceptable. Be patient enough to bring in sufficient applicants to give yourself a good chance of finding high-scoring applicants. This will increase the probability of success.

The implications of this illustration are as follows:

- Employment methods that are far less than perfect can nevertheless be very effective if you can demand high enough applicant scores.
- High applicant scores are more likely to occur if you recruit effectively. Your advertising, working conditions, pay rates, and so on must help attract many qualified applicants.
- The value of finding high-scoring applicants must be balanced against the cost and time involved in evaluating larger numbers of applicants.

WHO SHOULD DESIGN YOUR SELECTION STRATEGY?

The selection strategy used for a job is critical to filling the position successfully and economically. It is very important, therefore, to devote your best thinking to the design of the selection strategy. If the strategy is to be developed in your organization, then your personal involvement is critical, or you must have an effective, well-trained personnel/human resources staff. If you don't feel fully confident in your organization's ability to develop a selection strategy, then retain a consultant.

Once a selection strategy has been designed for a job, it can be used again for that job. In this way, over time selection strategies will be acquired for all jobs. These strategies need not change unless the content of jobs change or there is some indication that the selection methods are not working properly, such as dissatisfaction with the quality of employees.

CASE APPLICATION: A SELECTION FAILURE

In retrospect, one of the biggest employment mistakes I made occurred when an applicant pool wore me down. As a result of bad luck, poor applicants, ineffective recruiting, or whatever, applicant after applicant failed to survive some critical part of the employment process. One particular problem was that many applicants were scoring at high levels on the Fake Good Scale of the California Psychological Inventory. A high Fake Good score may mean that the applicant is trying to present a false impression on the test. It would be reasonable to assume that such an applicant might well have problems with honesty and sincerity on the job.

Unfortunately, the high Fake Good applicants generally performed better than others in the interview and on the various ability tests. In effect, the Fake Good Scale was the only thing keeping the medical practice from hiring a business manager. The physician was growing more anxious as applicant after applicant was rejected. I explained the problem to the physician, and we jointly chose to conclude that the Fake Good Scale wasn't working properly. With the Fake Good Scale no longer an impediment, I recommended an applicant who, although well into the questionable range on that scale, otherwise had excellent testing and interviewing results. Needless to say, the employee's subsequent job performance was marked by covering-up problems, deception, manipulation of employees, and outright mendacity. The personal and financial costs of searching for a few more days or weeks would have been far less burdensome than the problems caused by hiring this applicant. This experience proved to me that there are times when one must "tough it out." Hire a temporary employee, use a contractor to cover, or do whatever is necessary, but don't easily compromise your hiring standards.

CASE APPLICATION: HIRING A BUSINESS MANAGER

The purpose of this case description is to provide you with an example of how selection methods and strategy can be applied in a real employment situation. It illustrates how to use the general guidelines presented above in a realistic and practical manner. The case also illustrates how to adjust your employment procedures to take advantage of the changing reality of the selection process.

A family practice employing six physicians was seeking a new business manager. The current business manager had fallen behind in collection and did not have the organizational skills, efficiency, or motivation to fix the problem. The job description for the position was organized into five technical skill factors, two interpersonal skill factors, and one personal trait, which were to be evaluated using resumes, interviews, work samples, psychological tests, and reference checks (Table 3–4). The sequence of selection methods was as follows:

1. resume review
2. telephone interview
3. face-to-face interview and psychological test
4. second face-to-face interview and work samples
5. reference check

Recruiting methods included word of mouth and two newspaper advertisements spaced one week apart. These generated 18 resumes. Exhibit 3–11 shows the resume of the applicant who was eventually selected for the position. This resume shows experience on most, if not all, of the selection factors. Ann's resume was well organized and contained appropriate language with correct spelling and grammar. The information was presented in a neat, logical, and concise manner. Her resume made an acceptable initial impression. It indicated that she was experienced in the following areas: revenue collection, developing systems to deal with business problems, efficiency, and interpersonal relations on the job. Their importance to her, however, did not guarantee that she did these things well. The time break between the last two jobs was accounted for in the initial telephone contact.

Next, Ann was interviewed on the telephone by Dr. Frederick, the managing physician. Dr. Frederick took on this task because the position reported directly to him and he considered this

---

Table 3–4 Job Description Factors, Selection Factors, and Selection Procedures

Job Description Factor	Selection Factor	Selection Procedure
Collections	Technical skill	Resume Work sample Interview
Insurance billing	Technical skill	Resume Work sample
Payroll	Technical skill	Interview Work sample
Taxes	Technical skill	Interview Work sample
Fee negotiations	Interpersonal skill	Work sample
Management reports	Technical skill	Work sample
Problem identification	Trait	Psychological test
Teamwork	Interpersonal skill	Psychological test

Exhibit 3–11 Resume of Business Manager Applicant

Ann Johnson

342 Main Street
Virginia Beach, Virginia 23456

(804) 555-1212

Experience

Andrew Carey, M.D., Surgeon
1867 Oats Road
Eastville, Connecticut 06387
Position: Business Manager (November 1984 to August 1988)
My objective, as an effective business manager, was to achieve a consistent income for the practice by utilizing proven, effective means of collection. With this end in mind, I initiated a turnover system so that within 12 hours after a patient's visit the insurance had been processed. By thoroughly understanding the mechanisms of different insurers, we were able to achieve a 100 percent collection rate month after month. By streamlining different tasks and implementing time management principles, much of the loose paperwork was eliminated, and fewer errors were made. Consistent with this objective was my desire to create a satisfying environment for all employees. All employees had their own sphere of importance and expertise, which afforded them some control over their work and resulted in higher productivity.

John Blanchard, M.D.
Professor and Chair
New England Medical School
Westville, Connecticut 06774
Position: Practice Manager–Executive Secretary (March 1982 to July 1983)
The position encompassed two areas: private practice manager and secretary to the Chair of OB-GYN. As practice manager, I was responsible for patient records, transcription, coding, charges, and patient scheduling. As secretary to the Chair, I was involved with the residency program for obstetrics and gynecology.

Nutmeg Roofing
87 Westover Street
Westville, Connecticut 06774
Position: Office Manager (September 1978 to June 1980)
I ordered supplies, maintained inventory, payroll, and accounts receivable and payable, and did the preliminary figures for the quarterly taxes.

Education

New England Business College: Eastville, Connecticut, 1986
Principles of Accounting, Business Management, English, Principles of Information Processing

Connecticut Community College: Eastville Connecticut, 1985
Biology, English, English Literature, American Literature

Smith Business School: Westville, Connecticut, 1981
Medical Terminology I, II, Physiology I, II, Medical Transcription I, II, Insurance I, II, Psychology, English, Typing I, II, Shorthand I, II

worth his time. His objectives were to acquire more detailed information about Ann's previous work experience, assess her verbal skills, familiarize her with the job description to clarify whether the job interested her, and determine whether the salary range for the job was acceptable. The telephone interview was organized so that the most fundamental qualification issues were discussed first. It also could thus be quickly ended if the applicant was not appropriate for the job.

The telephone interview began by verifying that Ann was still in the job market. Next, the job was described to her in considerable detail. She was encouraged to ask questions at any point during the interview. After the job description had been reviewed, she was once again asked whether she was interested in the position. Benefits were then discussed, including the salary range, vacation time, sick leave, the retirement plan, and medical insurance. Once again, she was asked whether she was still interested in the position. Finally, she was told that the next step would include a face-to-face interview and testing. She was informed that testing was included in the next step, so that she could drop out if that was a problem for her. An evaluation of her performance in the telephone interview is included in Exhibit 3–12.

Dr. Frederick decided that Ann was a very promising candidate, so he scheduled her for an interview. He stated his reasons for immediately scheduling interviews with promising candidates as follows:

> When I conclude during the telephone interview that the applicant is a very good candidate, I schedule the next step in the employment process before I end the call, so that I don't waste time recontacting the applicant. This can be advantageous for three reasons. First, we can easily lose a day or two trying to recontact and schedule an applicant who is in demand. Second, the selection process works two ways. The applicant is also making decisions. I am in competition with other employers, and if the applicant is tied down tomorrow morning interviewing with me, then she *can't* be interviewing with my competition! Finally, scheduling the next step will shake out the serious from the nonserious applicants. The danger in scheduling the applicant at the end of the telephone interview is that she may not be as good as the next two or three that I will assess on the tele-

Exhibit 3–12 Structured Telephone Interview Format and Evaluation

1. Ask applicant to identify himself or herself.
2. Ask applicant whether he or she is still in job market.
3. Describe the position to applicant, and tell applicant to ask questions at any point during this interview.
4. Ask what applicant is looking for.
   (*Ann:* Position with responsibility, enjoys getting the money in, place where she fits in, long-term relationship)
5. Ask applicant to describe previous work experience.
   (*Ann:* Handled accounts to $650,000 by herself without computer; stressed her ability to organize, look for efficient ways of working; has done insurance billing, posting, collections; no experience with local CHAMPUS, some with state BC/BS)
6. Discuss salary and benefits.
   (*Ann:* No problem)
7. Next step is interview and testing.

Evaluation of skills

Language was always appropriate. No observable mistakes in grammar or syntax. Asked relevant questions at several points—possibly indicates good problem-solving ability. Technical skills appear to be appropriate. Overall, she appears to be intelligent, qualified, and interested.

phone, but I can always call back and cancel. . . . In reality, deciding whether to immediately offer the second step or postponing that decision is usually not difficult. Those applicants who are really good stand out.

The next step in the selection procedure consisted of a structured interview and administration of the California Psychological Inventory (CPI). The interview focused on technical questions related to insurance billing and collection. The object was to explore the depth of the applicant's knowledge and assess her ability to make the shift into another medical field. Exhibit 3–13 presents selected interview questions and the interviewer's notes, although not the scoring categories into which he subsequently classified her answers. The first five questions were used with all applicants. The sixth question was specific to this applicant because her last job had been in another state and her previous experience had been in another medical field.

The most important consideration on this job was collection, so the interview questions focused on this factor. Obviously, it was impossible for Dr. Frederick to assess every facet of Ann's collection knowledge, so he identified particularly important areas that would give an indication of the depth and degree of her knowledge. In addition, he used the structured questions as points of departure. If the applicant said something that raised another question or made a comment that didn't seem quite right, Dr. Frederick followed up until he felt confident that he had satisfactorily resolved any uncertainties.

The CPI is a 463-item questionnaire that assesses 24 traits related to psychological adjustment, work attitudes, and interpersonal skills. It takes about an hour to complete, and it is self-administered, so that it doesn't consume any staff time during administration. Computer scoring is available, or the CPI can be interpreted using the test manual and other reference resources. Exhibit 3–14 lists the CPI traits that were scored on applicants for this job. Dr. Frederick forwarded Ann's completed CPI to a consultant for scoring and interpretation. Examination of Ann's profile indicated that she had many traits that would contribute to success on the job. Exhibit 3–15 shows Ann's CPI interpretive report.

The interview took 45 minutes to complete, and the CPI took 65 minutes. Dr. Frederick, however, was only present during the interview. As a result of Ann's superior performance in the interview, her CPI results, and her stated interest in the position, it was decided to suspend assessment of other applicants until a decision could be made about her. It made sense, therefore, to change the ordering of assessment procedures and to proceed immediately with the telephone reference checks because these would consume less time than the second interview. The reference's comments were positive and Ann was asked back for a second interview and work sample testing.

The work sample testing was designed to end any remaining doubts regarding Ann's knowledge of revenue collection and insurance. The applicant was presented with a real account that had a large outstanding balance. She was told to analyze the account and identify any problems with it. She analyzed the account by identifying copayments, insurance payments, and write-offs for each procedure, and she then assembled personal and insurance balances. When asked what she would do regarding the personal balance, she stated "I'd call the patient on the telephone because the balance is large and long overdue." Because that type of conversation had already been role played in the first interview (Question 2, Exhibit 3–14), there was no need to role-play it again. Her ability to bill insurance companies successfully was assessed by presenting her with several insurance forms containing errors, such as a missing diagnosis code and undercoding that would have resulted in the practice receiving lower payment than was necessary. She responded by correctly noting the additional pieces of information that needed to be entered on the insurance forms.

The second interview focused on specifying the needs of the practice's director, Dr. Fred-

Exhibit 3–13 Structured Interview Questions and Responses

1. What is the procedure that you use when a patient has more than one insurance carrier?

   Answer indicated that she would identify the primary, hold billing on the secondary until the primary had paid. Addressed some of the difficulties of identifying the primary. Overall, an informed answer, quickly given.

2. How do you handle a delinquent account? (Follow with role play)

   Answers indicated the necessity to act quickly but with reason. If patient is in office, meet face to face. First, ask if there are any personal circumstances to account for not paying. Depending upon the situation use humor, sternness, etc. to achieve the goal. Obtain a partial payment on credit card if necessary. If patient is not present, use telephone call first, then short series of letters. Indicated that she did not like to use form letters. This was then role played. I stated, "O.K., I'm the patient. Talk to me." She was direct and courteous and asked me to make behavioral commitments. Overall, appropriate answers given quickly. Answer stressed reason, control, logic, need to be systematic, etc.

3. How do you handle a delinquent insurance company?

   Answer given with humor. Stated that she really "liked to go after them." When pushed on how you identify outstanding insurance claims, she stated that she assumed that there would be some aging reports available. Also indicated that she has simply looked through patient files. When pressed about how she would identify slow payers, she indicated that the key was systematic review of accounts, ideally on a weekly basis. When asked how she would review 800 accounts in a week, she stated that she would separate out the bad ones based on an aging and review them regularly. Overall, her answers were adequate. She seemed somewhat hampered or frustrated by not knowing our procedures.

4. What do you consider an acceptable standard for accounts receivable?

   Previously indicated a standard of 2 × current as the upper end of what would be acceptable, implying that this was marginally not acceptable. Body language and verbalizations indicated that she thought our accounts were out of control.

5. How would you go about reducing this practice's accounts receivable?

   She didn't have a particular strategy and seemed somewhat confused or surprised by the question. Her first response was that it would take long, hard work. She then asked if there was anyone else in the practice who could assist. This indicated to me a standard thought process of looking for available tools that could be utilized on a project. She then asked how long she would have to get the "AR plug" fixed. I indicated that it should all be gone, as well as current accounts properly handled, in six months. She stated and/or indicated through expressions that this was a reasonable if not generous time period.

6. Your background is in working in a surgical practice in Connecticut. What problems do you anticipate in doing billing in a family practice in Virginia?

   She indicated that there were differences between fields but that they were not major—related to knowing what codes to use, what diagnoses would be paid for, etc. In regard to the insurance companies, she stated that it was just a matter of getting on the phone, calling, and asking a lot of questions. She didn't minimize the shift across medical fields or in having to deal with new insurers, but she clearly was not intimidated by it, nor did she express overconfidence. A very appropriate and reasonable answer.

erick, and providing Ann with a realistic preview of the job and the personnel with whom she would work. Salary and benefits were discussed in detail, and a job offer was made. This second interview and the work sample testing took two hours. The telephone reference checks took 15 minutes. The time expended by practice personnel for Ann's selection is shown in Table 3–5.

Exhibit 3–14 CPI Factors

Dominance (Do): Self-confidence and assertiveness

Capacity for status (Cs): Need for success, ambition, and independence

Sociability (Sy): Friendliness and liking to be with people

Social presence (Sp): Self-assurance, spontaneity

Self-acceptance (Sa): Opinion of self

Independence (In): Self-sufficiency, resourcefulness, self-confidence

Empathy (Em): Understanding the feelings of others

Socialization (So): Ability to conform, acceptance of rules, etc.

Self-control (Sc): Control of emotions, self-discipline

Good Impression (Gi): Trying to do what will please others

Communality (Cm): Ability to "fit in" with others

Well-being (Wb): Optimism about the future

Tolerance (To): Tolerance for others' beliefs and values

Achievement via conformity (Ac): Drive to do well, ability to work in situations where there are rules and standards

Achievement via independence (Ai): Drive to do well, ability to work in unstructured work settings

Intellectual efficiency (Ie): Efficient use of intellectual abilities

Psychological mindedness (Py): Interest in the reasons why people act the way that they do

Flexibility (Fx): Liking change and variety

Femininity/masculinity (F/M): Sensitivity to criticism, feeling vulnerable, action orientation

Work orientation (Wo): Sense of dedication to work, strength of work ethic

Management potential (Mp): Talent and desire for management role

Leadership potential (Lpi): Foresight and decision-making ability

Fake Good Scale: Designed to identify protocols that were faked to look overly favorable

Source: Data from H.G. Gough, *California Psychological Inventory Administrator's Guide,* © 1987, Consulting Psychologist Press and L.W. McAllister, *A Practical Guide to CPI Interpretation,* © 1988, Consulting Psychologist Press.

In this instance, the entire selection process was directed by Dr. Frederick, the practice's managing physician. Dr. Frederick described his job as 80 percent clinical work and 20 percent administration. He felt that the business manager position was so important that he should personally assume the responsibility for filling it. In this regard, this case is not typical. Most physician managers will not take the lead in applying a selection process, as did Dr. Frederick. They would, however, have direct involvement at critical phases, such as interviewing, employment system design, and final applicant selection, for employees with whom they will work directly.

This case illustrates how a small medical practice can fill a critical position in a timely, cost-effective manner and at the same time obtain an employee with an excellent chance of success. The same principles can be applied to selection in a hospital, HMO, large clinic, or any other medical setting.

SELECTING PHYSICIANS AND OTHER PROFESSIONAL EMPLOYEES

Hiring a physician is one of the biggest management challenges faced by physician managers in group practices and large health care systems.[25] The right decision can enhance the organization's professional reputation, the quality of services provided, cost control, and profitability. A wrong decision can lead to frustrating interpersonal problems, difficulty in recruiting other physicians, and financial catastrophe. When the stakes are this high, you need to ask

Exhibit 3–15 Interpretation of CPI

CPI Overall Conclusions

A dominant theme is a strong sense of obligation and a need to meet the expectations of others. She wants to fit in and meet the needs of those whom she values. There is a strong need to be needed, but there is also evidence of assertiveness and perhaps aloofness and detachment. She is perceptive of others' needs and abilities, likes to be with other people and work with them, and is competent in interpersonal situations, but ultimately trusts her own ability to get things done more than she is willing to delegate to others.

She is serious, proper, stable, competent, rational, able to accept constructive criticism, disciplined, and concerned about her performance. There is a desire for structure and predictability and to stick to plans, which probably results in an aversion to risk taking.

Her behaviors are always appropriate, she strives for competence, and ascribes to the Protestant work ethic. She works hard, intelligently, and efficiently, and this effort is characterized by planning, setting of priorities, and anticipation of consequences. Overall, her personality and work are characterized by optimism and a positive attitude. Her pattern is opposite to that of a passive-aggressive behavior pattern.

Response Set Evaluation

Fake Good Scale was within normal limits. No indication of an attempt to fake good.

Class Evaluation

The high degree of consistency within classes indicated that class interpretation was appropriate. Class I scales indicate a self-confident person who is outgoing, competent in interpersonal situations, and interpersonally oriented. The *relatively* low self-acceptance score may indicate that she tries to put her evaluation of her own capabilities into a reasonable perspective, if not consciously minimize them, so as not to appear self-aggrandizing.

Class II scales suggest a person who has a sense of duty, behavioral control, and a dislike of taking risks.

Class III scales indicate that she is achievement oriented and uses an intellectual strategy as opposed to a brute force strategy to approach problems.

Class IV scales are mixed and cannot be interpreted as a set.

Structure Evaluation

Structural Scale characteristics indicate that she is a weak Alpha, which is an ambitious, action-oriented, productive type of person, a doer who does socially acceptable things and feels comfortable in interpersonal relationships. At their worst, Alphas can be self-centered, opportunistic, and manipulative. She has an exceedingly high v.3 score. This indicates that she has a superior development of the positive aspects of the type. This indicates a high degree of self-reflection and optimism regarding the future.

Selected Individual Scale Interpretations

Responsible level of dominance (Do), indicating that she is not overbearing but can be assertive when necessary.

Capacity for status (Cs) indicates that she aspires upward, should be sensitive to management's perspective, and can handle stress and pressure.

Sociability (So) indicates an ability to relate to people in an appropriate manner, enjoys interpersonal reactions, but is not a "backslapper" or inappropriately boisterous.

Social presence (Sp) indicates enthusiasm and ties in well with So, indicating a comfort with social situations.

Self-acceptance (Sa) is inconsistent with the previous two scales. This may indicate a conscious attempt to keep her own self-impression under control, to be modest, and to be socially appropriate regarding her own skills.

Independence (In) is at levels indicating appropriate goal-oriented behavior and an appropriate level of assertiveness.

Empathy (Em) indicates insight regarding her interpersonal behavior. As a result, her behaviors are viewed as reasonable by others.

continues

Exhibit 3–15 continued

Responsibility level suggests a sense of responsibility and a desire to follow through on obligations.

Sociability (So) is at levels associated with sincerity, honesty, and compliance with social norms.

Self-Control (Sc) indicates a preoccupation with detail, a tendency toward compulsiveness, and a reliance on facts as opposed to her intuition. She plans ahead and is good at developing systems and procedures for getting things done. She thinks before she acts but may also repress feelings and occasionally explode.

Tolerance (To) indicates a nonjudgmental, tolerant appreciation for differences and a trust of others.

The achievement scales suggest that she is comfortable working in organized structured situations, but at the same time she can act independently and still need a minimum of supervision.

Intellectual efficiency (Ie) indicates that planning, anticipation of events, and establishing priorities are very important to her. She does not act impulsively.

Psychological mindedness (Py) suggests that she is more comfortable in dealing with concepts and abstracts than in delegating responsibility. She is perceptive of others' needs and empathic. She would rather do something herself than delegate it.

Flexibility (Fx) level is consistent with someone who is deliberate and determined. She is not afraid of change but probably has a realistic concern with and skepticism of it.

Femininity/Masculinity (F/M) level indicates a balance between being tough minded and sensitive to the needs of others.

Special Scales

Her level of work orientation is very high. This is consistent with a person who is reliable, disciplined, and dependable. Similarly, managerial potential is well above average. This indicates that she creates a good impression and is confident, socially effective, emotionally stable, mature, realistic, optimistic, and well-organized; shows foresight; and gets things done.

yourself "Are the evaluation methods that I'm using simply giving me an excuse to select one applicant over another, or are they *really* able to identify the better candidate?"

Unfortunately, resumes, references, and unstructured interviews don't work any more effectively with physicians and other professionals than they do for the administrative and technical positions described above. If your evaluation is limited to interviewing physician

Table 3–5 Time Consumed To Select Applicant

Procedure	Time (hours)
Resume review	0.10
Telephone interview	0.50
Interview and testing	0.75
Reference check	0.25
Second interview and work sample	2.00
TOTAL	3.60

applicants and perhaps talking with their references, then you are overlooking several important sources of information that could help you make a better decision. Certainly, very few Fortune 100 companies would fill an equivalently important management or technical position on the basis of an unstructured interview and references. Why? Because there are important job performance issues that can be better measured using the other assessment methods that were discussed above, including structured interviews, work samples, and, in some cases, psychological testing.

As with any job, the place to begin is the job description. Some physician performance issues may include diagnostic ability, several types of technical clinical skills, interpersonal skills, and teamwork. Just as with any job, it is very unlikely that unstructured interviews will reveal much information that will allow you to separate physician applicants based on their abilities in these areas. Structured interviews, as we have seen, are more promising. Here, for example, is a sample structured interview question that assesses physician teamwork and respecting collegial boundaries:

> While covering for Dr. Jones, you notice that Mrs. Smith is receiving a drug that in your opinion is inferior to the drug that you routinely prescribe. How would you handle this situation?

- *Characteristics of an effective answer:* Review patient history and response to drug. Change medication only if clinical outcome has been less than satisfactory. If clinical outcome is satisfactory, don't change drug.
- *Characteristics of an ineffective answer:* Any expression of passive-aggressive tendencies toward colleague, such as comments that might subtly undermine the patient's confidence in the colleague. Failure to take into account prior clinical outcome when making prescription decision.

Work samples and other procedures that mirror the complexity of the job have great potential. Perhaps one of the best "work samples," if it can be arranged, is a visit to the applicant at his or her current location. A cardiology practice uses this approach as a final screen before making a selection, when this is feasible given the applicant's current work setting. One retired partner commented that generally it had been the interpersonal issues that created problems. He noted that it was possible for someone to create a facade for a short period of time, a few hours or a day. When you have been in the operating room with someone for several days, however, you can see indicators of how he or she will really interact with others. Roughly quoting one of the physicians who conducted this work sampling: "You really learn how a surgeon feels about quality when you see him put in a stitch that isn't *quite* right. What does he do? Does he take it out and replace it correctly?"

If this process isn't feasible, it may be possible to have an applicant pair with a physician.

In a family practice, for example, this could involve doing several joint consultations, with the evaluating physician retaining ultimate responsibility for all clinical decisions. During the process, the evaluating physician can observe the quality of the clinical decisions and the nature of the patient–colleague interaction. A locum tenens arrangement is another possibility. Working with someone for six months to one year is certainly an extended work sample. Would it be inconvenient or expensive then to part ways? Certainly. But what are the financial and interpersonal costs of a faulty hire?

Finally, you may want to consider obtaining a psychological test profile on finalists. This can provide information about issues such as personality, work attitudes, values, and ethics. The profile can highlight areas to be investigated further with interviews and work sample observations. Often, it is these less tangible issues that make or break a professional relationship. This type of testing should be performed by a testing professional, such as an industrial or clinical psychologist with experience in personnel selection.

Might some good physician applicants resist these "unorthodox" methods? Perhaps. These ideas, however, are not unorthodox in most other industries and are in fact the norm. As health care organizations grow in size and increasingly rely on proven business methods to improve quality and reduce costs, we will see more of them adopting these tactics. Are the costs in terms of dollars and time worth it? Only you can answer that question. As you are considering your answer, however, you might also ask yourself "What would AT&T do?"

EQUAL EMPLOYMENT OPPORTUNITY

You should use all your selection methods without regard to the race, religion, sex, national origin, or age of applicants. In addition, you cannot allow applicants' medical conditions or medical histories to affect your employment decisions, unless this directly affects their ability to perform on the job and you cannot make any reasonable accommodation to their condition. The employment methods described in this chapter provide health care organizations with greater legal defensibility than traditional unstructured interviews. This is a consequence of basing employment decisions on job-relevant issues that have been assessed through demonstrably valid methods. Specific guidelines for complying with federal Equal Employment Opportunity requirements are discussed in Chapter 14.

CONCLUSION

You should now understand that there are many tools, procedures, and methods for selecting and hiring employees. By beginning with a good understanding of job content and using the methods discussed in this chapter, you will be able to develop and implement selection methods that will assess job-related skills in a timely, cost-effective manner for all jobs, including physician positions. This approach to employment will greatly increase the chance of hiring employees who will perform satisfactorily. You should also have enough information about how the employment process should work to define your appropriate physician manager role in the process as well as the roles of your staff and consultants.

REFERENCES AND NOTES

1. Courts have held that inadvertent or minor misstatements may not be reason for termination. For example, misspelling an address or transposing a telephone number would be very questionable reasons for dismissal.

2. S. Kahn, B. Brown, and B. Zepke, *Personnel Director's Legal Guide: 1988 Cumulative Supplement* (Boston, Mass.: Warren, Gorham, and Lamont, 1988), s2-19–s2-20.

3. W. Cascio, *Applied Psychology in Personnel Management*, 3d ed. (Englewood Cliffs, N.J.: Prentice-Hall, 1987), 264.

4. J. Hunter and R. Hunter, Validity and Utility of Alternative Predictors of Job Performance, *Psychological Bulletin* 96 (1984): 72–98.

5. W.H. Weisner and S.F. Cronshaw, The moderating impact of interview format and degree of structure on interview validity, *The Journal of Occupational and Organizational Psychology* 61 (1988): 275–290.

6. The coefficient of determination is the square of the correlation, or $(0.20 \times 0.20) = 0.04$ for the unstructured interview, and $(0.63 \times 0.63) = 0.397$ for the structured interview.

7. Equal Employment Opportunity Commission, Uniform Guidelines on Employee Selection Procedures, *Federal Register* 43 (1978): 38290–38315.

8. R.C. Sweetland and D.J. Keyser, *Tests: A Comprehensive Reference for Assessment in Psychology, Education, and Business* (Austin, Tex.: PRO-ED, Inc., 1983).

9. J. Conoley and J. Kramer, *The Mental Measurements Yearbook* (Lincoln, Neb.: University of Nebraska, 1989).

10. Test prices change over time and with the number of tests purchased.

11. Generally, test prices go down substantially with larger volume. For example, the cost of the Wonderlic Personnel Test is about $1.25 each when 100 tests are purchased.

12. Industrial Psychology, *Judgment Test Examiner's Manual* (Champaign, Ill.: Industrial Psychology, Inc., 1981).

13. Both the EI and the CSI are published by Personnel Decisions, Inc., 2000 Plaza VII Tower, 45 Main South Seventh Street, Minneapolis, MN 55402.

14. Personnel Decisions, *PDI Employment Inventory and PDI Customer Service Inventory Manual* (Minneapolis, MN: Personnel Decisions, Inc., 1994).

15. Parts of this section first appeared in R. Solomon, Integrity Testing Can Help You Avoid Hiring a Thief. *American Medical News*, 18 October, 1993, p. 26.

16. L. Saxe, D. Dougherty, and T. Cross, The Validity of Polygraph Testing, *American Psychologist* 40 (1985): 355–366.

17. Some employers are still permitted to use the polygraph to screen applicants. These include employers with national defense contracts, parts of the nuclear power industry, businesses with access to highly classified information, and city, state, and federal governments.

18. J. Hogan and R. Hogan, How To Measure Employee Reliability, *Journal of Applied Psychology* 72, no. 2, (1989):273–279.

19. S.O. Lillienfled, G. Alliger, and K. Mitchell. Why Integrity Testing Remains Controversial. *American Psychologist* 50, no. 6, (1995):457.

20. D.S. Ones, C. Viswesvaran, and F.L. Schmidt, Integrity Tests: Overlooked Facts, Resolved Issues, and Remaining Questions. *American Psychologist* 50, no. 6 (1995): 456–457.

21. For an examination of the issues involved in *providing* references, see the discussion of the tort of defamation in Chapter 14.

22. J. Wareham, *Secrets of a Corporate Headhunter* (Chicago, IL: Playboy Press, 1981), 213–225.

23. Some very large companies will hire applicants at random to test new employment methods. As a result, they will be able to observe how applicants whom the selection procedure predicted would fail actually perform on the job. This strategy for evaluating the predictiveness of a selection procedure is called predictive validation.

24. Few health care organizations would hire the number of applicants in the position represented in Figure 3–2. The same phenomenon could be observed, however, by plotting the performance of applicants hired over a very long period of time. Even though a practice may only be filling one position, the same forces illustrated by this example will be at work.

25. Parts of this section first appeared in R. Solomon, There Are Ways to Check Skills before Hiring a Doctor, *American Medical News*, 25 April 1994, p. 41.

CHAPTER 4

Compensating Employees

Chapter Objectives

An effective compensation plan will help you to hire, retain, and motivate good employers, while at the same time keeping your payroll costs under control. The objective of this chapter is to provide you with a strategy and procedures for determining how much to pay each of your employees. Although compensation is largely dispensed in the form of direct wages, many employers also provide some benefits, including life insurance, health insurance, a retirement plan, vacation time, sick leave, educational benefits, and profit sharing. Benefits will be discussed as a means of fine-tuning your compensation plan to best meet your needs and those of your employees.

Obtaining compensation skills is important for physician managers working in all types of health care organizations. The methods that are presented in this chapter can be most directly applied in larger health care organizations because these organizations have to deal with many more positions and compensation decisions than smaller organizations, such as small group practices. Nevertheless, the same compensation concepts that are used by larger organizations are relevant to physician managers working in smaller health care and private practice settings.

Physician managers in practices and larger health care organizations will find that basing a compensation plan solely on intuitive judgments of appropriate salaries for positions will create personnel and compensation problems. In particular, employees might become dissatisfied with their pay, which can manifest itself in such symptoms as absenteeism, tardiness, productivity problems, and turnover. Alternatively, the size of your payroll might become excessive. If you notice either of these conditions, you should take a closer look at your compensation plan.

Physician managers working in large practices or health care organizations, such as hospitals and health care systems, will want to use either a consultant or their professional personnel staff to build a compensation plan. The information contained in this chapter will help you more effectively utilize these compensation professionals and apply the results of their work.

Physician managers in smaller practices may conclude that use of the methods described in this chapter for determining salaries for their limited number of positions is overkill. If that is the case, you can improve the results you obtain from an intuitive approach to compensation by applying the theory of compensation discussed in this chapter. Seeing how this theory translates into procedure in larger organizations will give you a model around which to build your intuitive compensation strategy. If you understand what compensation should be based on and the goals that any compensation plan, either large or small, should achieve, you will be able to make better intuitive judgments and arrive at more equitable salaries. Physician managers in smaller practices will find that they can determine salary rates for front office personnel without the use of a consultant, although whether this is a cost-effective use of their time is problematic.

EQUITY: A THEORY AND STRATEGY FOR DETERMINING COMPENSATION

The goal of any compensation plan is to achieve equity in the minds of employees. Equity is a judgment made by the employee regarding the fairness of compensation. Equity judgments are comparative, not absolute. An employee judges the equity of compensation by making a comparison of his or her rewards and the work performed with the rewards of and work performed by others. Equity is therefore a personal, cognitive ratio of rewards to performance compared with the ratio of rewards to performance for significant others. Three equity conditions can be expressed conceptually as formulas:

$$\frac{R_e}{I_e} = \frac{R_o}{I_o} \quad \text{Equity}$$

$$\frac{R_e}{I_e} < \frac{R_o}{I_o} \quad \text{Inequity due to underreward}$$

$$\frac{R_e}{I_e} > \frac{R_o}{I_o} \quad \text{Inequity due to overreward}$$

where R_e represents the rewards received by the employee, I_e is the inputs made by the employee, R_o is the rewards received by the other person, and I_o is the inputs made by the other person.

The reward component in these equations includes all rewards associated with the job. In ad-

dition to salary, retirement plan, vacation leave, and health insurance, this would include non-monetary considerations such as friendships, status, working conditions, and the like. The work inputs, similarly, would include all items that the employee perceives himself or herself as contributing, including items that may not be mentioned in the job description. These could include loyalty and willingness to adapt to the employer's needs (e.g., overtime, adjusting work hours, changing projects, etc.).

An important point to remember throughout this discussion is that equity is ultimately judged by the *employee*, and the employee's judgment regarding what is equitable may differ substantially from the conclusions of an independent, unbiased observer. This is significant because the equity of your compensation plan ultimately will be judged through your *employees'* eyes, not yours.

Employees do not consciously calculate mathematical equity ratios for themselves and others. Although some equity judgments may result from conscious comparisons, most equity judgments are based on semiconscious or unconscious evaluations. In addition, many of the data that the employee uses to form an equity judgment are "messy." For example, although John, your business manager, has good data regarding the rewards you provide, he may somewhat distort his input by over evaluating the importance of his job. Also, suppose John compares his rewards and inputs to those of Jane, a business manager at another practice. His data regarding Jane's rewards may or may not be accurate. He may be drawing his conclusions, for example, based partly on the clothes Jane wears, the car she drives, the neighborhood in which she lives, "hints" she has dropped during conversations indicating satisfaction with her compensation, and so on. The data regarding Jane's inputs might also be questionable. These might include self-serving remarks made by Jane, a halo effect based on the reputation of the other practice, comments made by a Blue Cross claims representative regarding the ease or difficulty of working with Jane, and so on. John then combines all these data at a semiconscious or unconscious level and forms an impression of the equity of his compensation.

Given these circumstances, there is a real possibility that what you perceive to be fair, just, and equitable may not be similarly perceived by your employees. The degree to which your employees will perceive their compensation as equitable will be affected by a number of issues besides salary, including:

- the general climate of employee relations in your organization
- the quality of your performance appraisal feedback
- the "reasonableness" of employees in choosing peers for comparison
- other characteristics of your compensation plan

The employee relations climate will have a pervasive impact on many aspects of your practice. If there is disharmony and unpleasantness, employees will add them to the I_e component. For example, suppose that, in your heart of hearts, you know that on occasion you can be an overbearing beast when working with Sally, your nurse. When Sally calculates her equity ratio, she adds "working with an overbearing beast" to the I_e component. To some degree, this will offset the value that you will be adding to the R_e component through your compensation package. The offset may be even greater if Sally has a friend who works for a physician who is always calm and reasonable and whom she uses to make her equity comparison. On the other hand, if you have very good employee relations with Sally and she prizes this, it can add value to the R_e component.

Performance appraisal feedback sets the stage for your employees' equity judgments. The quality and truthfulness of your performance appraisals will also have a profound impact on your employees' perceptions of equity. Suppose that you have a laboratory director with some serious performance problems that you choose not to address in the performance review. Given the lack of criticism, the laboratory director will assume that his or her performance is at least adequate. If you then give the director a small pay raise based on your recognition of the inadequate performance, he or she probably will perceive this reward as inequitably low. Similarly, providing a glowing appraisal for an employee who is competent but certainly not outstanding will result in an average pay raise being viewed as inequitably low.

An employee's perception of equity is partly based on comparisons with peers. The peers whom your employees choose will certainly have an impact on the evaluation of your compensation plan. Unfortunately, this matter is largely out of your control. If you have an employee who makes unreasonable comparisons, there is little that you can do. Generally, employees do not discuss these comparisons with their employer, and, as you have seen, they may only be vaguely aware of the comparison process.

This brings us to your compensation plan, something over which you *do* have considerable control. By using the methods discussed in this chapter, you will be able to determine equitable compensation rates based on your market and develop a compensation plan that creates equitable compensation differences corresponding to the various jobs and employees in your organization. You can also increase the fairness of the plan by talking with your employees to understand better the types of compensation that they desire.

Sometimes organizations can provide, in lieu of direct wages, benefits that are of great value to employees and of little or no additional cost to the organization. For example, a cafeteria style benefits plan that allows an employee to choose among similarly costed packages of increased health insurance coverage or additional vacation time can have a significant impact on equity perceptions, at little or no additional cost to the organization. Other benefit options might include child day care services or education. Similarly, offering an employee a reduced salary coupled with higher benefits that the employee could not otherwise purchase can also increase equity. Using information about desired benefits to determine the characteristics of your compensation plan will increase the probability that the plan will be perceived as equitable.

USING EQUITY TO CONSTRUCT A COMPENSATION PLAN

To use equity concepts effectively, it is important to make a distinction between compensating jobs and compensating employees. Jobs have value to your organization irrespective of the job incumbent. For example, no matter how well a secretary performs, the value of the job has an upper limit. This is why secretaries are not paid $75,000 per year. No matter how well the incumbent performs, and regardless of the employee's years of service, dedication, and commitment, *the work itself* simply does not merit this level of compensation. Similarly, the value of each job has a lower limit. Assuming that the incumbent is competent enough to retain in the position, the duties dictate that the incumbent be paid at least a minimum amount. There is a pay range, therefore, that exists for each job irrespective of the characteristics or performance level of the incumbent.

To establish an effective compensation plan, therefore, you first must think of the pay for each job as being composed of an equitable pay range that is associated with the *position,* independent of the job incumbent. For example, you may determine that the pay range for a training specialist is $25,000 to $34,500, for a level I secretary from $12,500 to $16,000, for a marketing director from $80,000 to $95,000, and for a family practice physician from $120,000 to $150,000. Next, you determine a specific employee's pay level from within this range based on job performance, seniority, experience, and so on. Perhaps, as a result, Fred Smith's pay as a training specialist will be $30,800, and Dale Yee's salary as a secretary will be $13,000.

Determining a reasonable salary for an employee requires consideration of three distinct types of equity: internal, external, and individual. These are summarized in Exhibit 4–1. Internal equity comparisons are comparisons among jobs within the practice or health care organization. The director of the physical therapy department, for example, might compare inputs and rewards associated with his or her job with the inputs and rewards associated with the department heads of

Exhibit 4–1 Internal, External, and Individual Equity

Concepts	Tools	Outcomes

Internal Equity
    Relationships Between & Among
    Jobs in the Organization
	Job Descriptions
	Job Analysis
	Job Evaluation
		Cost Control

Individual Employee Equity
    Relationships Between & Among
    Individuals Within a Job
	Performance Appraisal & Merit
	Seniority
		Attract Competent
		    Employees
		
		Retain Competent
		    Employees

External Equity
    Relationships Between & Among
    Jobs in the Labor Market
	Wage & Salary Survey
	Anecdotal "Going Rate"
	    Information
		Motivate Competent
		    Employees

nursing, radiology, various hospital laboratories, and so forth. He or she will also probably compare the salary with subordinates' salaries in the department and with the boss's salary. Once again, the data regarding the contributions and rewards of each of these positions and the people who occupy them may vary in accuracy and will certainly be subjective in nature. Nevertheless, each employee will make internal equity comparisons. To achieve internal equity, jobs that are generally recognized as having lower value, being less demanding, or requiring less training should, all other things being equal, be paid less, whereas the opposite should be true for more difficult, higher-value jobs. Your compensation plan, therefore, must have a mechanism to ensure logic and consistency between and among jobs in your organization.

This can be a particular problem for health care systems that have been acquiring physicians and putting them on salaries. These physicians' initial salaries are generally related to their productivity prior to acquisition. As a result, the health care system may have a wide range of salaries within a specialty, such as family practice or cardiology. At some later point in time, however, this could become a problem as performance differences between physicians change and as the relative market value of various specialties adjusts to the changes resulting from managed care. One effect, for example, is that the value of primary care physicians increases relative to specialists, such as cardiologists. As a result, the health care system needs a mechanism to adjust for the changing relative value (internal equity) across specialties.

External equity comparisons are made between the jobs in your organization and jobs in other organizations. External equity is the perception of the so-called going rate or market rate for a job. A compensation plan with external equity allows you to attract and retain qualified employees. The positions in other organizations that employees use as the "comparison other" can be medical, nonmedical, or both. For example, employees may evaluate the equity of compensation for clerical, business, and man-

agement positions by making comparisons with banks, law firms, construction companies, and so on because these are other viable employment alternatives. Physician employees will make comparisons with peers in other health care organizations, such as other health care systems, health maintenance organizations (HMOs), medical schools, private practices, and practices managed by physician management companies. Once again, the accuracy of the perceptions of the rewards and inputs of the "comparison others" may be questionable. The process will vary from fully conscious investigation to semiconscious and unconscious ruminations. Nevertheless, employees make these comparisons and in part act on them.

Both internal and external equity comparisons are essentially comparisons among *jobs*. Individual equity comparisons are comparisons among *employees*. In its simplest form, individual equity relates to the differences in pay received by different incumbents on the same job. For example, if you employ several family practice physicians, then pay differences between them will be subject to individual equity judgments. Once again, one or all physicians may be operating on the basis of poor or inaccurate information. Nevertheless, they will make inferences and take actions based on their assessments. Each, individually, will subjectively discount experience, training, seniority, and job performance differences and form a conclusion about whether his or her pay is equitable. Sometimes, employees will make individual equity comparisons across jobs. For example, a nurse might compare him- or herself with a secretary by discounting job and performance differences. Similarly, a physician may do the same with a top level administrator. If they can account for all the perceived salary differences as being due to job and performance differences, then they will conclude that their pay is equitable. If there is a discrepancy, they will perceive themselves as either underpaid or overpaid.

Employees combine their internal, external, and individual equity data to form conclusions about the fairness of their compensation. For example, a secretary might go through the following cognitive exercise (not necessarily consciously):

I'm making $15,500 per year. I think that is pretty good. I saw an ad in the newspaper last month that offered $14,500 for a medical secretary over at Dr. Brown's practice. I know that Dr. Brown doesn't have automated scheduling, so you don't have to be as computer capable as I am. On the other hand, that probably means that his secretaries have to work harder to do the same amount of work. I prefer to work in a more automated office anyway. (external equity comparisons)

Susie, our business manager, is probably paid about $10,000 more than I. I've been here almost two years. She just bought a new Ford Taurus with all the options—those cars cost about $18,000! Her being single and all, why she must be making $25,000 or $26,000. Also, she always dresses very well. Not terribly expensive, but stylish and up to date. Yeah, she's probably making about $25,000 or $26,000. She's responsible for collecting all the money, making certain that all the bills are paid, and supervising the rest of us. She also has to train us on all the computer programs used in the office, and she knows them all really well. (internal equity comparisons)

I've heard, however, that she's not a superstar; she issued six incorrect W-2s a few months ago. Also, insurance collections have been slow, and I know that Dr. Simpson is not happy about that. He also knows that sometimes she has problems getting along with some of the rest of us. (individual equity comparisons)

Dr. Simpson always tells me that I am doing a super job and in my last performance review, Susie gave me the highest evaluation possible in four of the five evaluation factors. My super performance should make up for some of the difference in the importance of our jobs. It would be fair if

Susie made $6,000 or $7,000 more than I, but not $10,000. She does have a more important job, but I am better at what I do than she is at what she does. (employee equity comparison)

I really think that she is being paid at least $25,000. That's not really fair. If she gets that much, then I should be making another $2,000 or $3,000. She just isn't worth that much more than me. I know that secretaries at some of the local offices of big companies like TRW and DuPont have salaries in the middle to upper teens. Steve works for DuPont, and he as much as told me that. (external equity comparisons)

Maybe I really put too much into this job. When I switched schedules to cover when Francis was sick, I didn't get anything for it other than a thanks from Dr. Simpson. If he really wanted to thank me, he would pay me more. He obviously has the money—look at what he's paying Susie! I guess I should stop putting myself out. I should do a good, competent job, but not anything extra. (equity decision)

This example illustrates how an employee can integrate several sources of information and combine external, internal, and individual equity data to reach an overall judgment regarding the fairness of compensation. It also illustrates one other very important point: Employees *always* achieve equity *one way or another*! When employees feel that their rewards are inequitably low, they will achieve equity by reducing inputs. When employees cannot reduce inputs enough to achieve equity, then they will take more extreme measures, including passive-aggressive behavior, noncompliance, open disobedience, sabotage, and ultimately resignation.

Employees who perceive that they are overpaid will also achieve equity. They will increase the quality or quantity of their work or will psychologically adjust their perceptions of their input or the rewards they receive until they perceive equity. Some physician managers may be tempted to increase the compensation of valued employees to inequitably high levels to "freeze" them and thereby deter turnover. This strategy is dangerous because it creates internal inequities relative to other employees, thereby causing dissatisfaction and motivating other employees to act out or to leave. Of course, the compensation of all employees could be raised to inequitably high levels, but this would inflate the size of the organization's payroll to unnecessary levels.

Generally, employees are less concerned about external equity than about internal and individual equity. This is because it is easier to rationalize working for somewhat lower compensation compared with someone across town than it is to rationalize differences compared with someone at the next desk. For example, "the work atmosphere is nicer here," "parking is easier," "this health care system will be the dominant one in the area," "Dr. Jones is a pleasure to work for," and so on are all justifications for working for somewhat lower compensation. If, however, the pay is less than that of another employee in the same organization, it is much more difficult to produce convincing rationalization because the comparison is with someone working under the same circumstances.

Because of internal and individual equity considerations, it is not sufficient simply to pay the going market rate to each employee. First, it is simply too time consuming and difficult to identify the market rate for all jobs, with the possible exception being the smallest practices. Second, using the average rates for jobs in your local labor market will not necessarily produce a pay plan that is internally equitable. The market rate for a job is based on an amalgam of below-average, average, and above-average performers in organizations with varying mixes of job content for a given job title. In effect, not all positions labeled Clerk/Typist perform the same tasks. Some clerk/typist positions are more demanding and require more skills and abilities than other positions with the same job title. Adopting the average or market rate across all positions in your organization won't take into account real performance differences between your employees or the mix of tasks as they exist in your organization. As a result, you need ways to build internal, individual, and external equities into your compensation plan based on the mix of jobs and performance levels *as they exist in your organization*. Column two in Exhibit 4–1 lists the methods that are used to achieve each of these equity goals.

JOB EVALUATION METHODS FOR ACHIEVING INTERNAL AND EXTERNAL EQUITY

Job evaluation is the process that compensation professionals use to build internal and external equity into their compensation plans. Although there are three major job evaluation methods and many variations on these themes, all these methods do two things. First, they order jobs based on their internal content and worth to the organization. This achieves the internal equity goal. Next, they identify the market rate for some of the jobs. These jobs are called benchmark jobs because they will be used to benchmark or anchor the internal ordering of jobs to outside market rates.

Generally, you will want to identify some benchmark jobs toward the top, middle, and bottom of the internal equity order. Once benchmark pay levels have been determined, then pay levels for jobs between the benchmark jobs can be resolved. These rates will be derived subjectively, through interpolation, or by calculation, depending on the particular job evaluation method that is used.

We will examine two job evaluation methods. The ranking method is the simplest and easiest to use. Simplicity and ease can be real advantages for a small organization. Its disadvantage is that it becomes cumbersome to use when there are many jobs to be evaluated or when the jobs are highly technical or complex. Smaller private practices and health care organizations will find that the ranking method may be sufficient to develop compensation plans for front office, technical, and professional positions.

The other method that we will cover is called a point plan. Point plans require more time, effort, and skill to create. They can, however, cover large numbers of jobs and jobs that are complex in their work content. Point plans are the most common job evaluation method used in the United States. Larger group practices and health care organizations, such as hospitals and hospital systems, will generally find the point system to be appropriate.

Before looking at how to use job evaluation methods, we must discuss who will do this. Because equity is the eventual goal, two considerations to remember are that the eventual plan must be understandable by those whom it covers and that these employees must accept the results as valid. As a result, larger organizations often use a committee to develop their compensation plans. Often, these committees span several employee groups, such as administrative, technical, professional, and medical. Using broader representation gives additional perspective to job content and provides more "real world" data on what employees really do on a job. In addition, participation often improves acceptance. If nurses know, for example, that they had representation on the team that developed the compensation plan covering their positions, then they are more likely to accept the results.

RANKING JOB EVALUATION METHOD

The object of a ranking method is to rank jobs on the basis of their overall value to the organization. The procedure works as follows:

1. Assemble all the job descriptions to be covered in the compensation plan.
2. Read all the job descriptions so that you are fully familiar with their contents. Validate that the descriptions are current, and resolve any questions regarding what employees really do on a job.
3. Considering all issues covered by the descriptions, identify the job that is most important to the organization.
4. Next, identify the job that is least important to the organization.
5. Of the jobs remaining, identify the one that is most important, then the one that is least important. Repeat this process until all jobs have been ranked.

The first two columns in Table 4–1 illustrate the outcome of this ranking process. This ranking expresses the internal equity ordering of jobs in this organization. Because we are using ordinal measurement, however, the "distances" between jobs are not meaningful. That is, the "importance difference" between Nurse Practitioner and Surgical Nurse will not be the same as between Surgical Nurse and Business Manager.

Using the ranking process obviously requires an ability to evaluate subjectively the composite of compensable factors possessed by each job. For example, the business manager position may require more experience and supervisory skills than a nursing position, yet the nursing position may require more formal education and have greater responsibility. Nevertheless, when there are a fairly small number of jobs and the evaluator or evaluating team really understands the jobs, the relative worth or value of the positions to the organization can be captured with the ranking process.

Next, benchmark jobs must be identified. The standard way of obtaining benchmark information is with a wage and salary survey. Table 4–2 is from a wage and salary survey published by the U.S. Bureau of Labor Statistics (BLS). Wage and salary surveys can be obtained in three ways. First, you can conduct a survey yourself. Some large companies conduct their own surveys. Larger health care systems, such as hospitals, may have personnel staff who are capable of conducting a local wage and salary survey.

Table 4–1 Rank Ordering of Jobs

Rank	Job Title	Benchmark Rate
1	Nurse Practitioner	$45,000
2	Surgical Nurse	
3	Business Manager	$28,500
4	Practice Nurse	
5	Laboratory Technician	
6	Clerk/Word Processor	$14,500
7	Receptionist	$12,500

Table 4–2 Bureau of Labor Statistics Wage and Salary Survey

Occupation and Level	Number of Workers	Average Weekly Hours (Standard)	Weekly Pay (In Dollars)			200 and Under 225	225 – 250	250 – 275
			Mean	Median	Middle Range			
Key Entry Operators								
Level I	463	38.4	$353	$340	$316–$377	—	2	4
Private industry	432	38.3	354	343	316–377	—	2	4
Goods-producing industries	51	39.5	309	305	273–324	—	12	16
Manufacturing	51	39.5	309	305	273–324	—	12	16
Service-producing industries	381	38.2	360	348	319–378	—		2
State and local government	31	39.7	346	—	— – —	—	—	3
Level II	179	39.3	408	421	353–462	—	—	1
Private industry	162	39.3	406	422	350–462	—	—	1
Service-producing industries	112	39.0	395	396	320–462	—	—	1
State and local government	17	40.0	425	411	357–519	—	—	—
Personnel Assistants (Employment)								
Level II	26	39.1	390	—	— – —	—	—	—
State and local government	7	37.5	393	—	— – —	—	—	—
Secretaries								
Level I	210	38.5	382	382	353–415	—	1	4
Private industry	116	38.4	391	394	360–417	—	—	3
Service-producing industries	107	38.4	386	392	358–417	—	—	4
State and local government	94	38.7	371	374	324–403	—	2	4
Level II	900	39.3	465	471	421–493	—	—	—
Private industry	378	38.7	475	462	414–534	—	—	—
Goods-producing industries	36	39.0	526	—	— – —	—	—	—
Manufacturing	32	38.8	522	—	— – —	—	—	—
Service-producing industries	342	38.7	469	461	414–524	—	—	—
State and local government	522	39.7	458	471	424–482	—	—	—
Level III	735	39.0	522	523	454–474	—	—	—
Private industry	655	38.9	519	520	450–565	—	—	—
Goods-producing industries	97	39.1	581	572	473–661	—	—	—
Manufacturing	96	39.1	580	572	470–660	—	—	—
Service-producing industries	558	38.9	508	515	445–548	—	—	—
State and local government	80	39.7	553	576	476–614	—	—	—
Level IV	365	39.3	564	539	515–615	—	—	—
Private industry	153	38.4	633	643	556–701	—	—	—
Service-producing industries	117	38.5	619	625	538–693	—	—	—
State and local government	212	40.0	514	527	493–539	—	—	—
Level V	42	38.9	700	672	656–779	—	—	—
Private industry	36	38.8	697	—	— – —	—	—	—
Service-producing industries	33	38.8	688	—	— – —	—	—	—
State and local government	6	40.0	720	—	— – —	—	—	—

Source: Reprinted from *Bureau of Labor Statistics Area Wage and Salary Survey—Richmond-Petersburg Virginia*, U.S. Department of Labor, August 1995, Washington, D.C.

Percent of Workers Receiving Straight-Time Weekly Pay (In Dollars) of —

275–300	300–325	325–350	350–375	375–400	400–425	425–450	450–475	475–500	500–550	550–600	600–650	650–700	700–750	750–800	800–900	900–1000	1000–1100
12	17	22	19	8	6	2	4	3	2	—	—	—	—	—	—	—	—
12	17	21	20	8	6	2	5	3	2	—	—	—	—	—	—	—	—
20	35	2	2	—	10	—	2	—	2	—	—	—	—	—	—	—	—
20	35	2	2	—	10	—	2	—	2	—	—	—	—	—	—	—	—
11	14	23	22	9	6	2	5	3	2	1	—	—	—	—	—	—	—
10	19	39	3	3	13	6	—	3	—	—	—	—	—	—	—	—	—
7	9	7	11	7	23	8	13	6	7	2	—	—	—	—	—	—	—
7	10	7	9	7	24	8	15	6	4	2	—	—	—	—	—	—	—
11	14	10	8	10	15	2	12	9	6	3	—	—	—	—	—	—	—
—	—	12	29	6	12	12	—	—	29	—	—	—	—	—	—	—	—
8	—	—	62	8	—	4	4	4	4	4	—	4	—	—	—	—	—
—	—	—	71	—	—	—	14	14	—	—	—	—	—	—	—	—	—
4	8	5	20	22	20	5	6	1	2	—	—	—	—	—	—	—	—
4	1	7	20	22	28	7	3	1	3	1	1	—	—	—	—	—	—
5	1	7	21	23	26	7	2	1	3	—	—	—	—	—	—	—	—
3	17	2	21	23	11	3	9	2	2	—	—	—	—	—	—	—	—
—	—	2	7	6	13	9	17	24	11	8	2	—	—	—	—	—	—
—	—	1	5	9	16	8	14	12	14	17	2	1	1	—	—	—	—
—	—	6	6	6	11	3	6	6	11	22	11	3	11	—	—	—	—
—	—	6	6	6	13	3	6	6	9	16	13	3	13	—	—	—	—
—	—	1	5	9	17	8	15	13	14	16	1	—	—	—	—	—	—
—	—	2	8	5	10	9	20	33	9	2	1	—	—	—	—	—	—
—	—	1	1	4	7	12	9	11	25	15	8	5	2	1	—	—	—
—	—	—	1	4	7	12	9	12	26	14	7	4	2	1	—	—	—
—	—	—	—	3	5	1	16	3	12	16	13	9	13	4	1	1	—
—	—	—	—	3	5	1	17	3	13	17	14	9	13	4	1	1	—
—	—	—	1	5	7	14	7	13	29	14	6	3	—	—	—	—	—
—	—	4	1	—	7	5	7	7	14	19	15	15	2	2	—	—	—
—	—	—	1	1	2	2	7	5	37	18	7	8	7	2	2	—	—
—	—	—	—	—	1	1	4	1	18	14	16	20	17	5	5	—	—
—	—	—	—	1	2	5	—	23	14	17	18	14	2	5	—	—	—
—	—	—	1	1	3	3	9	8	50	21	1	—	—	—	—	—	—
—	—	—	—	—	—	—	5	—	7	12	38	10	19	5	2	2	—
—	—	—	—	—	—	—	6	—	6	14	39	11	17	3	3	3	—
—	—	—	—	—	—	—	6	—	6	12	42	12	18	—	—	3	—
—	—	—	—	—	—	—	—	—	—	17	—	33	—	33	17	—	—

This approach is not a cost-effective alternative, however, for most health care organizations, even large hospital systems.

A second alternative is to commission a consultant to conduct a wage and salary survey. This option provides accurate, current data for jobs that are comparable to the ones in your organization. The disadvantage of this approach is the relatively high cost of conducting a private study. Once again, larger health care organizations that have a continuing need for current data may find this to be a cost-effective alternative. This is not the case, however, for most private medical practices.

A variation on this theme is to use a consultant who conducts ongoing wage and salary surveys in the medical field. Generally, these consultants provide survey data for a subscription fee. This approach often provides the most feasible source of wage and salary survey data for health care providers that are looking for market rates for jobs specific to health care, such as medical secretaries, radiation technologists, respiratory therapists, and the like.

Another source of wage and salary data can be your local or state medical association, which could commission a one-time or ongoing survey for the use of its members. Generally, each organization that wants a copy of the survey results pays a nominal fee, perhaps $100, and also completes a survey questionnaire. The consultant collects, analyzes, and interprets the data and then provides a written report to the association and to participating organizations. Each organization is identified in the report by a code number. In this way, physician managers can examine the data to see how their organization compares with others and with group statistics, yet complete anonymity is maintained for all the participants. An example of this type of survey report for a business manager position is found in Exhibit 4–2.

Other possible sources of published wage and salary data include your state Employment Commission or Department of Labor, your local Chamber of Commerce, and local trade and professional associations in both medical and nonmedical fields. The problem with these sources is that generally their surveys don't contain data on medical jobs. Nevertheless, you may be able to get some good data on selected other jobs, such as clerical and business-related positions, that are not unique to medicine.

Irrespective of the source of your survey, remember that the data it contains will to some degree be approximate because of the data collection method. When employers receive a request for data from the BLS or any other surveying organization, they also receive a set of job descriptions. Each employer selects the jobs in his or her organization that most closely match the job descriptions provided by the surveyor and then reports the salary and benefits data for those jobs. Therefore, the salary data reported across a number of employers will be a blend of data for jobs that vary in their degree of closeness to the survey job descriptions. *Thus you should appreciate the need to use the survey's salary figures as a starting point.* You may conclude that it is best to establish benchmark job rates at levels somewhat above or below the survey rates, based on your judgment of how similar the survey job descriptions are to your jobs.

A final method of obtaining external equity data that would be appropriate for a smaller practice is to contact a few major hospitals and colleagues in your area to obtain salary information about selected jobs. *This is not the same as conducting a survey.* Your data have none of the precision of data collected from a representative sample of employers. Because the data are not representative of the population of practices, you should not attempt to subject these data to any statistical operations, such as calculating a mean. Nevertheless, if you have a small practice, need data on only a few jobs, understand the concept of external equity, and can make some good intuitive inferences, this method can provide useful information. It certainly can be a cost- and time-effective way of collecting information. Many hospitals conduct or purchase wage and salary surveys. Some hospitals may be willing to provide affiliated physicians and practices with these data, especially if you routinely hospitalize there. Others may consider these data

Exhibit 4–2 Coded Wage and Salary Survey for Business Manager (Direct Wages Only)

Job Description: The business manager handles the major day-to-day financial and supervisory duties in the practice. These include responsibility for at least three of the following: accounts receivable, accounts payable, insurance collection, checkbook, negotiation of patient payment arrangements, payment of taxes, and supervision of clerical staff.

Rank	Code	Annual Salary ($K)	Rank	Code	Annual Salary ($K)
1	XO37	28.9	25	ER77	18.5
2	EK94	25.2	26	LL49	18.5
3	JK23	24.9	27	KK34	18.5
4	OI38	24.9	28	IO38	18.3
5	FI34	23.0	29	UT44	18.1
6	KL99	22.5	30	RR67	18.0
7	OF39	22.5	31	TW78	18.0
8	HL81	22.1	32	IQ37	18.0
9	JG88	22.0	33	OO99	17.7
10	BB12	22.0	34	PU38	17.3
11	CM31	21.7	35	HH78	17.0
12	XM44	21.5	36	RQ56	16.8
13	VM55	21.5	37	UT48	16.4
14	MM21	21.0	38	OW60	16.0
15	NN39	20.5	39	UW29	16.0
16	ZX94	20.5	40	NV39	15.9
17	AQ51	20.3	41	AQ29	15.8
18	PL81	20.0	42	QP51	15.5
19	PP79	20.0	43	XZ37	15.5
20	PU42	19.7	44	YT38	15.2
21	YT30	19.3	45	UW11	15.0
22	TT28	19.0	46	QQ55	15.0
23	YT23	18.8	47	LK38	14.8
24	UZ39	18.5			

Mean = 19.30
Standard deviation = 2.86
Interquartile range = 21.5–16.8

proprietary and will not share them. You have nothing to lose, however, by asking.

As a result of using one or several of the methods discussed, you will be confident that you have good market rate data on some of your jobs. You will also realize that you are less confident about the market rates of other jobs, and you will have no data at all on some of your jobs. That is fine. Even large organizations do not try to obtain market data for all jobs. As we have seen, given the mechanics of conducting a survey, this would be an impossible task. Those jobs where you have obtained good market data will be used as your benchmark jobs. In Table 4–1 benchmark rates are listed in the third column for those jobs where the organization felt confident about the data. These jobs will then be used to anchor the compensation plan.

Next, base compensation rates are determined for the nonbenchmark jobs through interpolation. For example, we know that the rate for a surgical nurse must be somewhere between the nurse practitioner's $45,000 and the business manager's $28,500. Similarly, we know that a practice nurse should be compensated less than the business manager. If the evaluators are knowledgeable about the jobs and rates in the field, they generally can make valid interpolation decisions. Is it possible for evaluators to make bad interpolation decisions that result in the perception of inequity? Certainly! But that is the disadvantage of this method and the other side of the ranking method's ease and simplicity.

POINT JOB EVALUATION METHOD

The ranking method treats jobs as wholes because they are evaluated based on their overall worth. Jobs, however, are composed of factors, such as education, responsibility for money, supervision, and the like. A more sophisticated job evaluation method will take this complexity into account when determining pay rates. For example, if one job is high in responsibility and moderate in complexity, and another is high in complexity and low in responsibility, then these relative differences should have an effect on each job's relative compensation. A point system is capable of dealing with the factorial complexity of jobs.

In a point system, jobs receive points based on how much they possess of each compensable factor. A compensable factor is an issue that you or the labor market is willing to pay for. Generally, for example, organizations are willing to pay positions more for supervision, responsibility, education required, and so forth. A point system begins with the identification of *all* the compensable factors that relate to *any* of the jobs to be covered in the compensation plan. It is not necessary for all jobs to load on all factors, but it is necessary to identify all the compensable issues that relate to any of the jobs. An example of a point system is found in Appendix 4A. It is designed to assess jobs based on those compensable factors that often occur in medical practice jobs. After examining the point system in Appendix 4A, you may conclude that developing a plan in your organization is not feasible. This question is directly addressed below.

Next, each factor is weighed based on its importance and is broken down into a number of different levels, which are called degrees. Point values are assigned to each degree, so that the value of the highest degree for a factor is the same as the factor's weight.

Jobs are then evaluated by comparing the job content with the degree definitions. Although the job description will be helpful, it is important to have a thorough knowledge of what job incumbents really do on a day-to-day basis. Once again, having a knowledgeable compensation person or committee use the job descriptions and point chart will greatly improve the outcome of the process.

It is important to remember that you are evaluating what is required by the job, not the characteristics of the particular incumbent. Many incumbents possess skills, education, or experience not required by the job. Because these are characteristics of the person and not job requirements, you should not pay for them, and they should not enter into the evaluation of the job. For example, look at the degree choices (1–9) for the factor Education in Table 4A–1 (Appendix 4A). Now, suppose that you have a clerical position in which the demands of the job require a high school education and some specialized courses. The incumbent happens to have a master's degree. Because the job only requires a high school education and some specialized courses, it would be evaluated at degree 2 and would receive 135 to 255 points, depending on the number of years of experience required to perform the job adequately. The important thing to remember is that you are evaluating the worth of *jobs*, not people. Paying for irrelevant skill or experience that contributes nothing to job performance is simply a waste of money and ultimately will reduce perceived equity.

Using the job description and your knowledge of the job, evaluate the job on each factor, and calculate a point total. For example, Table 4–3 contains an evaluation for the job of computer operator/secretary (see Exhibit 3–1 in Chapter 3 for the job description). The job requires a high school education with experience of less than one year, so it receives 110 points for the knowledge factor. The amount and nature of the job's nonsupervisory responsibility is best described by degree 3C, so the job receives 185 points for this factor. Given the evaluations for the other three factors, the job receives a total of 780 points. A similar evaluation of the business manager position produces a total of 1,235 points. *The point totals represent the relative worth of the jobs in terms of the compensable factors.* This is the internal equity determination process.

The next step is to convert points into dollars. This is accomplished once again by identifying benchmark jobs as described above for the ranking job evaluation method. Table 4–4 contains data on the benchmark jobs of computer operator/secretary, business manager, and nurse practitioner. You can now derive the point–pay relationship in two ways:

1. Use regression analysis to derive the straight line formula for the relationship between points and pay.[1] In Table 4–4, this results in a *y* intercept of $3,106.83, with each point worth $12.34. *Warning*: Regression analysis is only appropriate if the data are essentially linear. If you plot the data on a graph and there is a clear bend or curve in the plot, do not use regression analysis. In this event, use the "eyeball" method described below.
2. Plot the relationship, and "eyeball" a line that fits the data (see Figure 4–1). If you decide to eyeball a line, remember that

measurement errors may cause your benchmark jobs not to line up perfectly. Sometimes, also the point–pay relationship is best described by a smoothly curving line. Once again, use your judgment. If you can eyeball a line that appears to do a reasonable job of describing the data, that will be sufficient.

Because the line (expressed either as a formula or on paper) is based on benchmark jobs, *which by definition represent the equitable relationship between points and pay*, any point on the line should represent equity. The line can be used, therefore, to calculate an equitable salary for other jobs. Table 4–4 illustrates this by showing a projected salary for a nurse position. The job description was evaluated using the point plan in Appendix 4A. The total was 835 points. Using either the regression formula or a graph results in a projected base pay of $13,410.73.

PAY RANGES

Having one pay rate for a job could create a number of problems. For example, if $15,000 represents equity for a job, you will want the flexibility to pay somewhat above or below this amount to take into account differences among employees, such as merit and seniority. Developing pay ranges will give you this flexibility. A pay range treats the equity level of a job as the midpoint of a range. Pay ranges can be applied

Table 4–3 Point Evaluation of Computer Operator/Secretary and Business Manager Positions

Factor	Computer Operator/Secretary		Business Manager	
	Degree	Points	Degree	Points
A. Education	2A	110	2A	120
B. Operating responsibility	3C	185	4E	320
C. Ingenuity	1B	115	3A	225
D. Administrative responsibility	1B	130	2B	140
E. Outside/patient relations	3B	240	4B	430
TOTAL POINTS		780		1,235

Table 4–4 Determining Base Pay Using a Point System

Benchmark Jobs	Salary	Points
Computer operator/Secretary	$13,000.00	780
Business manager	$18,000.00	1,235
Nurse practitioner	$40,000.00	2,985
Nurse	$13,410.73 (projected)	835

Salary = $a + $b (points)
Salary = $3,106.83 + $12.34 (points)

to compensation rates derived through either ranking or point job evaluation methods.

There are no incontestable ways of determining the correct size of a pay range. Generally, rules of thumb are applied. At the low end of a pay scale, spreads may vary from 10 percent to 20 percent of equity. At higher pay levels, spreads may vary from 20 percent to 40 percent. Judiciously applying these rules of thumb to the positions listed in Table 4–4 might result in the salary structure found in Table 4–5. Obviously, this can result in some overlap between posi-

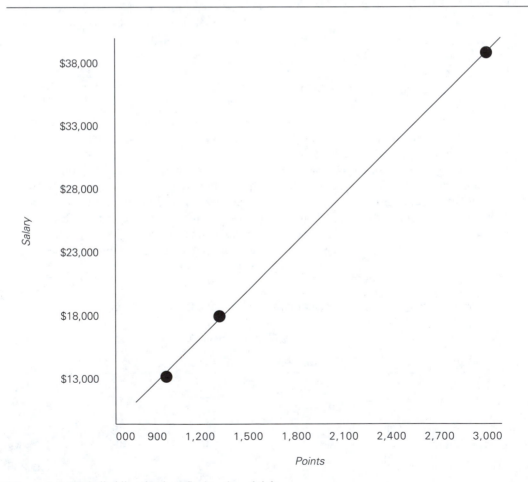

Figure 4–1 Eyeballed line that best fits benchmark jobs.

Table 4–5 Job Salary Structure

Job Title	Salary Midpoint	Range Percentage	Range Salary
Computer operator/secretary	$13,000	±10%	$11,700–$14,300
Nurse	$13,500	±10%	$12,150–$14,850
Business manager	$18,000	±15%	$15,300–$20,700
Nurse practitioner	$40,000	±25%	$30,000–$50,000

tions. That is, a high performer or very senior employee occupying a lower position may actually make somewhat more money than a low performer or very junior employee occupying a higher position. Generally, these overlaps are perceived by employees as equitable. It is generally advisable, however, to develop pay ranges so that salaries for supervisors and subordinates don't overlap, or will do so only in extreme and rare cases.

Realistically, pay levels substantially below equity will not be used very often because of the difficulty of recruiting at these levels. Labor markets, however, are not perfect, and the combination of job evaluation and wage and salary survey data provides you with only an estimate of equity. Employees and applicants will form their own equity judgments. As a result, you probably can hire some applicants at below-midpoint salary levels. If you find resistance to these lower levels, then you will have to raise your salary offer. You may find, however, that some well-qualified applicants will accept below-midpoint offers.

Once you have a pay range associated with a job, the next task is to decide where an employee fits within that range. This decision should be based on job performance, seniority, or some combination of the two. It is essentially a subjective decision, and in making it you will have to rely on your evaluation of the employee's performance and the employee's value to the organization. The discussion of performance appraisal in Chapter 2 gives you a number of ideas about how to obtain the performance data you need to make salary decisions on the basis of merit. Some organizations use a salary matrix that is based on the outcome of the performance appraisal (Table 4–6).

If you decide that you want to give merit pay increases, it is important to have wide enough pay ranges to make meaningful distinctions among employees. A merit system will be counterproductive if employees perceive that meaningful differences in performance result in trivial compensation differences. This can be a particular problem at the low end of the compensation plan, where the spread between low and high for a job might only be 20 percent. Under these circumstances, it is particularly important to make allowance in your pay ranges for increases in the cost of living. The problem is compounded by the fact that most people expect an annual salary increase. You probably will find that it is best to base pay raises on a combination of seniority and merit. The seniority component might account for 1 percent to 3 percent, and it should be used to address the cost of living/inflation issue. The merit component might account for an additional 1 percent to 10 percent. For example, a health care system decides that each department will get a 7.5 percent increase in wages based on total salaries of all positions below executive level, to be distributed as follows: 2.5 percent based on seniority, and 5.0 percent based on merit.[2] If the physician manager of the Physician Services Office wishes to give one employee a 10 percent raise on the merit component, he or she will on average have to give several other employees merit raises of less than 5 percent to achieve the 5 percent merit average.

The range above equity can be very effective as a control for excessive payroll expenses. When an employee hits the top of a pay range, he or she cannot receive any additional increases because of the job that he or she occupies. When

Table 4–6 Performance Appraisal–Salary Matrix

Current Salary Level (Percentage of Pay Grade Midpoint)	Overall Performance Level				
	Outstanding	Excellent	Satisfactory	Fair	Poor
110%	6%	4%	2%	0%	0%
100%	8%	6%	4%	0%	0%
90%	10%	8%	6%	0%	0%
80%	12%	10%	8%	6%	0%

employees start to approach the top of the range for their job, it is time to do one of the following:

- Increase the employee's duties and responsibilities to justify a higher salary. This option may be limited by the ability or willingness of the job incumbent to take on different duties or by the degree to which these changes would make sense given other jobs in your organization.
- Prepare the employee for a shift into another position. This option may be limited, once again, by employee ability and interest and by the availability of an appropriate, higher-paying position. In a larger organization, such as a hospital or hospital system, this career path approach to staff development can be a powerful selling point to job applicants and a real incentive to successful employees.
- Tell the employee that, with the exception of cost of living adjustments to the whole salary structure, he or she will not be able to make more money in this job. If you do this, the employee may leave. Depending on other considerations, such as staff morale and the employee's job performance, it may be reasonable to risk the employee's resignation because it could provide an opportunity to hire an acceptable replacement at a significantly lower pay level.
- Continue to give the employee pay raises, fully recognizing that you are overpaying for the job. You may be able to justify this on the basis of staff morale or simply because it makes your life easier. Overpay-

ment, however, should be the result of a conscious, informed decision, and you should be aware of the probable effects on your payroll and the potential for creating internal equity problems. At some point, the overpaid employee will become costly enough in terms of payroll expenditures and equity problems that the inconvenience associated with turnover becomes more desirable than continuing to grant pay increases.

INFLATION

Irrespective of how you derive your pay rates, you should consider the effects of inflation. A year from now, your equitable rates may no longer be perceived as equitable because of inflation. You can adjust your salary line by some percentage of the inflation rate to keep your compensation plan current. It is not advisable, however, to raise the salary line by the full cost of living increase because you will have difficulty lowering salaries if the cost of living actually goes down. Cost of living adjustments, therefore, should lag cost of living increases by several points. If the cost of living increases 5 percent, you might adjust your salary line upward by 1 percent. Any increase that an employee receives above this level should be based on job performance or seniority.

COMPENSATION PLAN COVERAGE

Generally, organizations have several different compensation plans. One plan may cover hourly and blue collar jobs. Another may cover administrative positions, and a third might cover medical and other professional positions. The reason for this is that the underlying job factors relevant to the different compensation plans will vary. For example, the job factors that medical and other health care professional positions load on would be different from those that would be appropriate for administrative positions. A separate compensation plan, therefore, is appropriate. The methods described above will work, however, for all these types of jobs.

Job evaluation procedures should allow you to achieve internal and external equity for most, but not all, positions in your organization. Occasionally you will encounter an "outlier." Outliers are jobs with unusually high or low compensation due to temporary fluctuations or historic inconsistencies in the labor market. For example, the market rate in many parts of the country for nurses is below what job evaluations would project as equitable. Geologists were paid at inequitably high rates by oil companies in the 1970s as a result of the OPEC oil crisis. Many jobs requiring MBAs were similarly overpriced in the 1980s and early 1990s, reflecting the temporary lack of applicants with this degree. Currently, management information system positions tend to be overpaid. Eventually, most of these market inequities work themselves out as the supply of candidates increases or decreases in response to prevailing salaries. Some physician specialties, such as anesthesiology and cardiac surgery, are outliers in some health care systems.

It is important, therefore, to know enough about the local market to know whether a job or profession is an outlier. If it is, don't use it as a benchmark job because this would bias your estimates for other jobs. Outliers must be dealt with idiosyncratically and paid either what you can get away with, as in the case of a low outlier, or what is necessary, as in the case of a high outlier.

For high outlier fields, the bottom line is that, unless you pay the going rate, you won't be able to fill a position, or the candidates whom you attract will be "bottom of the barrel." Don't allow these few exceptions, however, to corrupt the remainder of your compensation plan. Base the first 85 percent to 90 percent of your compensation decisions on your job evaluation methods, and deal with the remaining outliers as what they are: exceptions.

PRACTICAL CONSIDERATIONS

The compensation process discussed in this chapter may sound like overkill for a small private medical practice. For most small practices, using a ranking method with limited investigation of benchmark rates is feasible. For example, a cost- and time-effective strategy for a small practice might include obtaining the regional BLS *Area Wage and Salary Survey* to acquire data on some generic jobs, such as secretary and computer operator positions. Phone calls to a few hospitals and colleagues might provide ideas about the going rate for medical jobs. A ranking system could then be used to determine rates for those positions for which you were not able to obtain market data. A "devil's advocate" pay line could be eyeballed. Salary spreads could be created and then adjusted based on your judgment of what makes sense for your practice.

At a minimum, this approach will cause you to ask yourself penetrating questions as you make compensation-related decisions. It almost certainly will give you a better outcome than using no system at all. It will provide an answer when employees ask how their pay was determined. Finally, it will probably save you money by controlling payroll costs.

Larger health care organizations may find it advantageous to form alliances to develop a point plan jointly. For example, several regional hospitals may use a joint task force to identify compensable factors, weight factors, and write degree definitions. Each individual hospital can then take the jointly developed point plan and use its own benchmark job data to create its own compensation plan. In this way, competitors can share common expenses to develop the point plan but go their own separate ways as they use it.

Irrespective of whether you run a small practice or a large health care organization, the compensation methods discussed in this chapter are best used as a means of forming hypotheses. Formal methods should never replace good, sound management judgment. Formal methods, however, can be used to stimulate you to think and consider alternatives. If a wage and salary survey gives you answers that you don't like, then ask yourself why you don't like them. Is it because you really don't want to hear that a fair salary for a position is $3,000 higher than you want to pay? Or is it because the survey was inaccurate or not really relevant? By forcing yourself to ask questions and investigate, formal compensation methods can help you make better compensation decisions.

WHO SHOULD CONSTRUCT YOUR COMPENSATION PLAN?

If you are a physician manager in a private practice who wishes to develop a compensation plan, you will have to do most of the work yourself or delegate it to a consultant. With the exception of some data collecting tasks, such as obtaining published wage and salary surveys, the tasks should not be delegated to subordinates in the practice. The need for judgment, as well as the potential for influencing their own salaries, makes these decisions inappropriate for your subordinates.

Hiring a consultant to construct a practice compensation plan can be an effective strategy for three reasons. First, and perhaps most important, contracting this work to a consultant gets you out of the compensation business and back into practicing medicine. Generally, physicians in private practice are more successful if they leave technical personnel issues to those with expertise. The physician manager assumes his or her traditional role of knowing enough about compensation to know when the contracted work is being competently performed. Second, hiring an experienced consultant will give you the benefit of knowledge and perspective in a task where these commodities are obviously of great importance. Finally, the objectivity that a consultant can provide will give your plan greater credibility with and acceptance from your employees and your partners.

If you do decide to use a consultant, be certain that you receive adequate training in the use and maintenance of the plan. As a physician manager, chief executive officer, or partner, one of your responsibilities is to be certain that the consultant is providing a quality product. In addition, you want a plan that is usable by you and your staff and will not require the consultant's constant attention.

Compensation plans in larger health care organizations should be developed either by experienced consultants or by personnel staff with compensation expertise. As a physician manager, your responsibility should be to use the concepts discussed in this chapter to ensure that the personnel constructing and utilizing the compensation plan are doing so in a thorough and professional manner. If, for example, a compensation committee is being formed to construct a point system that will cover jobs that affect physicians, then it would be important to ensure that physicians are on the committee.

Some consulting firms have their own proprietary point plans that they utilize, with minor adaptations, for all clients. Large national compensation firms, such as Hay Associates, use plans that have been developed and refined over many years. Generally, these plans do a very good job. In addition, these firms maintain large databases that can be very helpful when establishing benchmark job rates and making comparisons between your compensation rates and those of other hospitals, HMOs, large multispecialty practices, and the like.

The physician manager working in a large health care organization can select a national firm with the knowledge that the work will be competently performed, even though this might not be the low-cost option. Using one of these plans, however, does involve a trade-off between the precise fit of a custom-developed plan that measures the specific factors relevant to your jobs as they exist in your organization and generalizability and access to national data offered by the more generic plans.

INCENTIVE PLANS

In an incentive plan, an employee receives compensation as a direct result of a change in some performance indicator. For example, a business manager who receives a percentage of the gross receipts as part of his or her compensation is receiving an incentive. A physician manager who receives a bonus as a result of an increase in the HMO's net income also is receiving an incentive.

Incentive plans appeal to most of us. After all, who can argue with the logic that employees will perform at their best if they directly benefit from their own performance? In addition, because the incentive payment is based on an objective index, both the employer and the employee have unambiguous commitments. There are no uncertainties, such as those that characterize performance appraisals and merit compensation decisions.

Incentive plans can be highly motivating, but unfortunately they can also be very dangerous. Employees will direct their performance toward maximizing their incentive payments. Often, this is detrimental to other job performance areas. For example, the business manager who receives a percentage of the gross receipts may neglect those duties that do not immediately affect the bottom line. Responding inadequately to patient inquiries, neglecting accounts payable duties, working on "easy money" accounts while avoiding more difficult accounts, and neglecting cost control responsibilities could all be dysfunctional outcomes of such an incentive plan.

It is important, therefore, to anticipate dysfunctional reward contingencies. Some organizations attempt to counteract dysfunctional behavior by creating several incentives, so that employees cannot neglect a major aspect of the job. This quickly can become a cumbersome arrangement in which crafty employees may meet the letter of the incentive agreement but still manage to avoid doing all that the job requires. Generally, front line positions in medical practices, such as collection clerks, receptionists, and business managers, should not be on incentive plans. There simply are too many possibilities to "game" behavior, which may adversely affect patients and other employees in ways that are not obvious to management.

It is also important to remember that most performance indexes can vary for many reasons. It may be very difficult to say with certainty that one person has made any contribution to an increase or decrease in a performance index, such as gross receipts, insurance collections, net income, and so forth. Additional capital investment, effective employee selection, good marketing, an increase in the quality of services, and hiring of additional physicians and employees can all contribute to raising objective indexes. As a result, employees may benefit even when their performance has not affected the outcome. Under these circumstances, an incentive arrangement will be unfair to the organization because employees will receive pay increases as a result of factors neither due to their efforts nor under their control.

It is critical, therefore, to think through thoroughly the possible consequence of an incentive plan. If you still feel that an incentive is valuable, then try to build an incentive plan that will protect you from possible dysfunctional consequences. For example, you may limit incentive payments to only those employees whose individual performance as noted on their performance appraisal exceeds some threshold level, such as adequate performance on *all* factors. Another alternative is to require that the organization achieve some productivity increase, such as an increase in net income of at least 10 percent, before any incentives are payable. Employees would then share in any increase over the 10 percent level.

Incentives are particularly important in health care systems that are trying to achieve organization integration (Chapter 11). Organization integration refers to getting the parts of the health care system to act in a coordinated manner that furthers the total organization's objectives. Sometimes, parts of a health care system will excel at its own objectives to the detriment of the whole organization. Incentive plans can be used to penalize this suboptimal behavior.

For example, Figure 4–2 illustrates a few of the divisions in a health care system with a matrix organization structure. Matrix structures are discussed in Chapter 11. The goal of this structure is to concentrate the focus of executives on critical success factors. The executive in charge of Hospital A has the job of integrating all services within the hospital to maximize quality and productivity for that facility. The director of Information Systems has charge of information systems across the complete health care system. His or her responsibility is to develop and operate information technology in the most effective manner across all system locations. The goal is to get both the hospital and information technology directors to work cooperatively. The danger is that if each is measured and rewarded only on the success of their own component, that each may optimize at the expense of the whole health care system.

For example, the Information Systems division may select an electronic medical record (EMR) that is relatively inexpensive and easy to maintain. This keeps acquisition and maintenance costs down and makes the Information Systems division look good, but if the EMR lacks decision support capabilities that could reduce wasted physician time and improve the quality of care this could be a bad decision from the health care *system* perspective. Similarly, the Director of Hospital A may push for doing open heart procedures in his facility, because they produce high margins and make his financial outcomes look better. In the process, however, he may simply be taking patients away from other system facilities that already have this capability. One way to reduce this dysfunctional behavior is to give executives incentives that provide a motivation to look beyond their own unit. For example, each of the executives in Figure 4–2 leading a row or column subunit could have an incentive plan with three components.

The first component is based on individual performance against personal goals. For example, one goal set by the health system CEO for the director of Information Systems might be to successfully bring a new EMR on-line that

provides physicians with the cost of medications as they are prescribed. A second component of this executive's incentive plan is based on the performance of the Information System division. Did they meet their cost budget? How do users, such as physicians, rate the quality of information system services? Is the automated pharmaceutical dispensing process in the hospitals actually resulting in cost savings? The final component of this executive's bonus is based on health care system performance, such as net income and return on total assets.

Usually, these three components are linked, so that the incentives received for succeeding personally and divisionally are greatly reduced unless the whole health care system meets or exceeds its goals. For example, the Director of Information Systems' incentive plan may be apportioned with 30 percent of the bonus based on individual performance, 40 percent based on the performance of the Information Systems division, and 30 percent based on overall health care system success. If, however, the health care system's net income is not 110 percent of last year's net income, then there is no system based bonus; if it is less than 105 percent of last year's net income, the personal and divisional incentives are reduced by 50 percent; if it is less than 100 percent of last year's net income, the divisional bonus is eliminated; and if system net income is less than 98 percent of last year's net income, the personal component is eliminated. Plans of this nature create an incentive for division heads to be concerned about how their unit's actions affect other parts of the health care system, and total organization performance.

Physicians who have sold their practices to hospitals and health care systems often find themselves working for the first time in their lives without productivity incentives. Previously, the more these physicians worked, the more they earned, whereas now they are receiving straight salaries with annual fixed percentage increases. Many health care organizations are finding that these physicians, who previously were working 50 and 60 hours per week, have turned into "clock punchers." They put in their 40 hours each week and go home.

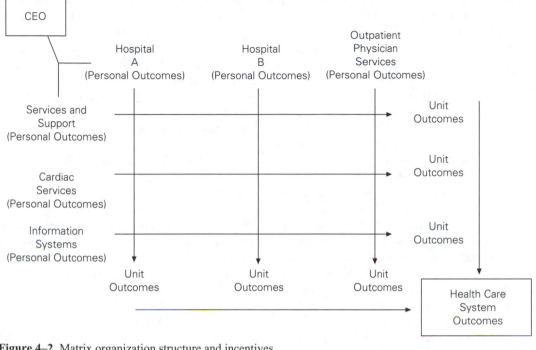

Figure 4–2 Matrix organization structure and incentives.

Profit and productivity estimates that were based on physician work habits and production levels before purchase have proven to be wildly optimistic. As a result, many health care organizations are rethinking how they compensate employed physicians. A consensus is developing that physician salaries need to be supplemented by bonuses or rewards based on performance. Once again, carefully specifying performance, so that perverse incentives are not created, is critical if the health care organization is going to achieve the type of performance it desires.

In summary, incentive payments can motivate behavior, but the behavior that is motivated may not be in the best interest of the organization. If you determine that you want to use incentives, do so with caution, and examine the arrangement from the employee's perspective to determine possible unintended consequences.

BENEFITS

Benefits are an important part of any compensation package. As with direct wages, the ben-efits you provide will affect the attractiveness of your organization to job applicants and will influence employee satisfaction and job performance. Some benefits, such as vacation time, are simple and generally available, whereas others, such as retirement plans, are complex and require the consultation of a specialist. Data on many benefits can be found in wage and salary surveys. These benefits include vacation time, sick leave, holidays, and insurance (health, life, disability, and dental).

When considering the selection of benefits, look closely at the operation of your organization. In a private practice, for example, is the day before Christmas normally a slow day? If it is, consider making this a holiday; you would thereby provide a benefit to employees at little cost to yourself. Do you really want to work the day after Thanksgiving? If you don't intend to work, close the office. Once again, it will be a relatively inexpensive benefit. Do you want to keep employees for a longer time, or do you prefer some turnover so as to keep salaries down? If the former, then you may want to offer better retirement and education benefits. If the latter, then offering these benefits would be counterproductive.

Health insurance and sick leave are benefits that can have an important effect on your employees' productivity. Employees who delay medical treatment don't take the time to get well. Those who are worried about their medical expenses will be less than fully productive. Good health insurance can also contribute to lower employee turnover because it will tend to tie employees to your organization.

Benefits are expensive. In 1995, they averaged $11,700 per employee, or 39 percent of payroll. When you are considering which benefits to provide, it is important to determine the needs of your employees. At a minimum, both large and small health care organizations should consider surveying their employees to find out what benefits they most desire. You are simply wasting money if you spend it on unwanted benefits. A survey can be as simple as a listing of potential benefits accompanied by a rating scale (e.g., extremely desirable, very desirable, somewhat desirable, slightly desirable, not desirable).

Some companies have adopted what is called a cafeteria plan. A cafeteria plan allows employees some flexibility in choosing a set of benefits to meet their needs. A cafeteria plan gives each employee a benefit budget based on his or her salary. Jobs with higher salaries have more benefit points to spend. Certain benefits are required, such as health insurance and a minimum number of vacation days. The employee may then use the remainder of the budget as he or she chooses. For example, basic health coverage may be through an HMO. Preferred provider organization (PPO) coverage, however, may be available at an expense in cafeteria points. Similarly, everyone may receive one week of vacation. Employees may purchase additional days from their cafeteria budget. Each employee can then choose among more choice in health care providers, vacations, life insurance, and so forth. A cafeteria plan has the added advantage of familiarizing employees with the full cost of providing benefits.

There are some disadvantages to cafeteria plans. Employees can make bad choices and find themselves exposed to predictable emergencies. Obviously, this is not your personal responsibility, but to the extent that an employee is distracted, his or her performance may suffer. Cafeteria plans do cost a bit more because of the extra management burden. Finally, employees will tend to select those benefits that they will use. For example, those with health problems may tend to select indemnity and PPO health options, and healthy employees remain with the HMO. This adverse self-selection may increase the overall cost of benefits to the organization.

Finally, the concept of a cafeteria compensation plan ties in nicely with the discussion of the expectancy theory of employee motivation. You may want to refer to that discussion in Chapter 5.

Retirement plans have a number of advantages for employers and employees. Not only do they provide a means of accumulating retirement funds, but they can also be used to defer taxation and allow accumulation of funds at tax-deferred rates. For most physicians, the retirement plan is one of the cornerstones of their personal financial plan. Because of tax and pension reform legislation, the provisions that govern contributions to physicians' retirement plans are inextricably tied to the benefits offered to other employees. This can make a retirement plan a very complex and expensive benefit.

Retirement plans can take on a number of different forms. A pension plan becomes a fixed obligation. Contractually, your organization is committed to making certain contributions to the plan. If you have agreed to a defined contribution plan, then you are obligated to make these contributions for all qualified employees, irrespective of the organization's profits, in good years and in bad. If you have a defined benefits plan, then you are obligated to make contributions that will support the benefits promised to employees upon retirement, once again in good years and in bad. The pension plan approach to retirement planning can be burdensome for a young private practice, where income may vary from year to year and substantial funds may have to be reserved for capital investment to support growth.

Profit-sharing plans provide some of the same retirement and tax advantages as pension plans. Contributions, however, are made out of profits. If there is no profit, there is no obligation to fund the plan. This is advantageous for young practices, for example, because it provides greater discretion in the use of corporate funds. Currently, however, the amount of funds that can be sheltered in a profit-sharing plan is less than in a pension plan. Physicians in a private practice setting should carefully analyze their practice's financial needs before making a commitment to a retirement plan. In addition, personal introspection regarding your need for predictability and flexibility is necessary before you can determine whether your retirement needs are best met by a pension or profit-sharing strategy.

Another option is a 401K plan. A 401K plan can be used to amend a profit-sharing plan to allow employees to contribute part of their salary to the plan. These contributions are deducted from the employee's taxable income and at the same time constitute a corporate expense. This can be advantageous because employees, including you, can make contributions even if there is little or no profit available to fund a profit-sharing plan. This flexibility is limited, however, by Internal Revenue Service (IRS) rules that govern the size of contributions and the ratio of contributions that can be made by high-salaried and low-salaried employees.

Retirement planning has developed into a profession. The taxation issues and the IRS rules that govern whether a plan qualifies for preferential tax treatment are very complex and change on an annual basis. It is *essential*, therefore, for smaller health care organizations to consult an advisor who specializes in retirement planning. In addition, you should remember that creating a retirement plan is like having a baby. It is going to be with you for the remainder of your corporate life. It will be constantly consuming time and resources. There are annual IRS statements and financial reports that must be assembled and filed in a timely manner. The plan will have to be updated from time to time to comply with current law. In addition, someone will have to administer the plan and make in-

vestment decisions. Employees will come and go, and some will leave their vested money in the plan, whereas others will withdraw it. In each case, documentation and management will take time and effort. Unless you are particularly interested and skilled in this area, you will have to pay someone to administer the plan and invest the funds.

Larger health care organizations should have a position, perhaps even a department, devoted to retirement planning and management. Physicians in closely held organizations, such as private practices, should obtain the advice of a professional who understands both their personal financial objectives and their organization's objectives.

CASE APPLICATION: DR. EARLY

Dr. Early was an internist with a growing group practice. After Dr. Garland joined the practice, the amount of clerical work in the front office began to increase dramatically. Dr. Early employed a business manager, Ralph, whose primary responsibilities were to handle the accounts receivable and accounts payable. Dr. Early also employed Louise as a full-time secretary. Her duties included typing, filing, transcribing, greeting patients, scheduling appointments, and answering the telephone. Finally, Brenda worked four hours each afternoon as a part-time receptionist. When she arrived, she replaced Louise at the front window and took over the role of greeting patients, scheduling appointments, and answering the telephone. Louise was then able to work uninterrupted on her other duties.

Within a few weeks of Dr. Garland's arrival, it became obvious that the clerical staff could not handle the additional work. Dr. Early decided that the best way to manage the increased front office workload was to change the part-time receptionist position into a full-time position and restructure the secretarial position. The secretary would no longer perform receptionist duties, such as greeting patients, answering telephones, and scheduling appointments. The secretary would instead concentrate on typing, correspondence, filing, recordkeeping, and other clerical duties.

Dr. Early offered the full-time receptionist position to Brenda at the same pay ($5.75 an hour) that she had been receiving for the past four months. She refused to take the job, stating that she was only interested in part-time work. Dr. Early now had to find someone to fill the position. He was worried about two issues. First, he was somewhat concerned that Brenda might have turned down the job because the pay was too low. He had assumed that, if Brenda was already working for $5.75 an hour, this would be fair pay for the same work done full time. Second, he was concerned about Louise's reaction if he reduced the pay differential between her job and the receptionist position. Because of both these issues, he undertook a compensation study.

First, he consulted a BLS *Area Wage and Salary Survey*. None of the job descriptions in the survey exactly matched either the secretary or the receptionist position. He felt, however, that two positions in the survey were close enough to allow him to work with the figures: The Secretary III position in the survey could be used as a basis for his secretary position, and the Secretary I position could be used for his receptionist position. The $5.75 an hour that he was currently paying his receptionist was well under the median of $8.01 an hour and even well under the low end of the midrange for Secretary I. Louise's salary of $17,100 was very close to the Secretary III median of $17,430 ($8.38 × 2,080 annual hours). In addition, Louise had been in the position for a little over two years. Her initial salary was $14,800. She received a $1,000 increase at the end of her first year and a $1,300 increase at the end of her second year. Dr. Early also thought that Louise's position had fewer responsibilities than the survey's Secretary III position.

Dr. Early could find no job in the BLS survey that was similar in content to his business manager position. He decided to ask three of his colleagues what they were paying their business managers. He wasn't certain how confidential his peers would regard this information, so he decided to ask them in terms of the following pay ranges: less than $18,000, $18,000 to $20,000, $20,001 to $22,000, $22,001 to $24,000, and more than $24,000. He also decided to ask for the number of years the incumbent had been in the position. Two colleagues stated that their business managers were in the $20,001 to $22,000 range. Both managers had more than two years of experience. The other colleague indicated that her business manager was in the $18,000 to $20,000 range and had three years of experience. Ralph had been Dr. Early's business manager for almost three years, and his current salary was $21,750.

Dr. Early formed some initial hypotheses. He felt that he was probably going to have to increase the salary for the receptionist. Although he had not previously considered the concept of a pay range for a position, it appeared that both the secretary and the business manager salaries were within reason. He concluded that if he did formally construct pay ranges for these two positions, the current salary of each incumbent certainly would be within the pay range.

He now attempted to validate his conclusions. Using a point system developed by a consultant, he evaluated the secretary, business manager, and newly defined receptionist positions. His results are reported in Table 4–7. The projected salary for the receptionist was $14,752.13. Eyeballing this result, he felt that this was a little high. A call to one of his colleagues, plus his increasing familiarity with the medical practice market, indicated that a fair rate would be closer to $14,000. In addition, he recalled that his secretary position seemed to carry fewer responsibilities than the BLS Secretary III position, so that in general his compensation rates appeared to be on the low side. Taking $14,000 as a midpoint, he decided to construct a devil's advocate pay range of ±10 percent. This resulted in a pay range for the receptionist position of $12,600 to $15,400. In addition, because he was only remixing duties that Louise already performed, he saw no need to change her pay as a result of the reorganization.

Dr. Early decided that the receptionist job required no special medical background, so he placed his advertisement in the general classified section of the local newspaper. Careful questioning of several of the best applicants revealed that the realistic market minimum was about $13,500. He hired the best of the applicants for a starting salary of $13,600. He did so with confidence that neither Louise nor Ralph would feel that the new receptionist's pay was unfairly high. This was very important to Dr. Early because both Louise and Ralph were good employees. They would be instrumental in the new receptionist's training, and turnover in either of their positions at that time would have been a serious problem.

Dr. Early drew several conclusions from this episode. He knew that he could have called a few colleagues, looked at some relevant want ads, and talked to his own employees to get an indication of what the receptionist salary level should be. In fact, he had done all these things. He concluded, however, that using survey and job evaluation data made him much more confident about his decision. The fact that several pieces of independent information all pointed in the same direction was very reassuring. He also liked being reasonably sure that by solving one problem he was not creating a whole new set of problems elsewhere. Finally, he felt a sense of satisfaction from knowing that he had done everything using the best tools and information available to him. This feeling was somewhat similar to how he felt when he combined several pieces of test and examination information to arrive at a clinical diagnosis.

Table 4–7 Point and Pay Evaluations of Dr. Early's Employees

Benchmark Jobs	Salary	Points
Business manager	$21,750	1,550
Secretary	$17,100	1,005
Receptionist	$14,752 (projected)	730

CASE APPLICATION: RAMONA'S EQUITY

Dr. Hendricks was an owner and the managing physician of a group family practice. He received a resume from Ramona for his vacant business manager position. Ramona had previously worked for Dr. Johnson's group radiology practice at a salary of $45,000. When Dr. Johnson retired, the remaining partners eliminated Ramona's position and her entire staff, with the justification that it would be more economical to "outsource" the function to a billing service. Ramona's experience appeared to be excellent, and at the interview she gave the impression of being a calm, mature 50-year-old woman who knew that she could do the job.

Dr. Hendricks had some reservations about hiring Ramona. The salary for his business manager position was $23,000, which he knew was a fair salary, perhaps even somewhat above the median salary for this type of position. Dr. Hendricks sensed that Ramona's real job at Dr. Johnson's practice had been to supervise an overstaffed office and that she hadn't been in the trenches actually billing insurance companies, posting payments, collecting fees from patients, and so on for many years. He knew that in his practice the business manager was in the front line and personally had to bill companies, follow up on problem claims, and negotiate payment plans with delinquent patients, among other things. Dr. Hendricks was concerned that the combination of more demanding work and substantially lower pay would result in perceptions of inequity, irrespective of the fact that he had given Ramona a realistic job preview and that she was voluntarily taking a job at a much lower salary than that of her previous job.

Ramona, however, insisted that she knew that she would have to take a pay cut wherever she went and that it was important to her to work for people with whom she felt comfortable. As a result of two interviews with Dr. Hendricks and his staff, she said that she would enjoy working at his practice. Ramona was the most qualified applicant in Dr. Hendricks' selection pool, and he needed to fill the position as soon as possible, so he hired her in spite of his reservations.

Ramona's tenure turned out to be unsettling to all involved. She quickly grew frustrated with the demands of the job. Her frustration manifested itself in temper tantrums and insubordinate comments and actions toward Dr. Hendricks and the other associates. She resigned after four months of employment. Dr. Hendricks had these comments:

> It started to go wrong right from the start. She was used to a country club atmosphere in which she was also overpaid. She quickly grew to resent realistic job demands at a realistic salary. She treated me like it was *my* fault that she was in this situation, that she was no longer employed by a Sugar Daddy practice! Toward the end, she even tried to manipulate me into firing her, so that she wouldn't have to take the responsibility for her circumstances!
>
> She never did get her equity equation readjusted to reality. Her "comparison other" was this image of herself at the previous practice, which had no grounding in the real world. How could I fight that? The answer is that I couldn't, and I should have realized this, despite her assurances to the contrary.
>
> Dr. Johnson's largess made Ramona largely unemployable. It would be a rare individual who has the self-awareness to be able to take a career step backward of this magnitude. Ramona couldn't do it, and I suppose that I shouldn't hold that too much against her. At the same time, however, I've learned that you can't fight unre-

alistic equity perceptions. In her mind her previous employment situation was equitable, and only she can change that perception. If she doesn't find another Sugar Daddy practice, she will eventually have to adjust her expectations. I have sympathy for any practice that she encounters between now and then. I'll never hire a person under these circumstances again. I've learned my lesson.

CONCLUSION

Making good compensation decisions is more of an art than a science. The most significant message of this chapter is the importance of achieving equity. The tools described are essentially aids for achieving equity. Some smaller practices may find that understanding the objectives of individual, internal, and external equity at the conceptual level will allow them to make good compensation decisions. Larger practices and other health care organizations will find it necessary to use compensation tools, such as wage and salary surveys, point job evaluation plans, and pay ranges, to achieve these objectives. You should be wary of incentive plans and always consult a knowledgeable professional regarding complex benefits, such as a retirement plan. Finally, consultants can be particularly useful in designing compensation plans because of the importance of experience in making good compensation decisions. In addition, they allow practice-based physician managers to assume their appropriate role of managing the outcomes of a technical process.

REFERENCES AND NOTES

1. Regression analysis requires a large enough sample size so that the resulting statistical conclusions are meaningful. The analysis presented in Table 4A–2 is presented for illustration purposes.
2. For example, if the Physicians Services employs two secretaries with current salaries of $15,000 and $17,000, and a computer analyst who is currently being paid $23,000, then the total salary basis is $55,000. The bonus pool with be $4,125, of which $1,375 will be based on seniority and $2,750 will be based on merit.
3. Mondy, R.W., Noe, R.M. *Human Resource Management.* Prentice Hall, Upper Saddle River, NJ, 1996, p. 396.

Point System of Job Evaluation

(This point plan is provided for illustrative purposes only. The factors that it contains, their weighting, and the degree definitions may not be relevant to your organization. If you wish to use a point system, contact a qualified compensation professional. If you decide to develop your own point system, you may find the point plan in this appendix to be a helpful starting point.)

KNOWLEDGE

Knowledge is the combination of education and experience that is required by the job. Education refers to knowledge that is normally acquired through formal schooling; experience is knowledge that is normally acquired through on-the-job training or work experience (Table 4A–1).

NONSUPERVISORY RESPONSIBILITY

This factor considers the degree of analytical ability, judgment, discretion, and timeliness involved in making decisions. It is concerned with how education and experience are applied to the job, but it does not cover responsibility for personnel administration, which is covered elsewhere (Table 4A–2).

Consider the following issues when evaluating the vertical scale of the chart:

- What decisions are made?
- What are the most difficult decisions and actions?
- Is independent judgment required, or are decisions based on precedent?
- How frequently are decisions made?
- Consider all the responsibilities for the position, even if some of them are delegated to

Table 4A–1 Factor: Knowledge

Education	Experience (Years)						
	<1	1–2	2–3	3–4	4–5	5–6	>6
High school degree	110	120	135	150	170	195	230
High school plus some specialized courses	135	145	160	175	195	220	255
High school plus many additional courses up to 1 year of college	160	170	185	200	220	245	300
Extensive courses beyond high school, 1 or 2 years of college, business school or technical training	210	220	235	250	270	295	350
Courses equivalent to 2 or 3 years of college	265	275	290	305	325	350	405
Bachelor's degree	325	335	350	365	385	410	465
Master's or equivalent graduate degree	385	395	410	425	445	470	525
Master's or equivalent degree plus other graduate degree or certification	445	455	470	485	505	530	585
Doctorate	510	520	535	550	570	595	650

Table 4A–2 Factor: Nonsupervisory Responsibility

This factor measures the degree to which making decisions and taking action are important on the job. It is composed of the degree of complexity of analytical ability, judgment, and the like when the employee is making decisions or taking actions; the degree of review provided; and the inconvenience and cost associated with inadequate performance.
- *Column A:* Decisions/actions reviewed regularly. Limited effect on operations.
- *Column B:* Decisions/actions reviewed regularly. Inadequacies would only result in minor problems.
- *Column C:* Decisions/actions usually reviewed. Inadequacies could cause moderate inconvenience or expense.
- *Column D:* Decisions/actions occasionally reviewed. Inadequacies could cause considerable problems or expense and could affect patient health.
- *Column E:* Decisions/actions occasionally reviewed. Inadequacies could cause extensive inconvenience or expense and could affect patient health.
- *Column F:* Decisions/actions rarely reviewed. Inadequacies could cause extensive inconvenience or expense and could affect patient health.
- *Column G:* Decisions/actions rarely reviewed. Inadequacies may affect long-range plans and strategies, and could affect patient health.
- *Column H:* Decisions/actions usually final. Inadequacies may affect long-range plans and strategies and could affect patient health.
- *Column I:* Decisions/actions usually final and may seriously affect long-range plans or patient health.
- *Column J:* Decisions/actions final and would seriously affect long-range plans or patient health.

	Degree of Review and Impact									
Degree of Independence	*A*	*B*	*C*	*D*	*E*	*F*	*G*	*H*	*I*	*J*
Operating procedures are well defined, and independent activity is limited.	120	140	165	195	245	315	415	560	765	1,060
Operating procedures are generally covered by clear rules, regulations, instructions, etc. Decisions/actions required are not complex.	140	160	185	215	265	335	435	580	785	1,080
Makes operating decisions and takes some actions of importance. Occasionally decisions are of considerable complexity.	165	185	210	240	290	360	460	605	810	1,105
Makes operating decisions and takes actions of moderate difficulty. Occasionally actions/ decisions are of considerable complexity.	195	215	240	270	320	390	490	635	840	1,135
Makes frequent operating decisions and takes actions of considerable										

continues

Table 4A–2 continued

Degree of Independence	A	B	C	D	E	F	G	H	I	J
					Degree of Review and Impact					
difficulty. Assists in the formulation of recommendations on difficult and important issues.	245	265	290	320	370	440	540	685	890	1,185
Assists in the formulation of, and on occasion independently formulates, recommendations on difficult and important matters.	315	335	360	390	440	510	610	755	960	1,255
In addition to the above, sometimes makes independent decisions and takes independent action on important matters.	415	435	460	490	540	610	710	855	1,060	1,355
Frequently makes independent decisions and takes independent action on important operating matters.	560	580	605	635	685	755	855	1,000	1,205	1,500
Continually makes independent decisions and takes independent action on very important operating matters.	765	785	810	840	890	960	1,060	1,205	1,410	1,705
Continually makes independent decisions and takes independent action on operating matters of the greatest importance.	1,060	1,080	1,105	1,135	1,185	1,255	1,355	1,500	1,705	2,000

Note: Cell entries are point values.

a subordinate. For example, an office manager may be responsible for collection even if some specific collection tasks are delegated to a billing clerk.

- Remember, making decisions is more important than making recommendations.

Consider the following issues when evaluating the horizontal scale of the chart:

- To what extent are decisions reviewed by superiors?
- What is the potential cost or seriousness of errors, and how often does the position re-

quire making decisions for which there is a chance of serious cost or consequences?

- What is the time span that could occur before an error is detected?
- Evaluate the job under normal day-to-day conditions. Don't place disproportionate weight on unusual or unlikely circumstances.

For both the horizontal and the vertical scales, if a subordinate position merits more points than the position being evaluated, assign the number of points associated with the subordinate position.

INGENUITY

This factor is concerned with the creativeness and resourcefulness required by the position. This can occur as a result of creative thinking or developing new ideas, plans, methods, and the like. Evaluate the job based on how much ingenuity is normally required, as opposed to overweighting unusual circumstances. The key issue is whether the job requires ingenuity, not whether a particular incumbent happens to be personally creative (Table 4A–3).

PERSONNEL MANAGEMENT RESPONSIBILITY

This factor assesses the job requirements for organizing, leading, coordinating, training, and controlling employees. This factor assesses both line and functional responsibilities. Line responsibilities are defined as organizing, selecting, training, promoting, dismissing, setting performance objectives, evaluating, and directing the actions of others. An example of a line relationship would be a business manager who directly controls the actions of a subordinate secretary.

Functional responsibilities are concerned with implementing programs and policies through employees, but the position does not have direct line authority over the other positions. An example of a functional relationship would be a business manager who must use secretaries to do collections, but the secretaries report on a line basis to the office manager (Table 4A–4).

Table 4A–3 Factor: Ingenuity*

Degrees	Point Values		
	A	B	C
Requires little original or independent thinking.	100	115	130
Requires occasional ingenuity in the refinement of ideas originated by others.	150	170	195
Ingenuity is definitely required but usually involves the refinement of established ideas, procedures, methods, etc.	225	260	300
Some original and independent thinking in originating and developing new or improved ideas.	350	400	475
Frequent application of a high degree of original and independent thinking in developing complex ideas in new, undefined areas.	550	625	700
Continuous application of a high degree of creativeness, resourcefulness, and inventiveness. Originates very complex creative ideas in new and undefined areas. Creativity has major effect on the practice.	800	900	1,000

*The B point values should be used when the definition closely matches the job. The A or C columns can be used for jobs that are somewhat above or below the definition but not to a significant enough extent to warrant selection of a higher- or lower-degree definition.

Table 4A–4 Factor: Personnel Management Responsibility

Degrees	Number of Line Subordinates Supervised				
	0	*1–5*	*6–10*	*11–15*	*16 or More*
Little or no line or functional responsibility.	120	130	140	155	170
Line responsibilities are primarily simple and routine, *OR* functional responsibility is limited to advice or guidance with no responsibility for control or follow-up.	130	140	150	165	180
Line responsibilities are generally routine and involve the same or similar activities *OR* some functional advice and guidance usually without responsibility for control or follow-up.	145	155	165	180	195
Line responsibilities are somewhat complex and occasionally difficult, involving the same or similar activities, *OR* frequent functional advice and guidance usually without responsibility for control or follow-up.	160	170	180	195	210
Line responsibilities are moderately complex and occasionally difficult, involving varied activities or work groups, *OR* frequent functional advice and guidance with some control responsibilities, or limited complexity, for upholding standards.	180	190	200	215	230
Line responsibilities are generally complex and difficult, involving varied, moderately complex activities or work groups, *OR* moderately complex functional control responsibilities for upholding standards.	205	215	225	240	255
Line responsibilities are complex and difficult and somewhat diversified, involving complex activities or work groups, *OR* complex functional control responsibilities for upholding standards.	235	245	255	270	285
Line responsibilities are highly complex and diversified, involving highly complex activities or work groups, *OR* highly complex functional control responsibilities for upholding standards.	275	285	295	310	325
Line responsibilities are of extreme complexity, involving activities and work groups of extreme complexity, *OR* functional control responsibilities of extreme complexity.	420	430	440	455	470
Line responsibilities are of maximum complexity, *OR* functional control responsibilities of maximum complexity.	790	800	810	830	860

The following issues should be considered when you are evaluating jobs on this factor:

- Only consider responsibility for managing people.

- It is important to determine whether the position has line responsibility, functional responsibility, or both.
- When evaluating line responsibility, consider the diversity of supervisory activities

involved, the type of people being supervised, and any extenuating or complicating issues.

- When evaluating functional responsibility, consider the diversity of activities, the types of employees with whom the incumbent must work, and any extenuating or complicating issues.
- It is often more difficult to get things done through people in a functional relationship than in a line relationship.
- If a subordinate position merits more points than the position being evaluated, assign the number of points associated with the subordinate position.

OUTSIDE RELATIONSHIPS

Outside relationships assess the extent to which the position must interact with others outside the health care organization. This could include insurance companies, patients, physicians, and the like. It is important to determine whether these outside contacts involve simply exchanging information or whether something more significant occurs, such as influencing the decisions of others. Consider the level of people being contacted, the frequency of contact, and whether the nature of the communication is to elicit or provide information (Table 4A–5).

Table 4A–5 Factor: Outside Relations*

Degrees	Point Values		
	A	B	C
Outside contacts are limited to the exchange of information with employees in other organizations who do not make decisions. Little tact or few negotiating skills required. Contacts are fairly infrequent.	50	65	80
Outside contacts are required that involve some tact and diplomacy, and on occasion they may influence decisions, OR contacts may occur frequently, but they only involve the exchange of information.	100	120	150
Outside contacts are a requirement of the position. They necessitate tact and diplomacy and frequently influence decisions that are of moderate importance. They could involve discussions with relatively high levels of management.	190	240	300
Outside contacts are a major job responsibility. They involve important decisions, require negotiation and tactical skills, and occur at high organizational levels.	360	430	500

*The B point values should be used when the definition closely matches the job. The A or C columns can be used for jobs that are somewhat above or below the definition but not to a significant enough extent to warrant selection of a higher- or lower-degree definition.

CHAPTER 5

Management Skills

Chapter Objectives

This chapter will help you understand how to manage employees and work groups. It will do this by discussing those management skills that will help you motivate and lead employees, partners, and peers. As a result, you will be able to:

1. understand how to identify the rewards that others desire
2. motivate others so they will work toward organizational goals
3. evaluate situational and work context issues, so that you can choose the most appropriate management methods
4. improve the performance of work groups and overcome problems that often occur in groups

---

The glue that holds an organization together is the people management skills of its managers. The effectiveness of a physician manager's financial, marketing, and strategic skills is greatly diminished if he or she cannot successfully bring them to fruition through the actions of subordinates, peers, and superiors. As a physician manager, much of your work will be performed through the actions of others.

Let's take an example. You have been given the job of evaluating the feasibility of starting an obstetrics triage center for your hospital. You are aware of the importance of constructing a financial model to evaluate the cost of the center, the degree to which it will improve acute obstetrical care, and how it will affect resident staff, who formerly provided treatment in the emergency department. After you identify the data that you want to examine, others will probably collect and assemble them into spreadsheets and reports. Next, you will probably discuss the fi-

nancial and medical implications with those who will be affected by this change, including emergency department staff, obstetrics staff, residents, administration, and so forth.

The success of this project will be due in no small measure to your ability to understand the incentives of the individuals involved, to create a vision of how the change will be beneficial, and then to galvanize others to help make the change a success. Leading and managing the process with subordinates, peers, and superiors and anticipating potential sources of resistance and overcoming this resistance will be as much a determinant of the project's success as properly evaluating the financial considerations.

Two skills that are essential to managing employees successfully are motivation and leadership. Motivating and leading employees are related but separate skills. Both are concerned with getting employees to work toward organizational goals. Motivation is the process of persuading employees, peers, partners, and others to work toward the organization's goals by giving them the rewards that they desire. When personal rewards are truly valued and contingent upon reaching organizational goals, then employees are motivated to attain them.

Leadership, on the other hand, is concerned with obtaining the voluntary cooperation of others. Leadership involves appealing to more than employees' self-interest. It is concerned with influencing behavior through inspiration, personal example, words, and actions.

Motivational and leadership skills can complement each other. For example, employees who are only moderately motivated by the nature of the financial rewards provided may still work very hard for an effective leader. Similarly, a well-designed reward system may compensate for a substantial lack of inspirational leadership.

MOTIVATION

Why does an employee work? You may have thought that this question was addressed in Chapter 4, on compensation. It was, but only partly. An organization's compensation plan, important as it is, only determines what an employee should be paid. It does not address such questions as these:

- What is the relationship between the rewards that an employee receives from the organization and the employee's personal goals?
- Does the employee think that he or she will be able to perform successfully?
- How does the employee perceive the relationship between performance and rewards?
- What things, in addition to money, does each employee desire?

You might respond to this list of questions by saying "Well, I really don't care!" You *should* care, because knowing the answers to these questions can help you obtain better employee job performance.

Obtaining the knowledge necessary to answer these questions requires taking the time to learn something about each employee. Time, of course, is one of your most valuable commodities. For physician managers who also practice clinical medicine, time is what you sell to generate revenues. You won't want to make the same time investment with all employees. Employees in less critical positions may merit little or no time investment. Employees in very critical positions may merit a substantial investment.

The questions listed above were not randomly selected. Rather, they relate to the elements of expectancy theory, a well-developed theory of motivation designed by Vroom at Yale University.[1] Expectancy theory has become one of the dominant theories for understanding and directing work behavior. Vroom observed that the rewards that we obtain from a job are intermediary benefits that will be used to satisfy other, more fundamental and personal needs. For example, a nurse works for a salary, which is then used to buy a car, go on vacation, continue education, contribute to a personal sense of worth, and so on. The nurse's motivation, or force to perform, is a function of the following components:

- *First-level outcome* (j) is an outcome that is directly related to the job. In this case, this could be developing new cost control procedures for disposable items (e.g., gowns, syringes, etc.), providing a high level of patient care, and so forth.
- *Second-level outcome* (k) is an outcome that is of larger significance in your life. It may be a direct function of your job performance, but it may also relate to your life in a larger sense, and it can express your most basic goals in life. In this case, a car, vacation, and continuing education are stated second-level outcomes
- *Valence* (V_j or V_k) is the expected value or satisfaction that should come from achieving a certain outcome. V_j indicates the anticipated satisfaction associated with a first-level outcome. V_k indicates the anticipated satisfaction associated with a second-level outcome. In both cases, the anticipated

value (valence) may be different from the eventual satisfaction that actually occurs.

- *Expectancy* (E_{ij}) is the likelihood that an action on the employee's part will result in receiving or achieving a given first-level outcome. It can be expressed as a probability, and therefore it is measured on a scale of 0.00 to 1.00.

- *Instrumentality* (I_{jk}) is the relationship between first- and second-level outcomes. It can be conceptualized as a correlation, and therefore it is measured on a scale ranging from –1.00 through 0.00 to +1.00. For example, if a first-level outcome is always associated with a second-level outcome, then $I_{jk} = 1.00$. If a first-level outcome is never associated with obtaining the second-level outcome, then $I_{jk} = -1.00$. If a first-level outcome is perceived as being unrelated to a second-level outcome, then $I_{jk} = 0.00$.

- *Force* (F_i) is the desire, predisposition, or motivation to act.

- *Action* (i) is something that you do on the job. In the case of the nurse, it might be those things that he or she would have to do to develop new cost control procedures. This could imply some rather remote activities, such as taking a statistics course to better implement total quality management. Normally, it would be the daily things that in sum constitute everyday job performance and accumulate into a level of overall success.

The following equations describe how these components relate to each other:

$$V_j = f \sum (V_k * I_{jk}) \text{ (5–1)}$$

$$F_i = f \sum (V_j * E_{ij}) \text{ (5–2)}$$

It is possible, therefore, to restate the nurse's motivation in the following manner: Effort or work level (F_i) is a function of both anticipated satisfaction from a pay raise and any other job-related rewards that may be provided (V_j) and subjective probabilities (E_{ij}) that, if the nurse acts in certain ways or tries to achieve the goals that have been given to him or her, he or she will in fact succeed. Effort or work level is equal to the sum of all the V_j and E_{ij} combinations for all the work outcomes that the nurse perceives.

What determines the nurse's valence (V_j) for a pay raise? That is a function of the instrumentality of the pay raise for satisfying other needs in his or her life and the valence (anticipated satisfaction) that he or she will derive from satisfying these other life needs, such as a car, a vacation, a master's degree, a personal sense of control over his or her life, and so on.

It is possible, therefore, to restate the nurse's valence (V_j) for a pay raise or any other first-level outcome offered by your organization as a function of both valences for second-level personal life goals sought (V_k) interacting with how instrumental (I_{jk}) the nurse perceives the first-level rewards that you provide for achieving second-level personal life goals. Restated more simply, if your rewards help employees achieve what they really want to achieve in their personal lives, then these rewards will motivate them. If your rewards don't tie in with employees' personal reward structures, then they will be as motivating as meat would be to a horse or oats would be to a dog.

Examination of equations 5–1 and 5–2 demonstrates that the ultimate value of any reward is related to second-level goals. If you offer rewards that contribute little toward achieving these second-level goals, they will have a correspondingly small motivational value. Your first objective, therefore, is to understand what an employee ultimately desires. The expectancies and instrumentalities define the paths that your organization provides to an employee to reach his or her personal goals. Once you understand the employee's personal goals and his or her perception of these paths, you can then influence the employee's motivation to perform.

Expectancy theory suggests several points at which you can influence an employee's motivation. First, however, you must have some understanding of the employee's second-level goals. Second-level goals are "big picture," personal, life objectives. Managers generally can't influence what an employee's second-level goals are. These are, after all, a very personal matter. Second-level goals often range from psychologically based issues, such as security, recognition, a sense of personal self-worth, and achievement, to materialistic concerns, such as a nice home, a car, financial security, and the like.

Because second-level goals are personal and out of your control, you must direct your efforts toward enhancing the perceived relationship between the rewards you do provide and the achievement of these goals. The equations given above provide the means to enhance an employee's motivation. This can be accomplished in three ways:

1. Provide first-level outcomes that more naturally relate to an employee's second-level outcomes.
2. Influence the employee's expectancy perceptions.
3. Influence the employee's instrumentality perceptions.

Before investigating how these three strategies can be used to affect motivation levels, let's first consider a few general observations that are useful for understanding the motivational implications of expectancy theory.

First, if either expectancy or instrumentality is low, then the employee's motivation for employees will be low. Even if you provide excellent rewards, there will be little or no motivation to act in ways that you want if they believe that they can't achieve the first-level outcome. For example, suppose that an employee understands that he or she will receive very desirable rewards for leading the project to develop a critical path for DRG uncomplicated vaginal delivery. He or she also believes that it is not possible to achieve this goal given the time available and the people whose cooperation is needed in order to complete the project. Referring back to Equation 5–2, the fact that expectancy is essentially zero means that F_i will essentially be zero.

Second, an employee is motivated by the *anticipated* satisfaction (valence) of a reward, not by the *ultimate* satisfaction received. All of us work for rewards based on what we imagine they will be like. Our actual satisfaction may be far different from what we anticipate. Your motivation, for example, to work hard so that you

can afford a new sports car is influenced by the satisfaction that you *think* you will experience. The reality may be different, with the actual satisfaction being either more or less than what you anticipate. The reality of receiving a reward only affects the perceptions of future valence judgments.

Providing first-level outcomes that are directly related to an employee's ultimate goal is an effective strategy for increasing employee motivation. For example, a retirement plan will have a high valence to an employee who has long-term financial security as an ultimate goal. On the other hand, a retirement plan that reduces immediate discretionary income would have a negative instrumentality for an employee whose life goals were strongly oriented toward satisfying present material needs.

Providing schedule flexibility or educational benefits could have a high valence for employees who view additional education as a means to reach a personal goal of increased competence or personal achievement (second-level outcomes) and a valence approaching zero for others. A four-day work week is a benefit that many employees can use to meet their own idiosyncratic second-level goals. In the case of any benefit, you must determine whether the expense or inconvenience of providing the benefit is too burdensome.

The variability of employees' second-level goals is responsible for a corresponding variability in the valences of first-level outcomes. Because salary can be used to satisfy so many different needs, it is a very powerful, safe motivational tool. Salary, however, is not the only requisite for achieving life goals. Many writers and behavioral scientists have discussed the nonmonetary reasons why people work. For example, Maslow discussed self-actualization, or the desire to grow and express creativity; McClelland described the need for achievement; and Herzberg and colleagues concluded that employees are motivated by a number of factors, including recognition and responsibility.[2–4] These nonmonetary motivators are very real, and they can be particularly attractive to employers because their nonmonetary nature means that they often don't cost anything that directly appears on an income statement. Stated very simply, it doesn't cost you a dime when you reward an employee by fulfilling his or her need for self-respect, accomplishment, recognition, or achieving the best of which he or she is capable.

Self-actualization, achievement, recognition, and responsibility certainly qualify as life goals and can therefore be second-level outcomes, as defined in expectancy theory. The nice thing about them is that you can directly help employees achieve these goals by providing appropriate first-level outcomes. Stated another way, the instrumentality of many nonmonetary rewards will be exceedingly high because they are so closely related to corresponding second-level outcomes. If an employee has the goal of feeling respected, then showing him or her respect on the job will "pass through" directly to satisfy second-level needs and will have very high motivating value.

Not all employees are motivated by nonmonetary rewards. It is important, therefore, to obtain a sense of each employee's need for these types of rewards. In addition, it is important to appreciate that even those employees who are motivated by nonmonetary rewards probably will also be strongly motivated by financial rewards. You cannot compensate for inadequate financial rewards by providing a sense of achievement and recognition. Appropriate use of nonmonetary rewards, when coupled with adequate financial rewards, can result in a highly motivating work environment.

EXPECTANCY

Expectancy is the employee's subjective estimate of the probability that his or her actions will lead to certain outcomes. One of the more effective motivational methods that a manager can use is to change an employee's expectancy perceptions. Perhaps the most important systematic way of influencing expectancies is by conducting thorough performance appraisals and providing training and other opportunities to improve. This provides a very real improvement in

ability, and therefore the employee's expectancy of succeeding realistically increases.

Sometimes, people have low expectancies for realistic reasons. Perhaps they need additional clerical or computer support. Perhaps others on whom they are dependent for information have been less than cooperative. As a manager, you can improve the real probability of success by intervening and changing the reality of the situation. Providing additional clerical and computer support and negotiating with roadblocks to pave the way for cooperation are real contributions that managers can make so that subordinates' expectancies will change.

Providing immediate feedback is another way of raising expectancies. If employees are routinely told when their performance is adequate or inadequate, this tells them that their performance is noticed and that it matters. When this is coupled with a merit compensation plan, all the parts are in place for very strong expectancy linkages between desired behaviors and rewards. Correspondingly, you will also establish weak expectancy linkages between undesirable behaviors and rewards. That is, employees will perceive that inadequate performance will have a low probability of being rewarded.

The valences of nonmonetary rewards are particularly susceptible to manipulation through expectancies. For example, you know that Ellen is especially desirous of personal recognition. You say to her, "I will consider it an outstanding personal achievement if you manage to solve our computer billing problem. In addition, the ideas that you have proposed to fix it seem as if they should work. All that it will now take is your hard work and concentration to fix this problem." You have in effect told Ellen that there is a high probability that her actions will lead to the desired work-related outcome. Your pep talk has encouraged her to give it a try. Upon successful completion of the task, you should then personally congratulate Ellen, document the incident in her critical incident file, and verbally recognize her achievement at the next staff meeting. Discussions in which you encourage employees or strengthen their confidence that they can achieve an objective increase their motivation through altering their expectancies. The Knute Rockne half-time pep talk is one example of this approach.

INSTRUMENTALITY

Instrumentality is the correlation that an employee sees between the rewards that you provide (first-level outcomes) and the life goals that the employee desires (second-level outcomes). If you understand what the employee ultimately seeks, you can point to how your rewards will facilitate the achievement of these goals. If the employee is logical and intelligent, he or she will have already discerned this relationship, and your ability as a manager, therefore, to influence motivation by exploring instrumentality may be inversely related to an employee's introspectiveness. Nevertheless, it does not hurt to point out the instrumentality relationships to an employee.

Another approach to using instrumentality to motivate employees is to make assignments based on the likelihood that they will have high instrumentalities for an employee. For example, suppose that a physician employee has very strong second-level achievement and recognition needs. By expanding the opportunities for the physician to obtain these on the job, you will increase the instrumentality of work outcomes, increase overall motivation, and coincidentally increase the chance that the job will be well done. You could do this by providing the physician with opportunities to work on high-visibility, "spotlight" projects. For example, this physician might perceive an assignment to a committee developing the specifications for and selecting a hospitalwide automated clinical record as an exceptional opportunity. Another physician might perceive the same assignment as a diversion (unlinked, noninstrumental) to achieving his or her primary goals, which relate to the satisfaction that he or she derives from practicing clinical medicine. In this instance, understanding the second-level goals of each physician and then looking for the natural linkages to existing projects (instrumentalities) will allow you to select the physician who will be naturally more motivated to work hard on the project.

FORCE

The eventual outcome of the equations stated above is force, or the desire to act in a particular way. Force is not necessarily equivalent to job performance. At least two issues intervene. The first is ability. Irrespective of how motivated employees may be to succeed, if they don't have the appropriate skills and abilities, their performance will be limited. Most of us could not hit a major league fastball, no matter how motivated we might be to do so. Another intervening variable is luck or chance. Sometimes, even the most skilled and motivated are thwarted by random, unpredictable events.

MOTIVATIONAL STRATEGIES

You motivate employees by understanding their ultimate goals in life and the contingent relationships between job performance, the rewards you can supply, and the employees' attainment of their goals. Obtaining the level of knowledge necessary to affect the motivation of employees may take some time. Talking with employees about their life objectives and how their work might lead to the realization of those goals is an important motivational strategy.

This strategy should be supplemented with a healthy dose of unobtrusive observation. Sometimes, idly made comments can also reveal an important second-level goal, instrumentality, or expectancy perception. A secretary who whimsically states that he or she has always wanted to go to college may be making a profoundly important statement. You may be able to use this information to structure organization rewards, so that you motivate the employee to achieve his or her objectives while simultaneously meeting organizational needs.

Correspondingly, you can also understand when you won't be able to motivate an employee. For example, you notice that Bill's performance is inadequate or marginal, and this does not result from inadequate training. You know from previous discussions with him that his most salient second-level objectives are inconsistent with the first-level outcomes that you can provide. Perhaps his primary unsatisfied need is to live in Colorado. Unfortunately, your hospital is in New York! Equation 5–1 predicts that, when the instrumentality is low (or perhaps even negative), the anticipated satisfaction with the first-level outcomes that you provide (V_j) is low (or aversive). If the anticipated satisfaction is low (V_j), then the force (F_i) in Equation 5–2 will be low. Under these circumstances, you will not be able to motivate Bill to meet your organizational needs. Pep talks will be a waste of time, and if progressive discipline fails to change his behavior, cut your losses and replace him.

One attempt to accommodate these individual differences in employee motivational needs is called a cafeteria compensation plan. Cafeteria compensation plans allow employees to individualize their benefits. In a cafeteria plan, all employees receive a core set of benefits. Based on their salary level, each employee receives additional credits that he or she can use to purchase benefits that he or she chooses. For example, the core health insurance benefit might be a health maintenance organization. For an additional 300 points, the employee could purchase a preferred provider organization plan, and an additional 500 points might purchase an indemnity insurance plan.

Getting to know your employees on a more personal level has some inherent dangers. It is important never to allow your interest in the goals and desires of an employee to develop into friendship. Employees can never be friends because the employer–employee relationship has adversarial aspects to it. If you begin to look upon an employee as a friend, you expose yourself to the risk of manipulation and disappointment when the employee acts in his or her own self-interest. Similarly, if the employee perceives you as a friend, he or she will inevitably be disappointed and resentful when you must act

as an employer or manager. Getting to know your employees' personal goals should take place, therefore, at arm's length. Successful managers have appropriate boundaries.

LEADERSHIP

Leadership is the process of getting subordinates and peers to work voluntarily toward your vision of the organization's goals. In late 20th century terms, this definition sounds overly organization centered. Leaders can also have a vision of work, however, that includes achieving the organization's goals through a team process, consensus, and delegation. This definition, therefore, encompasses a wide range of leader styles that vary from autocratic to democratic.

Leadership has three aspects to it. Vision involves an intuitive ability to see where the organization, employee, or group needs to go. Inspiration is being able interpersonally to motivate others to follow your lead. Although both these aspects of leadership can be important, neither one is particularly learnable. A final aspect of leadership, however, is quite learnable and focuses on how to involve others in the decision-making process. This last element of leadership is the primary focus of this discussion.

Sometimes, it is easier to identify a successful leader than it is to understand what he or she does to be a successful leader. Bennis has noted that successful leaders seem to have the following four characteristics in common[5]:

1. They use exceptional communication skills to make ideas and visions tangible to others.
2. They generate trust through clear, consistent behavior.
3. They have a realistic sense of their limitations.
4. They reject the notion of failure.

As broad themes, these four points are interesting and may even be helpful, but how do they translate into things that you can do to lead more effectively? Originally, management scientists thought that leadership was a combination of personal or personality characteristics. Effective leaders were expected to have more or less of some combination of personal traits and characteristics, such as intelligence, charisma, decisiveness, strength, bravery, self-confidence, extroversion, height, attractiveness, and so forth. When research studies found too many exceptions to this approach, it was then proposed that leadership was a set of behaviors. For example, researchers at Ohio State University concluded that leaders exhibit varying amounts of concern for employees' welfare, which they called consideration, and concern for getting the task accomplished, which they called initiating structure. Once again, too many exceptions were found to conclude that particular behaviors or behavioral strategies per se are the essence of leadership.

A more recent approach to understanding leadership focuses on examining leader attributes and behaviors in the context of specific situations. This approach to understanding leadership has been the most successful to date. Successful leaders seem to be able to choose certain behaviors or decision-making styles that are appropriate given the situation at the time. This is called a situational approach to leadership. Sometimes a leader has to make autocratic decisions, whereas at other times delegating decisions to subordinates will produce the best results. There are also many situations in which a leader will be most effective if he or she uses methods somewhere between these two extremes. The successful leader knows, for example, when to delegate and when to make decisions himself or herself.

There is considerable research and practical evidence supporting the validity of this situational approach to leadership. Imagine, for example, the model Marine Corps drill instructor. He or she certainly would typify the directive leader. Imagine, however, if this very successful leader of Marines was to direct the efforts of a volunteer church organization using the same behaviors used with recruits! It is obvious that the result would be a disaster. Conversely, lead-ership behaviors that would bring success to the volunteer church organization would be equally inappropriate for leading Marine recruits.

The key is to match the leadership style to the situation. There are very few organizations in which a leader can be successful using only one leadership style. The truly successful Marine Corps sergeant will recognize that, when the nature of the work changes, delegating decisions and involving others in a participative decision-making process are necessary for success. Once again, the skill is to know *when* to choose a particular decision-making style.

The following discussion presents a way of thinking about leadership. It is based on a line of research begun by Vroom at Yale University.[6] Vroom's approach to understanding leadership was based on observing successful leaders. Based on these observations, he reached several conclusions about the strategies that successful leaders use. Successful leaders make decisions that:

- *protect the quality of the decision*—Effective leaders are concerned with the specific outcome. If the decision involves developing a critical care pathway for pneumonia, then producing a pathway that provides effective clinical care, controls costs, and coordinates personnel and facilities is of primary concern and an effective leader will ensure that these goals are achieved.
- *protect the acceptance of the decision*—Effective leaders understand that a high-quality decision that others will resist, will fail to implement, or don't understand will not produce an effective outcome. Effective leaders, therefore, use a leader style that will result in others accepting the decision.
- *are timely*—Effective leaders understand that late decisions may be irrelevant.
- *develop the skills and abilities of their subordinates*—Effective leaders understand that many daily decisions are made by subordinates and peers in their name. As a result, they try to develop their coworkers' leadership and decision-making abilities, so

that the overall level of organizational decision making improves.

Vroom found that quality and acceptance are of the greatest importance to effective leadership. Timeliness and employee development are also very important, but somewhat less so than quality and acceptance. This order of priorities is important to appreciate. It suggests that leaders should not sacrifice quality and acceptance to make a decision "on time." Instead, effective managers appear to emphasize quality and acceptance and then manage the time issue as a secondary, although still important, consideration. Similarly, if it is feasible to use an event to develop others' decision-making skills, such as by delegating the project to them or consulting with them, this is also achieved, but not at the sacrifice of quality or acceptance.

Vroom also found that effective leaders use a range of leader behaviors or decision-making styles (Exhibit 5–1). If the decision has implications for only one other person, then the individual styles are appropriate; the group styles are appropriate for decisions that will affect more than one other person. Vroom's nomenclature used an A to indicate a variation on the autocratic theme, a C to indicate a consultative theme, a G to indicate a group process, and a D to indicate delegation.

Vroom's research also indicates that effective leaders follow certain rules about when to use specific leader styles or, more specifically, when *not* to use particular leader styles. These rules, based on Vroom's observational research, are given in Exhibit 5–2. It is also important to consider that many effective leaders probably use these rules at an unconscious or semiconscious level. Intuitively, they grasp the essential elements of a situation and have a "sense" about how to respond. It is this unconscious or semiconscious decision making that Vroom tried to capture by deducing the rules that effective leaders seem to follow.

Let's examine a few of these rules. Rule 1, for example, states that, if you have insufficient information or skill to make a high-quality decision, then don't use AI, which is an autocratic decision-making style. This certainly reflects common sense. Obviously, if you don't know what you are doing, you shouldn't act! The fact that research and theory validate our observations should provide some confidence in the paradigm's validity.

Rule 3a says that, if a subordinate's goals are not consistent with the organization's goals, then don't delegate the decision making to him or her. The implication is that subordinates will work toward their own agendas as opposed to the organization's goals. This certainly is consistent with the preceding discussion of motivation. Once again, when stated this way, the rule describes common sense. Often, however, in the "heat of battle" we get confounded in the details and miss the big picture.

These rules can help clarify the most important issues when you are considering how to involve others in decisions. Notice also that the effect of the various rules is to *exclude* decision-making styles from the "feasible set." In effect, leaders begin with a complete palette of leadership style choices. Depending upon the situation, some leader styles may not be appropriate.

As a way of integrating all the decision-making styles into one easy-to-understand paradigm, Vroom assembled a flowchart (Figure 5–1). Before discussing the flowchart, let me tell you where I am *not* going with this discussion. I am *not* going to suggest that you make a copy of the flowchart and put it in your back pocket or purse. Then, the next time that you have to make a decision, perhaps in a meeting, you stand up and say "Excuse me! I'll be right back!" You leave the room like Clark Kent looking for a telephone booth, pull out your flowchart, identify the "ideal" decision-making style, return to the meeting, and then calmly issue a statement such as "Well, doctors, I think that this is one decision that we need to handle through group consensus."

The flowchart is far too mechanical and requires simplistic, dichotomous (yes–no) decisions in situations that are generally problematic.[7] The flowchart is, however, a useful

Exhibit 5–1 Decision-Making Processes

For Individual Problems	For Group Problems
AI You solve the problem or make the decision yourself, using information available to you at that time.	AI You solve the problem or make the decision yourself, using information available to you at that time.
AII You obtain any necessary information from the subordinate, then decide on the solution to the problem yourself. You may or may not tell the subordinate what the problem is, in getting the information from him. The role played by your subordinate in making the decision is clearly one of providing specific information which you request, rather than generating or evaluating alternative solutions.	AII You obtain any necessary information from subordinates, then decide on the solution to the problem yourself. You may or may not tell subordinates what the problem is, in getting the information from them. The role played by your subordinates in making the decision is clearly one of providing specific information which you request, rather than generating or evaluating solutions.
CI You share the problem with the relevant subordinate, getting his ideas and suggestions. Then *you* make the decision. This decision may or may not reflect your subordinate's influence.	CI You share the problem with the relevant subordinates individually, getting their ideas and suggestions without bringing them together as a group. Then *you* make the decision. This decision may or may not reflect your subordinates' influence.
GI You share the problem with one of your subordinates and together you analyze the problem and arrive at a mutually satisfactory solution in an atmosphere of free and open exchange of information and ideas. You both contribute to the resolution of the problem with the relative contribution of each being dependent on knowledge rather than formal authority.	CII You share the problem with your subordinates in a group meeting. In this meeting you obtain their ideas and suggestions. Then, *you* make the decision which may or may not reflect your subordinates' influence.
DI You delegate the problem to one of your subordinates, providing him with any relevant information that you possess, but giving him responsibility for solving the problem by himself. Any solution which the person reaches will receive your support.	GII You share the problem with your subordinates as a group. Together you generate and evaluate alternatives and attempt to reach agreement (consensus) on a solution. Your role is much like that of chairman, coordinating the discussion, keeping it focused on the problem, and making sure that the critical issues are discussed. You do not try to influence the group to adopt "your" solution and are willing to accept and implement any solution which has the support of the entire group.

Source: The *Decision Sciences* journal is published by the Decision Sciences Institute, located in the College of Business Administration at Georgia State University, Atlanta, Georgia.

training tool to acquaint you with how a situation interacts with leader style to produce a feasible set. It is useful as a tool to get you to think about how situation should influence how you involve others to make decisions. The lines in the flowchart solve for the first two considerations that were discussed above, that is, quality and acceptance. The questions that are listed at the top of the flowchart take the rules in Exhibit 5–2 and recast them as operational questions. By addressing these questions you define the situation.

For example, let's assume that you are directing a project for the renovation of a patient wait-

Exhibit 5–2 Leader Decision-Making Rules

1. *The Leader Information Rule*

    If the quality of the decision is important and the leader does not possess enough information or expertise to solve the problem by himself, then AI is eliminated from the feasible set.

2. *The Subordinate Information Rule*

    (applicable to individual problems only)

    If the quality of the decision is important and the subordinate does not possess enough information or expertise to solve the problem himself, then DI is eliminated from the feasible set.

3a. *The Goal Congruence Rule*

    If the quality of the decision is important and the subordinates are not likely to pursue organizational goals in their efforts to solve this problem, then GII and DI are eliminated from the feasible set.

3b. *The Augmented Goal Congruence Rule*

    (applicable to individual problems only)

    Under the conditions specified in the previous rule (i.e., quality of decision is important, and the subordinate does not share the organizational goals to be attained in solving the problem) GI may also constitute risk to the quality of the decision taken in response to an individual problem. Such a risk is a reasonable one to take only if the nature of the problem is such that the acceptance of the subordinate is critical to the effective implementation and prior probability of acceptance of an autocratic solution is low.

4a. *The Unstructured Problem Rule (Group)*

    In decisions in which the quality of the decision is important, if the leader lacks the necessary information or expertise to solve the problem by himself and if the problem is unstructured, the method of solving the problem should provide for interaction among subordinates. Accordingly, AI, AII, and CI are eliminated from the feasible set.

4b. *The Unstructured Problem Rule (Individual)*

    In decisions in which the quality of the decision is important, if the leader lacks the necessary information to solve the problem by himself and if the problem is unstructured, the method of solving the problem should permit the subordinate to generate solutions to the problem. Accordingly, AI and AII are eliminated from the feasible set.

5. *The Acceptance Rule*

    If the acceptance of the decision by subordinates is critical to effective implementation and if it is not certain that an autocratic decision will be accepted, AI and AII are eliminated from the feasible set.

6. *The Conflict Rule*

    (applicable to group problems only)

    If the acceptance of the decision is critical, an autocratic decision is not certain to be accepted and disagreement among subordinates in methods of attaining the organizational goal is likely, the methods used in solving the problem should enable those in disagreement to resolve their differences with full knowledge of the problem. Accordingly, AI, AII and CI, which permit no interaction among subordinates, are eliminated from the feasible set.

7. *The Fairness Rule*

    If the quality of the decision is unimportant, but acceptance of the decision is critical and not certain to result from autocratic decision, the decision process used should permit the subordinates to interact with one another and negotiate over the method of resolving any differences with full responsibility on them for determining what is equitable. Accordingly, AI, AII, CI, and CII are eliminated from the feasible set.

8. *The Acceptance Priority Rule*

    If acceptance is critical, not certain to result from an autocratic decision and if (the) subordinate(s) is (are) motivated to pursue the organizational goals represented in the problem, then methods which provide equal partnership in the decision-making process can provide greater acceptance without risking decision quality. Accordingly, AI, AII, CI, and CII are eliminated from the feasible set.

continues

Exhibit 5–2 continued

9. *The Group Problem Rule (Group)*

If a problem has approximately equal effects on each of a number of subordinates (i.e., is a group problem) the decision process used should provide them with equal opportunities to influence that decision. Use of a decision process such as GI or DI, which provides opportunities for only one of the affected subordinates to influence that decision, may in the short run produce feelings of inequity reflected in lessened commitment to the decision on the part of those "left out" of the decision process and in the long run be a source of conflict and divisiveness.

10. *The Individual Problem Rule (Individual)*

If a problem affects only one subordinate, decision processes which unilaterally introduce other (unaffected) subordinates as equal partners constitute an unnecessary use of time of the unaffected subordinates and can reduce the amount of commitment of the affected subordinate to the decision by reducing the amount of his opportunity to influence the decision. Thus CII and GII are eliminated from the feasible set.

Source: The *Decision Sciences* journal is published by the Decision Sciences Institute, located in the College of Business Administration at Georgia State University, Atlanta, Georgia.

ing area. One decision is what color to paint the walls. Using this model, the first question that you would ask yourself is "Is there a quality requirement, such that one solution is likely to be more rational than another?" It is largely irrelevant to the room's function whether the walls are white, beige, or tan, so the answer is no. Question D on the flowchart is "Is acceptance of decision by subordinates critical to effective implementation?" Your subordinates don't care, so you answer no. This leaves you with feasible set 1.

You can see that, based on your analysis of the situation, all the leader styles for both group and individual situations remain in the feasible set! In effect, leadership style is *unimportant* in this situation in regard to the quality and acceptance considerations. The styles, however, are listed in a particular order. The style farthest to the left in each feasible set generally will be the fastest, and the style farthest to the right will generally be the slowest. Similarly, the style farthest to the right will generally provide the greatest potential for developing subordinate skills, and the one farthest to the left generally has the least potential for subordinate development.

Returning to our short example, if you looked at the waiting room paint decision as simply a

step to move through quickly to get to more critical decisions, then make the decision yourself (AI). If you saw this as an opportunity to develop your assistant's understanding of working with contractors and having to make choices or meet a deadline, then you might choose to use GI (GII for a group).

The flowchart in Figure 5–1 can be used in several ways. First, the questions themselves should sensitize you to issues that merit consideration in your day-to-day relations with your peers, subordinates, team members, and others. Second, when you are confronted with a major decision requiring considerable thought, you may want to use Figure 5–1 to play devil's advocate vis-à-vis your natural inclination regarding how to involve others in the process. If, for example, the chart says to delegate but your gut intuition is to be autocratic, then you have the basis for a dialogue with yourself regarding the two approaches. No matter what you finally choose to do, your decision will be based on considerable thought.

By becoming more aware of the issues that should be considered when you are determining how to involve others, you will sharpen your decision-making and leadership abilities. The situ-

A. Is there a quality requirement such that one solution is likely to be more rational than another?
B. Do I have sufficient info to make a high quality decision?
C. Is the problem structured?
D. Is acceptance of decision by subordinates critical to effective implementation?
E. If I were to make the decision by myself, is it reasonably certain that it would be accepted by my subordinates?
F. Do subordinates share the organizational goals to be attained in solving this problem?
G. Is conflict among subordinates likely in preferred solutions? (This question is irrelevant to individual problems.)
H. Do subordinates have sufficient info to make a high quality decision?

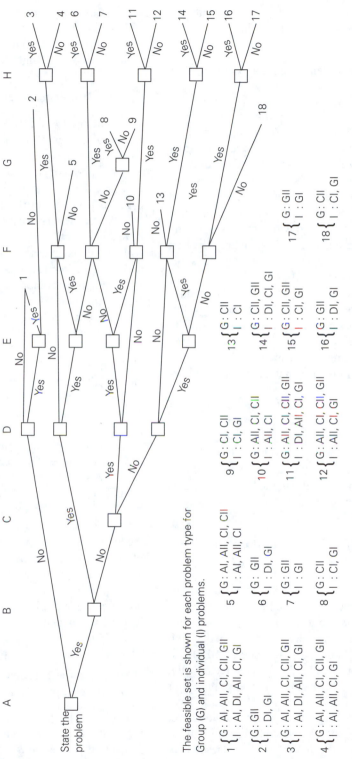

The feasible set is shown for each problem type for Group (G) and individual (I) problems.

1 { G: AI, AII, CI, CII, GII
    I : AI, DI, AII, CI, GI

2 { G: GII
    I : DI, GI

3 { G: AI, AII, CI, CII, GII
    I : AI, DI, AII, CI, GI

4 { G: AI, AII, CI, CII, GII
    I : AI, AII, CI, GI

5 { G: AI, AII, CI, CII
    I : AI, AII, CI

6 { G: GII
    I : DI, GI

7 { G: GII
    I : GI

8 { G: CII
    I : CI, GI

9 { G: CI, CII
    I : CI, GI

10 { G: AII, CI, CII
     I : AII, CI

11 { G: AII, CI, CII, GII
     I : DI, AII, CI, GI

12 { G: AII, CI, CII, GII
     I : AII, CI, GI

13 { G: CII
     I : CI

14 { G: CII, GII
     I : DI, CI, GI

15 { G: CII, GII
     I : CI, GI

16 { G: GII
     I : DI, GI

17 { G: GII
     I : GI

18 { G: CII
     I : CI, GI

Figure 5-1 Decision-making flowchart and feasible leader style sets. *Source:* The *Decision Sciences* journal is published by the Decision Sciences Institute, located in the College of Business Administration at Georgia State University, Atlanta, Georgia.

ational questions that are presented in Figure 5–1 are discussed in more detail below.

A: Does the Problem Possess a Quality Requirement?

This question concerns the importance of identifying a high-quality solution irrespective of the need for subordinates to accept the solution. If a problem does not possess a quality requirement, you would be indifferent to any proposed solution. Generally, if a problem does not possess a quality requirement, this means that there are two or three obvious solutions and no technical or rational means for picking the best solution. The primary consideration is that some solution be implemented.

Most problems do possess a quality requirement, and generally you will answer yes to this question. Problems (or processes) with quality requirements include developing a marketing plan, determining which brand of radiography equipment to purchase, and making clinical decisions. In the extreme, one could argue that all problems have some quality requirements. For example, it would be possible to paint the reception area in the discussion above in a color that is so horrible that it becomes distracting. Generally, however, determining the paint color of a reception area has minimal quality issues and is probably more an issue of taste.

B: Do You Have Sufficient Information To Make a High-Quality Decision?

This question concerns whether you have sufficient technical information to solve the problem yourself without consulting your subordinates or peers. The main issue is whether you have enough knowledge to understand all aspects of the problem and to solve it technically, not whether you have more knowledge than your subordinates. It is also possible for you to have the most knowledge of any one individual yet lack sufficient knowledge to produce a good solution without the information possessed by others.

This question is a critical fork in the road. If you answer no, then this automatically means that you will have to involve others in some way in the decision making.

C: Is the Problem Structured?

A structured problem is one in which the alternative courses of action and the criteria that will be used to evaluate whether you are making progress on a course of action are obvious. For example, once you have identified the selection methods to be used in filling a secretarial position, the problem is structured. At that point, you have a plan of the methods to use and how they will be utilized to assess a group of applicants to make a selection decision.

Developing a comprehensive community care system for patients with acquired immunodeficiency syndrome, including family, medical, and financial issues, would be an unstructured problem because there is no existing "game plan" indicating all the issues to be considered, their relative importance, and potential sources of funding. Once the plan is developed, implementing it would then become a structured problem.

Often, it is helpful to think of situations on a scale of structure. A patient who is on a critical pathway is in a highly structured situation. The treatment plan is specified, including medications, expected test values, and a plan for where the patient will be at each hour of treatment for the length of the pathway. If the patient falls off of the pathway, perhaps because of a laboratory test that falls outside of pathway parameters, then the situation is far less structured. There is no longer as clear an expectation of what will happen, when, and by whom.

D: Is Acceptance of the Decision by Your Subordinates Important or Critical for Effective Implementation?

Even a technically correct solution can fail if those who must implement it are resistant or opposed to it. The issue is whether, *irrespective of how the decision is made*, subordinate acceptance of what is to be done is critical to implementing the decision.

When judging whether a solution has an acceptance requirement, consider whether your initiative, judgment, or thinking will affect the execution of the plan and whether others are likely to disapprove strongly enough to actively oppose the solution. The question here is whether they will do what you want, not whether they like it. If a problem does not require your subordinates to be involved in the execution of the decision, there is no acceptance issue. Similarly, if subordinates are likely to be indifferent, there is also no acceptance issue.

E: If You Were To Make the Decision Yourself, Are You Reasonably Certain That It Would Be Accepted by Your Subordinates?

If subordinate acceptance as defined by question D is important to the successful implementation of the solution, then you certainly want to use a decision-making process that will increase the chance of acceptance. If you allow subordinates to participate in the decision, this can further their acceptance. On the other hand, if you are viewed as the person who legitimately *should* make the decision or as someone who has the *expertise* to make the decision, then autocratic methods also may be acceptable. Once again, having knowledge of those with whom you are working is critical.

F: Do Your Subordinates Share the Organizational Goals To Be Obtained by Solving This Problem?

Others' self-interests can be incompatible with organizational goals. Our discussion of motivation makes it clear that people may work for many reasons that have nothing to do with the goals of your organization. Employees are not altruistic. If their personal goals are incompatible with your goals, they will work to achieve their personal goals if they can.

Once again, this question is a fork in the road. If others do not share the organization's goals,

then this automatically rules out delegating the task. To delegate under this condition could easily result in others achieving their goals at the expense of the organization's goals.

G: Is Conflict among Subordinates Likely To Arise in Preferred Solutions?

This question concerns whether employees are likely to disagree on the best way to solve a problem. This is different from question F, because it is possible for employees to share organizational goals but to disagree on how best to realize them.

H: Do Subordinates Have Sufficient Information To Make a High-Quality Decision?

This question parallels question B but focuses on subordinate, team member, partner, or peer information.

CASE APPLICATION: LARRY JOHNSON, M.D.

Larry Johnson owns a radiology practice. He has one associate, Phil Downs, who shares expenses but does not yet own part of the practice. Both Larry and Phil are doing very well, their appointment slots are usually filled, and it is Larry's intention to have Phil become a partner in the future. Recently, Larry decided that he would bring in a new associate. He was uncertain how much he should involve Phil in the selection process.

Probably the most fruitful way to approach this case is to think about the issues raised by the leadership model's questions. Two questions have particular significance. First, if Larry makes the decision himself, is Phil likely to object? This question strikes to the core of the relationship between Larry and Phil. Larry must consider whether Phil expects to be part of the decision-making process and how he will react if he is excluded. Finally, does Phil share the same organizational goals as Larry?

Introspectively, Larry believed that Phil would feel excluded, hurt, and disenfranchised if Larry totally excluded him from the employment process. Larry also felt, however, that his goals and Phil's were not aligned. Because Phil was not a partner, Larry felt that Phil might be more short term and personally focused than a partner would be. The first question logically excludes the A styles from consideration, and the second question logically excludes the DI style. Larry adopted a decision style that could best be described as "heavy" CI or "light" GI.

Larry informed Phil before the interview process that he would be consulted but would not participate equally in the final hiring decision. Larry decided that he would do all the initial screening himself and eliminate those applicants whom he did not like for one reason or another. Phil then interviewed four candidates. Larry and Phil met after all the interviews and discussed their conclusions. Both agreed on whom to hire. Larry, however, stated to the case writer that he would not have acquiesced to hiring one of the applicants.

Parenthetically, Larry analyzed the decision-making situation by using the flowchart in Figure 5–1 and provided the following answers:

- *Question A:* Yes—He could hire someone with inadequate professional or personal skills.
- *Question B:* Yes—He knew more about the hiring process than Phil, and he believed that he knew enough to make the decision himself (after all, he did hire Phil!).
- *Question D:* Yes—If he hired someone who was incompetent or whom Phil disliked, there was the chance that Phil would become dissatisfied and leave. It was important to Larry for Phil to like the new associate.
- *Question E:* No—Larry felt that, as the sole owner and the most knowledgeable of the two, he had the prerogative to make the hiring decision. He sensed, however, that excluding Phil from the decision-making process might jeopardize their relationship.

- *Question F:* No—Phil, as an associate, may have more of a short-term view of the decision. As an associate, Phil's long-range concerns might be more personally focused than practice focused.

Larry had this to say about his choice of leadership style:

> Vroom's model of thinking about how to lead was helpful, because it made me think about important considerations related to *how* I make a decision. I might well have come up with the same decision-making process on my own. At least I like to think that I would. At a minimum, this process gave me confidence that my gut intuition regarding how to proceed was valid.

EMPOWERMENT

The preceding discussion suggests that there will be times when it is appropriate to involve subordinates in decision making. *Empowerment* is a relatively new term that captures the notion of giving subordinates increased involvement and decision-making responsibility.[8] Empowerment, however, goes beyond selectively delegating to or consulting with subordinates. Instead, it is a more pervasive and encompassing management philosophy that routinely pushes decision making down to front line employees. It is being practiced by a number of successful service organizations including Marriott, Four Seasons Hotels, Scandinavian Airlines Systems, and Federal Express.

By freeing employees from the tight controls of rules, regulations, and policies, they have the freedom to exercise their own discretion. The potential advantages offered by empowered employees include quicker response to customer needs and quicker recovery with dissatisfied customers. In addition, proponents of empowerment contend that empowered employees have higher job satisfaction, generate more service improvement ideas, increase customer retention, and provide excellent word-of-mouth advertising.

There are, however, potential costs associated with empowerment that physician managers should balance against its advantages to determine whether it is appropriate in their organization. Jobs that are empowered generally require higher skill levels because employees will be making decisions and balancing competing interests that previously were accomplished by supervisors. Therefore, effectively using employment methods, including structured interviews, tests, and work samples, becomes more important because you now must be able to identify applicants with decision-making and prioritizing skills that previously were not needed on the job.

Training becomes critical so that employees can fully comprehend and balance various perspectives, such as the patient's, the organization's, and their own. Previously, management would do this. Finally, because more power will reside at a lower organizational level, it becomes even more important to create reward systems in which everyone's self-interests are aligned.

Empowered employees can create equity problems. Many patients associate rules and procedures with fairness. How do you feel, for example, when you are a customer and you see someone "getting a deal?" In addition, changing or creating rules on the spot takes time. The empowered physician assistant who spends 10 minutes satisfying Mrs. Smith may be angering the waiting Mr. Jones.

We also need to remember that empowered employees can make *bad* decisions! There may be a certain romance in imagining that subordinates with power and control mystically become Super Employees. The perhaps apocryphal story of the hotel doorman, who upon seeing that a guest had forgotten his briefcase personally took the next flight to return it to him, should give us pause. Bottom line: How many of your consult fees are being given away by an empowered employee who may not *really* comprehend the big picture? How many times does a scheduler make more problems and create more overall patient dissatisfaction by fitting in a late arriving patient?

Given that the empowerment sword clearly has two edges, what evidence do we have that it really works? Aside from volumes of anecdotal stories, there is little hard scientific evidence to support or refute the value of empowerment. Conclusive research findings simply aren't available. If you decide to utilize this elixir, you are at least forewarned.

Empowerment, as a way of providing employees with more discretion in decision making, seems very close to the definitions of the GII and DI leadership styles. In fact, it is appropriate to think of empowerment as a special case of delegated leadership. As such, this raises the question of whether empowerment, like leadership, is situational. That is, are there some circumstances where it is more appropriate to empower and others where it may be less appropriate?

Research conducted by Bowers and Lawler suggests that this is the case.[9] In addition to recognizing different situational variables that seem to affect the appropriateness of empowerment, these investigators have also defined three levels of empowerment or empowerment styles:

1. *Suggestion involvement* allows employees to contribute ideas through formal programs, such as suggestion programs, quality circles, and the like. Day-to-day discretion and activities are not empowered. In effect, empowerment is limited to making *recommendations*.
2. *Job involvement* gives employees considerably more freedom to decide how to do their work. Job involvement is often characterized by the use of work teams. Often, duties and responsibilities are rotated at the team's discretion, so that members get a sense of the whole job. Decisions that relate to how the team conducts its work are decided by the group. Decisions, however, that relate to the organization's structure, such as how many work teams will there be, compensation and reward decisions, and so forth, are still retained by management. Generally, performance

information will be team specific and will not encompass the whole organization. Often, patient-focused units are characterized by job involvement. Employees decide how to improve service, schedule work, and perform across functions to improve the nature of the service to the patient.

3. *High involvement* allows employees to share in all aspects of decision making. In for-profit settings, reward systems will often involve profit sharing. Employees have access to total organizational performance data. Employees in high involvement settings need skills that go beyond teamwork, to include looking at the larger organization and considering how change can affect the whole medical organization.

Exhibit 5–3 contrasts empowerment with a traditional production line approach to employee management. Under a production line approach, control is hierarchical, top down, and driven by rules and procedures. In contrast, empowerment achieves control through involving employees in the decision-making process. It utilizes horizontal coordination and employee discretion. Supposedly, the doorman in the hotel anecdote didn't leave his post unattended. He went into the kitchen and found a kitchen worker who had been cross-trained in his function. She determined that, given the current kitchen workload, the kitchen could make do without her for a few hours. The two employees quickly made the decision without involving supervisors. The employees between them made the decisions that, in a production line organization, would be made by two supervisors.

The production line mentality leads to scripted behavior, where employees learn the script (job description), and their job is then to follow the script. Changing the script is left to others. In contrast, empowered employees are self-motivated and self-managed, so they can change the script to suit the circumstances.

Finally, the goal of the customer contact employee in the production organization is to "sell" the product. Determining what the customer wants is someone else's job. In contrast, the whole structure of empowerment is focused on providing discretion to satisfy the customer. It provides employees with the flexibility to modify the job, product, or service to improve it from the customer's perspective.

Historically, health care organizations have possessed many of the characteristics of a production line organization. Consider, for example, most of the work that is performed in a hospital. Supervisors tell subordinates what to do and how to do it, if not personally then through scripts, such as procedures and job descriptions. Nursing, laboratory, and technical jobs are driven by rules and procedures. Finally,

Exhibit 5–3 Comparison of Empowerment and Production Management Styles

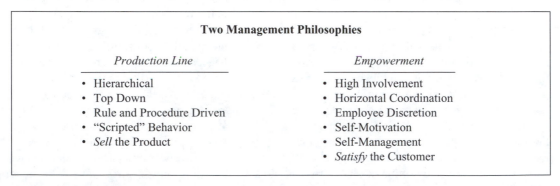

Two Management Philosophies	
Production Line	*Empowerment*
• Hierarchical	• High Involvement
• Top Down	• Horizontal Coordination
• Rule and Procedure Driven	• Employee Discretion
• "Scripted" Behavior	• Self-Motivation
• *Sell* the Product	• Self-Management
	• *Satisfy* the Customer

Source: Data from D. Bowers and E. Lawler, The Empowerment of Service Workers: What, Why, How, and When, *Sloan Management Review*, Vol. 33, No. 3, pp. 31–39, © 1992, Sloan School of Management.

the outcome is to sell the patient on why he or she needs to like the service that is provided.

Exhibit 5–4 provides a means for considering which philosophy may be most appropriate given five situational considerations:

1. business strategy
2. tie to customer
3. technology
4. business environment
5. type of employee

Exhibit 5–4 Evaluating Empowerment's Situational Fit

Basic Business Strategy

Production Line	1	2	3	4	5	Empowerment
High volume						Tender Loving Care
Lowest cost						Personalized service
Cheap						Customized service
Quick						
Reliable						

Tie To Customer

Production Line	1	2	3	4	5	Empowerment
Short time period						Managing a relationship
Transaction performance						Build loyalty
Tangible oriented						Selling intangibles

Technology

Production Line	1	2	3	4	5	Empowerment
Routine						Non-routine
Simple						Complex

Business Environment

Production Line	1	2	3	4	5	Empowerment
Predictable						Unpredictable
Few surprises						Uncertain

Types Of People

Production Line	1	2	3	4	5	Empowerment
Lower growth needs						High growth needs
Weaker or undeveloped interpersonal skills						Strong interpersonal skills
Limited range or undeveloped leader abilities						Flexible, adaptable

Score	Situation
5–10	Production Line
11–15	Suggestion Involvement
16–20	Job Involvement
21–25	High Involvement

(This is a very rough guideline!)

Source: Data from D. Bowers and E. Lawler, The Empowerment of Service Workers: What, Why, How, and When, *Sloan Management Review,* Vol. 33, No. 3, pp. 31–39, © 1992, Sloan Management Review Association.

For example, where in health care is the business strategy characterized by high volume, low cost, cheap, quick, and reliable? One place would be urgent care and "doc in the box" clinics. Some health maintenance organizations have built their primary care strategy around these characteristics. In contrast, where in health care is the strategy characterized by tender loving care, personalized service, and customized service? Cosmetic plastic surgery, pediatrics, and psychiatry are specialties where these strategy characteristics are prevalent. Other medical niches where the path to success is best characterized by the production line or the empowerment philosophy probably quickly come to mind.

Where in health care is success predicated on the tie to the customer being short time period, transaction performance oriented, and focused on the tangible? The emergency department is generally one location that relies on these characteristics. Others might include hospital-based laboratory and diagnostic radiology. Urgent care centers once again come to mind. In contrast, many primary care practices, pediatrics, dermatology, psychiatry, and cosmetic plastic surgery often have ties to the customer that are more closely aligned with empowerment characteristics.

The issue regarding technology is the nature of the employee–technology interaction. For example, the AT&T operator has a relatively simple interaction with technology, even though the technology behind the control console that he or she operates is one of the most complex in the world. In determining the appropriateness of empowerment, we are concerned with the nature of the interaction that the employee has with the technology, not the complexity of the technology itself. When that interaction is routine and simple, as it is in the conduct of laboratory tests, for example, then the formula for success is probably found in a production line approach. Do we really want our laboratory and radiology technicians getting creative and experimenting on the job? In contrast, when the employee really has to understand the workings of the technology, then empowerment is more appropriate.

For example, when developing the information systems to support a coronary artery bypass graft critical path, we want people to be able to focus on the job and not be constrained by rules, procedures, and job boundaries.

The business environment for health care as a whole has shifted toward unpredictability and uncertainty. Although there are pockets of refuge, in general most administrators of health care organizations feel that they are living in a much more chaotic and uncontrolled world than they formerly faced.

Finally, I would like to discuss the "Types of People" issue from a different perspective. Let's begin with the observation that many health care organizations have historically operated as production organizations. As a result, many of the people whom they have attracted to lower and middle positions are often characterized by low growth needs, less developed interpersonal skills, and a limited range of leader abilities. They prefer consistency and feel less comfortable defining new ways of approaching a problem. These are the people who were sought and who felt comfortable sticking around.

Now the world changes. Suddenly, hospitals and other health care organizations are saying "We need people with strong interpersonal skills, who are flexible and adaptable, and who take pride and satisfaction in changing the way we think." Obviously, the person whom we formerly sought is not going to feel comfortable in this new, empowered environment.

This presents a problem to health care organizations that are suddenly changing what they expect their employees to do. At a minimum, it often means that, when a health care system decides to empower positions, it should devote considerable thought and training to developing employee interpersonal and leadership abilities. On occasion, however, it means that some employees will have great difficulty in changing to a more fluid, discretionary environment. These employees may have to be transferred or replaced.

The paradigm that Bowers and Lawler have developed suggests that organizations can vary in their need for empowerment across the five situational considerations.[10] In addition, large organizations, such as hospitals, health care systems, and even practices, will have positions, units, and departments that vary in their suitability for empowerment. Bowers and Lawler suggest scaling the organization, department, job—whatever the unit of analysis is—across the five situational issues. A score between 5 and 10 suggests considering a production line approach, between 11 and 20 a suggestion involvement approach, and so on.

As with other tools that we have discussed, I suggest that you use this paradigm with moderation, as a point of departure to *think* about the appropriateness of empowerment. Consider the employees who would be empowered. How might they react to empowerment, and what training would be necessary? Discussing this with them to obtain their reaction often is appropriate if your initial speculation is that empowerment may be beneficial. Think about the other situational issues, and consider how empowerment might result in change and whether these changes are truly beneficial to the organization and your customers. Consider, also, the effect that might be felt by others who are not empowered. Finally, consider the level of empowerment that would be appropriate and that you and your organization would feel comfortable with. Often, empowerment means changing the organization's culture. Big changes often generate strong resistance. Consider starting with the less aggressive forms of empowerment, gaining some experience, and then perhaps incrementally increasing employee discretion.

I want to stress the point that we are not dealing here with science so much as with a philosophy and strategy of human resources management based on the nature of the organization's business. Empowering employees is neither right nor wrong, good nor bad. It is simply more or less consistent with other aspects of your organization. As a physician manager, you should consider empowerment one of your possible choices.

One last anecdote. People Express, the pioneer in cut-rate air fares, was also an empowerment company. Many feel that its initial success was largely a result of its empowered employees. Throughout People Express's short life, it was chronically understaffed. People Express understood that it needed a very different type of employee if the airline was to succeed using an empowered management system. It never was able to find enough employees with the necessary skills. The employees, who gave the company incredible effort and devotion in return for opportunity, job variety, and freedom to do their work unencumbered by traditional management restrictions, eventually burned out from overwork.

The lesson for physician managers is that effective hiring and training methods become critical to success in an empowered environment. People Express never successfully solved this problem, and many feel that this was a major reason why it eventually failed. If you are considering empowering your employees, also consider the selection and training implications. Exactly how will you identify those applicants who have the necessary decision-making and judgment skills? Until you can answer this question, don't empower. In addition, take a close look at your current employees. Have they shown you indications that they have the necessary skills? You shouldn't assume that they will "grow" to meet an empowered environment if they haven't shown you signs of this growth in the past.

CONCLUSION

Most of the work performed in health care organizations is dependent on the success of individuals working in groups and teams. Knowing how to search for the life goals of others, as well as their expectancies and instrumentalities, can help you motivate them to perform at higher levels. This chapter has outlined a strategy for motivating employees by thinking about and structuring monetary and nonmonetary incentives, so that employees achieve their own personal goals in the process of working toward achieving the organization's goals.

Leadership involves conveying a vision of what you want and then inspiring employees to work toward that vision. The way in which you make leadership decisions will have a profound effect on the willingness of employees to follow. This chapter has provided a method of examining decision-making situations and determining how best to lead. By considering the situational issues discussed in this chapter and recognizing that effective leaders choose a leader style based on the situation, you can work more effectively with subordinates, partners, and peers.

Finally, empowerment can be a powerful tool for harnessing and utilizing the creativeness of employees. As with leadership and motivation, it is a contingent process that is not appropriate for all organizations or all parts of an organization. By considering where empowerment is appropriate, you can selectively use this management philosophy to improve customer satisfaction.

REFERENCES AND NOTES

1. V. Vroom, *Work and Motivation* (New York, N.Y.: Wiley, 1964).

2. A. Maslow, A Theory of Human Motivation, *Psychological Review* 41 (1943):370–396.

3. D. McClelland, *The Achieving Society* (New York, N.Y.: Free Press, 1961).

4. F. Herzberg, B. Mausner, and B. Snyderman, *The Motivation to Work* (New York, N.Y.: Wiley, 1959).

5. W. Bennis, The Four Competencies of Leadership, *Training and Development Journal* 15 (1984):15–19.

6. Vroom, *Work and Motivation*.

7. One possible exception would be to use the flowchart to generate "devil's advocate" solutions that you could compare with the results of a more thoughtful process.

8. Parts of this section originally appeared in R.J. Solomon, Watch Training Needs When Empowering Employees, *American Medical News*, 24 January 1994, p. 42.

9. D. Bowers and E. Lawler, The Empowerment of Service Workers: What, Why, How, and When, *Sloan Management Review* 33, no. 3 (1992): 31–39.

10. Bowers and Lawler, The Empowerment of Service Workers.

CHAPTER 6

Financial Management

Chapter Objectives

The goal of this chapter is to help you become an informed *consumer* and *user* of financial and accounting information. When you have completed this chapter, you will be able to:

1. use financial information to help you make decisions, such as a hospital or practice expansion or acquisition
2. assess the financial health of your organization and determine how well it is doing in comparison with past years
3. utilize cash and accrual accounting information to understand better the financial status of your organization
4. evaluate the financial impact of capital decisions, such as the decision to purchase additional equipment
5. determine whether you should lease or purchase equipment
6. use a budget to help you plan, evaluate, and guide performance

Physician managers are in a unique position in the health care system. By virtue of their medical training, they are capable of understanding the medical implications of management decisions. Physician managers who have acquired financial skills can then combine this medical perspective with their understanding of the financial implications of a decision. This ability to balance the medical and financial components of a decision is unique to the financially informed physician manager. These physician managers can use their nonmedical colleagues' financial language and logic to communicate and provide support for their medically informed decisions.

One of physician managers' most critical responsibilities, therefore, irrespective of whether they are in a practice, hospital, or health care system, is to understand the financial implications of decisions and then to act on this information. All too often, health care providers use financial information as if it were an autopsy. Two years after the expansion was undertaken, or after the new physician was hired, or after the pain management program was initiated, the financial reports are examined, and the conclusion is "Oops! This sure isn't working well, is it"? Physician managers need to use their financial skills *proactively*. That is, they should consider the financial implications and risks *before* proceeding with a project or decision. This not only reduces the chance that a poor decision will be made, but it also will help identify what things must occur for both the financial and medical outcomes to be achieved.

To use financial data proactively, physician managers need to know what financial information is needed to make an informed decision. Consistent with the physician manager's appropriate role, assembling data, constructing spreadsheets, and undertaking other data collection and basic analysis tasks generally should be done by others. Physicians should not be replacing their accountants or chief financial officers. There is a direct analogy here to the physician's clinical role, which includes identifying tests to be performed but does not encompass personally conducting the laboratory analysis on a patient's blood. Similarly, the physician manager's critical financial role is to know what financial information to ask for, understand how to interpret the data, and make medically and financially informed recommendations and decisions.

The emphasis in this chapter is to describe financial tools and show how they apply to decision-making situations that physician managers routinely encounter. The primary financial skills used by physician managers are the following:

1. *cost-volume-profit (CVP) skills*—these methods provide an understanding of costs and how different types of costs along with volume affect profit.
2. *capital asset planning*—evaluating the financial impact of major capital acquisitions, such as buildings, office equipment, and medical equipment, and using payback period and time value of money concepts, such as net present value (NPV) and internal rate of return (IRR) to evaluate capital projects.
3. *statements, reports, and systems*—understanding the use and significance of standard financial statements, such as the income statement, balance sheet, and cash flow statement, and understanding the appropriate uses of cash accounting and accrual accounting.
4. *control and budgeting*—developing financial plans and using them to evaluate the performance of operations, using budgets to benchmark or set standards for financial performance instead of as a rigid constraint, and understanding the difference between static and flexible budgets.
5. *short-term financial and cash control*—accounting for cash, so that it is not diverted; converting receivables into cash; knowing what reports to examine so that the organization meets its cash obligations.

Physician managers in all settings should be proficient in the first four categories. The fifth category is covered in Chapter 7, and may have more direct applicability to physician managers who are working in a practice setting or who have overall financial responsibility for an organization.

CVP ANALYSIS

CVP analysis examines how different kinds of costs interact with the volume of business to affect profit. It can help you to answer such questions as the following:

- How many procedures will have to be conducted for a new magnetic resonance imager (MRI) to break even or to hit a targeted profit level?
- How would combining several primary care practices into a group affect profitability?
- What would happen to profitability if a partner were to leave the practice?
- What would happen to an integrated health care system if it were to sell its psychiatric hospital?
- If a managed care company enters our market and takes 20 percent of our inpatient volume, how might this affect costs and profitability?
- If I make an investment in educational cost and equipment to learn a new procedure, how many procedures will I need to conduct to break even or to reach a profitability target?

As you can see, the issues raised in these questions are critical to the financial viability of any health care organization. CVP is, therefore, one of the most powerful financial analysis tools available, and it should be routinely performed whenever decisions will be made that may affect cost, volume, or profitability.

To perform a CVP analysis, you must understand the nature of costs. Costs are expenditures of cash, such as for supplies, personnel, interest, and rent. Costs, however, can behave in different ways. Some costs vary with the amount of service provided. As more patients are treated or hospital beds are filled, these costs change. This type of cost is called a variable cost. Other costs remain the same irrespective of the number of procedures conducted, patients treated, hospital beds filled, and so forth, and they are referred to as fixed costs. Mixed costs have features of both fixed and variable costs. Understanding these distinctions is important because the nature of a cost has a profound effect on how you manage it and on the profitability of any health care organization.

Fixed costs remain stable as services vary. Typical examples include rent, salaried personnel, interest on equipment (e.g., computers and laboratory equipment), and taxes. This notion of a cost being truly fixed, however, is a convenient convention. In reality, no cost is truly fixed. Over a period of years, rent may increase, salaries may change as personnel come and go, loans may be paid off, and taxes may increase. In addition, if volume changes enough, fixed costs may change. For example, if a health maintenance organization (HMO) obtains a new contract covering an additional 20,000 lives, new physicians, nurses, and nonmedical personnel may have to be hired. As volume increases beyond a certain level, a hospital may have to build an additional wing, which will generate many additional fixed costs. Similarly, if volume decreases substantially, a hospital may be able to close a wing, downsize its personnel, and thereby reduce its fixed costs. Within a broad range of business activity, however, which is called the relevant range, fixed costs will remain the same.

Fixed costs represent the risk of doing business. Irrespective of whether the patients come, the fixed costs will be there. Procedures, practices, programs, hospitals, and health care systems that have high fixed costs, generally speaking, have high risk. When you are negotiating the terms of a contract, for example, one of the important issues to consider is who has the fixed cost. Often, a negotiating objective will be to try to get the other party to take the fixed cost and, with it, the risk.

There are two strategies for controlling fixed costs. The first is procurement. The maxim "Don't buy a Mercedes if a Ford Escort will do the job" is appropriate. This statement assumes that the job to be done is basic transportation, getting from point A to point B. If the job, however, was defined as "doing this in a safe manner in the event of an accident, providing superior comfort (because we have a lot of work to do and need to arrive rested), and conveying a certain image (because that communicates a message of success, and success begets success)," then a Ford Escort would be the wrong procurement decision. By effective procurement, I mean that we don't waste money on attributes that don't relate to our mission.

The second strategy for controlling fixed costs is "*Use it, use it, use it!*" Keep salaried personnel busy, keep treatment rooms full, expand office hours, and so on. All these tactics get more use out of costs that will be there anyway. This strategy is the economic driver behind the increasing number of group practices, the growth in the size of group practices, and the subsequent decline in the number of solo practitioners. One secretary, one nurse, one computer, and often one office suite can all service more than one physician. As the second physician is acquired, *the fixed costs remain the same*, but the second physician is generating additional revenue, so the *fixed cost as a percentage of revenue generated* is obviously lower. In effect, the practice has become more efficient.

Graphically, fixed costs plot as a series of stair steps, such as in Figure 6–1. Here, salary remains the same for the first 300 patients. Once

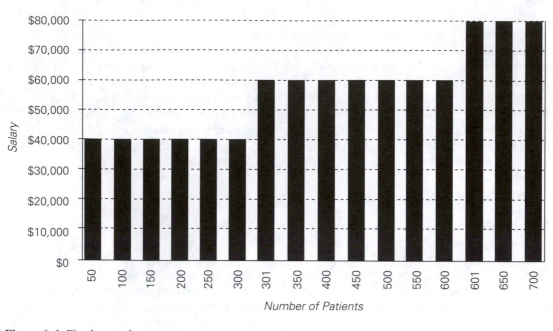

Figure 6–1 Fixed cost relevant ranges.

this relevant range is exceeded, additional salary cost is incurred, and we go up to a new cost plateau. When you examine this fixed cost–volume relationship, it is clear that you always want to be at the far right side of any plateau because this will give you the most revenue generated for the given level of fixed cost. In fact, it should be apparent that your net income (net revenue minus costs) will probably go *down* as a result of taking on the 301st patient and the associated additional fixed cost. Obviously, you would not want to take on the 301st patient and move to the higher cost plateau if you didn't have good reason to believe that you could push the volume up well beyond this level.

This relationship between fixed cost and volume underlies the failure of many businesses and projects. Take, for example, the restaurant that, given the opportunity to expand into adjacent space, does so to address overbooked weekends during the summer. As a result, it greatly increases its fixed costs. These costs are present during weekdays and in slower seasons. The

owner never comprehended that the expansion was perhaps tantamount to moving from the right end of a lower cost plateau to the left end of a higher cost plateau. Uninformed decisions such as this may mean that you are betting the business on a large increase in volume. Sometimes ill-informed decisions such as these translate into working harder just to stay in place. Sometimes they lead to lower profits and even failure.

Variable costs vary in total as activity varies. Typical examples include medical supplies, office supplies, postage, X-ray film, and the salaries of hourly personnel who can be called in or not called based on need. When more patients are treated, total variable costs increase; when fewer patients are treated, total variable costs decrease. Because total variable costs are obviously affected by volume, we need to think of them in terms of variable cost per unit, such as the variable cost per procedure, per patient, per diagnosis-related group (DRG), or per minute of machine time. The unit of analysis (procedure, patient, DRG, etc.) is often referred to as a cost driver because this variable drives the total variable cost up or down. Another way to think of this is as the cost driver being an independent variable, with the variable cost being a dependent variable. Once I know the level of the independent variable, I can predict the level of the dependent variable. If my variable cost per patient is $30, then I know with some certainty that if I treat 100 patients my total variable cost will be $3,000.

As with fixed costs, there are two fundamental strategies to control variable costs. The first is procurement. The goal is to purchase at the lowest per unit cost. To do this, however, I must clearly specify the quality and characteristics that I need. Otherwise, suppliers will translate "lowest possible cost" into "cheap." A low variable cost that changes the nature of your product or service in ways that are unfavorable to the customer or the health care organization is a false economy. On the other hand, reducing variable costs that don't affect real or perceived quality is a legitimate cost control.

For example, Sutter Health in Sacramento, California and Piedmont Hospital in Atlanta, Georgia evaluated the cost of vegetables served to patients.[1] The cost of vegetables ranged from $2.22 per pound for asparagus to $0.69 per pound for baby carrots. Quality was controlled by specifying USDA Grade A frozen vegetables. An analysis of the costs showed that the annual expenditure for frozen vegetables was $45,468, of which $26,707 was for asparagus. By completely eliminating asparagus and consolidating all frozen vegetable purchases into a mix, they achieved a 54 percent savings while maintaining the prescribed quality standard. In addition, patients, who were not expecting a five-star meal anyway, indicated equivalent levels of satisfaction on opinion surveys.

In this case, the hospitals used three aspects of effective procurement to control variable costs. They specified a quality standard, they eliminated unneeded cost, and they used their purchasing power to purchase a standard mix at the lowest possible cost.

Another strategy for controlling variable costs is conservation. The goal is to eliminate waste and unnecessary usage. The cardiologist who, without thinking, asks to have an extra package of balloons opened "just in case we need them" is a case in point. For example, an analysis of sutures used for total abdominal hysterectomy at Memorial Hospital in Houston, Texas indicated that 27 percent of the sutures pulled were not used.[2] By developing a conservation plan and appropriately educating physicians, the hospital reduced the rate of unutilized sutures to 8 percent, for an annual savings of $5,625 for this *one* procedure.

With both fixed and variable costs, we should be very concerned with purchasing wisely and clearly specifying the quality that we need. Once we acquire the cost, however, the prescription for utilizing fixed and variable costs is diametrically opposite. When we incur fixed costs, the goal is "use it, use it, use it," whereas with variable costs, the goal is to conserve, eliminate waste, and restrict usage to when it is really necessary.

We have discussed fixed and variable costs as though items were intrinsically in one category or the other. Often, this is not the case. Employees can be compensated on the basis of an annual salary (fixed) or on a commission or for hours worked (variable). In fact, some employees receive both forms of compensation. Similarly, rent can be fixed for a time period or taken as a percentage of sales. One of the goals of good financial management is to try to take costs in their most favorable form. For example, if you believe that you can get high volume, then it may be to your advantage to take costs such as salary and rent as fixed. If, however, you are uncertain of your volume level, then you can pass the risk to others by negotiating salary and rent as a percentage of revenues collected. Other examples of gaining efficiency by choosing how you take your costs include making local telephone calls (generally a fixed cost) instead of mailing letters (generally a variable cost) and using E-mail (generally a fixed cost) instead of making long-distance telephone calls or using U.S. mail (generally variable costs).

Finally, some items have characteristics of both fixed and variable costs. These are called mixed costs. A telephone bill often has a fixed local component and a variable long-distance component. Employee compensation may be composed of a fixed salary plus a commission based on volume. Similarly, rent can be a fixed monthly base plus a percentage of sales. Mixed costs must be broken into their fixed and variable components to control them effectively and to perform the calculations described below.

Contribution margin is defined as the excess of net revenue per unit over variable costs per unit:[3]

$$\text{Contribution margin} = \text{Net revenue per unit} - \text{Variable cost per unit}$$

For example, if a hospital collects average net revenue of $170 on a panel of outpatient diagnostic tests, and if its variable cost for consumable supplies (e.g., reagents, disposable syringes, report paper, etc.) is $20, then the contribution margin is $150. This contribution margin of $150 is not profit! Remember, we still haven't paid for the fixed costs (e.g., the building, salaries, etc.). The contribution margin can then be used to *contribute* to paying these fixed costs. Once the fixed costs are paid, then the contribution margin goes to the bottom line, meaning that it all becomes profit.

Different products and services have different margins. A flexible sigmoidoscopy generally has a higher margin than an office visit. We can see the variability of margins in all industries. In the fast food industry, the biggest margins are on soft drinks, and the margins on hamburgers are much smaller. When the order taker asks you whether you want fries and a deep-fried pie with your burger, that question is not necessarily directed at achieving a nutritionally balanced meal. The fries and the pie each add margin to your order, with no increase in fixed costs.

The portfolio of services offered by a health care organization or a practicing physician has varying margins. A health care system's outpatient chemotherapy center may have higher margins than the emergency department or maternity center. As a physician or health care system, you need to offer those services that are medically necessary. As a business, however, you need to understand *where* the margins are and be certain that the mix produces a financially acceptable outcome. For example, immunizations may have negative margins (variable cost is greater than net revenue), especially if they are administered by a physician. This is not to suggest that you should stop providing immunizations. This service, however, must be balanced somewhere else in your portfolio. Similarly, you might want to examine your portfolio of services and their margins and see how the services that are being promoted relate to their margins. Do you really want to develop a high-profile promotion campaign around a low-margin service? Correspondingly, is there something that you could do to variable costs to change a low-margin service that must be provided into one with more favorable margins?

Once we understand which costs are fixed and variable and what our contribution margin is for a service, we can make some calculations that will tell us the volume necessary to break even and the volume necessary to achieve a stated level of profitability. We will do this with a form of CVP analysis called break-even analysis:

$$\text{Break-even (in units)} = \frac{\text{Total fixed costs}}{\text{Contribution margin}}$$

For example, if a dialysis center received on average $150 for a dialysis, and variable costs averaged $40 per dialysis this would result in a contribution margin of $110 per dialysis ($150 − $40). If monthly total dialysis center fixed costs were $40,000, then the break-even point would be 363.64 patients per month ($40,000 ÷ $110). If each patient on average received 13 dialyses a month, this would mean that the facility would break even with 28 (363.64 ÷ 13) full-time equivalent (FTE) patients per month.

Conducting a break-even analysis is appropriate when you can make the following assumptions: You can determine whether a given cost is fixed or variable, and you can break mixed costs into their fixed and variable components; and there is a consistent linear relationship between costs and some measure of activity, such as the number of patients treated or the amount of revenue.

Generally, we are in business not just to break even, but to achieve a certain profit level. Target analysis allows you to state the volume level that must be achieved to achieve a net income target:

$$\text{Target volume} = \frac{\text{Fixed costs} + \text{Net income}}{\text{Contribution margin}}$$

In the above dialysis center example, if the center wished to make $10,000 of net income per month, then this would be achieved with 454 dialyses or 35 FTE (454 ÷ 13) patients:

$$\text{Target volume} = \frac{\$40,000 + \$10,000}{\$110}$$

$$= 454$$

Case: General Hospital MRI System

General Hospital is the flagship hospital in a system that includes four other hospitals.[4] Early in 1989, the staff of General Hospital was asked to evaluate a proposal to acquire a second MRI system. At the request of the hospital president, the following financial data were accumulated.

Equipment Cost and Useful Life

The estimated total cost of the installed system is $2,800,000. The expected useful life is five years, and depreciation is accounted for by recording one fifth of the system cost each year (the straight line method). Warranty coverage for equipment maintenance and repairs includes the first 2 years of operation. Repairs and maintenance costs for year 3 are projected at $248,000.

Revenue Projections

The average gross revenue per MRI scan before subtracting bad debt and contractual adjustments is expected to be $625. Based on past experience, bad debt and contractual adjustments

average 25 percent of gross revenue. Volume projections take into consideration that volume for the first year of operation will be unusually high because of an existing backlog. The estimate for the first year of operation is 2,260 MRI scans from new demand plus 940 scans from the existing backlog. After the first year, volume is projected to grow at the annual rate of approximately 15 percent. Thus, year 2 volume is projected to be 2,600 (115% × 2,260), year 3 volume is projected to be 3,000, year 4 volume is projected to be 3,450, and year 5 volume is projected to be 4,000.

Operating Costs

Supplies and film. These expenses are based on historical expense information and include film, developer, contrast media, chemicals, and other miscellaneous expenses. In year 1 the cost is estimated at $30 per MRI scan.

Salaries. Salary expense for year 1 is projected at $120,000 based on four technicians and one receptionist for 10 hours per day, 5 days per week. Additional staffing costs of $20,000 are required when the volume approaches 3,800 MRI scans. Employee benefits, including the employer's share of payroll taxes, health insurance, life insurance, and other benefits, are estimated at 25 percent of wages.

Cryogens. Cryogen expense is based on historical information. For year 1, the cost is estimated at $40,000.

Indirect expenses. Indirect expenses are allocated to the MRI facility by General Hospital. Indirect expenses are charges to the MRI facility for costs that don't directly relate to treatment, such as hospital administration, parking lot, cafeteria, and the like. The allocated indirect expenses for year 1 are $142,000.

Inflation

Based on past experience, cash operating costs, with the exception of salaries, are expected to increase at the rate of 5 percent per year. Salary costs include a provision for inflation and merit raises that are expected to total 8 percent per year.

Case Analysis: Building and Using a CVP Model

This case describes a typical situation in which physician managers may be asked to participate in making a decision that has both financial and medical implications. Without a way to organize the information, you may find the task to be confusing, if not overwhelming. Without an idea of how to use the information, you may not answer, or even ask, the important questions. The CVP model provides a way of organizing the information and provides answers to some of the most critical financial questions. To construct the model, the following data are required:

- net revenue per MRI scan
- variable cost per MRI scan
- projected volume
- total fixed costs

The model that we will build will provide a description of the cost, volume, and profit relationships within the MRI project. We can use the model to compute the break-even point, determine a safety margin, perform target analysis, and gain a better understanding of the financial risks involved.

We will begin building the model (Exhibit 6–1) by calculating net revenue. The gross fee per MRI scan is $625, which is reduced by contractual adjustments and bad debt to result in a net revenue per MRI scan of $469. Next, we identify our variable cost, which in this case is $30 per MRI scan. We then calculate the contribution margin by subtracting variable cost per scan from net revenue per scan, for a contribution margin of $439. This $439 is now available first to cover fixed costs and then, once they are paid, to contribute to net income.

Exhibit 6–1 MRI Facility CVP Analysis

1	Gross Fee per MRI Scan	$ 625
2	Less: Adjustments (25%)	156
3	Net Fee per MRI Scan	$ 469
4		
5	Variable Costs per MRI Scan	$ 30
6	Contribution Margin per MRI Scan	$ 439
7		
8	Fixed Costs	
9	Salaries	$120,000
10	Benefits	30,000
11	Cryogens	40,000
12	Indirect Expenses	142,000
13	Depreciation	560,000
14	Total Fixed Costs	$892,000
15		
16	Break-Even Calculation	
17	Units at Break-Even	2,033
18	Net Revenue	$952,991
19	Total Fixed Cost	$892,000
20	Total Variable Cost	$60,991
21	Total Cost	$952,991
22	Net Income	$0

Source: Copyright © William T. Geary, Ph.D., and Robert J. Solomon, Ph.D., used with permission.

Cells B9 through B13 in Exhibit 6–1 list the fixed costs, which total $892,000. We can now calculate the break-even point by dividing cell B14 by cell B6. If we have $439 left over after we pay the variable costs for each MRI scan, then we must conduct 2,033 scans to break even.

Exhibit 6–2 uses the CVP model that we have developed to project the outcome for the first year when we anticipate a total of 3,200 MRI scans. The projected net income (profit) is $512,000, with a safety margin or cushion above break even of 1,167 MRI scans.

Exhibit 6–3 contains a projection for the third year. We can see that fixed costs have increased as a result of salaries, benefits, and cryogens, with a large increase due to maintenance. As a result, the break-even point has increased to 2,717 MRI scans, and the safety margin is down

Exhibit 6–2 MRI Facility Year 1 Projection

Projected MRI Scans	3,200
Fee Per MRI Scan	$625
Gross Fees	$2,000,000
Less Adjustments	$500,000
Net Fees	$1,500,000
Variable Cost per MRI Scan	$30
Total Variable Cost	$96,000
Contribution Margin	$1,404,000
Fixed Costs	
Salaries	$120,000
Benefits	$30,000
Cryogens	$40,000
Indirect Expenses	$142,000
Depreciation	$560,000
Total Fixed Costs	$892,000
Projected Net Income	$512,000
Break-Even Point	2,033
Safety Margin	1,167

Source: Copyright © William T. Geary, Ph.D., and Robert J. Solomon, Ph.D., used with permission.

Exhibit 6–3 MRI Facility Year 3 Projection

Projected MRI Scans	3,000
Fee per MRI Scan	$625
Gross Fees	$1,875,000
Less Adjustments	468,750
Net Fees	$1,406,250
Variable Cost per MRI Scan	$30
Total Variable Cost	$99,225
Contribution Margin	$1,307,025
Fixed Costs	
Salaries	$139,968
Benefits	34,992
Cryogens	44,100
Indirect Expenses	156,555
Depreciation	560,000
Maintenance	248,000
Total Fixed Costs	$1,183,615
Projected Net Income	$123,410
Break-Even Point	2,717
Safety Margin	283

Source: Copyright © William T. Geary, Ph.D., and Robert J. Solomon, Ph.D., used with permission.

to 283 scans over the projected volume. At this level of operation, the projected net income will be down to $123,410.

Once this model has been built in a spreadsheet, it is then easy to do "what-if" analysis, which is also called sensitivity analysis. For example, what if increased managed care and other market factors increased the adjustment to gross fees from 25 percent to 35 percent in year 3? The answer is that projected net income would be a *negative* $64,090. In effect, we sensitize the spreadsheet to alternative scenarios and see what happens. Using our model, we can see how susceptible this project is to changes in fees, fixed costs, variable costs, and volume.

If we decide that we don't want to purchase an additional MRI machine unless we can generate $500,000 of net income per year by the third year, then we can conduct a target analysis using the formula presented above to determine that this would require conducting 3,592 MRI scans:

$$(\$1,183,615 + \$500,000) \div$$
$$(\$625 - \$156) = 3,592$$

CVP analysis and its variants break-even analysis, target analysis, and sensitivity analysis are fundamental to understanding the finances of any health care organization irrespective of its size or mission. For example, suppose a physician in a solo practice was considering enlarging his or her facility, hiring an additional secretary, and bringing on an associate. By adding the projected additional fixed costs to current fixed costs and using current variable costs to estimate the variable costs associated with the new associate's production, the physician could then project how much revenue the new associate would have to produce for the practice to break even or to reach a profit goal.

As the product mix becomes more complex, the calculations may become longer, but they remain fundamentally the same. For example, if fixed costs are common to a range of services with different contribution margins, then a weighted average variable cost must be calculated. Suppose that fixed costs for three procedures are $100,000. The procedures are provided in the ratio of 5:3:1, and their contribution margins are respectively $100, $75, and $25. The weighted average contribution margin is $[(\$100 \times 5) + (\$75 \times 3) + (\$25 \times 1)] \div 9 = \$83.33$. The break-even point would be calculated by dividing the total fixed cost of $100,000 by $83.33, or 1,200 procedures.

Once again, as a physician manager, generally you will not be performing these calculations.[5] You should, however, be examining the analyses and asking for "what-if" sensitivity analyses to understand better the financial impact of varying conditions. Your role is to *use* the financial data, along with your knowledge as a physician, to make decisions.

CAPITAL ASSET PLANNING

Capital purchasing is the process of acquiring equipment, buildings, and other items with lives

longer than one year. Examples include laboratory and diagnostic equipment, a building to locate a practice, computer equipment, a new wing to a hospital, or a new hospital. Capital asset planning methods are used to evaluate the consequences of these purchase decisions. Consistent with the focus of this book, the physician manager's goal is to anticipate these consequences before making the purchase decision.

Asset decisions are particularly important because, by definition, they often involve major expenditures with long-term commitments. Resources that are unwisely invested in one area are unavailable for opportunities in another. Because most asset decisions in health care systems have both financial and medical consequences, asset planning is an area in which physician managers can make a major contribution. Once again, the unique ability of financially skilled physicians to consider both medical and financial outcomes offers their organizations a uniquely insightful perspective. We will use three tools to evaluate the financial consequences of a capital decision: payback analysis, net present value (NPV), and internal rate of return (IRR).

Payback Analysis

This method asks the very simple and direct question: How long will it take to recover the original investment? To calculate the payback period, you must first estimate the annual net revenue flow. This is then compared with the initial capital investment to determine the year and month in which it would be repaid. If the income stream is equal over the life of the project, the calculation is easy. For example, a surgery suite that costs $800,000 to construct and is estimated to generate $200,000 of net income per year has a payback period of four years ($800,000 \div $200,000 = 4$). If the revenue stream is projected to be uneven, the calculation is somewhat more involved. For example, Exhibit 6–4 contains a payback analysis of the General Hospital MRI facility. Payback will be reached at approximately three years one month.[6]

Exhibit 6–4 MRI Facility Payback Analysis

	Projected Net Revenue	Net Payback
Year 1	$1,072,000	$1,072,000
Year 2	$787,650	$1,859,650
Year 3	$683,410	$2,543,060
Year 4	$1,078,434	$3,621,494
Estimated Capital Cost	$2,800,000	
Year 4 Revenue to Payback:	7.09%, or approximately 1 Month	
Payback Period	3 Years 1 Month	

Payback analysis is a very limited analytical tool because it does not take into account the *time value of money*. A dollar you receive a year from now is worth less to you than a dollar in hand today because the latter can earn interest during the year. In addition, payback tells you nothing about profitability.

Payback analysis is useful, however, to gain a sense of risk. If a piece of equipment has a useful life that is not much longer than it takes to pay it off, then this would indicate a high level of risk. In the MRI machine example, there appears to be about a two-year window of opportunity. Payback analysis can be useful, therefore, for a first, quick, but limited analysis of a project's financial implications.

NPV and IRR

NPV uses the time value of money concept to compare, or net, the projected financial benefits of a project against its projected financial costs. IRR is the interest rate that a project returns when financial benefits are exactly balanced by the financial costs. Because it is unlikely that two or more investment alternatives will have the same capital requirements, the IRR provides a way of comparing two otherwise disparate projects.

Both the NPV and the IRR concepts are based on the notion of present value (PV). PV is the value today of money received in the future. Money received in the future can't generate rev-

enue for you between now and then, so the PV of the sum must be *discounted* to account for the value of owning the money over time. The present value of an amount received in the future is a function of the interest rate you could earn if you could invest the money and the length of time between now and the receipt of the money.[7]

Table 6–1 is used to calculate the PV of an amount. A hand-held calculator or computer spreadsheet program can be used to do the calculations that follow. The tables are presented to help you understand how the financial numbers are derived. The columns in Table 6–1 are for various interest rates, and the rows are for various time periods. The entries in the table tell you the present value of $1.00 given the time period and the interest rate. For example, you receive an offer today for a lot you own that would net you $48,000 after transaction costs. Your cousin Phil has told you that he will buy it from you in one year for $50,000, once again, net of all costs. The land market has been flat, so you have no reason to believe that your lot will increase in value during the next year. What should you do?

Family issues aside, first you need to determine an interest rate. You look at alternatives. A one-year certificate of deposit from a bank will net you five percent. Your mutual fund has averaged 13 percent over the last five years. You feel confident that you could safely invest the money in a AAA corporate bond at 8 percent. You choose to use the 8 percent interest rate. You enter Table 6–1 in the 8 percent column and the

Table 6–1 PV Figures

Periods	6%	7%	8%	9%	10%	11%	12%
1	0.9434	0.9346	0.9259	0.9174	0.9091	0.9009	0.8929
2	0.89	0.8734	0.8573	0.8417	0.8264	0.8116	0.7972
3	0.8638	0.8163	0.7938	0.7722	0.7513	0.7312	0.7118
4	0.7921	0.7629	0.735	0.7084	0.683	0.6587	0.6355
5	0.7473	0.713	0.6806	0.6499	0.6209	0.5935	0.5674
6	0.705	0.6663	0.6302	0.5963	0.5645	0.5346	0.5066
7	0.6651	0.6227	0.5835	0.547	0.5132	0.4817	0.4523
8	0.6274	0.582	0.5403	0.5019	0.4665	0.4339	0.4039
9	0.5919	0.5439	0.5002	0.4604	0.4241	0.3909	0.3606
10	0.5584	0.5083	0.4632	0.4224	0.3855	0.3522	0.322

one year row. The factor 0.9259 indicates that $1.00 that you have to wait a year to receive is worth 92.59¢ today. Stated another way, if you invest 92.59¢ at 8 percent today, you will have $1.00 in a year. Therefore, $50,000 that you must wait a year to receive is equivalent to $46,295 today ($50,000 × 0.9259). The current $48,000 offer is worth more than the anticipated selling price in one year, so if selling price is your only consideration, you should take the current offer.

The concept of an annuity is also useful for evaluating capital investments. An annuity is a series of equal payments that are received periodically. For example, how much would you be willing to pay right now for the right to receive $1,000 cash annually for three years? Let's as-

sume that the prevailing interest rate is 10 percent. The value of this income stream would be equivalent to the PV of the stream of payments. Table 6–2 is a PV annuity table. It is used in a similar manner to the PV figures table. The columns are for various interest rates, and the rows are for the number of payments. In the example just stated, each dollar invested has a PV of 2.4869, so the $1,000 revenue stream for three years has a present value of $2,486.90. Stated another way, $2,486.90 invested today at 10 percent is equivalent to three annual payments of $1,000. An annuity calculation is a shorthand way of doing a series of PV calculations. In fact, you will notice that the entries for a single time period (the top row) are the same in both Tables 6–1 and 6–2. In effect, the PV of an amount is

Table 6–2 PV Annuities

Periods	6%	7%	8%	9%	10%	11%	12%
1	0.9434	0.9346	0.9259	0.917	0.9091	0.9009	0.8929
2	1.8334	1.808	1.7833	1.759	1.7355	1.7125	1.6901
3	2.673	2.6243	2.5771	2.531	2.4869	2.4437	2.4018
4	3.4651	3.3872	3.3121	3.24	3.1699	3.1024	3.0373
5	4.2124	4.1002	3.9927	3.89	3.7908	3.6959	3.6048
6	4.9173	4.7665	4.6229	4.486	4.3553	4.2305	4.1114
7	5.5824	5.3893	5.2064	5.033	4.8684	4.7122	4.5638
8	6.2098	5.9713	5.7466	5.535	5.3349	5.1461	4.9676
9	6.8017	6.5152	6.2469	5.995	5.759	5.537	5.3282
10	7.3601	7.0236	6.7101	6.418	6.1446	5.8892	5.6502

equivalent to a one-period annuity. In addition, the entry in Table 6–2 for any given interest rate and number of payments is equal to the sum of the entries for an equivalent number of time periods in Table 6–1. For example, the sum of the entries in Table 6–1 for four periods at 10 percent is 3.1698 (0.9091 + 0.8264 + 0.7513 + 0.6830), which is the same as the entry for a four-period annuity at 10 percent (the difference, 3.1698 versus 3.1699, is due to rounding error).

It is also possible to calculate the future value of a dollar received today. For example, suppose that you invested $10,000 today in a certificate of deposit that pays 10 percent annually for three years. A future value table provides a factor of 1.3310, so the future value of the $10,000 is equivalent to $13,310 in three years at 10 percent interest. Generally, future value calculations should *not* be used for making capital acquisition decisions because, psychologically, we tend to have difficulty judging the effects of inflation. Stated another way, you have a better sense of what a dollar is worth today than tomorrow. Therefore, the methods that we will use to evaluate capital decisions will "bring back" future financial effects into today's dollars.

Let's now use these time value of money concepts to evaluate an investment in new equipment. This equipment will require an initial investment of $30,000. You estimate that its useful life is five years and that you may then be able to resell it for $4,000. In addition, you must keep $5,000 worth of parts and supplies available to keep the machine in operation. These parts and supplies, however, can be easily resold, so when you sell the machine you can recover your parts and supplies inventory costs. Finally, you estimate that, if you purchase the machine, you will be able to generate an additional $12,000 in net revenue each year as a result of providing additional services. Is this a desirable investment from a financial perspective?

A payback analysis indicates that payback will be achieved in 2.5 years ($30,000 ÷ $12,000). Another simple analysis that does not take into account the time value of money indi-

cates that the equipment will generate $64,000 of revenue ($12,000 × 5 years plus $4,000 for the resale of the equipment) and $35,000 of costs, for a net revenue of $29,000 and a total return of 183 percent ($64,000 ÷ $35,000).

We will now use NPV and IRR to gain a better understanding of the financial consequences of this decision. Exhibit 6–5 lists the various elements of this problem as either a benefit or a cost. Some of the elements, such as the $12,000 of net revenue (gross revenue – expenses) that the machine will generate each year, are currently stated in future value terms and will have to be "brought back" to the present. Other elements, however, such as the initial capital investment of $30,000, are currently stated in PV terms.

To evaluate this investment, all the elements should first be converted into PV terms. This also has been done in Exhibit 6–5 in the "PV Equivalent" column.[8] Let's examine the benefits first. We will assume that the going interest or discount rate is 10 percent. The $12,000 annual revenue for five years has been treated as an annuity at an interest rate of 10 percent. This is the equivalent of $45,489.60 in today's dollars. The resale price of $4,000 will not be realized for five years, so this number is currently being expressed as a future value. It is necessary, therefore, to convert this into today's dollars, which is accomplished by calculating the PV of $4,000. At 10 percent interest, each dollar is worth 0.6209 of today's dollars, which equates to $2,483.60. The PV of the total benefits is, therefore, $47,973.20.

Examining the costs, the capital investment of $30,000 is already expressed as a PV because the equipment is being purchased today. The $5,000 for parts and supplies inventory is currently expressed as a PV because these must be purchased when the machine is purchased. The resale of these parts and supplies in five years when the equipment is sold is currently expressed as a future value and must, therefore, be converted into PV terms. The PV of $5,000 in five years at a discount rate of 10 percent is $3,104.50. The PV, therefore, of the total cost is

Exhibit 6–5 NPV IRR Analysis of Equipment Acquisition

	Amount	PV Equivalent
Benefits		
Net Revenue ($12,000 per year)	$60,000.00	$45,489.44
Resale of Equipment	$4,000.00	$2,483.60
Total Benefits	$64,000.00	$47,973.04
Costs		
Capital Investment	$30,000.00	$30,000.00
Parts and Supply Inventory	$5,000.00	$5,000.00
Inventory Recouped 5 Years	($5,000.00)	($3,104.50)
Total Costs	$30,000.00	$31,895.50
PV of Total Benefits	$47,973.04	
PV of Total Costs	$31,895.50	
NPV	$16,077.63	
Discount Rate	10%	
IRR	27.47%	

$31,895.50.

The NPV of this investment, $16,077.54, is defined as the PV of the total benefits ($47,973.04) minus the PV of the total costs ($31,895.50). Because the NPV is positive, this indicates that the investment will exceed the 10 percent hurdle rate. If the NPV had been negative, that would mean that the investment would not meet our 10 percent criterion.

The IRR is the discount rate at which the PV of the projected benefits is equal to the PV of the projected costs. It is calculated through trial and error by using different discount rates and observing the effect on NPV. When NPV is zero, the IRR has been found. Alternatively, computer spreadsheet programs and hand-held calculators can determine IRR using this same trial and error approach. In this example, the IRR is 27.47 percent. The IRR is useful if you are comparing this project with other projects and trying to determine which one to finance. If, for example, you had an office expansion alternative with an IRR of 20 percent, this would tell you that it would be an inferior *financial* investment compared with the project generating a 27.47 percent

IRR.

Given that you have no other projects with a more favorable IRR and the NPV of this investment is a positive number at a hurdle rate that you find acceptable, purchasing the equipment is worthy of consideration. Remember, however, that as a physician manager the financial considerations are only one aspect of your total decision-making process. For example, you might decide to purchase the equipment for ethical, convenience, or quality of care considerations even if the financial return is projected to be lower than another alternative. This thinking strikes back to one of the advantages of having physician managers involved in the decision-making process. Performing the financial analysis first will tell you what your ethics, quality, or convenience considerations would be costing you.

Next, we will apply these tools to a more complex problem by revisiting the General Hospital MRI facility case. Exhibit 6–6 contains an evaluation of the MRI facility based on expected volumes. With a discount rate of 12 percent, the NPV is $371,023.31, and the IRR is 17.33 per-

Exhibit 6–6 NPV and IRR Analysis of MRI Machine Purchase

	Year 1	Year 2	Year 3	Year 4	Year 5	Total
Volume	3,200	2,600	3,000	3,450	4,000	16,250
Average Charge	$625	$625	$625	$625	$625	$3,125
Gross Revenue	$2,000,000	$1,625,000	$1,875,000	$2,156,250	$2,500,000	$10,156,250
Less Bad Debts and Contractual Adjustment (25%)	$500,000	$406,250	$468,750	$539,063	$625,000	$2,539,063
Net Revenue	$1,500,000	$1,218,750	$1,406,250	$1,617,188	$1,875,000	$7,617,188
Less Variable Expenses						
Supplies and Film	$96,000	$81,900	$99,225	$119,814	$145,861	$542,800
Contribution Margin	$1,404,000	$1,136,850	$1,307,025	$1,497,373	$1,729,139	$7,074,388
Less Fixed Expenses						
Salaries	$120,000	$129,600	$139,968	$151,165	$183,259	$723,992
Employee Benefits	$30,000	$32,400	$34,992	$37,791	$45,815	$180,998
Cryogens	$40,000	$42,000	$44,100	$46,305	$48,620	$221,025
Indirect expenses	$142,000	$149,100	$156,555	$164,383	$172,602	$784,640
Maintenance	$0	$0	$248,000	$260,400	$273,420	$781,820
Fixed Expenses before Depreciation	$332,000	$353,100	$623,615	$660,045	$723,715	$2,692,475
Cash Generated by Operations	$1,072,000	$783,750	$683,410	$837,329	$1,005,424	$4,381,913
Less Depreciation	$560,000	$560,000	$560,000	$560,000	$560,000	$2,800,000
Net Income	$512,000	$223,750	$123,410	$277,329	$445,424	$1,581,913

Discount Rate	12%					
Cash Flows	($2,800,000)	$1,072,000	$783,750	$683,410	$837,329	$1,005,424
IRR	17.33%					
NPV	$371,023.31					
Break-Even Point		2,033	2,088	2,717	2,811	2,970

Source: Copyright © William T. Geary, Ph.D.

cent. This indicates that the project passes our hurdle of 12 percent, and that the PV of the benefits exceeds the PV of the costs by $371,023.31. Once a model like this is created on a spreadsheet, it becomes easy to test the project's sensitivity to various assumptions.

For example, an analysis at 85 percent (Exhibit 6–7) of projected volume paints a very different picture. A drop of 15 percent in volume results in a decrease of more than 41 percent ($210,600) in net income in year 1. The reason that a 15 percent volume reduction can cause a 41 percent drop in net income is that this operation has a high proportion of fixed to variable costs. Each dollar in the contribution margin is therefore very important. The NPV at the 85 percent volume level is –$368,232.58, which indicates that the costs exceed the benefits by this amount if we need to obtain a 12 percent return on our investment. In addition, the IRR is now 6.39 percent, which is the return that we will receive when benefits equal costs at the 85 percent volume level.

Finally, Exhibit 6–8 shows the analysis at 115 percent of expected volume. NPV is $1,107,442.06, with an IRR of 27.21 percent. Once again, a modest change in volume has a large impact on net income, NPV, and IRR.

After an examination of these statistics, it becomes very clear that the financial success of this project is highly dependent upon the volume level. A physician manager working on a committee considering this project should question very closely how the volume projections were derived. In addition, he or she should look at the marketing plan to see whether there is a concrete strategy to obtain the needed volume. The model could also be sensitized to other critical assumptions, such as the average charge and bad debt assumptions. We would expect that, given the sensitivity to changes in net revenue, controlling these other two variables also would be critical to the project's success. Once again, making certain that the business plan for this project made reasonable fee and collection assumptions and that there was a plan to manage these variables after project implementation would be critical to

the project's success. The physician manager who asks these questions, who ensures that reasonable assumptions are being made, and who ascertains that the business plan has taken them into account is making a very positive contribution to his or her organization.

Another capital asset decision that health care organizations often need to make is whether to purchase equipment outright or through a lease. Once again, the technique of pulling all financial considerations back to the present through a PV analysis provides a method of addressing this problem. For example, suppose that you could buy a computer for $10,000 or lease it with the following terms: an initial payment of $1,000, three annual payments of $2,500 at the end of each year, and an option to buy the computer at the end of the lease for $3,500. In addition, you feel that the value of the computer in three years will be $4,000. Under both arrangements, you will have to maintain the computer. The prevailing interest rate is 10 percent.

Exhibit 6–9 contains a PV analysis of this problem. The real cost of the lease can be determined by looking at the PV of the three annual payments, which can be treated as an annuity. The PV of a three-year annuity at 10 percent with annual payments of $2,500 is $6,217 ($2,500 × 2.4869). Assuming that you want to keep the computer at the end of the lease, the PV of the $3,500 payment is $2,630 ($3,500 × .7513). Adding the initial $1,000 payment already stated in PV terms, the total PV for the lease comes to $9,847 ($6,217 + $2,630 + $1,000). The purchase alternative costs $10,000, so that leasing the computer is $153 less expensive.

If you do not buy the computer at the end of the lease, the PV analysis in Exhibit 6-9 indicates that leasing will be $222 more expensive than purchasing. This analysis has excluded the risk of obsolescence. It is possible that in three years the computer will be worth less than $4,000. The analysis also excludes the cost and inconvenience of selling the computer. The analysis, however, could be repeated for any level of anticipated equipment value, and the

Exhibit 6–7 NPV and IRR of MRI Machine Purchase at 85 Percent of Volume

	Year 1	Year 2	Year 3	Year 4	Year 5	Total
Volume	2,720	2,210	2,550	2,933	3,400	13,813
Average Charge	$625	$625	$625	$625	$625	$3,125
Gross Revenue	$1,700,000	$1,381,250	$1,593,750	$1,832,813	$2,125,000	$8,632,813
Less Bad Debts and Contractual Adjustment (25%)	$425,000	$345,313	$398,438	$458,203	$531,250	$2,158,203
Net Revenue	$1,275,000	$1,035,938	$1,195,313	$1,374,609	$1,593,750	$6,474,609
Less Variable Expenses						
Supplies and Film	$81,600	$69,615	$84,341	$101,842	$123,982	$461,380
Contribution Margin	$1,193,400	$966,323	$1,110,971	$1,272,767	$1,469,768	$6,013,229
Less Fixed Expenses						
Salaries	$120,000	$129,600	$139,968	$151,165	$163,259	$703,992
Employee Benefits	$30,000	$32,400	$34,992	$37,791	$40,815	$175,998
Cryogens	$40,000	$42,000	$44,100	$46,305	$48,620	$221,025
Indirect expenses	$142,000	$149,100	$156,555	$164,383	$172,602	$784,640
Maintenance	$0	$0	$248,000	$260,400	$273,420	$781,820
Fixed Expenses before Depreciation	$332,000	$353,100	$623,615	$660,045	$698,715	$2,667,475
Cash Generated by Operations	$861,400	$613,223	$487,356	$612,723	$771,053	$3,345,754
Less Depreciation	$560,000	$560,000	$560,000	$560,000	$560,000	$2,800,000
Net Income	$301,400	$53,223	($72,644)	$52,723	$211,053	$545,754
Discount Rate	12%					
Cash Flows	($2,800,000)	$861,400	$613,223	$487,356	$612,723	$771,053
IRR	6.39%					
NPV	($368,232.58)					
Break-Even Point	2,033	2,088	2,717	2,811	2,912	

Source: Copyright © William T. Geary, Ph.D.

Exhibit 6–8 NPV and IRR Analysis of MRI Machine Purchase at 115 Percent of Projected Volume

	Year 1	Year 2	Year 3	Year 4	Year 5	Total
Volume	3,680	2,990	3,450	3,968	4,600	18,688
Average Charge	$625	$625	$625	$625	$625	$3,125
Gross Revenue	$2,300,000	$1,868,750	$2,156,250	$2,479,688	$2,875,000	$11,679,688
Less Bad Debts and Contractual Adjustment (25%)	$575,000	$467,188	$539,063	$619,922	$718,750	$2,919,922
Net Revenue	$1,725,000	$1,401,563	$1,617,188	$1,859,766	$2,156,250	$8,759,766
Less Variable Expenses						
Supplies and Film	$110,400	$94,185	$114,109	$137,786	$167,740	$624,220
Contribution Margin	$1,614,600	$1,307,378	$1,503,079	$1,721,979	$1,988,510	$8,135,546
Less Fixed Expenses						
Salaries	$120,000	$129,600	$139,968	$171,165	$184,859	$745,592
Employee Benefits	$30,000	$32,400	$34,992	$42,791	$46,215	$186,398
Cryogens	$40,000	$42,000	$44,100	$46,305	$48,620	$221,025
Indirect expenses	$142,000	$149,100	$156,555	$164,383	$172,602	$784,640
Maintenance	$0	$0	$248,000	$260,400	$273,420	$781,820
Fixed Expenses before Depreciation	$332,000	$353,100	$623,615	$685,045	$725,715	$2,719,475
Cash Generated by Operations	$1,282,600	$954,278	$879,464	$1,036,935	$1,262,795	$5,416,071
Less Depreciation	$560,000	$560,000	$560,000	$560,000	$560,000	$2,800,000
Net Income	$722,600	$394,278	$319,464	$476,935	$702,795	$2,616,071
Discount Rate 12%						
Cash Flows ($2,800,000)	$1,282,600	$954,278	$879,464	$1,036,935	$1,262,795	
IRR 27.21%						
NPV $1,107,442.06						
Break-Even Point	2,033	2,088	2,717	2,869	2,974	

Source: Copyright © William T. Geary, Ph.D.

Exhibit 6–9 PV Analysis of a Lease Purchase Decision

Item	Amount	Lease PV Equivalent	Purchase PV Equivalent	Difference
Purchase after Three Years				
Initial Payment	$1,000	$1,000	$10,000	
Three Annual Payments @ $2,500	$7,500	$6,217		
Purchase at End of Lease	$3,500	$2,630		
Total		$9,847	$10,000	($153)
Do Not Purchase after Three Years				
Initial Payment	$1,000	$1,000	$10,000	
Three Annual Payments @ $2,500	$7,500	$6,217		
Purchase at End of Lease	$3,500	$0		
Sell Computer	$4,000		$3,005	
Total		$7,217	$6,995	$222
Discount Rate	10%			

physician could then make a decision to lease or buy based on the subjective probability of various resale values.

FINANCIAL STATEMENTS, REPORTS, AND ACCOUNTING SYSTEMS

Three financial statements form the basis for describing the financial status of any organization, whether it is a solo private practice or a large health care system. They are the balance sheet, income statement, and cash flow statement. They provide a standard, accepted way of presenting and summarizing important and fundamental financial information. They are informative in their own right, but they can also be used as the basis for additional analyses.

The balance sheet is a listing of the organization's assets and claims against the assets at a point in time. The income statement compares the wealth generated by the organization against the expenses incurred as a result of generating that wealth during a time period. The cash flow statement describes cash receipts and cash disbursements that have occurred during a time period.

Exhibit 6–10 contains a balance sheet for a private practice as of December 31, 19XX. A balance sheet shows the financial condition of an organization on a given day, and it is based on the following financial model:

$$Assets = Liabilities + Owner's\ Equity$$

The items in Exhibit 6–10 under the heading "Assets" delineate all the wealth owned by the practice. This can be cash, office equipment, medical equipment, receivables, and the like. Generally, they are listed in order of their liquidity, or the ability to turn the asset into cash. The liabilities are a listing of the claims against the assets. Examples include accounts payable (unpaid bills), salaries owed, taxes due, and loans payable. Owner's equity is that part of the assets that exceeds the liabilities. In effect, the owner(s) own whatever is left over after creditors have been assigned their claims against the assets.

Owner's equity can occur in various ways. Retained earnings represent the earnings over the life of the organization that have not been distributed to the owners. When the organization generates earnings but keeps them in the company, perhaps in anticipation of financing additional growth, this constitutes retained earnings. Contributed capital is wealth that the owner has put into the organization in the form of cash, equipment, or some other asset. In this case,

Exhibit 6–10 Balance Sheet: Arnold Bennett, M.D., P.C.

ASSETS			
	Current Assets		
	Cash	$40,589	
	Accounts Receivable ($145,664 less allowance for participating write-offs and 10% allowance for bad debt)	$101,965	
	Marketable Securities	$3,572	
	Prepaid Expenses	$7,325	
	Inventory of Medical and Office Supplies	$3,589	
			$157,040
	Property and Equipment		
	Building and Leasehold Improvement	$109,237	
	Land	$40,896	
	Medical and Office Equipment, Office Furniture	$87,567	
	Less Accumulated Depreciation and Amortization	($23,879)	
			$213,821
	TOTAL ASSETS		$370,861
LIABILITIES			
	Current Liabilities		
	Accounts Payable	$14,897	
	Refunds Due Patients	$879	
	Commissions Due Providers	$29,875	
	Prepaid Patient Fees	$527	
	Payroll Taxes Due	$5,010	
	Commissions Due on Accounts Receivable	$61,179	
	Salaries Due Employees	$13,582	
			$125,949
	Long-Term Debt		
	Loan from Sovran for Capital Equipment	$40,500	
			$40,500
	TOTAL LIABILITIES		$166,449
OWNER'S EQUITY			
	Contributed Capital at Start-up	$20,000	
	Retained Earnings	$184,412	
	TOTAL OWNER'S EQUITY		$204,412
TOTAL LIABILITIES AND OWNER'S EQUITY			$370,861

most of the owner's equity has resulted from retained earnings ($184,412) due to operational activity, and only $20,000 is due to contributed capital. If the situation were reversed, it would provide a very different economic picture. In a private practice, retained earnings are usually distributed to the owner each year to avoid double taxation.[9]

Balance sheets always must balance. The sum of liabilities and owner's equity always must be equal to assets. Someone always has a claim against the assets, whether it is creditors or owners of the organization. If liabilities exceed assets, then there will be a negative owner's equity. A negative owner's equity would indicate that the organization is insolvent.

At this point, it is appropriate to say a few words about depreciation. Depreciation is an adjustment for capital items, such as office equipment, surgical lasers, computers, buildings, and so forth, that are consumed through their use. All capital except land wears out with use and over time. An estimate is made of an item's useful life, and its cost is depreciated on that basis. If a lithotripsy machine has an expected useful life of 6 years and costs $300,000, then we would take $50,000 ($300,000 ÷ 6) each year if we were using straight-line depreciation.[10]

If depreciation of capital equipment is not provided for, then it is possible that, when the equipment does wear out, there will not be cash available to purchase a replacement. Imagine, for example, a self-employed trucker who does not set aside cash every year for the day that his rig wears out. If this trucker makes no provision for depreciation and treats all his net income as profit available for spending, he may well be living off his depreciation. When the inevitable happens and the rig does wear out, he may not have the cash available to purchase a replacement.

Depreciation appears on the balance sheet as a negative value under assets. This indicates that the full value of assets is being reduced by the amount of the depreciation. Because the net value of assets declines, owner's equity will also decline by this amount.

Cities, such as New York in the 1970s, and countries, such as Great Britain after World War II, found themselves in the predicament of not being able to tax their citizens at a sufficiently high rate to renew their capital infrastructure and pursue all the other initiatives that were politically desirable. As a result, both these entities did to some degree live off their depreciation, which ultimately resulted in near bankruptcy for New York, along with potholed roads and crumbling bridges, and the economic decline of Great Britain.

The income statement compares the wealth generated by an organization with the expenses incurred as a result of generating the revenue. Exhibit 6–11 contains an income statement for a private practice. The income statement is built on the following financial model:

$$Income = Revenues - Expenses$$

Revenues reflect the acquisition of wealth. They can be generated by clinical service, laboratory fees, patient beds, the gift shop, consultations, or any other product or service that the organization provides. Expenses are all the costs incurred by the organization to generate those revenues. These could include clerical and professional salaries, rent, medical supplies, and so on. Net income is what is left over after expenses have been subtracted from revenues.

Both the balance sheet and the income statement are examples of *accrual basis accounting*. Accrual accounting records events when wealth is generated, as opposed to when cash is received. Similarly, it records expenses when the wealth that they are associated with is generated, as opposed to when a check is written to pay for the expense. By pairing the wealth generated with the expense of generating that wealth, it is possible to determine whether the practice, program, or hospital, is operating at a profit or loss.

This should be contrasted with cash basis accounting, in which revenues are recorded when they are received and expenses are recorded when they are paid. With cash basis accounting, there is no attempt to match revenues with the specific expenses that they generated to determine income. As a result, if cash disbursements lag or precede the collection of cash, you cannot determine your true profit or loss position.

The cash flow statement is a cash-based analysis of cash receipts and cash disbursements for a given time period. Exhibit 6–12 shows a cash flow statement. It begins in the first column with the current cash balance. Cash receipts and cash disbursements for the period are then noted,

Exhibit 6–11 Income Statement: Arnold Bennett, M.D., P.C.

January 1, 19XX To December 31, 19XX
REVENUES

Clinical Services	$1,056,825	
Bad Debt and Adjustments	($264,206)	
Consultation Fees	$12,587	
Speakers Fees	$8,655	
NET REVENUE		$805,206

EXPENSES

Clerical Salaries	$103,667	
Professional Compensation	$296,438	
Payroll Taxes	$118,575	
Rent	$48,000	
Advertising	$8,995	
Office Supplies	$37,889	
Medical Supplies	$56,551	
Interest Expense	$1,229	
Local Taxes	$4,670	
Insurance	$67,899	
Education	$8,997	
Telephone		
Fixed	$2,400	
Variable	$6,595	
Depreciation	$14,278	
TOTAL EXPENSES		$776,183

NET INCOME $29,023

and a net income for the period is calculated. This is then added to the entering cash balance to calculate an ending cash balance. This ending cash balance then becomes the entering cash balance for the next month.

The cash flow statement tracks cash, which is very important because creditors have to be paid in cash. An organization can have wealth, but if it is not present in the form of cash when the bills need to be paid, it can have a serious problem. Also, we could have two organizations with the same cash position but very different financial positions if, for example, one also had $100,000 in receivables and the other only had receivables of $10,000.

Organizations need both cash and accrual basis information. Each serves a different purpose.

Cash accounting is necessary to pay the bills. It is the financial minimum that all organizations need. Cash management is important because bills have to be paid with cash, checking accounts need to be balanced, and cash needs to be managed so that it is in the most favorable place to earn interest and be available to pay expenses.

Accrual-based accounting information is used for making decisions. It provides a more complete picture of your financial situation by controlling for when bills happen to be presented and when payments happen to be received. Both cash information and accrual information are necessary to effectively manage an organization's finances.

For example, suppose that you pay an annual liability insurance premium of $12,000 in April.

Exhibit 6–12 Cash Receipts and Disbursements

	January	February	March	Year to Date
ENTERING CASH BALANCE	$10,237.67	$49,434.44	$27,328.36	$10,237.67
CASH RECEIPTS				
Fees Collected	$60,046.06	$33,082.35	$68,746.74	$161,875.15
Interest Income	$61.49	$59.73	$48.56	$169.78
TOTAL INCOME	$60,107.55	$33,142.08	$68,795.30	$162,044.93
CASH DISBURSEMENTS				
Salaries–Management	$0.00	$6,812.22	$7,322.70	$14,134.92
Salaries–Administrative	$1,735.79	$4,016.14	$6,429.97	$12,181.90
Salaries–Physician	$7,536.15	$30,723.40	$22,976.23	$61,235.78
Temporary Help	$401.85	$619.20	$0.00	$1,021.05
Employee Benefits	$236.98	$445.70	$440.00	$1,122.68
Building Rent	$5,789.95	$7,021.41	$5,492.48	$18,303.84
Equipment Rental	$0.00	$836.74	$418.37	$1,255.11
Utilities	$447.95	$381.69	$626.91	$1,456.55
Maintenance and Repairs	$0.00	$46.25	$40.50	$86.75
Advertising	$0.00	$570.25	$407.34	$977.59
Office Overhead	$1,409.03	$656.80	$1,804.09	$3,869.92
Professional Services	$500.00	$700.00	$250.00	$1,450.00
Billing Service	$0.00	$0.00	$321.00	$321.00
Insurance	$1,060.01	$455.06	$877.99	$2,393.06
Interest	$0.00	$0.00	$0.79	$0.79
Credit Card Discounts	$30.50	$84.29	$53.53	$168.32
Bank Service Charges	$0.58	$0.39	$0.61	$1.58
Dues and Subscriptions	$97.47	$58.00	$51.47	$206.94
Auto and Travel	$0.00	$0.00	$178.00	$178.00
Meals and Entertainment	$626.49	$146.35	$318.99	$1,091.83
Taxes and Licenses	$739.03	$1,375.27	$1,969.83	$4,084.13
Fines and Penalties	$0.00	$0.00	$10.00	$10.00
Depreciation	$294.00	$294.00	$294.00	$882.00
Amortization	$5.00	$5.00	$5.00	$15.00
TOTAL DISBURSEMENTS	$20,910.78	$55,248.16	$50,289.80	$126,448.74
NET INCOME	$39,196.77	($22,106.08)	$18,505.50	$35,596.19
ENDING CASH BALANCE	$49,434.44	$27,328.36	$45,833.86	$45,833.86

You need to record the full amount in a cash disbursements journal in April because it reflects the reality that your checking account has $12,000 less in it. If, however, you are using only cash basis information, then this disbursement could be misleading. If total disbursements for April were $50,000 and total monthly receipts were $45,000, then on a cash basis you would be showing a $5,000 loss for the month.

The insurance payment, however, is an annual premium, and you are distorting the April results by allocating all the insurance expense to that month. To gain a better understanding of how the practice really performed in April, you should recognize that you really only used one twelfth of the premium ($1,000) during April. The accrual analysis found in Exhibit 6–13 indicates a net income of $6,000 as opposed to a cash basis loss of $5,000. In a similar way, the cash picture for May also would be misleading unless you make an adjustment for one twelfth of the annual insurance expense because, with cash-based accounting, you would allocate none of the annual insurance premium to May.

Both perspectives are important. You need cash accounting to be certain that the cash is available to pay the insurance premium. You need accrual information to understand the financial position of the organization and for planning purposes.

Accrual-based accounting utilizes the following adjustments that otherwise would distort the financial picture:

- *Revenue collected in advance but not yet earned (deferred revenue)*—Mr. Johnson sees you on January 23 for a sinus infection. You treat him and tell him to return in two weeks. Mr. Johnson pays a $25 copayment for today's appointment and an additional $25 copayment to cover the future visit. In this case, the cash that was collected for the future visit preceded the recognition of revenue because you have not yet provided the service. Mr. Johnson's payment for the future appointment would appear as a balance sheet liability because it is a debt or obligation that you owe to Mr. Johnson. It might appear under a category such as "Prepaid Patient Fees." This second $25.00 payment would not affect the income statement because the activity that generates the recognition of wealth (the follow-up visit) has not occurred. Both $25.00 transactions would be logged as a cash receipt in the cash flow statement, because cash was received.

Prepayment of capitated fees to cover a panel of patients for a future time period also falls into this category. Failure to treat the capitated payment in this manner could lead to disbursements of cash to physicians because cash would be available and the balance sheet would indicate retained earnings. Unfortunately, the expenses (patients coming in for services) would then follow. In addition, the fixed expenses associated with these future time periods would also become payable. The result could be that cash might not be available to cover these expenses.

- *Revenue earned but not yet collected (accrued revenue)*—When you provide services today but patients or insurance carriers pay at a future time, the moneys are recorded *now* as revenue. Revenue is recorded when you provide the service irrespective of whether the service is paid for immediately in cash, whether you extend credit in the form of a promise to pay, or whether you bill an insurance company. Some revenue will translate into future cash, and some will not (e.g., such as revenue that will be written off as bad debt or insurance company contractual adjustments). Revenue that will be paid at a future time can be listed as an asset in the form of an accounts receivable item, such as on the balance sheet in Exhibit 6–10. Notice also that this balance sheet makes a provision for bad debt and contractual write-offs.

Exhibit 6–13 Accrual and Cash Comparison

April 1–April 30	Cash Analysis	Accrual Analysis
REVENUE		
All Sources	$45,000	$45,000
EXPENSES		
Noninsurance	$38,000	$38,000
Allocated Insurance	$12,000	$1,000
Total	$50,000	$39,000
Net Income	($5,000)	$6,000

Wealth in this category will appear on the income statement under revenue. Once again, it would be appropriate to make an adjustment for expected bad debt and contractual write-offs. Items in this category would not affect the cash flow statement because no cash has been received.

- *Expenses paid in advance but not yet incurred (deferred expenses)*—Expenses that are paid in advance must be deferred to the future time periods to which they apply. These prepaid items appear as assets on the balance sheet. Prepaid expenses could include annual insurance premiums, computer service contracts, rent, and so on. Usually, you will have no choice regarding the prepayment of these items. The insurance company, for example, may want the whole annual premium now. From a cash receipts and disbursements perspective, this can create real cash flow problems. Examining this situation from an accrual perspective will not make the insurance company's "bite" any less painful. It will put it into perspective, however, so that you can see the real relationship between your assets and your liabilities and between your revenues and expenses. Obviously, from a time value of money perspective, this category of expense should be avoided.

Prepaid expenses do not affect the income statement, Once again, the activity that generates wealth, and therefore its associated expenses, has not occurred yet. Prepaid expenses *do* appear on the cash flow statement. In this case the whole prepayment is entered because that was the actual amount of cash that was disbursed.

- *Expenses incurred but not yet paid (accrued expenses)*—Expenses in this category must be recorded in the time period in which they were incurred irrespective of when you actually pay them. For example, suppose your local government assesses a 0.58 percent tax on gross receipts in arrears. Your cash analysis will show no local tax payments for 12 months and one large payment in the 13th month. Accrual-based ac-

counting, however, would allocate 0.58 percent of gross receipts to each month because you are accruing the tax and incurring the debt monthly. Once again, cash-based accounting would be deceptive, and if you had not made a provision for the tax you may incur a cash flow problem at the end of the year.[11] Accrued expenses affect both the balance sheet and the income statement. They do not affect the cash flow statement because no cash has been disbursed.

- *Allocation of the cost of long-term assets considered used up in the current period to help generate revenues*—An example is the requirement that a hospital record monthly depreciation charges (expenses) for a portion of the property, plant, and equipment that is considered to be consumed each month. The balance sheet effect is to reduce an asset account, such as capital equipment, along with retained earnings on the liability side. This item also affects the income statement, since the asset has been consumed or depreciated in value in the process of generating revenue. It does not affect the cash flow statement, because no disbursement of cash has taken place.

Case Analysis: Angus McLeod, M.D.

Angus McLeod, M.D., was perplexed.[12] "I can't figure it out," he said. "I've run my own practice for almost a year now, and I have more patients by far than I have ever had. Yet here I am, just before Christmas, and I don't have enough cash in the bank to pay for that new computer for my family. What has gone wrong?"

Dr. McLeod started his own practice on January 1, after leaving a seven-physician group psychiatric practice, where he had worked for three years. He left the group because he did not like the "politics." He took $80,000 from savings, rented office space, purchased the necessary furniture and supplies, and hired a secretary/business manager.

By midyear, his practice had grown substantially, and he hired a clinical psychologist to take his overflow. He also hired an insurance/collection clerk to deal with the volume, purchased a computer system for billing and word processing, and signed a lease for adjacent office space for the new staff. "Other than this, I don't recall any other major changes," he added. It seemed to him, however, that the better his practice became, the less cash he had in the bank.

Dr. McLeod was confident that his December work would bring in enough cash to meet the December 31 payroll. Even so, he had far less cash in the bank at the end of the year than when he started his practice. This disturbed him because, as he put it:

> I have sunk a lot into this practice—given up the security of a large group practice, and have worked day and night to make a go of it. If this isn't going to pay off, I'd like to know it soon, so that I can make other plans. Recently, for example, an HMO asked me if I would like to join them in a salaried position. I've made a lot of sacrifices in this past year, and I'd like to know whether it was all worthwhile.

A balance sheet for Dr. McLeod's practice dated 1 October 19XX is shown in Exhibit 6–14. The top row of data in the spreadsheet in Exhibit 6–15 is the same as the data in the balance sheet in Exhibit 6–14, but turned on their side so that we can use them more easily to do calculations. We will use this spreadsheet to construct a new income statement, balance sheet, and cash flow statement based on the following events that occurred in October. The numbers of the following items pertain to the items in Exhibit 6–15:

1. The total revenue generated through therapy sessions, medication evaluations, hospital rounds, and his employed psychologist is $60,000. Of this amount, $10,000 is received in cash or check, and the remainder is billed. *Effect*: We add $10,000 to the cash account and $50,000 to the receivables account. Because balance sheets always must balance, we must add $60,000 to the retained earnings account. *Notice that all the wealth is recorded at the time it was generated*, not when it happens to be converted into cash.

Exhibit 6–14 Balance Sheet: Angus McLeod, M.D.

Balance Sheet: October 1, 19XX
Assets

	Cash	$10	
	Accounts Receivable	$60,000	
	Prepaid Insurance	$1,000	
	Equipment	$24,000	
			$85,010
Liabilities			
	Accounts Payable	$2,000	
			$2,000
Owner's Equity			
	Contributed Capital	$80,000	
	Retained Earnings	$3,010	
			$83,010
Liabilities and Owner's Equity			$85,010

Exhibit 6–15 Spreadsheet Analysis: Angus McLeod, M.D.

Transactions for October, 19XX

		Assets					Liabilities			
Item	Cash	Accounts Receivable	Prepaid Insurance	Equipment	=	Accounts Payable	Contributed Capital	Retained Earnings	=
	$10	$60,000	$1,000	$24,000	$85,010	$2,000	$80,000	$3,010	$85,010
1	$10,000	$50,000						$60,000	
2	$38,000	($38,000)							
3	($6,000)		$6,000						
4	($8,000)							($8,000)	
5	($22,000)							($22,000)	
6	($8,000)			$8,000					
7	($3,000)							($3,000)	
8			($800)					($800)	
8				($500)				($500)	
9		($15,000)						($15,000)	
	$1,010	$57,000	$6,200	$31,500	$95,710	$2,000	$80,000	$13,710	$95,710

Note: Item numbers refer to description in the text.

Source: Copyright © William T. Geary, Ph.D., and Robert J. Solomon, Ph.D., used with permission.

2. $38,000 in cash is collected on old accounts. *Effect*: Add $38,000 to the cash account and subtract $38,000 from the receivables account. Notice that nothing needs to be done to the right side of the spreadsheet because the wealth was recorded at the time that it was generated.

3. Dr. McLeod pays an annual insurance premium, due 15 November, of $6,000. *Effect*: We move $6,000 from cash into prepaid insurance. Once again, nothing needs to be done to the right side of the statement because we are simply changing how we are holding wealth that has already been accounted for. Note also that none of the value of the insurance has been consumed yet.

4. $8,000 cash is paid for monthly operating expenses exclusive of salaries. *Effect*: Cash is disbursed, so the cash account is reduced by $8,000. The balance sheet must remain in balance, so retained earnings must also be reduced by $8,000. The distinction between this disbursement and the preceding one is that this time the disbursement is for items that have been consumed in this month. Retained earnings represent the wealth retained in the organization. The $8,000 cash is gone as is the value of what it purchased. Retained earnings, therefore, must be reduced by this amount.

5. Cash is paid to employees for salaries of $22,000. *Effect*: Once again, we have a disbursement for work that was fully utilized in this month, so both the cash account and the retained earnings account are reduced by $22,000.

6. $8,000 cash is paid for new computer equipment and upgrades in office furnishings. *Effect*: This transaction simply changes the form in which we are holding this wealth. As a result, we decrease the cash account by $8,000 and increase the equipment account by $8,000. Our balance sheet remains in balance.

7. Dr. McLeod pays himself $3,000 in salary for the month. *Effect*: We reduce the cash account by $3,000. Because this is a transfer of wealth outside the practice, we

must also reduce the retained earnings account by $3,000, and our balance sheet remains in balance.

8. Monthly adjustments are made of $800 for expired insurance and $500 for depreciation. *Effect:* We reduce the prepaid insurance account by $800 and the equipment account by $500 because we have consumed a month's worth of insurance and equipment life. The retained earnings account must also be reduced by these amounts because this wealth has been consumed. The balance sheet remains in balance.

9. During this month, Dr. McLeod writes off $15,000 of his outstanding receivables as uncollectable. *Effect:* Both the accounts receivable and retained earnings accounts are reduced by $15,000. The balance sheet remains in balance.

If we now examine our final spreadsheet, the bottom row constitutes our new balance sheet. We can construct an income statement for October 19XX by looking at the new revenues and expenses that have been incurred during October 19XX. This information is contained in the assets side of the spreadsheet. Finally, we can construct a cash flow statement from the cash account by noting the beginning balance, the cash transactions that occurred, and the ending balance.

A new set of financial statements is given in Exhibit 6–16. What conclusions can we draw about Dr. McLeod's practice? We can see from the cash flow statement that he is short on cash. Things are better, however, than they were at the beginning of the month. The income statement tells us that he had a very good month for generating wealth. Unfortunately, much of the wealth is not in cash but in receivables. The balance sheet tells us that his assets are largely in receivables and equipment. In addition, the retained earnings are largely due to his original investment, not economic growth. The last month, however, has seen his retained earnings due to economic growth increase by $10,700. This is hopeful.

In summary, Dr. McLeod has put the pieces in place to generate wealth. The question now is whether he can convert the wealth that exists in his receivables and equipment into cash. The cash picture is not rosy. He must manage his cash very carefully, stop all spending on equipment unless it is absolutely essential, perhaps use leasing, and motivate his staff to collect on the accounts effectively.

This case illustrates how financial information can help describe the financial status of an organization. It also illustrates how financial information can be used to guide management decision making. The financial data from the balance sheet, income statement, and cash flow statement tell Dr. McLeod where he needs to focus his attention in his management capacity as a physician manager. Finally, they also provide him with some insight into his decision about the HMO offer. This practice clearly needs management attention, specifically Dr. McLeod's attention. If he decides that the management part of being a physician manager is not for him, then he probably will be best off to accept the HMO's offer.

The use of financial information to aid in making management decisions is further illustrated by the case of Oregon Sports Medicine, which is discussed at the end of this chapter.

Ratio Analysis

Data from the balance sheet and the income statement can be used to assess an organization's liquidity, solvency, and profitability by constructing ratios. Ratios can also be used to help examine an organization's financial performance over time and observe developing financial trends.

Liquidity is the ability to use assets to meet currently maturing debts. Tests of liquidity evaluate the degree to which an organization's current liabilities can be met using its current assets. Current liabilities are defined as obligations or services that a practice owes or will have to fulfill within the next year. Examples include wages payable, income taxes payable, and credit

Exhibit 6–16 October 19XX Financial Statement: Angus McLeod, M.D.

Balance Sheet: October 31, 19XX

Assets

Cash	$1,010	
Accounts Receivable	$57,000	
Prepaid Insurance	$6,200	
Equipment	$31,500	
		$95,710

Liabilities

Accounts Payable	$2,000	
		$2,000

Owner's Equity

Contributed Capital	$80,000	
Retained Earnings	$13,710	
		$93,710
Liabilities and Owner's Equity		$95,710

Income Statement: October 1–31, 19XX

Revenues

Cash	$10,000.00	
Receivables	$50,000.00	
		$60,000.00

Expenses

Operating	$8,000.00	
Salaries	$22,000.00	
His Salary	$3,000.00	
Insurance	$800.00	
Depreciation	$500.00	
Bad Debts and Write-Offs	$15,000.00	
		$49,300.00
Net Income		$10,700.00

Cash Flow Statement: October 1–31, 19XX

Opening Balance		$10
Cash Received	$10,000	
Cash Collected on Account	$38,000	
Insurance Premium	($6,000)	
Operating Expenses	($8,000)	
Employee Salaries	($22,000)	
Computer, Etc.	($8,000)	
His Salary	($3,000)	
Closing Balance		$1,010

card balances. Current assets are resources owned by the organization that are currently in cash form or could be converted into cash within the next year. Examples include cash savings, shares in publicly traded common stock, and a reasonable (defined as likely to be collected) proportion of accounts receivable. Examples of ratio analyses will use the balance sheet (Exhibit

6–10) and income statement (Exhibit 6–11) for Dr. Arnold Bennett's practice.

Liquidity Ratios

A commonly used test of liquidity is called the current ratio, which is defined as follows:

Current ratio = Current assets ÷ Current liabilities

Referring to the data in Exhibit 6–10, the current ratio for Dr. Bennett's practice is:

Current ratio = $157,040 ÷ $125,949 = 1.25

This indicates that Dr. Bennett has $1.25 of current assets for each dollar of current liabilities. Stated another way, this indicates that Dr. Bennett has a 25 percent "cushion" to deal with his liabilities. This cushion is helpful given that cash may flow unevenly into his practice. If Dr. Bennett's current ratio was 2.00 at this time last year, then he should consider investigating the change.

A more demanding test of a practice's liquidity is called the quick ratio or the acid test ratio:

Quick ratio = Quick assets ÷ Current liabilities

Quick assets are cash or other current assets that can be easily converted into cash, such as stocks, bonds, certificates of deposit, and accounts receivable. Dr. Bennett's quick ratio is as follows:

Quick ratio = $146,126 ÷ $125,949 = 1.16

All Dr. Bennett's current assets, except his inventory and prepaid expenses, are considered quick assets because they could be readily converted into cash. Dr. Bennett's quick ratio indicates that his practice has $1.16 worth of readily available assets for each dollar of current debt.

An additional perspective on liquidity is gained by considering how quickly a practice's receivables are turned into cash. An index of this can be calculated by examining the average daily billings and the average collection period, which are defined as follows:

Average daily billings = Net billings ÷ 365 days

Average collection period = Accounts receivable ÷ Average daily billings

By using the data in Exhibits 6–10 and 6-11, we can calculate these ratios for Dr. Bennett's practice:

Average daily billings = $792,619 ÷ 365 = $2,172

Average collection period = $101,965 ÷ $2,171 = 47 days

This indicates that, on average, Dr. Bennett collects his receivables in 47 days. This figure can be used in two ways. First, it can help determine whether the collection performance is acceptable. What is required is a qualitative evaluation in which Dr. Bennett examines the 47-day average in the context of his revenue sources. If, for example, he does a large amount of insurance work, then an average collection period of 47 days might indicate acceptable effectiveness. On the other hand, if a large proportion of Dr. Bennett's patients are capitated, or are supposed to pay at the time of service, then 47 days might indicate a collection problem.

A second use of the average collection period ratio is as a gauge of liquidity over time. By tracking this ratio over the years, Dr. Bennett can assess how his practice's liquidity is changing and examine whether changes in his clientele, the services he provides, insurance company policies and procedures, HMO participation, capitation participation, and so on may be affecting its liquidity.

Solvency Ratios

An organization's solvency is its ability to meet its debt obligations. A common statistic used to assess solvency is the debt-to-equity ratio (DER). The data used to compute the DER are contained in the balance sheet (Exhibit 6–10). The ratio is computed as follows:

DER = Total liabilities ÷ Owner's equity

Both current and long-term practice liabilities are included in this ratio. Dr. Bennett's DER is as follows:

$$DER = \$166,449 \div \$204,412 = 0.81$$

This means that, for every dollar of equity owned by Dr. Bennett, there are 81¢ worth of liabilities. The use of debt may involve risk because interest will have to be paid on some of it, and eventually the principal must be repaid. Typically, young organizations have high DERs because large capital expenditures are required for equipment, and revenue levels are relatively low at start-up.

Profitability Ratios

Return on owner's investment (ROI_o) is a measure of an organization's profitability. It indicates how well the owner's equity is being used to generate income. Stated another way, the equity that an organization has could be "cashed in" and invested in other ways, such as in treasury bills or the stock market. Given that this money is invested in your organization (practice, hospital, etc.), what return are you receiving on this investment? In a sense, evaluating your profitability involves taking off your physician's hat and looking at your organization as a stockholder. Are your investment funds being well used? Return on owner's investment is calculated using the following formula:

$$ROI_o = \text{Pretax income} \div \text{Owner's equity} =$$
$$\$29,023 \div \$204,412 = 14.2\%$$

It is important to remember, when examining Dr. Bennett's return on investment, that his salary and his net income are inversely related. If Dr. Bennett increases his salary, then the net income of his practice will decline. To evaluate the profitability of a practice as a *business*, a fair market rate must be paid to the physician/owner for professional and administrative services. Looking at it another way, Dr. Bennett wears two hats. Wearing one hat, he is an employee-physician-administrator; wearing the other, he is a stockholder-investor. To evaluate his success as a stockholder-investor, he must compensate himself fairly as an employee, just as he would fairly compensate any other employee who would perform the same administrative and medical duties with the same level of competence. Dr. Bennett's return on investment of 14.2 percent is meaningful only to the extent that his compensation as an employee-physician-administrator is equitable.[13]

Another way of assessing profitability is to examine the relationship between total assets and the income used to generate them. This ratio is called return on total investment (ROI_t) and is defined as follows:

$$ROI_t = (\text{Pretax income} + \text{Interest expense}) \div$$
$$\text{Total assets}$$

Dr. Bennett's return on total investment is:

$$ROI_t = (\$29,023 + \$1,229) \div \$370,861 = 0.082$$

Stated another way, Dr. Bennett's practice earned 8.2 percent on the total resources that it used during the year. Conceptualized in this manner, investment is defined as the total resources provided by both the owner(s) and the creditors.

Another gauge of profitability is the profit margin. The profit margin is defined as follows:

$$\text{Profit margin} = \text{Net income} \div \text{Total net revenue}$$

Dr. Bennett's profit margin is as follows:

$$\text{Profit margin} = \$29,023 \div \$805,206 = 0.036$$

This says, in effect, that for each dollar of service provided by Dr. Bennett's practice, the practice makes an average of 3.6¢ profit. It is important to remember when evaluating the profit margin that this statistic does not take into account the amount of resources invested to generate this profit. Obviously, a practice that has a 3.6 percent profit margin but has required only a $20,000 investment is in one sense performing better than a practice that has the same profit margin but has required a $60,000 investment. Profit margin is a part of the profitability picture, but because it omits the very important investment component, it should be considered in conjunction with return on investment statistics.

Summary

After examining the above ratios, you may well be wondering how to use them. Ratios are useful as screening devices to highlight possible problems and strengths. They are particularly useful for making internal comparisons over time. If you notice, for example, that your profit margin has declined from the previous year, this should stimulate you to investigate why this happened. Have expenses risen without an adjustment to fees? Is your product mix changing so that you are conducting a greater proportion of lower-profit procedures? Is this a result of taking more managed care contracts? Correspondingly, is this a result of losing market share as a consequence of bidding unsuccessfully on managed care contracts?

If you find that your quick ratio is more favorable this year than it was last year, then you might give yourself a pat on the back. On the other hand, perhaps your quick ratio is too high! You might conclude that you could be investing your funds in other, more profitable ways, which might make the funds less liquid and could reduce your quick ratio.

Ratios, therefore, are useful tools for stimulating thinking. They do not provide answers by themselves. Instead, they allow you to focus and direct your inquiries.

CONTROL AND BUDGETING

Control is the process of measuring, evaluating, and correcting actual performance to ensure that goals and plans are accomplished.[14] The control issues that will affect a physician manager will vary depending upon the physician manager's job description. Physician managers working in larger health care organizations will be working on control issues in response to plans and budgets. For example, the financial analysis of the MRI scanner acquisition decision can be used as a basis to generate a budget and evaluate subsequent performance against that budget. Based upon how results compare with projections, the MRI project could be modified to bet-

ter achieve target net income, NPV, and IRR goals.

Physician managers working in smaller organizations, such as solo and small group practices, similarly will use plans and budgets to implement controls. In addition, they will also be interested in cash control to deter theft and to be certain that office operations are complying with practice policy and guidelines.

Using a Postacquisition Analysis To Achieve Control

We will revisit the General Hospital MRI facility case to demonstrate how the financial projections already discussed can be used as the basis of a control process for the project. Exhibit 6–17 contains a postacquisition analysis performed one year after the new MRI machine was put into operation. The data in Exhibit 6–17 indicate that net income is 5.76 percent above projections. Examination of the volume level, however, provides some disturbing information. Volume was 242 (7.56 percent) MRI scans lower than expected. Fortunately, the average gross charge had a favorable variance of $115, or 18.40 percent above expectations. The collection rate was 28 percent ($612,898 ÷ $2,188,920) versus a projected 25 percent. Variable costs were expected to average $30 per MRI scan, but actually were more than $41 ($121,870 ÷ 2,958) per scan. Fixed costs were about what was expected.

The fact that the volume estimates were below expectations is very disturbing because our previous analyses have demonstrated the high volume sensitivity of this project. In addition, the unfavorable variable cost variance compounds the problem for a volume-sensitive project. As a result of the first-year experience, the projections for years 2 through 5 were revised. The primary changes are a reduced volume level and an increased variable cost to $40 per MRI scan, plus inflation. The effects of these changes on NPV and IRR are disconcerting. NPV is now negative, which means that we will miss our 12 percent profit goal by $355,534. The IRR is now at 5.98 percent.

Exhibit 6–17 MRI Facility Postacquisition Analysis after Year 1

Executive Summary*
A postacquisition analysis was performed for MRI system 2 for the year ended 30 June 1991, after the first year of service. Net income exceeded projections for year 1 by $29,514, and cash generated by operations exceeded plan by $47,514. Volume, however, was 242 MRI scans fewer than projected. Downward revisions for years 2 through 5 result in a corresponding downward revision of the internal rate of return to approximately 6 percent.

GENERAL HOSPITAL
MR Imaging System 2
POSTACQUISITION ANALYSIS for the year ended June 30, 1991

	Actual Year 1	Projected Year 1	Fav Var (Unfav Var)	% Change
Volume	2,958	3,200	−242	−7.56%
Average Charge	$740	$625	$115	18.40%
Gross Revenue	$2,188,920	$2,000,000	$188,920	9.45%
Less Bad Debts and Contractual Adjustment (25%)	$612,898	$500,000	($112,898)	−22.58%
Net Revenue	$1,576,022	$1,500,000	$76,022	5.07%
Less Variable Expenses				
Supplies and Film	$121,870	$96,000	($25,870)	−26.95%
Contribution Margin	$1,454,153	$1,404,000	$50,153	3.57%
Less Fixed Expenses				
Salaries	$121,300	$120,000	($1,300)	−1.08%
Employee Benefits	$33,964	$30,000	($3,964)	−13.21%
Cryogens	$40,825	$40,000	($825)	−2.06%
Indirect expenses	$138,550	$142,000	$3,450	2.43%
Maintenance	$0	$0	$0	
Fixed Expenses before Depreciation	$334,639	$332,000	($2,639)	−0.79%
Cash Generated by Operations	$1,119,514	$1,072,000	$47,514	4.43%
Less Depreciation	$578,000	$560,000	($18,000)	−3.21%
Net Income	$541,514	$512,000	$29,514	5.76%

Revised Projections

	Year 1-Act.	Year 2-Proj.	Year 3-Proj.	Year 4-Proj.	Year 5-Proj.
Volume	2,958	2,200	2,420	2,662	2,928
Average Charge	$740	$740	$650	$625	$625
% Collectible	72.00%	75.00%	75.00%	75.00%	75.00%

continues

Exhibit 6–17 continued

Net Revenue		$1,576,022	$1,221,000	$1,179,750	$1,247,813	$1,372,594
Variable Costs		$121,870	$92,400	$106,722	$123,264	$142,370
Fixed Costs before Depreciation		$334,639	$353,100	$623,615	$660,045	$698,715
Cash Generated by Operations		$1,119,514	$775,500	$449,413	$464,504	$531,509
Discount Rate	12.00%					
Cash Flows	($2,890,000)	$1,119,514	$775,500	$449,413	$464,504	$531,509
IRR	5.98%					
NPV	($355,534)					

Notes To Accompany the First Analysis

1. The cost to acquire and install the equipment was $90,000 more than plan (total cost, $2,890,000). This results in an increase in the annual depreciation charge of $18,000.
2. The rate of growth in volume projections for years 3 through 5 has been revised downward from 15 percent to 10 percent.
3. Projected average charges reflect recent experiences and current expectations. For the year ended 30 June 1991, the bad debt and contractual adjustment were 28 percent of gross revenue.
4. Variable costs for supplies and film averaged $41.20 during the year ended 30 June 1991.

*This case written by William T. Geary, PhD.

Source: Copyright © William T. Geary, Ph.D.

At this point, management has the opportunity to change this unfavorable outcome. The postacquisition analysis has pointed out where the problem areas are and indicates where management must make changes to turn this project around.

A second postacquisition analysis was conducted after the second year of operation (Exhibit 6–18). It contains more bad news. The volume of 1,909 MRI scans was, once again, below the original projection of 2,600 scans and also below the revised projection of 2,200 scans. Average variable cost has risen again. Fixed costs are almost 30 percent above expectations, due largely to cryogens, which were 293 percent above expectations. The impact on NPV is dramatic. Given the desire for a 12 percent return, we project that we will miss this mark by $737,294. The IRR is a dismal 0.83 percent.

We might also note that the project now has been extended out to seven years. If we retained the original five-year payback, the projected NPV would be under the target 12 percent return by $1,057,134.84, with a *negative* IRR of 10.07 percent. Over five years the MRI facility is projected to generate net cash of $2,293,306 versus the initial projection of $4,381,913 (Exhibit 6–6). Once again, we can see the volume sensitivity of this project.

At this point management has another opportunity to intervene. One major problem is volume. Devoting more marketing resources and restructuring management positions to emphasize critical parts of the marketing mix (Chapter 9) are options that could increase MRI volume. A second major problem is cost control. Fixed costs are 30 percent above expectations by year 2. Since volume is down, there should be excess capacity, and management needs to think creatively of ways to reduce fixed costs. One strategy would be to try to convert some to variable costs. Perhaps there are some positions that could be changed from full-time to part-time on-

Exhibit 6–18 MRI Facility Postacquisition Analysis after Year 2

GENERAL HOSPITAL
MRI System 2
POSTACQUISITION ANALYSIS for the year ended June 30, 1992

	Actual Year 1	Projected Year 1	Fav Var (Unfav Var)	% Change	Actual Year 2	Projected Year 2	Fav Var (Unfav Var)	% Change
Volume	2,958	3,200	–242	–7.56%	1,909	2,600	–691	–26.58%
Average Charge	$740	$625	$115	18.40%	$810	$625	$185	29.60%
Gross Revenue	$2,188,920	$2,000,000	$188,920	9.45%	$1,546,290	$1,625,000	($78,710)	–4.84%
Less Bad Debts and Contractual Adjustment	$612,898	$500,000	($112,898)	–22.58%	$448,424	$406,250	($42,174)	–10.38%
Net Revenue	$1,576,022	$1,500,000	$76,022	5.07%	$1,097,866	$1,218,750	($120,884)	–9.92%
Less Variable Expenses Supplies and Film	$121,870	$96,000	($25,870)	–26.95%	$82,278	$81,900	($378)	–0.46%
Contribution Margin	$1,454,153	$1,404,000	$50,153	3.57%	$1,015,588	$1,136,850	($121,262)	–10.67%
Less Fixed Expenses								
Salaries	$121,300	$120,000	($1,300)	–1.08%	$118,700	$129,600	$10,900	8.41%
Employee Benefits	$33,964	$30,000	($3,964)	–13.21%	$33,236	$32,400	($836)	–2.58%
Cryogens	$40,825	$40,000	($825)	–2.06%	$165,231	$42,000	($123,231)	–293.41%
Indirect Expenses	$138,550	$142,000	$3,450	2.43%	$141,650	$149,100	$7,450	5.00%
Maintenance	$0	$0	$0		$0	$0	$0	
Fixed Expenses before Depreciation	$334,639	$332,000	($2,639)	–0.79%	$458,817	$353,100	($105,717)	–29.94%
Cash Generated by Operations	$1,119,514	$1,072,000	$47,514	4.43%	$556,771	$783,750	($226,979)	–28.96%

continues

Exhibit 6-18 continued

Less Depreciation	$578,000	$560,000	($18,000)	-3.21%	$578,000	$560,000	($18,000)	-3.21%
Net Income	$541,514	$512,000	$29,514	5.76%	($21,229)	$223,750	($244,979)	-109.49%

Revised Projections

	Year 1-Act.	Year 2-Act.	Year 3-Proj.	Year 4-Proj.	Year 5-Proj.	Year 6-Proj.	Year 7-Proj.
Volume	2,958	1,909	2,100	2,310	2,541	2,795	3,074
Average Charge	$740	$810	$650	$625	$625	$625	$625
% Collectible	72.00%	71.00%	75.00%	75.00%	75.00%	75.00%	75.00%
Net Revenue	$1,576,022	$1,097,866	$1,023,701	$1,082,761	$1,191,037	$1,310,141	$1,441,155
Variable Costs	$121,870	$82,278	$92,606	$106,959	$123,538	$142,687	$164,803
Fixed Expenses before Depreciation	$334,639	$458,817	$748,615	$785,045	$823,715	$864,901	$908,146
Cash Generated by Operations	$1,119,514	$556,771	$182,481	$190,756	$243,784	$302,553	$368,206
Discount Rate	12.00%						
Cash Flows	($2,890,000) $1,119,514	$556,771	$182,481	$190,756	$243,784	$302,553	$368,206
IRR, 7 Years	0.83%						
NPV, 7 Years	($737,294)						
NPV, 5 Years	($1,057,134.84)						
IRR, 5 Years	-10.07						

Notes To Accompany the Second Postacquisition Analysis

1. Growth in volume for years 4 through 7 is projected at the rate of 10 percent.

2. Projected average charges reflect recent experiences and current expectations. The bad debt and contractual adjustment for the year ended 30 June 1992 was 29 percent of gross revenue.

3. Variable costs for supplies and film averaged $43.10 during the year ended 30 June 1992.

4. Fixed costs included in the projections for years 3 through 7 include an annual increase of $125,000 to reflect the expected increase in costs associated with meeting refrigeration requirements (cryogens). Fixed costs in years 6 and 7 are based on year 5, with an adjustment of 5 percent for inflation.

5. The useful life of the project was extended from 5 years to 7 years.

Source: Copyright © William T. Geary, Ph.D.

call. The major fixed cost variance has been cryogens. Greater efficiency in purchasing has to be examined. Perhaps General Hospital can form a purchasing alliance with other hospitals to gain purchasing power and a lower price.

The sudden rise in the cost of cryogens was largely due to federal regulation of ozone-depleting chemicals. One must question why this somewhat predictable event was not considered in the original financial analysis. It turns out that radiologists, who might well have been more aware of this issue, were not an integral part of the original financial analysis. This illustrates the importance of having financially literate physicians fully involved in the decision-making process.

Using Budgets for Financial Control

A budget is simply a formal statement of your financial plans for a specific time period. It is a statement about what should happen financially to your practice or health care organization. You can then compare actual events with the budget to see whether you are behind, matching, or exceeding your expectations. Often, budgets are viewed as constraints. Viewed more positively, however, they can be an important part of a control process to identify when the unexpected has occurred and how to deal with it.

Budgets are not essential to the operation of a small medical practice. They are a step above the minimum financial cash accounting methods that often characterize small private practices. Budgets, however, can be important for even a small practice if it must demonstrate a degree of financial planning so that a lending institution will lend you money.

The sophistication that budgets can add to the process of identifying financial problems early enough to take effective action must be balanced against the time that they take to construct and utilize. Budgeting is very consistent, however, with the notion that as a physician manager you are a consumer of accounting information and will use it to plan and make management deci-

sions. Budgets are most useful when they stimulate you to think ahead, anticipate future conditions, prepare for them, and take action if things are not going according to plan. Budgets are universally used in larger health care organizations.

Budgets can be established for virtually any quantifiable issue, including cash receipts and disbursements, procedures, DRGs, revenues, and expenses. Some organizations may find the budgeting process useful for tackling very specific financial problems. For example, if an evaluation of office supply expenses indicates substantial waste, then budgeting for office supplies and closely following up on variances would be an effective cost control procedure. Similarly, other expense or revenue items can be selectively targeted and brought into line through the budgeting process.

Let's examine how a budget could be used to help manage a group practice. Dr. Brandon Jones has two colleagues. He is undertaking the budgeting process because he expects that his practice will be growing. He wants to plan for this growth so that it takes place in an orderly, efficient manner. As a result, he has decided to construct a budget for the next three months.

Because many costs vary with the activity level of a business, the budgeting process often begins with the development of an index of sales. Dr. Jones asked his two colleagues to estimate the number of procedures that they would conduct and their revenues for each of the next three months. The physicians' revenue forecasts are shown in Exhibit 6–19.

Next, Dr. Jones projected the following expenses:

- Rent, interest, and insurance expenses were fixed, so he simply carried over the monthly amounts from the previous year.
- Clerical salaries would remain the same for the first three months because all performance appraisals and probable pay raises should occur in the second half of the year.
- Professional compensation would remain proportionally the same, so Dr. Jones took the percentage of revenue paid to physi-

Exhibit 6–19 Static Budget: Dr. Jones

	Budget Jan. - Mar.	Actual	Variance	Direction
REVENUES				
Dr. Jones	$100,000	$95,468	($4,532)	U
Dr. Warren	$80,000	$85,684	$5,684	F
Dr. Stewart	$90,000	$75,698	($14,302)	U
Total Clinical	$270,000	$256,850	($13,150)	
Consultation Fees	$1,000	$1,000	$0	
Speakers Fees	$500	$500	$0	
Total	$271,500	$258,350	($13,150)	U
EXPENSES				
Clerical Salaries	$39,057	$39,057	$0	
Professional Compensation	$118,800	$113,674	($5,126)	F
Payroll Taxes	$14,207	$13,746	($461)	F
Rent	$12,000	$12,000	$0	
Advertising	$2,249	$2,732	$483	U
Office Supplies	$10,500	$9,375	($1,125)	F
Medical Supplies	$14,138	$13,903	($235)	F
Interest Expense	$307	$307	$0	
Local Taxes	$1,575	$1,498	($76)	F
Insurance	$16,975	$17,250	$275	U
Education	$2,249	$2,800	$551	U
Telephone				
Local	$471	$471	$0	
Long Distance	$849	$785	($64)	F
Cellular	$929	$929	$0	
Total	$234,305	$228,527	($5,778)	F
NET INCOME	$37,195	$29,823	($7,372)	U

cians in the previous year and multiplied the projected net revenue by this percentage.

- Payroll taxes would remain proportional to compensation.
- Dr. Jones reviewed the expenditures for office supplies for the previous year with the practice business manager. He concluded that supplies were not being wasted. He assumed that supplies would be used at the same rate as last year, so he budgeted for 25 percent (three months) of the previous annual supply expenditure. If he thought that there had been waste, he could have used the budget to try to reduce the utilization of supplies by budgeting at a level below the previous year's expenditures.

- Education expenses were calculated by estimating the amount Dr. Jones and his colleagues were likely to spend at the conferences they were planning to attend during the three-month period.
- Telephone expenses were fairly consistent across the previous year, and Dr. Jones saw no reason for there to be a change. In addition, he reviewed the long-distance charges and determined that they were reasonable. As a result, he budgeted 25 percent of last year's telephone bill for each month.
- Advertising consisted of two display ads each month in the "Science and Medicine" section of the daily newspaper plus Yellow Pages listings. Dr. Jones planned to continue this practice for the next three months.

These known fixed costs were entered in the budget.

- All other expenditure categories were entered into the budget at the rate of 25 percent of the previous year expenditure.

The "Actual" column in Exhibit 6–19 is a performance report comparing first quarter revenues and expenses with the budgeted amounts. Favorable variances occur when actual costs are less than budgeted costs, whereas unfavorable variances occur when actual costs exceed budgeted costs.

The data indicate that the practice had lower net income than had been planned for the first quarter. Fortunately, total expenses were also lower than the budget. Advertising, insurance, and education had unfavorable variances. They were compensated for, however, by favorable variances in professional compensation (although Dr. Jones might not take pleasure in this "favorable" variance), office supplies, medical supplies, payroll taxes, and long-distance telephone calls.

Dr. Jones could now use the performance report to examine the causes of this situation. After talking with Dr. Stewart, Dr. Jones determined that his variance was due to a faulty revenue estimate. Examination of the unfavorable variances in advertising and education both revealed acceptable but costly explanations. The advertising variance resulted from a display ad in a local newspaper during a local high blood pressure awareness week. Dr. Jones felt, after a review, that advertising in this edition of the paper was well justified. The education variance was explained by Dr. Warren exceeding his budgeted education amount. Dr. Jones concluded that Dr. Warren's actual expenditures were questionable.

Dr. Jones may encounter some difficulties, however, in evaluating some of the other variances. For example, office supplies and medical supplies both show favorable variances. The practice's activity level, however, was below expectations, so it really isn't clear whether the lower utilization of office and medical supplies was due to treating fewer patients or to more efficient operations. Unfortunately, such questions cannot be easily answered with the static budget used by Dr. Jones. They *can* be addressed, however, with a flexible budget.

A flexible budget utilizes a budget formula to express the relationship between variable costs and an index of the activity level, such as revenue or number of procedures. Flexible budgets adjust to reflect the *actual* volume as opposed to the *projected* or budgeted volume. Based on the previous year's data, Dr. Jones expected that the following budget items would vary with physician revenues:

- professional compensation, because Dr. Jones and his colleagues pay themselves a percentage of the revenues
- payroll taxes, because these are a function of professional and clerical compensation
- office and medical supplies, because their consumption should vary with the practice's activity level
- local taxes and licenses, because these are a direct function of the amount of revenue
- long-distance telephone calls, because these should be related to patient activity

Dr. Jones determined the flexible budget amounts by examining the relationship between these variables and clinical revenue for the previous year. Each dollar of clinical service revenue resulted in the generation of 44.0¢ of professional compensation expense, 9.0¢ of payroll tax expense, 3.8¢ of office supply expense, 5.2¢ of medical supply expense, and so forth. These relationships are indicated in the "Flexible Formula" column in Exhibit 6–20. Items that do not vary with the level of practice activity are labeled *fixed* in this column. The budgeted amounts for these fixed items are the same as in the static budget (Exhibit 6–19). Flexible budgets, therefore, adjust to changes in revenues and variable costs while allowing fixed costs to remain static over the relevant range.

Differences between flexible budgets and static budgets are due to variance in activity

Exhibit 6–20 Flexible Budget: Dr. Jones

	Static Budget Jan. - Mar.	Actual	Static Budget Variance	Flexible Formula	Flexible Budget	Flexible Variance	Flexible Direction
REVENUES							
Dr. Jones	$100,000	$95,468	($4,532)			($4,532)	U
Dr. Warren	$80,000	$85,684	$5,684			$5,684	F
Dr. Stewart	$90,000	$75,698	($14,302)			($14,302)	U
Total Clinical	$270,000	$256,850	($13,150)			($13,150)	U
Consultation Fees	$1,000	$1,000	$0			$0	
Speakers Fees	$500	$500	$0			$0	
Total	$271,500	$258,350	($13,150)			($13,150)	U
EXPENSES							
Clerical Salaries	$39,057	$39,057	$0	Fixed			
Prof. Compensation	$118,800	$113,674	($5,126)	44% × Total Rev.	$113,674	$0	
Payroll Taxes	$14,207	$13,746	($461)	9% × Total Comp.	$13,746	$0	
Rent	$12,000	$12,000	$0	Fixed			
Advertising	$2,249	$2,732	$483	Fixed			
Office Supplies	$10,500	$9,375	($1,125)	3.8% × Total Rev.	$9,817	($442)	F
Medical Supplies	$14,138	$13,903	($235)	5.2% × Clin. Rev.	$13,356	$547	U
Interest Expense	$307	$307	$0	Fixed			
Local Taxes	$1,575	$1,498	($76)	0.58% × Total Rev.	$1,498	$0	
Insurance	$16,975	$17,250	$275	Fixed			
Education	$2,249	$2,800	$551	Fixed			
Telephone			$0				
Local	$471	$471		Fixed			
Long Distance	$849	$785	($64)	0.3% × Clin. Rev.	$771	$14	U
Cellular	$929	$929	$0	Fixed			
Total Fixed	$74,237	$75,546	$1,309				
Total Variable	$160,069	$152,981	($7,087)		$152,862	$119	U
Total	$234,305	$228,527	($5,778)				
NET INCOME	$37,195	$29,823	($7,372)				

level and are, therefore, an index of effectiveness. Differences between flexible budgets and actual results are due to efficiency, if the amount of inputs used for a given level of output is less than expected, and price variance, if the cost or price of a unit of service differs from that expressed in the flexible budget formula.

The relationship between effectiveness and efficiency is important to understand. For example, you may have an objective of generating $30,000 in revenues in a month. You only generate $25,000, but you do this with the inputs specified in the flexible budget. Your production has been ineffective, but it has also been efficient. Alternatively, you could have a $30,000 revenue month but have unfavorable variances on several flexible budget items, in which case you have been effective but inefficient in those areas.

After examination of both Dr. Jones's flexible and static budgets, several conclusions can be reached:

- Revenues were $13,150 less than expected. Expenses, however, were $5,778 less than expected, for a net income of $7,372 below expectations. Even taking into account this lower volume level, variable expenses were still $119 more than would be expected.
- Office supplies were efficiently used because actual consumption was less than that in the flexible budget (–$442).
- The cost of medical supplies was less than what had been statically budgeted, but not as low as would be expected in the flexible budget. This implies inefficient utilization ($547). This also, however, could have resulted from an unexpected change in procedure mix.
- Long-distance telephone calls were marginally higher than would be expected for the volume level. Given the small variance, however, perhaps the safest conclusion is that this category was about at expectations.
- Dr. Jones needs to reevaluate the issue of discipline. Advertising and education had unfavorable variances because someone

chose to exceed the budget. These choices could have been good decisions or wasteful decisions. A budget should not be viewed as inviolate because situations change and organizations must have enough flexibility to adapt. On the other hand, a lack of discipline will almost always be clad in the armor of necessity. The effective manager will be able to determine when a variance is truly in the organization's best interest and when it is simply the result of extravagance.

The concept of flexible budgeting can be applied to the MRI facility year 1 postacquisition analysis (Exhibit 6–21). Volume and charge are drivers. One flexible formula evaluates actual average charge to expected average charge ($740 – $625), which indicates a $115 favorable efficiency variance. This results in a gross revenue favorable efficiency of $340,170, meaning that *for the volume achieved*, the facility efficiently generated revenue from the 2,958 MRI scans. Overall effectiveness, however, is an unfavorable $151,250, which is due to lower than expected volume. These two effects net to a favorable gross revenue variance of $188,920.

Of the $112,898 unfavorable collection variance, $65,668 was due to inefficient collection as a result of exceeding the 25 percent uncollectable target. The remaining $47,230 was due to the higher than expected gross revenues. This finding indicates that, if management could improve the efficiency of collection (i.e., get it back down to a projected 25 percent rate), then about 58 percent of the unfavorable collection variation could be eliminated. Finally, it can be seen that the unfavorable supply variance (–$25,870) was actually worse than it first appears. There was an inefficiency of –$33,130 that was partially obscured by the positive ineffectiveness variance ($7,260) of conducting 242 fewer than projected MRI scans.

In summary, the budgeting process can be used to help evaluate whether an organization is proceeding according to plan. It comes, however, at a price in both effort and time. This issue is especially relevant for smaller health care orga-

Exhibit 6–21 MRI Facility Flexible Budget Analysis

	Actual Year 1	Projected Year 1	Variance	% Change	Flexible Formula	Flexible Efficiency	Flexible Effectiveness
Volume	2,958	3,200	–242	–7.56%			
Average Charge	$740	$625	$115	18.40%	740 – 625	$115	
Gross Revenue	$2,188,920	$2,000,000	$188,920	9.45%		$340,170	($151,250)
Less Bad Debts and Contractual Adj.	$612,898	$500,000	($112,898)	–22.58%	25% × Gross Rev.	($65,668)	($47,230)
Net Revenue	$1,576,022	$1,500,000	$76,022	5.07%			
Less Variable Expenses Supplies and Film	$121,870	$96,000	($25,870)	–26.95%	$30 × Volume	($33,130)	$7,260
Contribution Margin	$1,454,153	$1,404,000	$50,153	3.57%			

nizations. In a practice setting, someone, such as Dr. Jones or his business manager, must construct the budget and look for and investigate variances. Only Dr. Jones can determine whether this was or will be worthwhile in his particular situation. Some might believe that the variances that Dr. Jones discovered hardly justify the effort expended. Dr. Jones, however, may feel that the budgeting process was worthwhile if it gives him some assurance that things are generally going according to plan and that he has the capability of identifying specific variances as they grow, thereby providing the opportunity to control them before they reach critical levels.

In larger health care organizations, the use of budgets and projections as controls is essential. The numbers are simply too large and the consequences too great to "fly by the seat of your pants" in an unforgiving managed care environment. We have seen how badly a project, such as the MRI facility, can go. To forego the opportunity to change the course of events in midstream would be foolish.

Finally, the budgeting process conveys an image of financial competence, if not sophistication. Both large and small health care organizations that are seeking financing will have to demonstrate their financial competence to lending institutions. Almost without exception, this will imply presenting a budget and a management plan to operationalize it.

ACTIVITY-BASED COSTING

One of the major challenges facing health care organizations at the turn of the century is determining what it costs them to provide a service. It is difficult to bid confidently on a capitated contract, for example, unless you know what it costs you to provide the service. Activity-based costing (ABC) is a method for attaching costs to activities. The activity could be a procedure, DRG, diagnosis, or the like. Once you know what it costs to provide the procedure or DRG or to treat a particular disease, then you can more knowledgeably negotiate to provide medical care in a cost constrained environment. If you know, for example, that it costs you on average $20,000 to provide a cardiac artery bypass graft, you can then add margin over this level to determine a price. The price at which you can offer the service may or may not be consistent with the current market price of the service. You may then have to make a decision about whether to provide the service at a lower, and perhaps even negative, margin or to decline the opportunity. You will, however, be making this decision from a point of knowledge as opposed to ignorance.

An effective ABC system captures both direct financial information and behavioral information that has financial consequences. Often in health care, the value that is added is provided by the human, such as when a nurse, laboratory technician, or physician provides a service. It is essential, therefore, to attach a cost to this activity. The difficulty arises when we observe that much of the human behavior that occurs in the health care system is quite variable.

For example, think of the activities of a nurse working in an outpatient oncology practice. Much of the activity involves responding to the needs of patients receiving chemotherapy. Some of this activity is quite predictable and easily assessed, such as preparing and administering an infusion. If nurses are paid at $15 per hour, and the preparation of an infusion takes 20 minutes for one nurse, and one nurse can monitor eight patients over a 2-hour infusion, then the cost per patient per infusion would be $8.70 based on approximately 35 minutes of patient contact time (Exhibit 6–22).

Exhibit 6–22 ABC Analysis of Nursing Time

Nursing Pay Rate per Hour	$15.00
Infusion Preparation Time (Hours)	0.33
Average Infusion Time (Hours)	2
Average Number of Patients Supervised per Hour	8
Average Patient Contact Time (Hours)	0.58
Average Nursing Cost per Patient per Hour	$8.70

A more difficult situation to cost, however, arises in assessing the "off the record" activity. Ms. Smith calls the next day. She is running a fever, doesn't feel well, and wishes to talk to a nurse about her symptoms. Nurse Able responds to the call and talks with the patient for nine minutes. Mr. Jackson calls later that afternoon. He received a similar infusion the previous day. Nurse Baker takes the call and talks with him for 26 minutes. Two things of significance just occurred. First, an additional 35 minutes of nursing time needs to be allocated to the cost of the procedure. Second, there was significant variance in the time allocated across patients and nurses. Unless we know enough about the procedure to understand that there will be nursing time consumed in subsequent days as a result of the procedure, and unless we know how much this time can vary, we may fail to capture a significant amount of the procedure's cost.

The process for capturing behavioral cost information utilizes interviews, questionnaires, and sampling methods to determine what activities are performed by particular jobs and how much time it takes to perform the activities. Obviously, this can be an intrusive process. In this example, nurses would fill out activity questionnaires or enter their time directly into a computer touch screen over a period of days or weeks to get an assessment of their activities. In addition, job analysts may observe nurses performing their tasks to be certain that the questionnaires were assessing the full range of activities.

The validity of the data will be influenced by the organization's internal climate. If employees perceive that the data will be used to affect their pay, their discretion to act as they see fit, or their ability to provide the quality of care that they feel is appropriate, then the data may be biased. In more extreme cases, employees may resist the measurement process. Generally, this resistance will be covert as opposed to overt, such as when assessment questionnaires aren't completed for a myriad of reasons, all of which are *somewhat* legitimate.

It should be apparent that developing ABC systems can be very expensive and time con-

suming and may require skills not currently possessed by the health care organization. Given the current state of the art, these systems are probably most appropriately applied to procedures and programs that are of high value. A practice, therefore, might develop ABC models of its most important procedures. A hospital might develop ABC models for the most important parts of its most financially important programs, such as coronary artery bypass graft, an autologous bone marrow transplant, normal delivery, Caesarian delivery, and so forth.

Exhibit 6–23 shows a case example of an ABC model developed by a gastroenterology practice. This model focuses on the practice's outpatient services. It was determined that the most appropriate way to organize the ABC process was around their most important procedures and procedure codes. These are the columns in Exhibit 6–23. The rows represent medical and business expenses. The medical and business expenditure totals for the prior year were already known because they were available from the income statement. The ABC task, therefore, was to allocate these costs fully across the expense categories.

Effectively Using Financial Advisors

The relationship that a physician manager has with financial professionals should be analogous to that between an architect and an informed client with opinions regarding the qualities and characteristics of his or her home. By having a very clear understanding of your specific financial needs, you will be able to work most effectively with financial advisors.

In practices and smaller health care organizations, the financial advisor may be a consulting accountant or perhaps an employed business manager with an MBA. In larger health care organizations financial information and support may come from a finance department headed by a chief financial officer.

Accounting data are to your health care organization what current and historical medical test data are to a clinician treating a patient. They in-

Exhibit 6–23 Case Example of Gastroenterology ABC Analysis

	New Patient Consultation	Follow Up Office Visits	43235 EGD	43239 EGD Biopsy	45330 Flex.Sig.	45331 Flex.Sig. Biopsy	45333 Flex.Sig. Polyp Rem	45378 Colon.	45380 Colon. Biopsy	45384 Colon. Polyp Rem	Computed	Actual
Number of services rendered in 1995	967	1287	9	32	169	66	4	23	17	15	2589	
Total time for procedure in minutes			95	110	35	50	50	65	80	80		
Physician time spent with patients in min. (see table 1)	20	10	10	12	5	10	15	25	35	35		
Nursing time spent with patient in min. (see table 1)	20	8	90	105	30	45	45	60	75	75		
MEDICAL EXPENSES												
Physician cost per procedure-min.*/cost per min. (see table 2)	$30.86	$15.43	$15.43	$18.52	$7.72	$15.43	$23.15	$38.58	$54.01	$54.01		
Nursing cost per procedure-min.*/cost per min. (see table 2)	$7.47	$2.99	$33.62	$39.22	$11.21	$16.81	$16.81	$22.41	$28.02	$28.02		
Medical supplies	$4.32	$3.75	$37.79	$41.47	$21.78	$25.46	$25.46	$35.99	$39.67	$39.67		
Equip maint. & rep. - cost per procedure (see table 7)	—	—	$8.06	$8.06	$8.06	$8.06	$8.06	$8.06	$8.06	$8.06		
Endo suite space rent-total time* rent per proc. min. (see table 6)			$46.69	$54.06	$17.20	$24.57	$24.57	$31.94	$39.31	$39.31		
Exam room rent cost per use (see table 4)	$2.96	$2.96										
Equipment cost (see table 7)			$21.95	$21.95	$0.98	$0.98	$0.98	$18.18	$18.18	$18.18		
TOTAL	$45.62	$25.13	$163.54	$183.28	$66.94	$91.31	$99.03	$155.17	$187.26	$187.26		
BUSINESS EXPENSES												
Administration and Advertising												
Administration-annual salaries (see table 9) / total number of services rendered	$13.53	$13.53	$13.53	$13.53	$13.53	$13.53	$13.53	$13.53	$13.53	$13.53		
Telephone/advertising cost per procedure-cost per year (see table 8) / total number of services	$5.61	$5.61	$5.61	$5.61	$5.61	$5.61	$5.61	$5.61	$5.61	$5.61		
Equipment rental cost per procedure-cost per year (see table 8) / total number of services	$1.50	$1.50	$1.50	$1.50	$1.50	$1.50	$1.50	$1.50	$1.50	$1.50		
Office space rent (see table 5)	$10.16	$10.16	$10.16	$10.16	$10.16	$10.16	$10.16	$10.16	$10.16	$10.16		

continues

Exhibit 6–23 continued

	New Patient Consultation	Follow Up Office Visits	43235 EGD	43239 EGD Biopsy	45330 Flex.Sig.	45331 Flex.Sig. Biopsy	45333 Flex.Sig. Polyp Rem	45378 Colon.	45380 Colon. Biopsy	45384 Colon. Polyp Rem	Computed	Actual
Billing and Collection												
Office supplies-annual cost (see table 8) / total number of services	$1.64	$1.64	$1.64	$1.64	$1.64	$1.64	$1.64	$1.64	$1.64	$1.64		
Postage-annual cost (see table 8) / total number of services	$1.85	$1.85	$1.85	$1.85	$1.85	$1.85	$1.85	$1.85	$1.85	$1.85		
Salary & benefit cost per procedure-cost per procedure (see table 9)	$5.80	$5.80	$5.80	$5.80	$5.80	$5.80	$5.80	$5.80	$5.80	$5.80		
Reception, Scheduling, Med. Records & Transcription												
Minutes per procedure	63	15	37	37	37	37	37	37	37	37		
Receptionists' cost per procedure-Reception wage per minute (see table 8)*/minutes per procedure	$9.06	$2.16	$5.32	$5.32	$5.32	$5.32	$5.32	$5.32	$5.32	$5.32		
Office supplies-annual cost (see table 8) / total number of services	$3.28	$3.28	$3.28	$3.28	$3.28	$3.28	$3.28	$3.28	$3.28	$3.28		
Postage-annual cost (see table 8) / total number of services	$0.87	$0.87	$0.87	$0.87	$0.87	$0.87	$0.87	$0.87	$0.87	$0.87		
Transcriptionist-annual cost (see table 8) / total number of services	$2.25	$2.25	$2.25	$2.25	$2.25	$2.25	$2.25	$2.25	$2.25	$2.25		
TOTAL	$55.55	$48.65	$51.81	$51.81	$51.81	$51.81	$51.81	$51.81	$51.81	$51.81		
Cost Per Procedure Rendered	$101.17	$73.79	$215.35	$235.09	$118.75	$143.12	$150.84	$206.98	$239.07	$239.07		

Source: 1997 by Sentara Health System, William T. Geary, Ph.D., Robert J. Solomon, Ph.D. All rights reserved.

dicate the current and past states of the organization and allow you to make rational management decisions about future courses of action. The goal of using financial information is to manage your organization proactively and to make appropriate changes that take into account both financial and medical considerations. A knowledgeable financial professional can further this goal by providing you with the appropriate information that you need to be part of the decision process.

Generally, it will be a misuse of your and your staff's time to perform specialized tasks in which accountants and financial professionals develop proficiency over a period of years. For example, use an accountant for tasks that require skilled or timely financial or accounting knowledge, such as the preparation of tax returns or the development of a pension or profit-sharing plan. Use financial professionals to build financial models in spreadsheets and to perform the initial analyses of the finances of a medical project, hospital expansion, practice acquisition, and the like. Use professionals to get an expert's perspective. Similarly, you will want to use a financial professional to create your financial procedures and set up your cash and accrual accounts, so that you produce accounting data in a form that is most useful for tax, reporting, and planning purposes.

Case Analysis: Oregon Sports Medicine

The use of financial information to aid in making management decisions is illustrated by the case of Oregon Sports Medicine. Performance appraisal and compensation issues are central to the concept of control, and these issues are at the heart of the challenge facing the physicians at Oregon Sports Medicine. The data that they will use to help them make the critical decision that they face come from their income statement. The analytical method they will use employs the CVP model. Finally, the projections that they make can be used to develop static and flexible budgets to monitor progress toward financial goals and to modify management actions to achieve these goals.

Oregon Sports Medicine is composed of three physicians, Drs. Able, Baker, and Cane, along with several nurses, secretaries, and assistants. Drs. Able and Baker are partners; Dr. Cane is an employed associate. Exhibit 6–24 contains an income statement at the top. Below the income statement is an analysis of each physician's net revenue. Dr. Able has generated 31.36 percent of the net revenue, Dr. Baker has generated 42.04 percent of the net revenue, and Dr. Cane has generated 26.60 percent of the net revenue. Next, they assign 40 percent ($250,822.33) of the total practice expenses ($627,055.22) equally to each physician ($83,607.44). They then take the remaining expenses and divide them based on each physician's percentage of net revenue. Baker, the high producer, therefore takes $158,176.18 of additional expenses based on her volume, Able takes $117,968.26, and Cane, the low producer, takes an additional $100,089.06 of expenses. Each physician's salary is the sum of his or her net revenue minus his or her assigned expenses.

This case is not presented as an endorsement of how to structure compensation and incentive arrangements. Rather, it is presented as a case study of how one practice wrestled with the issues of how to tie work to rewards, control expenses, create equity so that those who incurred expenses would pay for them, and create incentives so that physicians would want to work harder and smarter.

As we examine this plan, it does have some logic to it. The sharing of a proportion of the expenses equally recognizes that some expenses are present irrespective of utilization. They are opportunity costs that occur as soon as the door is opened, and they will be there largely irrespective of the number of patients who walk in the door. In effect, these are fixed expenses given the practice's current relevant range. Intuitively, the physicians seemed to have an appreciation of the concepts of fixed and variable expenses.

Recognition that some expenses are tied to activity level, and that those who use more should pay more and those who use less should

Exhibit 6–24 Oregon Sports Medicine: Income Statement, Revenue Analysis, and Salary Calculations

	A	B	C
1	*Income Statement January–December 19XX*		
2	NET REVENUE		
3	Dr. Able	$390,109.27	30.58%
4	Dr. Baker	$523,072.85	41.00%
5	Dr. Cane	$362,506.86	28.42%
6	Total	$1,275,688.99	100.00%
7			
8	EXPENSES		
9	Non-Physician Gross Payroll	$151,943.11	11.91%
10	FICA (Includes Physicians)	$26,699.61	2.09%
11	Advertising	$26,601.83	2.09%
12	Maintenance	$6,619.63	0.52%
13	Telephone	$8,415.60	0.66%
14	Radiology	$12,106.81	0.95%
15	Postage	$6,942.50	0.54%
16	Licenses	$175.00	0.01%
17	Janitorial	$3,400.00	0.27%
18	Contributions/Gifts	$16,800.05	1.32%
19	Petty Cash	$3,132.76	0.25%
20	Accounting/Legal	$10,847.10	0.85%
21	Taxes - Corporate	$0.00	0.00%
22	Personal Property	$2,920.07	0.23%
23	State Unemployment	$76.02	0.01%
24	Fed. Unemployment	$2,288.80	0.18%
25	Gross Receipts	$6,872.54	0.54%
26	Office Supplies	$25,103.24	1.97%
27	Medical Supplies	$35,498.29	2.78%
28	Dues	$10,540.50	0.83%
29	Books	$8,775.59	0.69%
30	Meetings	$18,239.11	1.43%
31	Insurance	$68,138.58	5.34%
32	Rent	$65,832.00	5.16%
33	Christmas Parties	$1,039.01	0.08%
34	Equipment Lease	$50,429.97	3.95%
35	Interest Bank Note	$7,488.87	0.59%
36	Interest To Owners	$10,265.79	0.80%
37	Electricity	$7,150.98	0.56%
38	Depreciation	$25,113.00	1.97%
39	Miscellaneous	$954.46	0.07%
40	Transcription Service	$6,645.00	0.52%
41	Total Expenses	$627,055.82	49.15%
42			
43	Net Income Before Physician Salaries	$648,633.17	50.85%
44			

continues

Exhibit 6–24 continued

	A	B	C
45	PHYSICIAN NET REVENUE ANALYSIS		
46	Dr. Able - Net Revenue	$390,109.27	30.58%
47	Dr. Baker - Net Revenue	$523,072.85	41.00%
48	Dr. Cane - Net Revenue	$362,506.86	28.42%
49	Total	$1,275,688.99	
50			
51			
52	DISTRIBUTION OF EXPENSES		
53	40% Equally	$250,822.33	
54	60% Based on Net Revenue	$376,233.49	
55	Total	$627,055.82	
56			
57		Equally	By Revenue
58	Dr. Able	$83,607.44	$115,053.26
59	Dr. Baker	$83,607.44	$154,267.64
60	Dr. Cane	$83,607.44	$106,912.60
61			
62		$250,822.33	$376,233.49
63			
64	PHYSICIANS' INCOMES		%
65	Dr. Able	$191,448.57	15.01%
66	Dr. Baker	$285,197.77	22.36%
67	Dr. Cane	$171,986.82	13.48%
68	Total	$648,633.17	50.85%

Source: Copyright © William T. Geary, Ph.D., and Robert J. Solomon, Ph.D., used with permission.

pay less, is also encompassed in their compensation formula. This notion of variable cost is operationalized by the 60 percent of expenses assigned based on physician net revenue. Net revenue in this instance is being used as a surrogate for activity, probably because it is easily measurable. It is a cost driver. Finally, this system creates an incentive for all to try to reduce both fixed and variable expenses because each physician will receive some portion of the cost savings back through a higher salary.

Where did the numbers 40 percent and 60 percent in the expense allocation formula come from? Who knows? But we are not in a position to be critical. If the physicians are happy with this division, if it creates equity in their minds, then that is good enough. An alternative, however, would be to go down the list of expenses and classify each one as fixed or variable (mixed expenses would have to be broken into

their fixed and variable components). The difficulty with changing a compensation formula such as this is that someone will be a winner and someone will be a loser. For example, if an analysis of the costs indicates that more than 40 percent is fixed, then Dr. Baker, the high producer, would gain at the expense of both Drs. Able and Cane.

Unfortunately, all is not going well at Oregon Sports Medicine. Drs. Baker and Cane do not get along. Although Baker has expressed concerns about some of Cane's treatment decisions, she is quick to admit that the fundamental problem is a personality conflict. As she put it, "The thought of working together and managing a practice together for the next 20 years is truly depressing. He is not collegial. It will be constant conflict. We just look at the world differently." Dr. Able is less critical of Cane. He describes the situation differently:

He can be tough to get along with on some days, but his manner doesn't really bother me that much. His technique is good. He has good clinical skills, and he is a competent diagnostician—not a superstar, but well within the bounds of accepted practice. The patients like him. He will do well. I certainly can live with him for a few more years.

Dr. Able comments on the difficulty of replacing Dr. Cane:

If we decide not to offer partnership, we will have a major problem replacing him in the short run. We are out of the recruitment cycle. It will probably take us at least 18 months to get a replacement in here. In addition, we may have to provide some significant financial incentives and subsidies.

Dr. Baker is a partner in the practice. She is young, raising a family, and still paying off education loans, and she has a significant mortgage. Dr. Able is the other partner. He is in his late 50s and he has been reducing his involvement with the practice. Because he would like to retire in three to five years, Dr. Able is concerned about the value of the practice and who will purchase his interest. Dr. Cane is in the third year of a four-year contract. A partnership decision must be made in the next two months. Dr. Cane has made it clear that, if he is not admitted to partnership, he will leave at the end of his contract.

Given the information in Exhibit 6–24 we can see that it would not be too difficult to develop a model to see what would happen if Cane were to leave. This model is presented in Exhibit 6–25 and a supporting spreadsheet is given in Exhibit 6–26.

The model construction began with the current income statement. It was assumed that all Dr. Cane's revenues would be lost because Dr. Baker was already full and Dr. Able was winding down and not interested in increasing his workload. Variable expenses were adjusted by using a flexible budget formula using total revenue as a cost driver. These adjustments were

made on the supporting spreadsheet (Exhibit 6–26). For example, current radiology expense was divided by total net revenue, so that radiology expense could be expressed as a percentage of net revenue, in this case, 0.97 percent. This factor could then be used to project the future radiology expense after Cane's revenues have been removed. Fixed expenses were adjusted by asking: Do we still need it? Could it be eliminated or at least cut back? For example, Irene's position (Exhibit 6–26) was eliminated.

After these adjustments were completed, a projected income statement was produced. The results are sobering. They indicate that Dr. Baker's salary is likely to drop by about $62,000 and Dr. Able is projected to make about $53,000 less. Examination of the projected income statement reveals why the salary decreases are so large. If Cane goes, he will take with him his variable expenses, but he will leave his share of the fixed expenses. Unfortunately, this is largely a fixed expense operation.

Once a model such as this is produced, it can easily be sensitized to other scenarios. If Drs. Able and Baker don't like the outcome, then they can try other "what-ifs." Perhaps one of the other radiology technician positions could be converted to part time. Perhaps other fixed expenses could be reduced or eliminated. Perhaps Dr. Baker may conclude that Dr. Cane is not so bad after all!

Modeling such as this does not solve the problem. It simply attaches a financial cost to the modeled outcome. It provides an opportunity to explore the financial consequences of alternative outcomes and attaches a cost to behavioral choices.

If Dr. Cane does depart, there will be little room for financial errors until he can be replaced. The projected income statement can form the basis for static and flexible budgets, so that Drs. Able and Baker can track how they are proceeding against expectations. This may allow them to detect unfavorable trends before they become crises and manage the practice through a time when there will probably be little margin for error.

Exhibit 6–25 Oregon Sports Medicine: What If Dr. Cane Leaves?

	A	B *WITH CANE*	C *WITHOUT CANE*	D *VARIANCE*
1				
2				
3	NET REVENUE			
4	Dr. Able	$390,109.27	$390,109.27	
5	Dr. Baker	$523,072.85	$523,072.85	
6	Dr. Cane	$362,506.86	$0.00	
7	Total	$1,275,688.99	$913,182.12	$362,506.86
8				
9	EXPENSES			
10	Non-Physician Gross Payroll	$151,943.11	$136,914.32	$15,028.79
11	FICA (Includes Physicians)	$26,699.61	$21,090.67	$5,608.94
12	Advertising	$26,601.83	$26,601.83	$0.00
13	Maintenance	$6,619.63	$6,619.63	$0.00
14	Telephone	$8,415.60	$8,415.60	$0.00
15	Radiology	$12,106.81	$8,666.47	$3,440.34
16	Postage	$6,942.50	$4,969.68	$1,972.82
17	Licenses	$175.00	$155.00	$20.00
18	Janitorial	$3,400.00	$3,400.00	$0.00
19	Contributions/Gifts	$16,800.05	$10,000.00	$6,800.05
20	Petty Cash	$3,132.76	$3,132.76	$0.00
21	Accounting/Legal	$10,847.10	$10,847.10	$0.00
22	Taxes - Corporate	$0.00	$0.00	$0.00
23	Personal Property	$2,920.07	$2,920.07	$0.00
24	State Unemployment	$76.02	$68.50	$7.52
25	Fed. Unemployment	$2,288.80	$2,062.41	$226.39
26	Gross Receipts	$6,872.54	$5,296.46	$1,576.08
27	Office Supplies	$25,103.24	$17,969.76	$7,133.48
28	Medical Supplies	$35,498.29	$25,410.90	$10,087.39
29	Dues	$10,540.50	$8,250.50	$2,290.00
30	Books	$8,775.59	$8,775.59	$0.00
31	Meetings	$18,239.11	$16,955.40	$1,283.71
32	Insurance	$68,138.58	$50,179.44	$17,959.14
33	Rent	$65,832.00	$65,832.00	$0.00
34	Christmas Parties	$1,039.01	$1,039.01	$0.00
35	Equipment Lease	$50,429.97	$50,429.97	$0.00
36	Interest Bank Note	$7,488.87	$7,488.87	$0.00
37	Interest To Owners	$10,265.79	$10,265.79	$0.00
38	Electricity	$7,150.98	$7,150.98	$0.00
39	Depreciation	$25,113.00	$25,113.00	$0.00
40	Miscellaneous	$954.46	$954.46	$0.00
41	Transcription Service	$6,645.00	$4,756.72	$1,888.28
42				
43	Total Expenses	$627,055.82	$551,732.90	$75,322.92
44				
45	Net Income Before Physician Salaries	$648,633.17	$361,449.23	$287,183.94
46				

continues

Exhibit 6–25 continued

	A	B WITH CANE	C WITHOUT CANE	D VARIANCE
47	PHYSICIAN NET INCOME ANALYSIS			
48	Dr. Able - Net Revenue	$390,109.27	$390,109.27	
49	Dr. Baker - Net Revenue	$523,072.85	$523,072.85	
50	Dr. Cane - Net Revenue	$362,506.86	$0.00	
51	Total	$1,275,688.99	$913,182.12	
52				
53				
54	DISTRIBUTION OF EXPENSES			
55	40% Equally		$220,693.16	
56	60% Based on Net Revenue		$331,039.74	
57	Total Expenses		$551,732.90	
58				
59			Equally	By Revenue
60	Dr. Able		$110,346.58	$141,419.40
61	Dr. Baker		$110,346.58	$189,620.33
62	Dr. Cane		$0.00	$0.00
63			$220,693.16	$331,039.74
64				
65	PHYSICIANS' INCOMES			
66	Dr. Able		$138,343.29	15.15%
67	Dr. Baker		$223,105.94	24.43%
68	Dr. Cane		$0.00	0.00%
69	Total		$361,449.23	39.58%
70				
71		Before	After	Variance
72	Dr. Able	$191,448.57	$138,343.29	$53,105.28
73	Dr. Baker	$285,197.77	$223,105.94	$62,091.83
74	Dr. Cane	$171,986.82	$0.00	$171,986.82
75	Total	$648,633.17	$361,449.23	$287,183.94

Source: Copyright © William T. Geary, Ph.D., and Robert J. Solomon, Ph.D., used with permission.

Cases such as Oregon Sports Medicine reinforce the importance of a number of other issues discussed in this book. The goal of management should be to prevent a situation such as this from occurring by carefully selecting partners and then guiding their development through a performance appraisal and goal-setting process, so that antagonisms such as have occurred at Oregon are managed, if not prevented.

CONCLUSION

The strength of the material discussed in this chapter is that it really does work. The problem,

however, is that it can work too well. Allowing managers motivated primarily by financial considerations to make critical decisions in an organization with a health care mission can result in the medical mission being subordinated to the financial mission.

The underlying message in this chapter is that financial considerations in health care organizations are too important to be left entirely to financial managers. Physician managers must intercede and contribute a medically based perspective to decision making. To do this, they must understand the financial mind set as well as how to use financial data as an aid to decision making.

Exhibit 6–26 Oregon Sports Medicine: Projection Calculation Worksheet

Personnel		Salary	Without Cane
Office Manager	Ann	$23,410.66	$23,410.66
Computer Input	Bryan	$20,207.85	$20,207.85
Receptionist	Charlotte	$18,100.39	$18,100.39
Insurance/Collections	Dean	$17,898.07	$17,898.07
Medical Secretary	Elvira	$14,600.00	$14,600.00
Radiology Technician (Dr. Able)	Georgina	$20,984.24	$20,984.24
Radiology Technician (Dr. Baker)	Harry	$21,713.11	$21,713.11
Radiology Technician (Eliminated)	Irene	$15,028.79	$0.00
		$151,943.11	$136,914.32
X-rays (Percentage of projected net revenue)		0.95%	$8,666.47
Postage (Percentage of projected net revenue)		0.54%	$4,969.68
Business Licenses			
Dr. Able	$60.00		$60.00
Dr. Baker	$20.00		$20.00
Dr. Cane	$20.00		$0.00
Oregon Sports Medicine	$75.00		$75.00
Total	$175.00		$155.00
Gross Receipts Tax	$7,399.00		$5,296.46
Contributions/Gifts (Estimated)	$16,800.05		$10,000.00
Office Supplies (Percentage of projected net revenue)1.97%	$17,969.76		
Meedical Supplies (Percentage of projected net revenue)		2.78%	$25,410.90
Dues			
Dr. Able	$4,173.50		$4,173.50
Dr. Baker	$4,077.00		$4,077.00
Dr. Cane	$2,290.00		$0.00
Total	$10,540.50		$8,250.50
Meetings			
Dr. Able	$6,221.58		$6,221.58
Dr. Baker	$9,836.78		$9,836.78
Dr. Cane	$1,283.71		$0.00
Staff	$897.04		$897.04
Total	$18,239.11		$16,955.40

Source: Copyright © William T. Geary, Ph.D., and Robert J. Solomon, Ph.D., used with permission.

Managed care has placed a premium on creating and operating financially sound health care organizations, hospitals, and practices. The financial orientation to managing health care organizations is analogous to the camel whose nose was under the tent and who now has every intention of moving in and taking over. Pretending that this is not happening by ignoring it will not work. Simply, leaving decisions totally up to financial professionals ignores the problem. If a health care organization's medical mission is to be well served, financially literate physicians must participate in the decision-making process.

REFERENCES AND NOTES

1. VHA, Inc., *Utilization: A Guide to Reducing Variations To Improve Outcomes* (Irving, Tex.: VHA, 1994), 9–10.

2. VHA, Utilization, 13–16.

3. Net revenue is being defined as the fee as stated in a fee schedule less contractual write-offs, adjustments, and an average provision for account delinquency. For example, the fee for a panel of laboratory tests might be $200, but the insurance company contract may specify a contractual write-off of 15 percent ($30). If the insurance company and/or the patient paid the $170, it would be called net revenue.

4. This case was prepared by William T. Geary, Ph.D., Graduate School of Business, College of William & Mary, Williamsburg, Virginia. Used with permission.

5. Some physicians really enjoy working with spreadsheets, doing the sensitivity analyses, and modifying the assumptions contained in the spreadsheet formulas. If this is true for you, I am not suggesting that you forgo this activity, only that you consider what is the best use of your time.

6. Spreadsheets for years 2, 4, and 5 were constructed reflecting the projections made in the case. Maintenance costs of $25,000 were projected for year 4.

7. The interest rate reflects three components: risk, the rate of inflation, and real profit that is needed to bring money into investment markets. For example, if inflation is 3 percent and U.S. government securities, which are generally considered risk free, are selling for 5 percent, then the cost of capital is 2 percent. A company selling bonds at 10 percent in this situation would be figuring in a 5 percent risk factor.

8. The problem also could be approached by converting all the numbers into future value terms, but it is generally easier to reframe all your thinking into current dollars.

9. Often, this is done as salary at the end of the tax year. One must be careful to justify this distribution based on job content, such as management responsibilities, or to show that the total salary is in line with the amount of clinical work performed. Otherwise, the Internal Revenue Service (IRS) might consider the distribution a dividend, in which case both the corporation and the recipient will be taxed on the distribution.

10. There are many ways to calculate depreciation. The IRS prescribes some given particular factual circumstances. Often, what is advantageous for tax reasons may not be the most descriptive of economic reality.

11. It is likely that you have an intuitive understanding of the concept of accrual-based accounting. For example, if during the course of the year you say to yourself "I've got a big insurance bill due at the end of the year, and I should reserve some cash each month so that I will be able to pay it," you are making a provision for an expense incurred but not yet paid.

12. This case was prepared in collaboration with William T. Geary, Ph.D., Graduate School of Business, College of William & Mary, Williamsburg, Virginia.

13. A tax reality is that many physicians will pay their practice's profit to themselves before the end of a tax year to avoid double taxation. To the extent that this occurs, the return on owner's investment can still be meaningful if the calculations are made taking this tax adjustment into account.

14. D.T. DeCoster, E.L. Schafer, and M.T. Ziebel. *Management Accounting: A Decision Analysis* (New York, N.Y.: Wiley, 1988), 13.

CHAPTER 7

Cash Control in Small Practices

Chapter Objectives

This chapter is intended for physician managers working in a private practice setting. The goal of this chapter is to review basic management reports that a physician manager should routinely examine in order to ensure the validity of a practice's financial data and to deter theft.

The items covered in this chapter pertain most directly to physician managers working in smaller private practice settings. The types of controls discussed in this chapter also are essential in larger health care organizations. Physician managers in these larger organizations typically are removed from this activity, although it is their responsibility to ensure that the appropriate controls are in place.

Short-term financial and cash control involves generating financial and production reports that tell the physician manager how well the organization is functioning. These reports are easily generated by computer directly from most medical office management software (MOMS), so that it is feasible to produce them on a routine basis. The following sections describe a number of reports that are helpful for maintaining financial control. Many of the reports will be used on a daily basis by the business staff. Nevertheless, physician managers must be familiar with their significance and use to ensure that subordinates are fully utilizing the available information that they provide as well

as to be able to use them personally to assist with management decisions.

The names that are used for the following reports are somewhat arbitrary and may differ from those in your specific office software. The important consideration is the information that they provide.

DAILY RECEIPTS/ADJUSTMENTS

This report (Exhibit 7–1) provides the information necessary to determine whether the posting of payments to patient accounts is accurate. It should be run either at the very end of each day or at the beginning of each day on the transactions for the previous day. It provides the information necessary to audit, or verify, the accuracy of the following critical pieces of information:

- the amount of each payment
- the type of each payment (e.g., insurance payment, check, cash, credit card)
- the totals for each type of payment

Exhibit 7–1 Daily Receipts and Adjustments

Number	Name	Chart #	Transaction		Amount
21-G	Mills Joe		» Check Payment		500.00
21-G	Mills Joe		» Cash Payment		310.00
21-2	Mills Candace	06/10/87	Full-thick. skin graft to lip/mouth		
21-G	Mills Joe		» Card Payment		600.00
21-3	Mills Jeff	06/10/87	Closure of nasal sinus fistula		
23-G	Hernandes Tim		» Positive Adjustment		150.00
23-G	Hernandes Tim	06/10/87	» Positive Adjustment		
23-G	Hernandes Tim		» Uncollectible Write-Off		191.80
23-2	Hernandes Christine	06/10/87	Corneal transplant-not other. spec.		
23-2	Hernandes Christine	06/10/87	Tattooing of cornea		
10-G	Snyder David		» Card Payment		85.00
10-1	Snyder David	06/10/87	Cisternal Puncture		
10-1	Snyder David		Δ Aetna Life & Casualty		210.00
10-1	Snyder David	06/10/87	Other diagnostic procedures on skull		
10-G	Snyder David		» Money Express		45.00
10-2	Snyder Shari	06/10/87	Other cranial puncture		
10-G	Snyder David		» Cash Payment		35.00
10-G	Snyder David		» Welfare Check		50.00
20-G	James Jim		» Check Payment		90.00
20-1	James Jim	06/10/87	Suture of corneal laceration		
20-G	James Jim		» Negative Adjustment		96.80
20-G	James Jim		» Welfare Check		126.55
20-1	James Jim	06/10/87	Thermokeratoplasty		
2-G	Prokesh David		» Cash Payment		55.00
2-3	Prokesh David Jr.	06/10/87	Myringotomy w/insert of tube		
2-G	Prokesh David		» Welfare Check		150.50
2-3	Prokesh David Jr.	06/10/87	Myringotomy w/insert of tube		
2-G	Prokesh David		» Negative Adjustment		90.00

Total Checks	590.00
Total Cash	400.00
Total Credit Cards	685.00
Total Insurance	210.00
Total Uncollectible Write-Offs	191.80
Total Adjustments (+)	150.00
Total Adjustments (−)	186.80
Coupon	45.00
Gift Certificate	327.05
Two-party Check	0.00
	0.00

Courtesy of HealthCare Communications Inc., Lincoln, Nebraska.

The contents of this report should be checked against the actual cash receipts for that day. Receipts must *exactly* match the totals reported in the daily receipts/adjustments report. If there is a discrepancy, it must be resolved immediately.

This report is important for several reasons. First, if the accuracy of accounts is secured on a daily basis, problems are more easily resolvable because the problem must have occurred on one date. If the report is run less frequently, such as every week, the auditing and correction tasks are much more complex.

Second, using this report on a daily basis acts as a deterrent to some types of theft. If cash, primarily currency and checks, is being diverted by the employee who receives it, this will be detected when the cash posted to accounts does not balance against the cash on hand. For this control to be effective, both the posting of cash and the verification of the posting must be separated from the task of receiving cash. This involves dividing these responsibilities across different front office positions. Running this report each day ensures that any employee whose theft could be detected by this report will only have access to cash from 1 day before it would be detected. This report should be run daily. The users will generally be front office personnel.

DAILY ACTIVITY BY PROVIDER

This report (Exhibit 7–2) provides a summary of clinical work performed each day. If your practice has more than one provider, this report also will ensure that the proper physicians have been credited for their work. This report should be run either at the end of each day or at the beginning of each day for the previous day.

This report should indicate the name of the patient, the procedure that was performed, the provider who performed the procedure, and the fee that was charged. The contents of this report should be validated against an independent record, such as a day sheet or encounter form, to ensure that all services have been properly entered.

This report can also be used to deter theft. An employee might try to cover up the diversion of cash by simply not entering the cash and the associated procedures that generated them into the computer. Comparison of this report with an independent record of procedures, such as encounter forms, could defeat this strategy.

For this control to be effective, the person reviewing the report should be someone other than the person who collects cash. Once again, carefully dividing duties across front office positions

can increase the difficulty of theft. Having providers receive their own production report will serve as a deterrent as well as a quality control check.

This report should be run daily. The users will generally be front office personnel. Ideally, physicians should receive their own reports for deterrence and quality control purposes.

GROSS RECEIPTS

This report (Exhibit 7–3) provides a summary of receipts for any given time period. The gross receipts report is primarily useful as another deterrent to theft. The practice gross receipts for a month should balance exactly against bank deposits over the same time period. If the gross receipts report does not reconcile against the deposits to the bank account as indicated on your monthly bank statement, then it is possible that the person responsible for managing your checking account or making deposits is diverting funds.

To make this reconciliation easier, the posting of payments to patient accounts should be coordinated with deposits into the bank account, so that all payments posted into the MOMS for a calendar month are deposited in a timely manner and will appear on the bank statement for the same month. If this goal is not achieved, the balance can be reconciled by adjusting the gross receipts or the bank balance for cash posted to MOMS but not deposited to checking or cash deposited to checking but not posted to MOMS.

This report should be run at the end of each month. The users will generally be front office personnel and the practice's physician manager. The physician manager should receive a copy of the checking account statement, the report as it is produced by the computer, and any reconciliation calculations.

DETAILED PRODUCTION REPORT

This report (Exhibit 7–4) provides details and a summary of all the procedures performed for a specific time period. The data contained in this

Exhibit 7–2 Daily Activity by Producer

Number	Patient Name	Chart #	Last Visit	Diagnosis	Procedure	Prd	Fee	Balance
21-4	Mills Heather	21-4		995.5	21.22	D6A6	250.60	250.60
21-4	Mills Heather	21-4		682.2a	21.71	D4A4	382.98	633.58
21-3	Mills Jeff	21-3			22.71	D1A1	600.00	600.00
21-3	Mills Jeff	21-3			22.11	D1A1	274.60	874.60
21-2	Mills Candace	21-2		781.2	27.55	D3A3	306.32	306.32
23-2	Hernandes Christine	23-2		303.93	11.60	D2A2	91.80	91.80
23-2	Hernandes Christine	23-2			11.91	D2A2	100.00	191.80
10-1	Snyder David			793.2	01.01	D3A3	83.75	83.75
10-1	Snyder David				01.19	D3A3	210.00	293.75
10-1	Snyder David				01.24	D3A3	150.00	443.75
10-2	Snyder Shari			781.2	01.12	D2A2	284.75	284.75
10-2	Snyder Shari				01.09	D2A2	45.00	329.75
20-1	James Jim			303.9	11.51	D5A5	89.25	89.25
20-1	James Jim				11.74	D5A5	126.55	215.80
20-2	James Bonnie			704.00	02.02	D5A5	471.00	471.00
2-3	Prokesh David Jr.			272.2	20.01	D2A2	205.50	205.50
2-3	Prokesh David Jr.				20.22	D2A2	390.00	595.50

Total for Producer(s)   4,062.10

D1A1 Joe Carter   874.60
D2A2 Carl Yates   1,117.05
D3A3 Stephen Webb   750.07
D4A4 Keith Jergens   382.98
D5A5 Joseph Harris   686.80
D6A6 Bob Lovette   250.60

Courtesy of HealthCare Communications Inc., Lincoln, Nebraska.

report should include the type of procedure, the number of times each procedure was performed, and the gross fees (gross revenue) generated by each procedure. The fees generated are a very important indicator of the financial status of the practice, especially if you do a lot of work that is billed to insurance.

These revenue figures tell you what you are putting into the "pipeline." Unless you put revenues into the pipeline, you cannot get cash out. This truism is important because it will allow you to spot changes in practice patterns well before their cash impact.

For example, if you are tracking revenues and notice that they suddenly decline, you can be certain that cash will decline several weeks later.

This lag can be predicted with some accuracy by knowing the normal delay in payment by your insurance companies. If you know that revenues are down now, then you can plan for the decline in cash by curtailing and delaying spending, arranging for credit, and so on.

A significant decline can be due to many different causes, and it should always generate an investigation. For example, revenues will decline if there has been a shift from higher-paying to lower-paying procedures. Similarly, a decline in the absolute level of work will also generate reduced revenues. One practice identified a software problem in its billing by noting a decline in revenues. The billing program was not recognizing some procedures as billable, and as a result it

Exhibit 7–3 Gross Receipts

Posted Date: 06/01/96–06/30/96

Description		Amount Received
Check		8,188.26
Cash		898.00
Credit Card		305.00
Insurance		11,054.03
User 1 Payment » Pender & Coward		0.00
User 2 Payment » Glasser & Glasser		0.00
User 3 Payment »		0.00
User 4 Payment »		0.00
Total Receipts		20,445.29
Uncollectible Write-Offs		2,483.80
Self Pay Write-Offs		0.00
Workers Compensation Write-Offs		0.00
Medicare Write-Offs		0.00
Medicaid Write-Offs		0.00
Other Federal Program Write-Offs		0.00
Commercial Insurance Write-Offs		0.00
Blue Cross/Blue Shield Write-Offs		2,426.94
CHAMPUS Write-Offs		1,043.11
Other Write-Offs		2,449.14
HMO Write-Offs		0.00
PPO Write-Offs		0.00
Group/Other Write-Offs		0.00
CHAMPVA/Other Write-Offs		0.00
FECA Black Lung/Other Write-Offs		0.00
Lab Write-Offs		0.00
Gramm-Rudman Write-Offs		0.00
Positive Adjustments		227.79
Negative Adjustments		232.25

Source: Courtesy of HealthCare Communications Inc., Lincoln, Nebraska.

did not send bills that would have generated an increase in revenues.

Lower revenues can also be a symptom of theft. If someone is diverting cash, they may try to hide the theft either by not entering procedures or by entering lower paying procedures in the medical management software, and then billing the procedures manually or with a personal copy of the software. The result may appear as a decline in revenue. If you have split the fee collection and posting duties, then a diversion scheme such as this may indicate collusion between two or more employees.

Revenue data can be assembled into a separate database to detect changes in revenue trends more easily. An example of a report produced from such a database is found in Exhibit 7–5. It can be seen that this practice is undergoing very rapid growth in terms of both revenues and procedures. The 90801 procedure is an initial evaluation. Because this code is only used for the patient's first visit, it is a precursor of growth in

Exhibit 7–4 Production Detailed by Producer

Fee Schedule 1

Procedure	Description	Cnt	% Cnt	Fees	% Fees	Lab	% Lab
01.01	Cisternal puncture	4	15.38%	336.79	8.64%	5.00	1.97%
01.02	Ventriculopuncture/implanted catheter	1	3.85%	83.21	2.13%	30.00	11.85%
01.09	Other cranial puncture	1	3.85%	45.00	1.15%	0.00	0.00%
01.11	Diagn. procedures/skull, brain, cerebr.	1	3.85%	268.96	6.90%	12.00	4.74%
01.12	Other biopsy of cerebral meninges	1	3.85%	269.00	6.90%	15.75	6.22%
01.14	Other biopsy of brain	1	3.85%	99.75	2.56%	31.50	12.44%
01.15	Biopsy of skull	1	3.85%	236.25	6.06%	10.50	4.15%
01.18	Other diag. proc./brain & cerebr. men.	2	7.69%	350.00	8.97%	26.00	10.27%
01.19	Other diagnostic procedures on skull	2	7.69%	424.44	10.88%	31.00	12.24%
01.22	Removal/intracranial neurostimulator	2	7.69%	585.00	15.00%	40.00	15.79%
01.23	Reopening of craniotomy site	2	7.69%	199.75	5.12%	10.50	4.15%
01.24	Other craniotomy	1	3.85%	150.00	3.85%	0.00	0.00%
02.02	Elevation of skull fracture fragment	1	3.85%	450.00	11.54%	21.00	8.29%
02.92	Cisternal repair	1	3.85%	92.58	2.37%	0.00	0.00%
03.31	Spinal tap	1	3.85%	100.00	2.56%	0.00	0.00%
03.92	Injection of other agent into spinal c.	1	3.85%	39.29	1.01%	20.00	7.90%
03.98	Removal of spinal thecal shunt	1	3.85%	78.00	2.00%	0.00	0.00%
04.03	Divis./crush. of other cranial nerve	1	3.85%	48.29	1.24%	0.00	0.00%
04.43	Release of carpal tunnel	1	3.85%	43.93	1.13%	0.00	0.00%
Totals		26		3,900.24		253.25	

D1A1 Joe Carter
D2A2 Carl Yates
D3A3 Stephen Webb
D4A4 Keith Jergens
D5A5 Joseph Harris
D6A6 Bob Lovette

Courtesy of HealthCare Communications Inc., Lincoln, Nebraska.

Exhibit 7–5 Revenue and Procedure Database Report

Revenue	90801	90844	90815	90853	All Others
$68,970	78	608	8	47	12
$74,050	84	652	17	49	5
$78,070	72	705	12	65	8
$85,210	96	751	16	59	8
$87,855	87	792	20	45	15
$93,255	97	823	28	57	14

other procedures. In this case, the practice's revenue growth is driven by an increase in demand for the 90844 procedure. The revenue growth could be predicted, however, by the 90801 growth. Similarly, revenue growth is a precursor to cash growth and a decline in revenue for a period will be a precursor to declining cash several weeks hence.

This database should be revised and examined each month. The users will generally be front office personnel and the physician manager.

UNCOLLECTIBLE WRITE-OFFS

An uncollectible write-offs report (Exhibit 7–6) will indicate the amount of bad debt written off in a given time period. Once again, the most important use of this report is to examine patterns over time. If write-offs are increasing, it could be a sign that you have truly incurred more bad debt. This could be due to a number of causes, including inadequate collection efforts on the part of your staff, a change in your clientele, or deteriorating economic conditions. On the other hand, an increase in write-offs could simply mean that you are doing more work. For example, you will certainly notice an increase in your write-offs if you are a participating physician with an insurance company and you agree to accept its usual and customary rate as payment in full for your service; if the insurance carrier's usual and customary rates are less than your standard fees; and if you are treating more

patients who insure with this carrier. Substituting health maintenance organization or preferred provider organization patients for indemnity patients also could increase write-offs. Once again, the numbers simply provide information to interpret.

Increasing write-offs can also be a sign of embezzlement. One strategy for diverting money, especially if it is paid in cash, is to write off the amount. Typically, this embezzlement strategy will result in lots of small write-offs across a large number of accounts. The difficulty of using this report to identify embezzlement is that a practice of any size will be generating hundreds of write-offs each week. This report, therefore, will be most useful as an embezzlement detector when there are other indicators of embezzlement, such as patients calling and asking for receipts or being asked to pay in cash instead of by check. In this case, the write-off report will indicate the accounts that were most likely to have been embezzled.

This report should be run monthly. The users will generally be front office personnel. The physician manager, however, should receive a copy of the report as a deterrent to theft.

CASH RECEIPTS AND DISBURSEMENTS

This report may be part of your MOMS, or it may be generated from separate accounting software. Cash receipts are the monies your practice

Exhibit 7–6 Uncollectible Write-Off Report

REPORT Date: 10/8/96						
Acct.	Guarantor	Home Phone	Work Phone	Write-off Date	Write-off Amount	Account Balance
4532	Smith, Francine	555-3254	555-6658	10/7/96	$52.28	$0.00
236	Jones, George	555-9876	555-6549	10/7/96	$10.00	$0.00
896	Stewart, William	555-6789	555-3367	10/7/96	$36.98	$123.95
1125	Johnson, John	999-6523	999-6669	10/7/96	$102.68	$55.67
458	Hendricks, Fred	888-6661	888-6543	10/7/96	$226.98	$1,023.96
					$428.92	

actually collects, and cash disbursements are the payments you make to others. Cash receipts and disbursements journals are records of original entries into your accounting software.

The receipts and disbursements can be tabulated into a number of separate accounts. Exhibit 7–7 contains a chart of accounts for a private practice. Typical disbursement accounts for a medical practice include office expenses (rent, electricity, water, etc.), advertising, office supplies, medical supplies, interest payments, laboratory fees, legal and accounting fees, payroll, payroll taxes, corporate taxes, insurance, and so on. Receipt accounts might include receipts for medical services, hospital services, and laboratory tests. Work with your accountant to develop a system of accounts that will provide you with the most useful reports. In addition, the Medical Group Management Association has developed a chart of accounts for medical practices, and most accounting software will come with a suggested chart of accounts.

Exhibit 7–8 contains an example of a practice's cash receipts journal. The document column is used to record the deposit slip number. The accounts column lists the accounts that have been debited and credited in the transaction.

All transactions always affect two sides of the accounting system, which always must be in balance. The left side is referred to as the debit side, and the right side is the credit side. Assets are increased by a debit and decreased by a credit; liability accounts are increased by a credit and decreased by a debit. Therefore, when you add funds to checking (an asset account), these funds are listed as debits, and they show as a credit in the liability account to which they are also posted. For example, for deposit 126, the checking account (1010 Cash in Checking) has been debited $1,102.00 because this amount was added to it, and the income account (4100 Hospital Income) has been credited for an equal amount.

Exhibit 7–9 contains a practice's cash disbursements journal. The documents column contains the check number, and the account column indicates the accounts that were credited and debited as a result of each transaction. For example, check 6043 was written on (or credited to) account 1010 (Cash in Checking) and used to pay (or debit) account 6800 (Office Supplies). Check 6051 once again was credited against cash and used to debit, or pay for, several tax liability accounts (2100, 2210, and 2220).

By classifying transactions in this manner, it is possible to track where your receipts and disbursements come from and go to. The accounts that you choose to use are entirely up to you. In the extreme you only need two accounts: receipts and disbursements. The goal, however, is to create a more precise set of receipt and disbursement classifications for greater understanding and control of your practice's finances.

Examining monthly cash receipts and disbursements can help you control the flow of cash through your practice by allowing you to see in detail the sources of your receipts and disbursements. A cash receipts and disbursements report (see Chapter 6, Exhibit 6–12 for an example) combines the cash receipts data and the cash disbursements data into one report. This report can be used to assess receipt and disbursement trends over time and to evaluate the cash position of the practice. A cash receipts and disbursements report tells you how well you are meeting your cash needs, and this determines whether you will be around long enough to collect your receivables.

There are many excellent personal computer–based cash accounting software packages available that will allow your business manager to track and manage your cash receipts and disbursements. As was previously discussed in Chapter 6, accrual level accounting can provide additional information that is beyond the scope of cash level accounting. When you are using accrual level software, cash-based reports are virtually a no-cost byproduct of paying bills and collecting receipts. If the person using the software is capable of making accrual decisions, or if the software is sophisticated enough to be programmed for accrual decisions, then useful accrual-based reports can be produced within a practice as part of the cash accounting process at virtually any time.

Cash receipt and disbursement reports should

Exhibit 7–7 Chart of Accounts

Current Assets		
	1010	Cash in Checking
	1020	Cash in Savings
	1100	Accounts Receivable
	1200	Prepaid Expenses
Fixed Assets		
	1600	Furniture
	1700	Medical Equipment
	1800	Accumulated Depreciation
Current Liabilities		
	2100	FICA Tax Payable—Employer
	2210	FICA Tax Payable—Employee
	2220	Federal Withholding Tax Payable
	2230	State Withholding Tax Payable
	2240	Federal Unemployment Tax Payable
	2250	State Unemployment Tax Payable
	2300	Employee Deductions
	2400	Stockholder Loans Payable
Owner's Equity		
	3000	Common Stock
	3100	Retained Earnings
Income	4000	Practice Income
	4100	Hospital Income
	4200	Capitated Income
	4300	Interest Income
	4400	Rental Income
	4500	Other Income
Operating Expenses		
	6100	Advertising—Marketing
	6150	Advertising—Personnel
	6180	Advertising—Yellow Pages
	6200	Credit Card Discounts
	6250	Bank Service Charges
	6275	Interest Expense
	6280	Tax Penalties
	6300	Conference Expenses/Education
	6350	Travel—Business Related
	6360	Travel—Not Business Related
	6370	Professional Dues
	6380	Licenses—Professional
	6390	Licenses—Business

continues

Exhibit 7–7 continued

Operating Expenses		
	6395	Other Taxes and Licenses
	6500	Business Meals
	6550	Food—Entertainment
	6600	Legal Expenses
	6625	Legal Expenses—Collections
	6650	Accounting Expenses
	6670	Other Professional Expenses
	6700	Rent—Office Space
	6750	Rent—Equipment
	6800	Office Supplies
	6801	Medical Supplies
	6802	Laboratory Fees
	6803	Pharmaceuticals
	6803	Transcription Services
	6810	Gifts
	6820	General Overhead
	6830	Computer Repair/Maintenance
	6835	General Repair and Maintenance
	6850	Payroll Taxes—Employer Total
	6860	Electricity
	6870	Cleaning
	6900	Postage
	7100	Health Insurance
	7150	Professional Liability Insurance
	7175	Insurance—Other
	7200	Repairs
	7300	Salaries—Professional Staff
	7400	Salaries—Front Office Staff
	7600	Payroll—Front Office Staff
	7700	Telephone—Bell Atlantic
	7750	Telephone—MCI
	7760	Telephone—Answering Service
	7770	Telephone—Cellular Services
	7800	Depreciation
	7900	Donations
	8000	Retirement Plan—Dr. Able
	8100	Retirement Plan—Dr. Baker
	8200	Retirement Plan—Dr. Cane
	8300	Retirement Plan—Staff

Exhibit 7–8 Cash Receipts Journal

8/1/96 to 8/31/96					
Document	Date	Acct	Item Description	Debits	Credits
126	8/1/96	1010	8/1	1,102.00	
		4100	8/1		1,102.00
130	8/7/96	1010	8/5	2,368.00	
		4100	8/5		2,368.00
131	8/7/96	1010	Reach Rent	52.95	
		4350	Reach Rent		52.95
132	8/12/96	1010	8/6	459.35	
		4100	8/6		459.35
133	8/12/96	1010	8/7	1,818.21	
		4100	8/7		1,818.21
134	8/12/96	1010	8/8	1,682.03	
		4100	8/8		1,682.03
135	8/15/96	1010	8/12	1,616.22	
		4100	8/12		1,616.22
136	8/15/96	1010	8/13	1,209.45	
		4100	8/13		1,209.45
137	8/15/96	1010	8/14	738.24	
		4100	8/14		738.24
138	8/15/96	1010	8/15	2,219.25	
		4100	8/15		2,219.25
139	8/15/96	1010	8/19	3,229.38	
		4100	8/19		3,229.38
140	8/20/96	1010	8/20	831.80	
		4100	8/20		831.80
1010	Cash in Checking			17,326.88	
4100	MediMac Income				17,273.93
4350	Office Rental				52.95
				17,326.88	
					17,326.88

be prepared each month. Front office personnel will use these reports operationally to manage your cash, pay bills, and balance your cash accounts against bank statements. The physician manager should also examine a cash receipts and disbursements report monthly as well as an income statement and balance sheet.

APPLIED PRACTICE CASH MANAGEMENT PROCEDURES

To some degree, the size of your front office staff and your own possible unwillingness to in-volve yourself in some of the cash management responsibilities may require that you compromise on some of the procedures that are proposed here. These proposed guidelines are offered, therefore, as objectives, and the impracticality of implementing some of them in your practice should not preclude you from implementing as many others as is feasible. At a minimum, however, you will understand where your cash control procedures are weak, and, one hopes, you will be especially vigilant in those areas.

The basic principle in controlling cash is to separate various functions and responsibilities

Exhibit 7–9 Cash Disbursements Journal

9/1/96 to 9/30/96					
Document	Date	Acct	Item Description	Debits	Credits
6043	9/9/96	1010	Polar Water Company		32.85
		6800	Polar Water Company	32.85	
6051	9/10/96	1020	NationsBank		5,502.94
		2100	NationsBank	1,048.07	
		2210	NationsBank	1,048.08	
		2220	NationsBank	3,406.79	
6052	9/11/96	1010	Our Own Community Press		162.00
		6100	Our Own Community Press	162.00	
6053	9/11/96	1010	Postmaster		75.50
		6900	Postmaster	75.50	
6054	9/12/96	1010	Fidelity Magellan		370.81
		8100	Fidelity Magellan	370.81	
	1010	Cash in Checking			641.16
	1020	Cash in Savings			5,502.94
	2100	FICA Tax Payable—Employer		1,048.07	
	2210	FICA Tax Payable—Employee		1,048.08	
	2220	Federal W/H Taxes Payable		3,406.79	
	6100	Advertising—Marketing		162.00	
	6800	Office Supplies		32.85	
	6900	Postage		75.50	
	8100	SEP—Jones		370.81	
				6,144.10	
					6,144.10

so that they are performed by different persons. In this way, you prevent theft by employees who also have the ability to hide their actions. Procedures that facilitate the internal control of cash include the following.

Keep the Physical Handling of Cash Separate from All Phases of the Accounting and Recordkeeping Function

The reason for this is obvious. If a person handling the cash also controls the function that can disclose a diversion, then hiding a theft becomes easy. This means, for example, that if your receptionist is collecting cash at the window, then he or she should not be involved in balancing the cash receipts against MOMS cash receipts. If your business manager manages your checking account and also posts insurance payments, then the posting should be done from the insurance company remits, and the manager should not have access to unendorsed checks. Similarly, the person posting payments to accounts should not open the incoming mail and thereby have access to unendorsed checks.

The practical reality in a small medical practice is that some cash handling and accounting functions may overlap as a result of the small staff size. In this case, you might want to institute procedures that create additional "audit trails." For example, you might inform patients and post a sign to the effect that anyone who pays in currency *must* receive a written receipt from a receipt book that leaves a copy. Require that all checks that come into the office be immediately stamped "For Deposit Only to Account # . . . ."

Separate the Posting of Procedures and Payments to Patient Accounts from Management of the Checkbook

Because checkbook receipts and the receipts as recorded in your patient accounts must balance, these functions must be separate if each is to serve as a control for the other.

Make Deposits to Your Checking Account on a Daily Basis

If cash is not physically present, then it cannot be stolen.

Make All Cash Disbursements with Prenumbered Checks from One Checking Account

Using several checkbooks to make disbursements makes it more difficult for you to determine quickly where your cash is at any given moment. In addition, if all disbursements are made by check, then your checking account contains a complete record, and there is no opportunity for funds to be "lost" in petty cash.

You may choose to have more than one cash account. For example, you may have a savings account to store operating cash at a more favorable interest rate but still keep it highly liquid. Cash can be easily moved from one account to another by check. This suggestion also pertains to cash disbursements outside the practice.

Establish a Petty Cash Account

Petty cash is the cash that you need to provide change for patient transactions. Keep this petty cash fund as small as possible, locate it in a lockable cash box, and always fund the petty cash box by cashing a company check. Do not use the petty cash fund for small expenses, such as stamps or a business lunch. Once the notion of making unrecorded withdrawals from petty cash as a convenience has been established, it will be impossible to reconcile this account. An unreconcilable account is an invitation to exploitation. In addition, include the petty cash account in your cash receipts and disbursements journals.

Keep Check Signing Authority in the Hands of a Practice Owner

Never give employees signature power on your checking account. Trustworthiness and loyalty are difficult to assess and liable to change. If an employee forges your signature, then you have possible recourse with the bank, because the bank is responsible for recognizing authorized signatures. If the employee has check signing authority, then the question of whether an employee issued a check for an appropriate reason can be problematic (e.g., "I bought copier paper last February as a convenience to you, and you never did pay me back."). In any event, the bank is off the hook, and all your recovery options will probably be lengthy.

Larger practices may find this suggested restriction to be cumbersome, and they may have to resort to giving an employee check signing authority. If this is the case, have the employee bonded.

If You Have More Than One Owner, Separate the Check Approval Process from the Check Signing Responsibility

This separation of responsibilities will protect the interests of all owners. It provides each owner with a deterrent against inappropriate use of practice funds and an assurance that each will not be wrongly accused because the actions of each will be routinely examined by a colleague.

All Employees *Must* Take Vacations

Often, cash diversion schemes rely on someone being present at the right time to cover the previous diversion of funds.

CASE ILLUSTRATIONS

The following cases illustrate the ease with which an employee can divert funds and cover it up if the proper controls are not in place:

- *Case A:* The business manager of a small practice posts all payments to patient accounts, manages the checkbook, and opens the mail. A cash payment is received for $100 on the Jones account. The business manager pockets the cash and writes off or adjusts $100 on the Jones account.
- *Case B:* The business manager has check signing authority as well as the responsibility for paying all the practice's bills. She issues a check to a fictitious creditor, such as an office supply store, and then cashes the check herself.
- *Case C:* A secretary posts all procedures to patient accounts and verifies his own work the next day by comparing postings to the appointment book. No one else validates his work. He fails to post some procedures and keeps the payments.
- *Case D:* A business manager posts all procedures and opens the mail. She posts a procedure, bills the insurance company, corrects the ledger to show a posting error, and then intercepts the insurance check when it arrives in the mail.
- *Case E:* The business manager collects patient payments and posts all payments to patient accounts. Accounts are loosely managed, and the physician manager normally doesn't get concerned about an account until it is 150 days old. Patient Smith pays off a $200 balance on her account, which is 30 days old. Patient Jones pays off a $100 balance on his account, which is 120 days old. The business manager posts $100 from Smith's payment to the Jones account and pockets the remaining $100. He then continues to post money across accounts, always covering diversions with new payments. Employees who use this strategy to divert funds don't take many vacations.

All the safeguards to theft that have been discussed can be overcome if employees act in collusion. The probability of collusion, however, is obviously less than the probability of having one employee who is willing to steal if the opportunity presents itself.

THE SMALL PRACTICE PHYSICIAN MANAGER'S ROLE IN CASH CONTROL

The physician manager's role in the accounting and financial affairs of a practice is crucial. This role will vary somewhat with the size of the practice. In smaller practices, the physician manager is regularly involved in cash control procedures. The physician manager, for example, should be the only one with the authority to sign checks, although an employee should prepare the checks for signature. The solo practice physician manager should also be ultimately responsible for managing the checkbook and reconciling it with the bank statement. Because balancing a checking account is almost certainly not a good use of a physician manager's time, this task should probably be contracted out to a bookkeeper or an accountant. Even if the task is contracted out, the physician manager retains the ultimate responsibility and should routinely review the consultant's work.

Physician managers in all practices, irrespective of their size, should use financial, accounting, and production data extensively in their role as practice managers. Physician managers are ultimately responsible for the financial health of the practice and have a duty both to themselves and to their employees to use these data to ensure that the practice will survive and prosper. The following suggestions concern the appropriate role for the physician manager:

- The physician manager should determine which financial tasks will be performed by the various front office personnel. The business manager should be consulted about appropriate roles, but the ultimate responsibility must reside with the physician manager. This is essential to ensure financial control and reduce the possibilities of embezzlement or collusion.

- The daily receipts and adjustments and daily activity reports should be forwarded to the physician manager each day after they have been reconciled. The degree to which the physician manager should examine these reports on a daily basis can vary. The most important thing, as far as cash control is concerned, is that the physician manager *has* the report and that employees *know* it. Spot checks by the physician manager on a random basis can be used to detect sloppy, misleading, or deceitful posting practices.

- Cash receipt and disbursement reports and various other reports, including gross receipt, write-off, and aging reports, should be examined by the physician manager. These reports should also be examined by the business manager, but this is never a substitute for close review by the physician manager. The business manager should be using these reports to direct day-to-day activities. Part of the physician manager's job, however, is to ensure that the business manager is performing adequately, which requires that the physician manager be personally familiar with the data in these reports. In addition, the physician manager should be using these data to provide guidance regarding practice growth and direction. Personal familiarity with practice finances is essential for the physician manager to make intelligent, rational choices. In this regard, it is always important to remember that the physician manager is the best guardian of his or her own welfare.

- Periodically, the physician manager should set aside time to reflect on the implications of the financial data and consider plans for changes and improvements to practice procedures. Some amount of reflection should occur as a result of the daily, weekly, and monthly reviews of the data. It is important, however, to set aside time for developing a perspective on where the practice has been, where it is now, and various directions in which it might go.

- The physician manager and the practice's accountant should review the financial status of the practice annually. A logical time for this review is after the accountant has prepared the annual tax return. The accountant may be able to provide a perspective on the practice's performance and make helpful suggestions regarding, for example, modifying the practice's retirement plan, financing a proposed expansion, or leasing new equipment.

- The physician manager should determine which of the various accounting and financial tools will be useful for management purposes. The physician manager should direct employees to gather the appropriate information so that it will be available when it is needed.

Unfortunately, the task of managing a practice's finances takes time, which will be obtained by working more total hours or by sacrificing clinical hours. Administrative responsibilities such as these are simply part of the baggage that goes along with any business organization. Furthermore, your work as an administrator will have an impact on your patients. It will assure them that you and your practice will be available when they need your services. Practices do fail as a result of mismanagement, fraud, and poor planning. Bankruptcy can occur even if you have first-rate clinical skills. Your role as a vigilant, involved administrator is essential if these problems are not to befall your practice.

Physician managers in private practice should remember that this is their practice and that they are the only ones who will consistently look out for their own welfare. As a result, they should routinely examine financial data. Relying on another party to examine the accounting data might be more efficient, but it might also be ineffective or even disastrous because the other party's point of view or self-interest might not be consistent with your own. For example, a business manager with an incentive compensation contract might benefit if you bring in additional colleagues and hence might interpret the financial data in a biased manner. Similarly, a business manager who is on a flat salary might have an interest in keeping the practice small to minimize work. Your bookkeeper might be diverting funds and would be only too pleased to tell you that the accounting reports indicate that all is well. An accountant may simply be *uninterested* in why expenditures for supplies have been steadily growing over the last two years. He or she might assume that it is a result of practice growth, whereas you would be more likely to wonder whether your staff has been wasteful.

CONCLUSION

It is important to remember that others may waste your wealth if it in some measure will increase their own wealth or decrease their work. Although easily obtainable accounting information can allow you to identify the consequences if others are wasteful, you probably will have to examine and interpret this information personally to secure your own interests.

CHAPTER 8

Collection of Receivables

Chapter Objectives

This chapter is directed at physician managers who are in private practice. It is also relevant to physicians who are working for large health care organizations and have incentive contracts based on collected revenues. It will help these physicians increase collection from both patients and insurance companies. This chapter covers:

1. the appropriate role for the physician manager in the collection process
2. what employees can do to increase collection effectiveness
3. tactics for increasing patient payments, including education and collection methods
4. tactics to manage insurance collection
5. selecting and using a collection agent
6. what to do if your collection process is in disarray

In addition, you will learn how your medical office management software can be used to guide collection activities so that you will obtain the greatest return from your efforts. Finally, you will learn how to construct a collection plan that will orchestrate the collection components into an effective, coordinated activity.

This chapter is not designed to teach you how to comply with the claim filing procedures of specific insurance companies. These procedures vary by state and company, and they can change at any time. Staying current with particular claim filing requirements is a daily task for the collection administrator, not the physician manager.

At a time when most physicians are concerned with how to adapt to managed care and in many cases capitated contracts, it may seem somewhat anachronistic to be discussing collection, the process of collecting receivables from insurance companies and patients. Nevertheless, most patients in most regions of the United States are not covered by capitated contracts, and many other incarnations of managed care still require filing claims with insurers and collecting copayments from patients. Even those patients who are covered by capitation generally can be charged a copayment. Copayments can account for anywhere from 3 percent of net revenue for some specialties up to 15 percent for primary care physicians.

Collection is relevant to any physician manager who has an equity involvement in a practice or any type of incentive arrangement based on net revenue or net income. A physician, for example, who is employed by an integrated health care system or health maintenance organization (HMO) and receives as a bonus a percentage of net income above projected levels has an interest in seeing that the collection process is effectively managed. The issue of collection, therefore, is relevant and will remain so for most physician managers for the foreseeable future.

Effective collection is the result of consistently applying a well-conceived collection process, learning from collection failures, and using these experiences to modify the procedure. In other words, effective collection is the result of applying total quality management (TQM) methods (see Chapter 12). The foundation for effective collection is having an effective collection plan. A collection plan describes in detail how delinquent accounts will be handled, what actions will be taken, when these actions will occur, and the reports and databases that will be used to manage the collection process. Once you have a formal written plan, failures to collect can be used to modify the plan, so that the plan over time continues to improve and adapt to new delinquency tactics on the part of patients and insurers and to changes in collection law.

COLLECTION ROLES AND RESPONSIBILITIES

A cornerstone of effective collection is having the right personnel undertaking the right collection activities. Table 8–1 describes how the responsibilities of the physician, collection administrator, and front office staff relate to problems in patient collection, insurance collection, and practice collection procedures. Each of these areas must be specifically addressed by the appropriate personnel, who then undertake the appropriate tasks. The ideas presented in Table 8–1 are a starting point that you should consider modifying based on your own experience and practice circumstances.

Let's begin with the physician's role. There are three themes to the physician manager's collection role. The first theme is to ensure that the practice has the appropriate collection proce-

dures in place. The process by which revenue is collected is far too important to delegate to others without physician input. The second theme is control. This means that the physician manager is instrumental in ensuring that collection activity is achieving desired results. This is achieved primarily through reviewing critical management reports and supervising the collection administrator. (The term *collection administrator* is used to refer to the front office position primarily responsible for revenue collection. This position may in fact be titled *office manager*, *accounts receivable manager*, or some other job title.)

The third theme to the physician manager's role is motivating employees to collect fees. Many employees think that they and the physician will be unaffected by a few dollars that are not collected here and there. It is important for employees to understand that this is not the case and that inattention to collection could jeopardize everyone's job. Many employees never seem to be aware of the linkage between their paychecks, their job security, and their role in collecting fees and turning revenue into cash. Physician managers reinforce this link through face-to-face meetings and practice documents, such as an employee handbook.

Physician managers can also affect employee motivation by making collection effectiveness an important factor in employees' performance evaluations. Revenue collection should be an evaluation factor for any position with a role in the collection process. This includes the secretary who takes payments at the front desk as well as the collection administrator. In addition, an employee's evaluation on this factor should be tied to subsequent pay raises, rewards, discipline, or promotions in the same manner as any other important evaluation issue. (This statement does not imply that you must implement a merit system in which pay is directly driven by the performance evaluation. It simply suggests that collection effectiveness should be considered in the same manner as any other important job performance issue.)

Physicians should have no involvement in day-to-day collection activities. Generally, phy-

Table 8–1 Collection Roles and Tasks

| Role | Problem Areas | | |
	Patient	Procedures	Insurance Company
Physician	No direct negotiation Determine billing strategy Design patient education information Monitor controls Supervise	Design collection plan Design controls Supervise	Monitor controls Supervise
Business manager	Design patient education information Provide patient education information Use collection plan Use controls Supervise Receive and give feedback	Design collection plan Design controls Supervise Receive and give feedback	Use collection plan Use controls Supervise Receive and give feedback
Front office staff	Use collection plan Provide patient education information Use controls Give feedback	Use collection plan Give feedback	Use collection plan Use controls Give feedback

sicians also should stay out of direct financial negotiations with patients. Physicians should not discuss payments with patients because:

- they usually aren't aware of all the financial considerations regarding a given case,
- they may allow their feelings for a patient to interfere with what is essentially a business matter, and
- their involvement is likely to be perceived as interference that may frustrate the collection administrator, who as a result may hesitate to act for fear of being overruled.

This does not mean that physicians can't be involved in particular cases, but it does mean that this involvement should occur behind the scenes and through the collection administrator.

The physician should be very involved in designing patient education information. A major reason for patient delinquency is ignorance of fi-

nancial responsibility, insurance benefits, and the like. Development of these materials is too important to delegate entirely to the collection administrator. Patient pamphlets, intake forms, and other materials about patient financial responsibilities should be reviewed by the physician manager for completeness and clarity.

Controls are reports and measures that provide information about whether a process, such as collection, is working according to plan. The physician manager needs to routinely review control reports that describe the state of patient collection. The aging analysis is the most critical report in this area. An example of an aging analysis is found in Exhibit 8–1. Each day, uncollected revenue becomes a day older. The aging analysis ages receivables so that the physician manager can get a picture of the state of accounts. Because a practice will probably have several hundred accounts in the aging process, most of which are not problem accounts, it is critical that your medical office management software (MOMS) be capable of sorting the accounts so that the worst ones stand out. The report in Exhibit 8–1 was exported from the MOMS directly into an *Excel* spreadsheet. A new column defined as 90+ days was created, which was the sum of the 90, 120, and 150 days columns. The cases were then sorted in descending order on the 90+ day column. This practice considered any account that reached 90 days a problem account, so this process highlights those accounts that need immediate attention.

An important point to consider is what constitutes an unacceptable aging. One way to address this consideration is to refer to external sources of data. Exhibit 8–2 illustrates data from the Medical Group Management Association. Comparing data from your practice with national or regional data is one way to address this consideration. This approach is not particularly relevant for several reasons. First, many of the databases have small sample sizes. Second, the data are generally national or regional at best, so their relevance to your local situation is problematic at best. Finally, why limit yourself to what your colleagues are doing?

A better strategy is to implement TQM thinking and techniques. Consider collection a process that is amenable to TQM methods, such as statistical analysis and continuous quality improvement. Start from where you are now, and manage against that performance level. Set specific improvement goals in target categories, such as 150+ days and 90+ days. When those are reached, look at the failed cases, and see where you can improve the process again. If 150+ gets down to 1 percent of receivables, what changes can be implemented to bring it down to 0.5 percent? Managing your collection process from where you are now is a far superior solution than using external and largely irrelevant statistics.

The sorted aging report will be used by both the collection administrator and the physician manager, but for different purposes. The collection administrator will use the report to identify

those accounts to work first. The physician manager will use the report as part of the control function and to supervise the collection administrator. The physician manager should meet on a regular basis with the collection administrator to discuss the collection process. During these meetings, the physician manager should ask for a synopsis of some of the worst aging cases. If it is obvious that the collection administrator is knowledgeable about these cases and is using the appropriate practice collection policy, then this is an indication that the collection process is being effectively managed. If, on the other hand, the collection administrator's response is frequently "I'll have to get back to you on that one," or if it appears that practice collection policies are not being consistently applied, then there is a job performance problem.

Each monthly aging analysis should be recorded as a row in an aging history database. The aging history database is used to track collection performance over time. Exhibit 8–3 contains an aging database that was assembled retrospectively for a practice that lost control of its collection process. The increase in the current column indicates that the practice grew in size, however, the out-of-tolerance column of 120 to 180+ days grew far more rapidly. In a situation such as this, it is possible for the practice growth to mask the collection problem because cash receipts may remain stable or even grow. If the practice had been keeping an aging history database, it would have seen that something was going wrong in September, if not before.

The aging history database is useful for seeing trends over time and judging whether the collection process is responding to changes in procedures and personnel. It and the aging analysis are the two most fundamental control reports that the physician manager has for managing the collection process. Generally, MOMS do not have aging history databases. They are easy to construct, however, using spreadsheet programs such as *Excel* and *Lotus*.

All too often, the physician manager will avoid the responsibility of looking at aging analyses, using the rationalization that it is really

Exhibit 8–1 Aging Analysis, March 31, 19xx

Acct.	Guarantor	Current	30 Days	60 Days	90 Days	120 Days	150+ Days	Total	90+ Days
2203-G	xxxxxxxxx	$0.00	$90.00	$0.00	$270.00	$90.00	$450.00	$900.00	$810.00
2189-G	xxxxxxxxx	$37.85	$165.00	$90.00	$360.00	$90.00	$320.00	$1,062.85	$770.00
2182-G	xxxxxxxxx	$25.00	$90.00	$153.74	$90.00	$127.48	$467.16	$953.38	$684.64
2163-G	xxxxxxxxx	$4,536.00	$90.00	$180.00	$532.30	$0.00	$0.00	$5,338.30	$532.30
1855-G	xxxxxxxxx	$235.68	$159.30	$0.00	$0.00	$0.00	$315.10	$710.08	$315.10
2208-G	xxxxxxxxx	$0.00	$111.00	$21.00	$201.00	$55.50	$0.00	$388.50	$256.50
2214-G	xxxxxxxxx	$0.00	$0.00	$22.50	$45.00	$165.00	$37.50	$270.00	$247.50
2262-G	xxxxxxxxx	$56.98	$0.00	$0.00	$180.00	$0.00	$0.00	$236.98	$180.00
2001-G	xxxxxxxxx	$0.00	$90.00	$90.00	$90.00	$90.00	$0.00	$360.00	$180.00
2134-G	xxxxxxxxx	$0.00	$0.00	$0.00	$0.00	$0.00	$180.00	$180.00	$180.00
945-G	xxxxxxxxx	$0.00	$0.00	$150.00	$175.00	$0.00	$0.00	$325.00	$175.00
1996-G	xxxxxxxxx	$366.57	$0.00	$0.00	$0.00	$0.00	$170.00	$536.57	$170.00
1979-G	xxxxxxxxx	$0.00	$0.00	$0.00	$0.00	$0.00	$168.00	$168.00	$168.00
2178-G	xxxxxxxxx	$0.00	$75.00	$150.00	$88.00	$75.00	$0.00	$388.00	$163.00
2157-G	xxxxxxxxx	$5,225.30	$0.00	$105.00	$130.00	$10.00	$0.00	$5,470.30	$140.00
2244-G	xxxxxxxxx	$10.00	$0.00	$0.00	$45.00	$90.00	$0.00	$145.00	$135.00
1858-G	xxxxxxxxx	$25.36	$0.00	$45.00	$0.00	$0.00	$126.00	$196.36	$126.00
2213-G	xxxxxxxxx	$687.36	$118.00	$0.00	$97.00	$0.00	$0.00	$902.36	$97.00
743-G	xxxxxxxxx	$0.00	$270.00	$41.40	$0.00	$90.00	$0.00	$401.40	$90.00
2266-G	xxxxxxxxx	$0.00	$45.00	$0.00	$90.00	$0.00	$0.00	$135.00	$90.00
2173-G	xxxxxxxxx	$0.00	$0.00	$0.00	$0.00	$0.00	$89.27	$89.27	$89.27
1268-G	xxxxxxxxx	$56.35	$243.60	$162.40	$86.20	$0.00	$0.00	$548.55	$86.20
2253-G	xxxxxxxxx	$56.36	$0.00	$0.00	$0.00	$80.00	$0.00	$136.36	$80.00
2097-G	xxxxxxxxx	$123.65	$247.20	$235.80	$74.80	$0.00	$0.00	$681.45	$74.80
2147-G	xxxxxxxxx	$274.35	$90.00	$27.60	$53.88	$13.80	$0.00	$459.63	$67.68
1862-G	xxxxxxxxx	$15.00	$65.00	$270.00	$65.00	$0.00	$0.00	$415.00	$65.00
2222-G	xxxxxxxxx	$3,623.36	$0.00	$67.50	$0.00	$45.00	$17.50	$3,753.36	$62.50
2227-G	xxxxxxxxx	$56.98	$0.00	$0.00	$0.00	$0.00	$62.50	$119.48	$62.50
1997-G	xxxxxxxxx	$98.67	$79.65	$0.00	$0.00	$6.59	$48.65	$233.56	$55.24
2180-G	xxxxxxxxx	$552.37	$270.00	$41.40	$53.88	$0.00	$0.00	$917.65	$53.88
2028-G	xxxxxxxxx	$65.98	$124.00	$152.00	$51.25	$0.00	$0.00	$393.23	$51.25

continues

Exhibit 8-1 continued

Acct.	Guarantor	Current	30 Days	60 Days	90 Days	120 Days	150+ Days	Total	90+ Days
1170-G	xxxxxxxx	$10.00	$0.00	$0.00	$0.00	$9.17	$40.95	$60.12	$50.12
1478-G	xxxxxxxx	$0.00	$0.00	$0.00	$0.00	$8.87	$39.31	$48.18	$48.18
Net Current	$24,697.36	48.33%							
Net 30 Days	$13,174.41	25.78%							
Net 60 Days	$6,429.80	12.58%							
Net 90 Days	$2,950.34	5.77%							
Net 120 Days	$1,162.69	2.28%							
Net 150 Days	$1,303.66	2.55%							
Net 180+ Days	$1,378.93	2.70%							
Net A/R	$51,097.19	100.00%							
Total Credit Balance	($2,282.89)								

Exhibit 8–2 Accounts Receivable and Collection Percentage for Larger Multispecialty Practices

Accounts Receivable Data and Collection Percentages	50 to 75 FTE Count	50 to 75 FTE Median	76 to 150 FTE Count	76 to 150 FTE Median	151 FTE or More Count	151 FTE or More Median
Total Accounts Rec. ($/FTE physician)	35	99,064.56	28	95,651.91	12	107,894.58
Total Accounts Rec. ($/FTE provider)	35	86,961.45	28	79,341.78	12	85,494.93
0 to 30 days % of total A/R	35	36.27	26	28.09	11	37.41
31 to 60 days % of total A/R	35	19.84	26	18.55	11	18.88
61 to 90 days % of total A/R	35	10.65	26	10.58	11	10.68
91 to 120 days % of total A/R	35	6.38	26	6.36	11	7.73
Over 120 days % of total A/R	35	27.7	27	31.38	10	26.02
Months Adj. FFS Charges in A/R	30	3.54	20	3.4	12	3.69
Gross Collection Percentage	31	76.65	22	77.94	12	69.71
Adj. Collection Percentage	30	95.68	21	96.45	12	97.88

Source: Reprinted with permission from the Medical Group Management Association, 104 Inverness Terrace East, Englewood, CO 80112–5306; 303-799-1111. Copyright © 1994.

Exhibit 8-3 Aging History Report

Date	Current	90 Days	120 Days	150 Days	180+ Days	120-180+ Days
19-Aug-95	$50,337.71	$10,848.94	$7,808.98	$7,367.05	$13,133.66	$28,309.69
1-Sep-95	$50,662.18	$12,553.90	$9,316.42	$5,821.28	$16,796.44	$27,691.60
8-Sep-95	$45,168.16	$11,917.86	$10,072.02	$6,188.59	$17,316.72	$33,577.33
16-Sep-95	$44,391.19	$11,100.43	$10,558.39	$6,448.95	$17,404.32	$34,411.66
23-Sep-95	$46,590.00	$11,261.68	$11,392.22	$7,220.92	$17,900.17	$36,513.31
1-Oct-95	$44,213.02	$12,888.17	$10,106.40	$8,144.31	$17,650.38	$35,901.09
8-Oct-95	$50,995.77	$13,960.67	$10,278.99	$8,887.63	$16,988.79	$36,155.41
20-Oct-95	$52,224.71	$15,564.54	$8,929.06	$8,673.35	$17,979.17	$35,581.58
31-Oct-95	$52,893.07	$13,872.83	$10,933.86	$7,764.96	$18,678.98	$37,377.80
11-Nov-95	$51,042.84	$11,861.86	$12,372.18	$8,545.72	$19,477.86	$40,395.76
16-Nov-95	$56,353.12	$11,233.73	$13,329.26	$7,880.51	$18,820.92	$40,030.69
23-Nov-95	$56,918.49	$10,269.26	$12,861.16	$5,818.36	$19,801.99	$38,481.51
30-Nov-95	$54,111.96	$10,368.25	$11,315.71	$7,339.91	$20,091.09	$38,746.71
7-Dec-95	$56,878.04	$9,530.61	$12,226.70	$7,419.02	$21,086.99	$40,732.71
21-Dec-95	$58,209.00	$9,699.90	$9,558.29	$9,991.87	$19,730.74	$39,280.90
28-Dec-95	$56,851.92	$10,561.54	$9,861.57	$9,251.78	$23,662.41	$42,775.76
11-Jan-96	$44,365.88	$15,368.72	$8,017.26	$8,312.27	$24,480.69	$40,810.22
25-Jan-96	$51,291.50	$17,920.38	$9,215.53	$7,672.12	$25,599.25	$42,486.90
2-Feb-96	$52,428.12	$19,180.18	$10,213.47	$7,690.16	$27,296.92	$45,200.55
22-Feb-96	$56,697.74	$15,610.55	$15,598.89	$7,075.35	$25,485.00	$48,159.24
8-Mar-96	$53,696.79	$16,538.98	$16,055.50	$9,189.50	$27,179.17	$52,424.17
11-May-96	$57,707.94	$11,786.93	$8,260.40	$10,561.27	$34,407.16	$53,228.83
24-May-96	$52,550.12	$12,584.63	$8,089.75	$9,761.48	$36,362.00	$54,213.23
20-Jun-96	$62,099.38	$13,994.78	$9,657.96	$6,154.00	$40,096.60	$55,908.56
6-Jul-96	$63,470.52	$14,751.89	$9,494.78	$7,456.28	$41,387.89	$58,338.95
10-Jul-96	$60,828.01	$16,570.60	$9,129.24	$8,190.20	$42,778.60	$60,098.04
19-Jul-96	$58,256.31	$14,958.84	$10,003.03	$7,688.08	$42,295.48	$59,986.59
11-Aug-96	$48,444.09	$11,753.63	$10,831.80	$5,795.95	$34,785.62	$51,413.37
19-Aug-96	$62,533.46	$14,226.72	$9,193.01	$6,449.50	$34,508.65	$50,151.16

the collection administrator's job to identify and resolve receivable problems. The physician's objective, however, is different from the collection administrator's. The collection administrator reviews aging analyses to determine which accounts need immediate action. The physician manager reviews aging analyses to determine whether the collection administrator is doing his or her job and to evaluate the overall collection success of the practice. This is a critical physician manager responsibility. Failure to perform this control function exposes the practice to collection failure and eventual cash problems that otherwise could have been easily detected and corrected.

On occasion, a collection administrator may not want the physician to regularly review aging analyses and other management reports. The collection administrator may pander to the physician's ego and imply that this task is beneath the physician. Reviewing these reports is critical, however, to the physician's ultimate responsibility, which is to ensure the financial soundness of the practice. A good collection administrator will be proud of his or her achievements, and these achievements ultimately appear in the collection and financial reports. Whenever a collection administrator in any way suggests that the physician should not routinely review collection and financial reports, the physician should immediately become suspicious.

The physician manager's responsibility regarding procedures is to work with the collection administrator to design a collection plan. This is an area that is too critical to delegate totally to the collection administrator. A reasonable division of effort might be for the collection administrator to create initial drafts of policies, procedures, and timetables and for the physician to respond to and modify the proposals. Similarly, the physician should be involved in the identification of controls that will be used to monitor the collection process. Once again, this task is just too critical to delegate completely to a subordinate. As with patient collection, the physician manager is responsible for monitoring controls and supervising the collection administrator re-

garding insurance company collection. Once again, this will generally translate into examining reports, such as an aging analysis by insurance carrier.

The collection administrator's responsibilities involve working with the physician manager to design the collection plan, patient education information, and control systems. In addition, this position is primarily responsible for using these systems on a daily basis. The collection administrator is also the primary conduit for information from front line personnel, such as secretaries and insurance clerks. In small practices, the business manager may also be the collection administrator. In this situation, the collection administration role is simply part of the business manager's job description.

In large practices, the collection administration tasks may be significant enough to justify a full-time position. This position generally should report to the business manager. Some practices will be in a state of transition. Collection activities might begin to take too much time for the business manager to attend to all collection and noncollection responsibilities. If this happens, consider hiring a part-time employee who reports to the business manager. This part-time employee would perform the simpler collection tasks under the direct supervision of the business manager. This part-time position would be eliminated if the practice grows sufficiently to justify a full-time collection administration position.

Finally, it is the responsibility of front office staff to put the collection policies and procedures into operation. Because two of the keys to effective collection are consistency and timeliness, we don't want a whole lot of unguided creativity going on in the front line. We do want the ideas of front line personnel to be evaluated and included where appropriate. It is important, therefore, to encourage front line employees to think creatively about collection problems and to communicate their ideas to the collection administrator. From the collection administrator's perspective, an important goal is to encourage communication, provide feedback, and put reasonable suggestions offered by front line personnel into operation. A suggestion involvement level of empowerment is generally appropriate for these front line jobs (see Chapter 5).

All employees with some collection responsibility must be held accountable for successfully completing their tasks. Accountability is achieved by ensuring that there are undesirable consequences for failing to collect fees as well as desirable ones when it is done effectively. Whenever there is a collection problem that can be traced back to a particular employee or job, it is important to analyze the reward contingencies. Does the employee benefit by a failure to collect? What happens when the collection does not take place?

The following case illustrates the application of these principles. Nan was a receptionist for a group family practice that was having difficulty collecting copayments and deductibles. She reported to the collection administrator. Nan's collection responsibilities consisted of collecting payments, copayments, and deductibles at the time of service. Nan knew how to read a Blue Cross card to determine a deductible, and she was also told to refer cases to the collection administrator if she felt uncertain. In addition, she had a copayment database for commercial insurance, HMO, and preferred provider organization (PPO) plans for patients who were returning for treatment.

On occasion, Nan simply did not collect the fees. Her excuses included "I didn't see the patient leave" and "The patient told me he forgot his checkbook." The collection administrator routinely responded to these collection lapses by sending a bill to the patient or calling the patient and asking for payment by mail. The net effect, however, was that the collection administrator was devoting time to collection tasks that properly belonged to Nan. When the collection administrator was asked why Nan's behavior was tolerated, she stated "Generally, Nan does a very good job. Revenue collection is an exception. Besides, once the patient leaves without paying, I can follow through faster than she can."

Nan suffered no bad consequences when a patient avoided payment. On the contrary, if Nan didn't do her job, the collection administrator would do it for her. In effect, the collection administrator was rewarding Nan for not doing her job.

Once the collection administrator understood that she was rewarding undesirable behavior, she changed Nan's responsibilities. She told her that she was responsible for one *effective* collection attempt for each visit. If a patient managed to leave unnoticed or Nan dealt ineffectively with a patient's unacceptable excuse, she would be responsible for contacting the patient by telephone that day and asking the patient to put a check in the mail.

Nan quickly learned that it was easier to collect from patients before they left the practice. This had two effects. First, Nan greatly improved her collection rate. Second, the collection administrator now had more time available to pursue other tasks.

COLLECTING FROM PATIENTS

One way to conceptualize collection from patients is as follows: There is a line of creditors at the patient's front door. Unfortunately, the patient does not have enough money to pay everyone in the line, and the line is growing longer day by day, week by week. Your practice must be assertive enough to jump to the front of the line, so that it will be one of the few creditors that will be paid.

Sometimes it is helpful to understand the reasons for delinquency when you are formulating a strategy to collect on an account. Patients don't pay bills for an almost infinite number of specific reasons. Almost all, however, are variations on four themes:

1. economic hardships or misfortune
2. perceptions of inequity
3. irresponsibility
4. extreme irresponsibility, possibly resulting from a personality disorder

Unexpected economic misfortune can befall anyone. Unfortunately, you are probably not the patient's only creditor. Moving to the front of the line is particularly important when you are dealing with this class of delinquency. You can do this in a number of ways:

- *Be assertive*. The squeaky wheel does tend to get greased first. If your practice is visible through letters, telephone calls, collection procedures, and so on, you will be paid before the creditor who blends into the background.
- *Give the patient a solution*. Remind the patient that he or she can use a credit card. Suggest that the patient get a part-time job or obtain a loan from a bank, sibling, or parent. Ask the patient about assets that could be converted into cash, such as an individual retirement account. Have the patient complete a new financial information form. This may reveal some previously undisclosed assets as well as help you develop a payment plan. Propose a plan that will pay off the debt over a short period of time. If the amount is small, try to get the patient to make a payment *now* and close the account with a second payment. The patient may not follow through with the plan, but you may collect some of the debt. Your suggestions may not be in the patient's best financial interests. This is, however, an adversarial situation, and solutions here are intended to maximize your revenue collection. You should assess these solutions in light of your views regarding what is ethical or socially responsible.
- *Consider giving the patient a deal*. For example, if Sarah has a $500 balance, tell her that it will be turned over for collection on Friday, at which time legal fees of $250 will be added to the balance. If, however, she pays $400 by Thursday, the account will be closed, thereby saving her $350. Once Friday arrives, the matter will be out of your hands. You might want to calculate the "discount" that you will offer by considering your legal fee if you place the account in collection and subtracting a portion of this from the patient balance.
- *Don't be intimidated by threats of bankruptcy*. If a patient truly is insolvent, then bankruptcy protects the creditor as well as the debtor. In addition, it is unlikely that asserting the patient's debt to you will be the final act that pushes the patient into bankruptcy.
- *Accept known financial hardship cases with open eyes*. Intake procedures should be designed to identify potential financial hardship cases. For example, patients without insurance or without a job are likely to be hardship cases. You can then decide whether to take potential hardship cases that are likely to require ongoing treatment. If you do, be certain that the payment terms are agreed to in writing. If you feel that you have an obligation to take house cases or treat some patients at reduced fees, be certain that you closely monitor the proportion of these patients in your practice. You also have an obligation to your employees, your other patients, and your family to stay in business.

Some patients don't pay because they feel that a fee is unreasonable given the quality or quantity of service. Equity problems can be reduced, although not eliminated, by providing sufficient information to patients. Be certain that patients understand that fees are for services rendered and *are not contingent upon the success of treatment*. Educating patients concerning fees, their insurance coverage, probable clinical outcomes, and so on will allow them to make informed decisions regarding whether to seek services. Generally, a patient is less likely to feel that a fee is unfairly high when all the facts are known and the patient seeks treatment fully apprised of the probable clinical outcomes and financial implications.

Some people are ineffective at managing their lives and their responsibilities. Generally, these peoples' lives are characterized by unorganized and inappropriately directed activity. Obligations are not responded to based on objective, rational considerations. A major debt, such as a

$300 gynecology fee, has no greater importance than a minor luxury, such as going out to dinner. Irresponsible patients fail to pay for a number of reasons, including the following:

- *Paying is inconvenient.* The inconvenience, however, may be perceived as trivial by most people. Watching a basketball game on television, for example, may be more important than paying two months of back bills.
- *Irresponsible patients are often disorganized.* Bills are lost, misplaced, or never opened. Payments may sit on a desk for weeks because there are no stamps or envelopes in the house.
- *They often don't plan ahead.* The end of the month may well reveal debts in excess of available cash. In addition, these patients are usually responsible for a disproportionate number of cancelations.
- *They impulse buy.* A patient with a $300 balance buys a "cute, irresistible" puppy for $500, even though your bill remains unpaid.
- *They devise reasons why they can't pay now.* Rationalizations such as "Physicians are rich anyway," "I'll pay after my next paycheck," and "It's inconvenient to draw money out of savings" provide sufficient justification in the mind of the irresponsible patient.
- *They tend to deny the significance of their debts.* Irresponsible patients often feel that their obligations will disappear if they can postpone them long enough. Unfortunately, this belief is grounded in reality. Some creditors do in fact go away, either out of exhaustion or as a result of disorganized or inefficient collection methods.

The irresponsible patient often responds to personal impulse and to the most immediate or salient force in the environment. Therefore, the primary objective when dealing with an irresponsible patient is to provide structure and consistency. When the irresponsible patient does address financial commitments, you want to be the first creditor to come to mind. Providing constant reminders is an effective strategy with the irresponsible patient. Collection letters with very direct messages and telephone calls will make you an imposing presence. It is also essential to provide structure by enforcing cancelation fees, late payment charges, and, ultimately, termination of treatment for failure to meet financial obligations (obviously, this last alternative needs to be done in a medically appropriate manner to avoid an abandonment tort).

People with personality disorders possess basic personality flaws. Patients with personality disorders may at first simply appear to be irresponsible. The distinction is one of degree, with the depth, persistence, and creativeness of the irresponsible behavior being indicators. Unfortunately, there are no clear predictors that will differentiate irresponsible patients who have personality disorders from those who do not.

There are several types of personality disorders, but all of them are characterized by a high degree of self-centeredness and limitless ability to deny personal obligations. Patients with personality disorders have either no conscience or only a minimally developed conscience. Some are incapable of feeling guilt, obligation, or remorse and tend to view the world as existing solely to meet their needs. If lying or deception is necessary to satisfy a personal need, then that is what will be done.

Another characteristic of people with personality disorders is that they have an uncanny ability to involve others in their disputes. They are adept at "triangling," or passing on their responsibility to another party. For example, the patient who manages to get your collection administrator to agree to charge her estranged husband for your services has adeptly removed herself from the collection process. The husband may or may not be estranged, and he may or may not have any legal obligations in the matter.

Case Example 1

Mrs. Phlegmatic brought her youngest child to Dr. Phillips for treatment of allergies. She was poor, but she had insurance, and she told Dr. Phillips' collection administrator that Social Services had agreed to cover the copayment and deductible. After several visits and no sign of payment from Social Services, the collection administrator contacted the agency and was informed that Mrs. Phlegmatic had already exhausted her benefits.

At her next visit, Mrs. Phlegmatic was told that she would have to make payments on the account. She made payments for two weeks, at which time they stopped, and the collection administrator received a call from Reverend Mooney. He told the collection administrator that Dr. Phillips was inhumane, uncaring, and trying to take advantage of this poor woman. Reverend Mooney then stated that he would try to obtain the money for Mrs. Phlegmatic. Several weeks passed, and the collection administrator had several additional discussions with Reverend Mooney regarding the account. During this time, Mrs. Phlegmatic's child continued treatment, and the personal balance approached $1,000. The contacts between the practice and Reverend Mooney became increasingly strained and adversarial. On several occasions, the collection administrator delayed calling Reverend Mooney because the conversations had become so unpleasant. Finally, Reverend Mooney informed the collection administrator that he would not be able to obtain the funds. The practice then looked to Mrs. Phlegmatic for payment, who responded, "I've paid enough, and I'm not going to pay anymore. I'm leaving, and I'm not coming back!"

Mrs. Phlegmatic was very successful at triangling the collection administrator. She also was no fool. She chose well when she selected Reverend Mooney to champion her cause. She deflected her responsibility to Reverend Mooney, who was more than happy to adopt her cause and confound it with his own agenda—trying to get physicians to behave in a more socially responsible way. Unfortunately, the collection administrator took the bait and focused his attention on Reverend Mooney instead of Mrs. Phlegmatic. The net result was that Dr. Phillips was not paid, Reverend Mooney had more fuel for his indigna-

tion, and Mrs. Phlegmatic had taught her child another valuable lesson regarding how easy it is to manipulate others and evade personal responsibility.

Logic, rationality, equity, and guilt are useless when you are trying to collect from a patient with a personality disorder. Success will depend on power. Sanctions, legal procedures, and collection attorneys are the only alternatives when such a patient does not want to pay.

Often, the personality disorder patient will threaten to file a malpractice suit if the physician attempts to collect on the account. If this happens, the physician must balance the outstanding fee and the principle of resisting what amounts to extortion against the time and effort that could be expended in a legal defense.

Case Example 2

Rose was a medical secretary for Dr. Jonathan, a general surgeon. When she needed surgery, Dr. Jonathan recommended her to Dr. Apple, who performed a septal rhinoplasty and billed Rose's commercial insurance carrier for $1,800. The carrier directly reimbursed Rose $1,000, but Rose never forwarded the payment to Dr. Apple. After several months, Dr. Apple sent her a collection letter. At that point, Rose forwarded Dr. Apple two bad checks for the insurance amount of $1,000. Finally, after a call from Dr. Apple's collection administrator, Rose forwarded a good check. Dr. Apple's office then attempted to collect the personal balance. After several fruitless phone calls and collection letters, the office obtained a warrant in debt on Rose, and she was served with papers by a uniformed sheriff at work. Rose immediately responded by calling Dr. Apple's office. She stated that Dr. Apple had not taken good care of her, that she had a poor clinical result, and that she was thinking about filing a malpractice suit. In addition, she conveyed this information using abusive and defamatory language. Dr. Apple decided to write off the account. Rose was obviously a "loose cannon," and her threat to file a malpractice suit was sufficient to intimidate him.

THE PATIENT INTAKE PROCESS

Successful collection begins with the patient intake process. The intake process will provide you with the legal authority to render treatment as well as the information and the legal standing necessary to pursue collection.

Insurance information may be taken over the telephone when the patient schedules the initial office visit. This task can be performed by a clerical employee after brief training by the collection administrator. Practices with high "no-show" rates may find it a waste of time to verify coverage before the initial appointment. These practices should conduct the verification at the time of service.

Upon arrival, the new patient should complete an intake form before receiving treatment that solicits biographical information that could be useful for collection purposes and for initially evaluating the patient's creditworthiness. This form should also contain wording approved by your attorney that commits the patient to:

- seek treatment voluntarily
- be responsible for the fee, including any copayments, deductibles, or insurance denials
- cooperate in the filing of insurance claims by providing any necessary information
- be responsible for any collection fees, court costs, legal fees, or finance charges if the account becomes delinquent

In many states, finance charges are not worth the bother to collect. They do have a deterrent value, however, and once again they represent a way to convey the message that the practice is serious about collecting its fees. Note that state laws vary regarding provisions of this nature, so it is advisable to consult your attorney to obtain appropriate language for the assignment of collection fees, court costs, and finance charges.

If the patient is going to receive some form of extensive or ongoing care, such as repeated psychiatric visits or cancer treatments, it is also desirable to have the patient sign a method of payment form. Patients undergoing recurrent treatment have more potential to incur large balances, so the additional educational value of a method of payment form makes it worthwhile. This form contains detailed information about specific payment arrangements, what the practice expects of the patient, and other patient responsibilities. It also contains any specific payment plans, including payment schedules and copayments (if known and applicable). A sample method of payment form is found in Exhibit 8–4. Any time a special payment arrangement is negotiated with a patient, it should be put in writing on a method of payment form or an equivalent. Placing provisions for legal fees, court costs, collection fees, and finance charges in the method of payment form achieves three objectives:

1. It puts the patient on notice that you have procedures for dealing with delinquent accounts.
2. It informs the patient that he or she will bear any costs of delinquency by creating a legal agreement that will allow you to pass delinquency costs on to the patient (the language required will vary with state law; consult your attorney for the most favorable language).
3. It communicates this information in a tactful and socially appropriate manner. Most of your patients will not become collection problems, and they will view this wording as a necessary condition of doing business in our times, not as specifically directed at them.

PATIENT EDUCATION

Educating patients regarding their financial obligations lets them make informed choices and avoid misconceptions and reinforces your legal standing if you eventually must resort to collection proceedings. At a minimum, patient education should include information about the patient's insurance coverage and probable fees and terms of payment. The practice should also indicate its expectations regarding payment and emphasize that the ultimate responsibility for settlement of the account lies with the patient.

Exhibit 8–4 Sample Method of Payment Form

Medical Associates Of Virginia, Inc.
123 Main St., Suite 123
Virginia Beach, VA 23456

STATEMENT OF FEE AND METHOD OF PAYMENT

This form is utilized to establish a clear understanding regarding the details of your financial account with this practice. Please read it, and do not hesitate to ask any questions. Your signature is an acknowledgment of your understanding and agreement with the provisions of this agreement.

Name of Patient: _____ Date: _____
Name of Responsible Party: _____ SSN: _____
Relationship to Patient: _____

I, _____, agree to be responsible for payment in full of the charges for professional services which have been rendered to the above mentioned patient by Medical Associates, Inc. I also understand and agree to the following provisions regarding the fee and method of payment:

1. Medical Associates, Inc. will file primary insurance claims on behalf of the patient for rendered services. Insurance payment shall be made directly to the practice. Should any payment be made to the Responsible Party or any other individual, the Responsible Party agrees to promptly forward payment to the Practice.

2. The patient or Responsible Party will supply to the Practice any insurance forms that may be necessary to expedite the insurance filing process.

3. The Responsible Party shall pay the co-insurance payment (co-payment) at the time of each service. The co-payment is that part of the fee which is not covered by insurance after the deductible has been paid, or it is the amount that your managed care company (HMO, PPO, etc.) specifies as your personal payment for each appointment.
   Based on the information provided by your insurance company, we estimate your co-payment to be $_____. Please call your insurance company to verify your co-payment.

4. The deductible is the amount that you must personally pay each year for covered services, before your insurance begins to provide coverage. Your insurance company has told us that your deductible is $_____. Please call your insurance company to verify your deductible.

5. The Responsible Party shall pay any outstanding balance which is not covered by insurance. The Responsible Party shall also pay claims or any part thereof which are denied or unpaid by an insurance company for any reason, such as for deductibles, co-payments, unfiled claims, preexisting conditions, etc. irrespective of who is responsible for the denied claim or the uncovered service. The patient or Responsible Party may receive a statement whenever there is an outstanding balance. *The Responsible Party, not the insurance company, is ultimately responsible for payment for the rendered services.*

6. It is understood that the usual and customary collection procedures may be initiated should the account become delinquent. It is also understood that any collection fees, including any reasonable court costs, and an attorney's fee of thirty-three and one-third percent (33 ⅓ percent) will be payable by the Responsible Party.

7. If for any reason the account becomes 90 days past due, the Responsible Party or the patient may be billed and expected to bring the account current. Please remember that we file insurance as a courtesy to our patients, and that your insurance contract is between you and your insurance company. We consider payment, therefore, to be the responsibility of the patient if a delay occurs from the insurance company. You will be expected to pay *any balance not paid by your insurance company, or which your insurance company delays beyond 90 days after the date of service.*

continues

Exhibit 8–4 continued

8. A fee of $15.00 will be charged for any returned checks. An interest charge of 18% per annum may be added to any balance which is not paid within 30 days of the date that it is billed to you.

9. You will be charged a minimum of $25.00 if an appointment is missed or canceled with less than 24 hours notice. Insurance will not cover this charge. Full payment for a late cancelation or a no show must be made prior to or at the time of your next visit. We do not accrue no show or cancelation fees. Monday appointments must be canceled no later than 12:00 noon on the preceding Friday, since we are closed over the weekend.

    A medical emergency requiring documented treatment by a physician or a death in the immediate family are the only exceptions to this policy. If you cannot come to the office for other reasons, you have the option of rescheduling your appointment for the same calendar week, if your physician has an available opening.

10. Only the business manager is authorized to modify this agreement, or to make any financial arrangements between the practice and the patient. Physicians are specifically excluded from making any financial arrangements with patients.

11. I hereby authorize Medical Associates, Inc. to provide my insurance company with any clinical or financial information which they may require.

12. Additional details or considerations regarding the method of payment may be outlined below:

_____

_____

_____

_____   _____
Signature of Responsible Party   Date

_____   _____
Signature of Business Manager   Date

Patient education can proceed somewhat differently for patients who will be receiving long-term or repeated treatment as opposed to walk-ins or patients who will receive infrequent treatment. Both infrequent and recurrent treatment patients should receive written patient educational material. Patients who are identified as infrequent should receive a standard patient education pamphlet. This pamphlet should describe billing methods, emphasize the patient's responsibility for the account, outline expectations (e.g., the practice's appointment cancellation policy), indicate where to call during an emergency, and so on. Infrequent treatment patients should also meet with the collection administrator if either party has any questions regarding insurance coverage or payment arrangements.

Recurrent treatment patients should meet with the collection administrator, who should review the topics covered in the patient education pamphlet; answer any questions regarding insurance coverage; discuss payment and copayment arrangements, deductibles, and so on; and review all appropriate practice policies. The collection administrator should also negotiate a payment schedule, if necessary and appropriate. All these arrangements should then be written into the method of payment form, which the patient should sign. The method of payment form then becomes a contract between the practice and the patient. It also gives the patient a written document to refer to regarding expectations and financial commitments.

Large fees should always be discussed with patients before treatment is provided. The physician may want to discuss a large fee directly with the patient. If this turns into a negotiation, however, the physician should turn it over to the collection administrator and orchestrate it from behind the scenes. If the physician feels uncomfortable discussing the fee, he or she should discuss the clinical aspects of the treatment and then direct the patient to the collection administrator, who will discuss the financial arrangements. If the procedure involves a standard fee, the collection administrator will be able to handle this as a routine matter. If the fee is not standard, the physician can explain the contingency issues to the collection administrator, who will then make payment arrangements with the patient. This approach has the added advantage that the collection administrator, who is knowledgeable about insurance matters and the patient's coverage, will handle all the financial arrangements.

BILLING STRATEGIES

A billing strategy is a plan for how and when to collect fees. In fee-for-service situations, there are two widely used strategies and several less frequently used strategies. Many practices still receive a portion of their revenues from traditional indemnity insurance plans. To the extent that this is true, the following discussion is relevant.

Insurance Pay–Patient Statement Strategy

This strategy is characterized by the following sequence of events:

1. The patient receives services.
2. The physician bills the insurance company.
3. When the physician receives an insurance company payment or denial, the patient is mailed a statement.

This is one of the most commonly used billing strategies. The advantage of this strategy is that it results in uncomplicated patient billing. Because the patient is not billed until the insurance company's obligation is resolved, the balance owed by the patient is clarified before the patient receives a statement. The patient receives statements on a regular basis, such as each month or each time that an insurance claim reaches resolution. This system is particularly effective when the physician's services are largely covered by insurance or when patients receive infrequent treatment.

This strategy becomes expensive and cumbersome when patients receive frequent treatment. When a physician supplies patients with weekly services or with several services per week over a period of time, the physician can be carrying large receivables on many patient accounts. This strategy also requires the mailing of a large number of statements. Because each mailing incurs postage, supply, and labor costs, this strategy becomes less efficient as the number of patients treated increases and as insurance coverage for typical services decreases. It also becomes complicated and time consuming when patients carry more than one insurance because the practice must then coordinate the payment of benefits among the carriers before issuing a statement to the patient.

This strategy can become inefficient and ineffective in practices that perform many high-fee procedures because a large fee can be under appeal with an insurance company for many months. As a result, the patient's first bill will be very old, thereby decreasing the likelihood that the personal balance will be collected.

Finally, this strategy may inadvertently suggest to patients that it is the physician's responsibility to collect from the insurance company and that, if the insurance company fails to pay, this is the physician's problem. Physicians who use this strategy should inform patients in writing that, insurance is a contract between the insurance company and the patient and that the patient is ultimately responsible for any unpaid fees.

Patient Payment–File Insurance Strategy

When this strategy is used, the patient pays for the estimated share of the fee or copayment, including any deductible, at the time of service, and the insurance company is billed simultaneously. Many managed care arrangements, including PPOs and some HMOs, fit into this category. In these cases, the copayments are often nominal and the same for all office visits, and there may be no deductible. This strategy is particularly appropriate when patients will receive continuing, frequent treatment. This approach is advantageous because the practice collects the copayment at the time of service, thereby taking advantage of the time value of money (see Chapter 6). In addition, this strategy reduces the expenses associated with mailing statements because statements are only mailed when the insurance benefit for a procedure has been overestimated or underestimated, when a patient misses a copayment, or upon termination of treatment, if the account closes with either a positive or negative balance.

To use this strategy, it is necessary to determine the patient's insurance benefits at or before the time of service. Exhibit 8–5 is a telephone referral information form. It can be used to collect the information necessary to verify insurance coverage. Benefits can then be confirmed by calling the insurance company before or at the time of the first appointment. This process of determining coverage at or before the onset of treatment works best in practices that use a fairly limited number of procedures and when most of a practice's patients use a small number of insurance carriers. Under these circumstances, it is relatively easy to determine insurance companies' usual and customary rates. Some MOMS has the capability of calculating probable usual and customary rates based on previous collection experience. As with the previous strategy, practices that use this strategy should make patients fully aware that insurance coverage is based on a contractual agreement between the insurance company and the patient. If the insurance company does not pay, the patient will be expected to settle the account.

Modified Strategies

With both of the above strategies, the practice assumes the risk that insurance companies will be slow to pay. In some cases, insurance companies will classify a claim as pending for several months. As a result, a medical practice's business office must constantly monitor the status of claims, refile lost or improperly denied claims, and call or send interrogatories regarding claims. Available cash is reduced because revenue is tied up in receivables. In addition, the eventual day of reckoning with the patient is delayed. Patients who do not receive a final statement for several months are less likely to pay and will consume more collection effort on the part of the practice.

Both of the first two strategies can become particularly burdensome to a practice when patients have more than one insurance carrier. When this occurs, all claims must be filed with the primary carrier, and copies of the explanation of benefits for each payment or denial from the primary carrier must accompany claims sent to the secondary carrier. Needless to say, this has the potential to become a protracted, paperwork-laden process. Unless the claims are large, physicians should not accept the responsibility of filing secondary insurance. This burden should be shifted to patients. When the primary carrier pays or denies a claim, the patient will also receive an explanation of benefits, at which time the patient can file the secondary claim.

Some practices have adopted a strategy in which they will try to collect from an insurance carrier for a stated period of time, such as 90 days. Delayed or denied claims are then billed to the patient irrespective of whether the practice could continue to pursue the claim with the insurance carrier. Patients are instructed to contact the insurance carrier if they have any questions. If the insurance company subsequently pays the claim to the practice, the practice then sends a refund to the patient. When practices use this approach they should inform the patient before the "90 day clock" expires on a claim. Often, including the patient in the process will get quick action from the insurer.

Full Payment Strategy

With this strategy, the patient is expected to pay the full fee at the time of service. Insurance

Exhibit 8–5 Sample Telephone Referral Form

Today's Date: _____   Clinician: _____

Patient Name (Parent if App.): _____ DOB _____

Sponsor SSN if CHAMPUS

Pt. Social Security Number: _____   _____

Home Telephone: _____ Work Telephone: _____

Referral Source: _____

Appointment Date: _____ Appointment Time: _____

Insurance Coverage ____ Yes ____ No   Carrier Name: _____

Checked Carrier against PPO/Managed Care List? Yes____ No____

If CHAMPUS: Active Duty: _____ Retired:_____ Rank:_____

Secondary Insurance ____Yes ____ No   Carrier Name: _____

If CHAMPUS, told patient to go to intake? _____ Yes _____ No

Primary Insured's Name:_____ Secondary Insured's Name:_____

Policy Number: _____ Policy Number: _____

Group Number:_____ Group Number: _____

Insd. Employer:_____ Insd. Employer: _____

Carrier Phone: _____ Carrier Phone: _____

Discussed Fee? _____ Yes _____ No

Told Patient To Bring Forms if Required? _____ Yes _____ No

Told Patient To Bring Ins. or I.D. Card? _____ Yes _____ No

Gave Directions to Practice? _____ Yes _____ No

Detect Problems with Account? _____ Yes _____ No

Made a Copy and Put Original on Board? _____ Yes _____ No

Person Who Handled This Intake: _____

*DIAGNOSIS CODE:*_____

WE CANNOT BILL THE PATIENT'S INSURANCE UNTIL YOU SUPPLY THE DX CODE!!!

may be filed as a courtesy to the patient, with the payment going directly to the patient (the practice, of course, can choose not to file insurance; filing the claim, however, is a reasonable act of goodwill toward the patient). This strategy has the advantage of increasing the practice's immediate cash flow and places the burden of insurance company collection on the patient. It is consistent with the idea that insurance coverage is based on a contractual agreement between a patient and an insurance carrier. It is also obviously the most advantageous strategy for the practice and the least favorable one for the patient.

The full payment strategy may be appropriate if there is more demand for services than a physician can supply. Even if this strategy is not feasible for most patients, it may be feasible for certain niches. Examples might include cosmetic plastic surgery, psychoanalysis, and foreign nationals who are willing to pay cash for high-quality immediate services.

A variation on this strategy is to use it for procedures below a certain amount, such as $300 for indemnity insurance patients. Fees above this amount are billed using the patient payment–file insurance strategy.

Patient Prepayment Strategy

In this strategy, the patient prepays for services. The prepayment can take a number of forms. For physicians in very high demand, the prepayment can be for reserving an initial appointment. Patients who have ongoing but standard treatment plans can prepay according to a regular schedule. For example, a patient who receives a routine course of allergy desensitization injections can be billed before treatment on a quarterly basis, with insurance being filed as a courtesy to the patient at the time of treatment.

Preventing Patient Payment Problems

One tactic that is essential for successful revenue collection is collecting personal fees at the time of service. Front office staff must be trained to respond appropriately to the typical payment excuses presented by patients. This training should be provided by the collection administrator. Appropriate responses include suggesting credit cards when checkbooks and cash are "forgotten" and giving the patient an addressed envelope with instructions to mail the payment today. In addition, the receptionist should approach the patient with the *expectation* of payment, not offer the patient excuses for failure to pay, and direct any patient who will be missing a second consecutive payment to the collection administrator. As we have seen, examination of the reward contingencies for those positions with cash collection responsibilities is also important.

Patients who repeatedly fail to make payments should meet with the collection administrator. Some patients test how far they can go before there will be consequences. Other patients may truly not have the funds. In either case, the collection administrator needs to ascertain the reasons for the delinquency and reiterate and enforce the agreement as stated in the method of payment form or patient pamphlet, negotiate new terms (taking into account any change in the patient's financial circumstances),

or recommend suspension of the patient's treatment to the physician.

COLLECTING OVERDUE BALANCES

Success in collecting overdue balances depends on consistency and timeliness. Consistency means that there is a plan and that it is followed in an automatic, relentless manner. The collection process should progress step by predetermined step with clockwork regularity. There should be *no* exceptions. Timeliness is important because as accounts age they become less collectible. This is true for a number of reasons, including these:

- *Patients move and thereby become difficult to locate.* If a patient moves to another jurisdiction or state, the collection mechanics become more difficult and expensive.
- *As a debt becomes older, you will move farther toward the back of the line in the mind of the patient.* The longer you wait, the more time the patient will have to go even further into debt. In addition, other creditors will have time to collect, thereby depleting the patient's assets and decreasing your chances of collecting.
- *Patients are more likely to consider older debts "ancient history."* The anxiety, fear, or pain you alleviated will become less salient with time, and thus any feelings of guilt and the associated motivation to pay the debt will be reduced.

Perhaps the simplest initial step, and the most appropriate one when failure to pay is truly an oversight, is to send a bill. The amount overdue, however, should be clearly indicated by being labeled as overdue. Computerized billing software normally ages balances, so that old debt is printed on the statement in an overdue or aged category, such as 60 days overdue. Alternatively, you can begin to send a series of collection letters.

Some physicians attach a special mystique to collection letters. They assume that, if they could only assemble the right combination of words, they would be able to convince even the most irresponsible patients to settle their accounts. This attitude is naive, especially when you consider that an irresponsible patient is probably well aware of the debt and has *chosen* not to pay. Unfortunately, there is no magic available to write collection letters.

Experience suggests that some messages may be more effective than others, however. Collection letters will be more effective if their contents follow these guidelines:

- A collection letter should be short. This will focus the patient's attention on the overdue balance.
- Don't dissipate your strength by giving the patient excuses or alternatives to payment ("I know that times are hard . . . ," etc.).
- The *initial* contact should assume that the patient is not malevolent. The overdue balance could be due to lost mail or to an oversight. Don't give excuses to the patient, but don't preclude them either. If the patient wants to save face and at the same time pay the bill, that shouldn't make any difference to you.
- Command the patient to action. Clearly state that the patient *must do something*, either pay the bill or contact the office, *by a stated date*.
- Always enclose a statement of the account with any collection letter.

Exhibits 8–6 and 8–7 are sample first and second collection letters. If the first letter is unsuccessful, it should be followed by the second (final) letter. The second letter should state that, if the bill is not paid within seven days, legal action will result. The contents of the second collection letter are based on a research study in which it was compared with other letters containing less direct content.[1] This letter produced statistically superior results compared with two other content strategies.

Both letters should command the patient to action by stating what to do and by when, as well as provide a reason why the patient should act. The time interval between the two letters should be short, such as 7 to 14 days. Do not waste time, energy, and resources by sending more than two letters. If a patient does not respond at this point, the account should be either written off or given to a collection attorney.

There are other techniques that should be used in addition to collection letters. The first and most obvious is to suspend services. This tactic is most effective when the patient is receiving continuing treatment because it creates immediate consequences for the patient. Naturally, termination must be done in a medically and legally appropriate manner to avoid a malpractice charge of abandonment (see Chapter 14). Physicians with high proportions of continuing patients, such as psychiatrists, gynecologists, family physicians, and allergists, should systematically apply this tactic using established rules. These rules should be communicated to patients through patient pamphlets or method of payment forms. For example, failure to make two payments or failure to pay two consecutive mailed statements will automatically result in the suspension of treatment. At a minimum, suspending services will put a cap on the outstanding balance. Once again, appropriately terminating treatment is absolutely critical to avoid a charge of abandonment.

The telephone is a very effective collection tool because it is both intrusive and selective. The telephone places your collection administrator in the patient's office, living room, bedroom, or kitchen (consult your attorney regarding state laws governing collection methods; some states have laws precluding collection calls outside certain hours). When the telephone rings, people stop whatever they are doing to answer it. Letters may be lost or opened and discarded by the wrong person. You may never know for certain whether a patient ever receives a letter. With the telephone, however, you can be sure you have reached the correct person.

Practices often delay using the telephone, either out of fear of a direct confrontation with the

Exhibit 8–6 Sample First Collection Letter

(Date)

(Guarantor Name)
(Billing Address)   Acct. # (Account Number)
(Billing Address)   (Patient Name)

Dear (Guarantor):

Recently, we sent you a bill for your outstanding personal balance of $(Balance). We asked for payment by this date, and we have not yet received it. I ask that you pay this balance, so that it is received no later than (Enter Date).

We have provided services in good faith, and we rely on the good faith of our patients to promptly pay their bills. If you have any questions regarding your account, please contact me at (Phone Number). Thank you for your attention to this matter.

Sincerely,

(Name Of Business Manager)
Business Manager

Enclosure: Account Statement

(*Note*: This letter is provided as an example. State laws vary regarding the methods that you can use in pursuing a delinquent account. Consult your attorney regarding specific content in your state.)

---

patient or because of a feeling that it is inappropriate to make such a personal intrusion except as a last resort. Instead, the telephone should be used *early* in the collection process because it lets the collection administrator evaluate why the patient is delinquent. If the patient has a grievance, this can be determined, and the collection administrator can begin resolving the problem. If there is an economic hardship, then it becomes possible to arrange a payment schedule. If the patient is irresponsible, then some structure can be applied to direct and motivate payment. If the patient's behavior suggests a personality disorder or simple intransigence, then aggressive collection strategies can be implemented more quickly than normally would be the case.

Here is a sequence of steps to follow when using the telephone:

1. *First, identify the answering party, and only talk to the patient (or whoever is responsible for the debt)*. If Mr. Smith is the guarantor of the account, then you are wasting your time discussing the matter with Mrs. Smith. In addition, talking to the wrong person may breach confidentiality.

2. *Try to determine the patient's state of mind regarding the debt*. The collection administrator needs to determine whether

Exhibit 8–7 Sample Second Collection Letter

(Date)

(Guarantor Name)   Acct. #: (Account Number)
(Billing Address)   (Patient Name)
(Billing Address)

Dear (Guarantor):

This is your final notification that you have an outstanding personal balance of $(Balance). As you will recall, you signed an agreement with this practice to pay for our services. We have provided services in good faith. We assumed good faith on your part, and that you would live up to your responsibility to pay for these services.

If complete payment is not received by (Date), your account will be turned over to our attorney for legal action, which can include a hearing in general district court, garnishment of wages, and attachment of bank funds. This will result in additional costs to you, since collection fees, attorney's fees, court costs, and finance charges will be added to your balance.

Once an account is turned over to our attorney for collection, we cannot call it back, and you will be assessed these additional charges.

Sincerely,

(Name Of Business Manager)
Business Manager

(*Note*: This letter is provided as an example. State laws vary regarding the methods that you can use in pursuing a delinquent account. Consult your attorney regarding specific content in your state.)

he or she is confronting someone who accepts this as a legitimate debt, who will be aggressive, or who will seek sympathy. One tactic for determining this is to identify yourself, state the nature of the debt, and then listen. Listen for both *what* the patient says and the *way* in which it is said.

3. *Control the conversation by offering the patient alternatives that meet your objectives.* Phrases such as "How large a payment can you make?," "When will you make your next payment?," or "What would be a good time for you to come to the office to discuss this?" convey weakness. Determine what *you* need. Make a proposal, and let the patient accept it or make a counterproposal. You can then accept or reject the counterproposal. The questions above could be replaced with "I need a payment of $200" (determine a level that will be satisfactory and propose it), "I expect to receive your final payment by Friday, February 18" (let the patient tell you if that is not possible), and "Let's meet this Friday at 10:00 A.M." (you can always state an alternative if the patient objects).

4. *Get to the point*. Brief conversations allow your collection administrator more time to contact more patients. Brief, no-nonsense contacts also communicate the serious business nature of the discussion.

5. *Obtain specific commitments from the patient*. Do this by getting specific agreements regarding amounts and time; "I'll send you a substantial payment in a few days" is worthless. In addition, the collection administrator should always restate the agreement to the patient and tell him or her that a note will be entered in the financial record (e.g., "You agree, then, that you will mail a check for $200 so that I will receive it by Monday, March 23, and I am noting this in your financial record"). Whenever a payment arrangement is negotiated over the phone, it should also be put into a letter and mailed to the patient.

6. *Be persistent, and follow through with your promises*. If a patient does not meet a commitment, immediately contact the patient. This tells the patient that you will not go away, and it also provides validity to future promises. For example, consider the following statement: "Mr. Johnson, I did not receive your payment for $200. If I don't receive it by Wednesday, I will turn your case over to our lawyer for collection on Thursday." Is Mr. Johnson more likely to respond to this message if it is communicated on the day that the $200 had been due or if it is communicated 3 weeks later? The telephone offers you the ability to provide immediate follow-through on broken promises.

PLACING AN ACCOUNT IN COLLECTION

Some patients will not respond to statements, collection letters, or telephone calls. When this happens, you will need to implement collection proceedings. The first step is to write off any account that will cost more to collect than it will generate in cash. The automatic write-off crite-rion for your practice should be determined by looking at the time, effort, and cost that are likely to be expended by your staff. Next, you must decide whether the practice will institute the legal process or whether you want to turn the account over to a collection agent.

If you are not faced with large numbers of accounts that must be placed in collection, you may want to consider undertaking collection in small claims court. The advantages of pursuing this course are that you will retain control over your cases and you will keep all the money that you collect. Generally, patients who are employed and for whom you have good addresses are good bets. In about 75 percent of these cases, obtaining a warrant in debt will result in a quick settling of the account.

The small claims process varies from state to state, but generally it proceeds in the following manner. The practice obtains a warrant in debt against the patient. Some jurisdictions will let a practice obtain a warrant by mail, whereas others require that this be done in person at the courthouse. The warrant specifies the delinquent amount and sets a court date. The cost is usually nominal (typically, $15 to $35), and it generally can be added to the patient's account. The patient is then served with a copy of the warrant by the sheriff and/or through the mail.

At this point, many patients contact the office and arrange to make payment. It is amazing how a legal notice delivered by a uniformed sheriff will get a patient's attention! When the patient contacts the office, negotiate payment arrangements that will close the account *before* the court date. This will leave you with the option to pursue legal action if the patient breaks the agreement.

If the patient does not arrange to make payment, the collection administrator will have to appear in court and present evidence that the services were provided and that the patient's account is still unpaid. The court will grant a judgment against the patient. If the patient still refuses to pay, you will then be faced with the challenge of collecting on the judgment. Once again, your options will be determined by state law, but the normal choices involve garnishing wages and attaching assets such as bank accounts, cars, and so on. Generally, these actions will require an additional legal action.

Medical practices should not routinely use small claims court. You "win" in those cases that pay off the account as a result of the warrant in debt because you will obtain payment with relatively little expenditure of time, effort, or money. The other cases, however, will require considerable collection effort.

Some patients will contest the case in court. Many patients, however, will simply fail to appear, and in essence they will challenge you to collect on the judgment. Most of these cases will be hard-core collection veterans. It will be difficult to locate their bank accounts and employers, and they may well have falsified some of the information on the intake form with the objective of misleading you.

These people can be abusive and vindictive. Your personnel are not trained to collect from these types of people, nor do they have the time or the resources available to track them down and force them to pay. As a result, the small claims procedure should only be considered for those cases in which there is a very high probability that the patient will pay as a result of receiving the warrant in debt. The collection administrator will have to make an educated guess based on the type of patient (hardship, equity, irresponsible, or personality disorder) and the patient's response to the initial collection attempts. With few exceptions, I endorse the practice of routinely sending all delinquent cases to a collection agent after two collection letters. Given the cost–benefit ratio of the small claims court process, this is a fully justified strategy.

The alternative to small claims court is to utilize a collection agent, which can be a collection agency or an attorney who specializes in this type of work. In either case, you should select a collection agent based on cost, recovery rate, and methods employed. Cost and recovery rate are interrelated. An agent with a recovery rate of 70 percent and a fee of 50 percent returns 35 percent of the revenue to the practice. An agent with a recovery rate of 50 percent and a fee of 40 percent only returns 20 percent of the revenue to the practice. Obviously, you must simultaneously consider both the fee and the recovery rate when selecting a collection agent.

Collection methods used by an attorney or agent are a legitimate concern. Generally, attorneys are less tempted to use abusive tactics because they have direct access to the court system and are more likely to pursue that route quickly than an agent who is not an attorney. An attorney or agent will be representing your practice to the community. Illegal or particularly inappropriate, inhumane, or disproportionate collection methods can damage your reputation. It is important, therefore, to contact several professional references when you are evaluating attorneys and agents. Question the references about customer or patient complaints, the actual level of recovered revenue, and the time that it takes to collect on accounts. Also, inquire about how cooperative and responsive the agent's staff have been in responding to clients' questions.

Generally, a collection attorney offers the best possibility of successful collection. Most patients who have refused to pay after receiving a bill, telephone call, and two collection letters are *choosing* not to pay. When an account reaches this point, the only thing that will get a patient to pay is force. An attorney has the ultimate weapon: access to the legal system and the ability to obtain a legal judgment. Even if a judgment cannot be collected upon immediately, it will sit out there for years like a mine floating in the ocean. It is not unusual for one to "go off" several years later. The routine credit checks associated with legal transactions, such as mortgages, house closings, car loans, and the like, will reveal the judgment, and suddenly the patient will be quite interested in settling the account.

Once you have retained a collection attorney, it is important to monitor results. Does the attorney successfully collect on your accounts, or have the accounts simply been moved into another black hole? If patients complain about collection methods, it is important to discuss this with the attorney. It is most likely that the patients will be objecting to legitimate, appropriate, successful tactics. It is important, however, for you to protect your reputation and to feel comfortable with the methods used by your attorney.

Another element of successfully using an attorney is to forward your delinquent accounts in a timely manner. If your final collection letter says that the account will be placed in collection if the balance isn't paid in a specific number of days, then be certain to turn the account over to the attorney on the day after the due date. Some attorneys will give you better terms for younger accounts, and there are good reasons for this. As we have seen, old accounts are more difficult to collect.

Once an account has been placed with a collection attorney, never take the account back from the attorney because a patient says that he or she will pay. Also, never accept a payment from a patient whose account is with an attorney. Some patients will contact the practice in an attempt to avoid collection fees or attorney's fees after the attorney has applied pressure. If you take a patient's payment, you may be responsible for these fees. In addition, the patient will invariably renege on promises made to you.

COLLECTING FROM INSURANCE COMPANIES

The most favorable payment arrangement for the physician is to collect fees at the time of service, with patients receiving payment from their insurance companies. Competition for patients, patient expectations, and the increasing incursion of PPOs and HMOs make this type of arrangement infeasible for most physicians. In fact, insurance collection probably will be the single largest revenue source for most independent practices for quite some time. Ensuring the validity and consistency of the insurance collection process is essential, therefore, to financial survival.

A particularly dangerous aspect of insurance collection, even within a PPO and many HMO settings, is the long period between the time that a claim is generated and the receipt of a payment or denial. This delay in feedback makes it possible for a significant problem to arise before it is perceived by the practice. Using efficient insurance billing procedures, monitoring insurance billing results, and identifying and correcting problems as early as possible are essential to protect the practice's revenue stream and its financial viability.

Effective insurance collection begins with effective insurance billing procedures. The objective should be to bill as often as possible, with daily insurance claim filing being the ultimate goal. Filing insurance daily or as frequently as feasible is analogous to dividing a ship into a honeycomb of compartments. A catastrophe in any one compartment can be localized and will not threaten the existence of the ship. Individual events, such as the post office losing a bundle of mail, e-claims software developing a bug, the power going off during an insurance billing run, an insurance check being lost, a hardware failure, or incompetence on the part of a particular claims agent, will then only affect a small and limited part of your revenue. If you file insurance claims on a weekly or monthly basis, then the same events might affect a week's or month's worth of revenues.

Some insurance companies are capable of processing electronically submitted claims. Electronic submission has a number of advantages, including faster payment, quicker error detection, reduced postage and mailing costs, and reduced clerical labor. Some electronic claims systems immediately indicate whether the claim will be paid or denied, which provides greater integrity to the billing process. Often, electronic claims must be filed through clearinghouses, which charge a fee. You should evaluate the total cost of electronic submission, including the cost of additional equipment and access fees. Some physicians, however, have concluded that immediate problem detection and reduced paperwork in the front office are worth the extra cost.

The next important consideration is to file your claims correctly and comply with any authorization procedures. Normally, there will be a provider support office to help practices deal with denied claims and comply with claim filing procedures. It is sometimes possible to have major carriers send a training representative to your office to train your staff in correct filing procedures. Many Blue Cross companies provide this service. This training can be particularly helpful if your office has had turnover in critical billing positions and you did not develop written procedure manuals.

Insurance companies are very large bureaucracies. One characteristic of a bureaucracy is that it solves problems by applying standards and rules. If you find that you are not getting your problems resolved, you have to get the ear of a person who is high enough in the bureaucracy to make exceptions to the standards and rules. The way to do this is to speak with a supervisor. If you don't get resolution to your problem, ask "If you agreed with my position, would you be able to . . . ?" If the answer is no, then you need to ask for *that* employee's supervisor. If the answer is yes, then you must determine whether continuing up the corporate ladder is worth the time and effort. Generally, ascending two levels of supervision above the normal claims representative will place you in middle management.

Some companies appear to go out of their way to make the billing process difficult. They require the use of company-specific forms, or they create their own procedure codes instead of using the standard Current Procedural Terminology codes. Unfortunately, there is not much that you can do about this, other than refuse to participate with these companies and not accept assignment of payment. Methods for dealing with nonstandard filing requirements include selecting flexible computer software, training employees to deal with requirements, and developing special office procedures. Unusual codes and forms generally result in higher claim error rates. By segregating these claims and working on them as a separate batch, employees can pay particular attention to the different codes and filing procedures required by these companies.

Some companies are very unresponsive to claim inquiries or take an unreasonably long time to process a claim or forward a payment. If a company is particularly unresponsive, you may want to consider filing a complaint with your state's insurance commission. Each state has an insurance commission or an agency that regulates insurance company operations. The power of the commission or agency, and therefore the degree to which insurance companies will be responsive to complaints filed with it, varies from state to state. If you feel that a claim has been unreasonably denied or has not been responded to in a reasonable amount of time *and* you have exhausted all internal remedies, you have little to lose by writing a letter to your state's insurance commission.

Generally, the most effective tactic for dealing with an unresponsive insurer is to involve the patient. This is particularly effective if your practice's education procedures have instilled in the patient the idea that unpaid claims will be the patient's responsibility. Contact the patient and let him or her know that the claim has been unreasonably denied or delayed. Tell the patient that he or she will be billed if the claim is not paid in 30 days as well as whom to call and what to do to get involved.

The physician manager should routinely review practice aging analyses and other management reports that relate to insurance collection. Other reports that may prove helpful for understanding the collection situation include the following:

- number of procedures per month
- revenue generated per month
- revenue by insurance company per month
- insurance receipts by company per month
- aging analysis by insurance company
- gross receipts per month
- write-offs and adjustments per month

Generally, most practices find that monthly reports reveal significant trends while being less subject to the random variations that make reports over shorter time periods more difficult to interpret.

The significance of an unpaid claim in an aging analysis is the most difficult to interpret because there is no overt message indicating that something is wrong. Unpaid claims are typically identified when money begins to move into older categories, such as 60 or 90 days past current. To discover this, the collection administrator must regularly run aging analyses, examine them, and then act upon the results.

Dealing with a rejected claim is arguably the collection administrator's *highest* priority. First, a rejected claim means that the wealth represented by the denied claim will *never* be paid unless action is taken, and it is therefore a higher priority than current claims, which may be paid. Second, the denial may be symptomatic of a larger billing problem. This may mean that many other claims for this patient and for other patients may be destined for denial. This circumstance can, if left unattended, threaten the financial soundness of the practice.

Any rejected claim must be immediately examined by the collection administrator to determine the cause of the problem. The collection administrator must always be thinking of the implications of a denied claim for other outstanding claims. If there are implications for other claims, the collection administrator must immediately address them. Often, the first indication of a software or a filing procedure problem will be a denied claim. If the symptom is not immediately detected, many additional claims will be denied. This not only delays the receipt of cash but also requires the refiling of more denied claims, which can add up to a substantial amount of additional work.

Case Example 1

MCCC, a large midwestern insurance company, is the carrier for about 10 percent of Dr. Feldstone's patients. It requires the use of its own procedure codes as well as patient information that Dr. Feldstone does not normally provide on claims filed with Blue Cross and other commercial carriers.

In August, Dr. Feldstone replaced his collection administrator. At about that time, MCCC supposedly mailed Dr. Feldstone a new set of procedure codes. The new codes either were never received or were lost as a result of the personnel transition. They were never entered into the practice's computerized billing system, and the practice continued to file claims with the ob-

solete codes. The new collection administrator was somewhat overwhelmed with her job, and consequently she did not attach great significance to the returned MCCC claims. They were placed in an in-basket, where they would receive attention when "things calmed down."

At about the same time, CCC, the insurance carrier for 40 percent of Dr. Feldstone's patients, changed one procedure code, which was used in about 15 percent of his billings for these patients. CCC had notoriously bad provider services, so it was unclear whether the information was never conveyed to the practice or was simply lost during the personnel transition. Once again, the new procedure code was not entered into the computer, nor were the billing personnel aware of the need for the code modification.

At about the same time, Blue Cross/Blue Shield's processing software began to have an intermittent problem that was limited to only a few practices, including Dr. Feldstone's. Claims would be randomly rejected for failure to have a diagnostic code when one was in fact present. The collection administrator attached no diagnostic significance to the rejected Blue Cross claims (this Blue Cross company did not return rejected insurance claims but forwarded a form requesting the additional or missing information). She simply assumed that the claims had been inappropriately submitted and proceeded to supply Blue Cross with new diagnosis codes. As a result, Blue Cross was unaware that it had a software problem.

MCCC, CCC, and Blue Cross together represented about 70 percent of Dr. Feldstone's monthly revenue. The new collection administrator did not appreciate the significance of the increasing proportion of rejected claims, and she continued to deal with them on a case-by-case basis. Over a three-month period, the revenues generated remained about the same, receivables in the current and current plus 30 days categories grew significantly, and cash receipts were down. After about three months, cash receipts were about 69 percent of normal levels.

Dr. Feldstone did not routinely review the practice's financial reports. He had noticed that cash receipts were down, but he attributed this to the new collection administrator's "learning curve." By the time Dr. Feldstone determined that he had a major collection problem, he was faced with:

- a cash crisis
- a backlog of MCCC rebilling, which could not begin until the billing personnel were trained in the use of the new procedure codes (average turnaround for this insurance company was about seven weeks)
- a backlog of CCC rebilling (average turnaround was eight weeks)
- a delay in Blue Cross cash of about eight weeks
- greater than normal vulnerability for the next several weeks to any other problem in the collections system, such as a hardware breakdown or software bug

Case Example 2

Field Psychiatric Association was a group psychiatric practice. In addition to providing psychiatric services, it employed several psychologists and clinical social workers, who were paid on the basis of monthly collections. Monthly collection figures were obtained from earned receipts reports for each producer. Dr. James, the practice administrator, was responsible for reviewing monthly management reports and attending to the business aspects of the practice.

On 3 March, the February earned receipts by producer reports indicated a large drop in collections, and as a result the subsequent payroll, which would be payable on the 10th of the month, would be roughly 60 percent of normal levels. The drop was uniform across all producers, with the exception of Dr. James, whose receipts were at normal levels. She did not participate with any insurance companies, and all her patients paid full fee at the time of treatment.

Dr. James was very concerned because her monthly fixed expenses would exceed the monthly gross receipts (see the section on break-even analysis in Chapter 6). She was also very concerned about the financial well-being of her employees. Dr. James's first reaction was panic. Where should she look for the cause of the problem? What information was available that could give her a clue regarding what had happened?

First, she focused her thoughts on the fact that this problem was not caused by magic or demons. It was soluble, and the answer, or at least some indication of the problem's source, would be found in the practice's financial data. Dr. James began the investigative process to determine the cause of the cash problem. She identified six hypotheses:

1. Cash receipts had been lost or stolen.
2. Insurance claims had not been mailed on a regular basis.
3. There had been a precipitous decline in procedures due to vacations during the holiday season, resulting in reduced receipts several weeks later.
4. Insurance claims had been improperly completed as a result of software or personnel problems.
5. Insurance receipts had been lost or stolen.
6. One or more insurance companies were having a problem processing claims.

Dr. James first determined that the cash shortage was approximately $15,000 by comparing a report of the practice's gross receipts for the month with the gross receipts for the previous three months. She then noted that the cash collections for February totaled $17,793, whereas the collections for the previous three months averaged $18,396. Because cash collections were stable, this largely eliminated hypothesis 1. It also suggested that the problem had to be associated in some manner with insurance collections.

Next, she examined hypothesis 2 by looking at a sample of accounts in the computer. Insurance claims were uniformly sent on either the day of treatment or the following day. In addition, all information relating to the patient computer accounts appeared to be correct. Finally, November through February monthly reports of revenues generated by insurance company did not indicate any substantial or unexpected monthly variability. These data in combination largely eliminated hypothesis 2. Wealth was being put into the pipeline, and the question was where and when it would come out, or even whether it would.

Revenue reports and reports on the number of procedures for December revealed less than a 10 percent decline. This eliminated hypothesis 3.

Hypothesis 4 could be time consuming to investigate fully. The collection administrator stated that she had not received an unusual number of returned claims. Her word was accepted at face value, although it was recognized that in theory she could be covering up a problem. Examination of a sample of accounts in the computer and a test running of the computer's claims filing program indicated that the practice was generating payable claims. A very unsettling hypothesis, however, was that the computer was *saying* that it was generating all the claims when in fact it was only generating a *portion* of the claims. To eliminate this hypothesis, it would be necessary to examine a sample of the patient business charts. If copies of claims were missing for dates on which the computer had indicated that a claim had been generated, then this would support hypothesis 4. Checking this would be a long, tedious task. As a result, Dr. James decided that she would postpone examining this hypothesis until after she had examined the others. Subsequent to this event, the practice discontinued using two-part claim forms. This had been a carryover from pre-computer days that no one, including the business manager or the managing physician, had rethought. Countless hours had been wasted filing copies of claims for no good purpose.

Hypothesis 5 would take time to investigate, although the strategy would be easy to implement. Insurers X and Y paid a large proportion of the practice's insurance claims. If insurance funds amounting to $15,000 were lost or diverted, at least some of the money would have to come from one or both of these carriers. These companies could be questioned by telephone about

claims that should have been paid by now. If there were funds that had been diverted or lost, then one or both insurance companies would indicate that they had paid on claims that the practice's computer indicated were still unpaid or had been covered with an adjustment or write-off. Once again, this would be a personnel-intensive process that could be addressed by sampling cases. Dr. James postponed further investigation of this hypothesis until other, more easily researchable alternatives had been eliminated.

Two sources of data would be used to examine hypothesis 6. An examination of an aging analysis by insurance company revealed that Insurer X's receivables in 30 days past current were much higher than normal. Reducing the revenue in this category by the approximate write-off and then guessing at the proportion in the category that might be old enough to be payable resulted in an estimate that could account for $15,000. An examination of insurance receipts by insurance company revealed that Insurer X's February receipts were $6,399, whereas they had averaged $22,118 for the previous three months. These data directly pointed to a problem with Insurer X's claims.

Dr. James now knew that the source of the problem was probably associated with Insurer X, although she still did not know with certainty whether the fault lay in the claims that her practice was sending, whether Insurer X's funds had been lost or diverted, or whether the problem was with Insurer X's claims processing. She decided that she would first test the hypothesis that would create the least difficulty for her. She called an administrator at Insurer X and stated that her 30 days past current claims were very high and that her cash receipts were down. She asked him whether there had been a problem in the processing of her claims. The administrator stated that someone would look at the practice's accounts. Later that day, a subordinate called back and told Dr. James that the processing department had gotten behind, that temporary and overtime help was being enlisted, and that the fault lay with the insurance company. The data that Dr. James had used to confront the insurance company were incontrovertible. Insurer X knew that if it denied that the problem existed, Dr. James would begin inquiring about specific accounts. To its credit, Insurer X quickly admitted the problem.

Dr. James stated that she and her employees should not have to suffer as a result of the insurer's problem, and she asked for a $15,000 advance against the outstanding claims. Insurer X's administrator countered with an offer to pull all Dr. James's claims and "put them on the top of the stack." Dr. James agreed, and three days later she began to receive payments.

PROBLEM ACCOUNT DETECTION AND TIMING

It is critical to have time standards and a sequence for collection activities. This ensures that the process moves along as rapidly as possible and that the most effective procedures are used in the most effective order. The most basic timing consideration is posed by the question: When is an account overdue? For a missed copayment or deductible, the answer is easy. It is overdue when the payment is missed. The first collection action should take place within one day. A more difficult circumstance is defining when a billed transaction is overdue. For example, when should action be taken on an unpaid insurance claim?

These less clearly defined billing questions can often be answered with enough precision from past data to set performance standards. For example, if most Blue Cross payments are received within 40 days of submission, then a reasonable standard that won't generate too many false positives might be to audit Blue Cross accounts that have moved into 60 days on an aging analysis. If another carrier has a turnaround that averages 21 days, then its accounts that have gotten into the 30-day category would be appropriate to audit.

The actions that are taken need to be part of a consistent plan that follows a set time standard. For example, the sequence on a patient collection might have five actions: statement, first collection letter, second collection letter with two telephone attempts, refer to attorney. The timing for this whole sequence should be standard for the practice and consistently applied to all cases. An example of aggressive but reasonable timing for a patient collection is found in Table 8–2.

Table 8–2 illustrates that it is possible to complete the collection sequence from initial delinquency to final action in 50 days. Although this process may seem fast, consider for a moment that the patient has received at least three communications (statement plus two collection letters) and has failed to respond. This is a clear indication that the patient has made a conscious *choice* not to respond. At this point, it is futile to make further requests. The account should be forwarded to the attorney for collection on the 50th day. The staff's time can be better utilized by working other accounts.

I cannot emphasize strongly enough the importance of actually following the time standards. If a first collection letter is to be sent on the 31st day, then this must occur on that day. It should not wait until the 32nd day. This consistency has two critical effects. First, it wrings slack out of your office operations. Once it becomes known that time standards are just rough guides, some accounts will get the second letter on the 31st day, and others may stretch out to the 51st day. You will have lost control over the process. Second, many patients and some insurance carriers test systems. They look for slack and take advantage of it. If you promise that you will

---

Table 8–2 Aggressive Patient Collection Sequence and Timing

Action	Act Day	Close Day
Personal payment missed	0	0
Send statement	1	30
First collection letter	31	41
Second collection letter	42	49
Telephone call*	42	49
Account to attorney	50	

*Business manager tries twice.

follow through on the 31st day and you do, then your adversary will take you more seriously than the practice across town that is not consistent. In effect, you just moved closer to the front of the line.

COLLECTION DATABASE

To operate a collection process using the rapid time frames illustrated above, effectively using collection reports and databases is critical. For example, if your collection administrator has 600 accounts to manage and 57 are in some stage of delinquency, how does he or she know that Fred Kringle should have responded to his second collection letter by today or that Anne Blert promised to get her payment in by yesterday?

The simplest solution to this problem is to use a daily calendar. Whenever an action is taken, a note is made of what should happen by the deadline date in the calendar. If Fred Kringle was given until 14 November to respond to a second collection letter, an entry to that effect is made for 14 November. On 14 November, the collection administrator will check the status of the account, and if Fred has not responded adequately, the collection administrator will *immediately* initiate the next collection step.

The same objective can be achieved, but with greater efficiency, by creating a collection database in a computer. This approach has the added advantage of allowing you to determine quickly the status of any account in the database and easily track each account's history. An example of a screen from a collections database is shown in Figure 8–1. Cases can be selected and sorted by any variable, so that it is easy, for example, to call up all accounts requiring action on or before 5 February that are being evaluated by a particular collection person and then sort them by last name and producer. The key to using a database such as this is that, when an action is taken, such as sending a second collection letter, the *next* action date and the *next action* that will be taken on that date if the patient does not comply are entered immediately into the database.

The collection database can be part of the MOMS. Most MOMS, however, do not possess an easy capability to segregate those accounts that are in the collection process based on an action that is due on a particular date. Often, it is easier to create a separate collection database by using a database program, such as Claris *Filemaker*. In this way, you can develop a screen that exactly tracks your collection sequence.

THE COLLECTION PLAN

The collection plan integrates all the parts of the collection system. Having a plan will help ensure that problem accounts are quickly identified and that revenue collection is pursued with consistency. An example of a collection plan is given in Appendix 8–A. The plan should provide an outline of the various parts of the collection process. At a minimum, the plan should cover the following eight areas:

1. patient intake process
2. patient education process
3. payment arrangement process
4. verification and preauthorization
5. copay and deductible collection procedures
6. insurance billing procedures
7. problem account detection
8. collection steps and sequencing

As indicated in Table 8–1, it is important for the physician manager and the collection administrator jointly to develop a collection plan that is reasonable to operate but fulfills physicians' needs. If the practice is large and collection is one of several front office functions that are assigned to different positions, then it may be necessary to have other functional leaders involved in the collection plan development. This will help ensure successful cross-function integration. Exhibit 8–8 contains a checklist that physician managers can use to assess the health of their collection process.

Last	Slopay
First	Arnold
Account Number	5662
Physician	Dr. Smith
Bill	Yes
Bill Date	2/1/97
First Letter Date	3/1/97
Second Letter	Yes
Second Letter Date	3/11/97
Last Action Date	3/11/97
Next Action Date	3/21/97
Next Action	Send Account To Attorney For Collection
BALANCE	360.00

Notes
Patient owes $350.00 deductible. Claims he has already paid this amount at other practices. Ins. Co. has no record of this. Told him this was between him and his Ins. Co.

Missed co-payment on 2/16/97. Said he would mail it in. Never did. This was noted in both collection letters.

Figure 8–1 Collection database screen.

WHAT TO DO IF YOUR ACCOUNTS ARE OUT OF CONTROL

"I don't know where to begin. The accounts are a mess. Some patients come and go and don't pay. I'm not even sure what some patients owe. It takes forever to collect from insurance companies. It seems like everything is out of control! What do I do?" At this point, some physicians throw their hands up in frustration, others fire the business manager, and still others hire a consultant[2] or subcontract the whole receivable function.

None of these responses is satisfactory. Pretending that the problem doesn't exist is a prescription for bankruptcy. Firing the business manager may be appropriate, if he or she is the source of the problem. *Assuming* that this is the case may make you feel better, but if it is not the case, then you have neither solved the problem nor delayed the ultimate consequences. Although a knowledgeable consultant can be helpful, simply handing the problem to a consultant and saying "fix it" is not a permanent solution. Someday the consultant will leave, and if the underlying causes are not fixed, collection problems will inevitably recur. Subcontracting can be effective if the subcontractor is effective.

Many, unfortunately, are not. At a minimum, you still must monitor performance closely.

What do you do? Begin by accepting your own personal responsibility for these circumstances. Whenever events get out of control, the ultimate source of the problem is top management, and that is *you*, the physician manager. It may be true that you hired others to run the front office and that, if they had performed better or more conscientiously, your financial problem would not have occurred. It is also true, however, that you are responsible for the actions of your subordinates. You may delegate to them the *authority* to bill and collect in your name, but you can never delegate ultimate *responsibility* for their actions.

The first step to turning around your practice's collection process is to accept that, as a physician manager, you are partly responsible. Your job is to know enough about all business aspects of your practice, so that you will know when things are going well and when they are drifting toward disorder.

All that is history, however. What should you do *now*? Here are some ideas:

- *Audit all overdue accounts*. Reassign secretaries, use overtime, or hire collection con-

Exhibit 8–8 Physicians' Collection Checklist

1. Have you recently evaluated your billing strategies for your mix of insurers?
2. Do your patient education materials discuss financial and collection issues, including patient responsibilities?
3. Does your intake process provide necessary legal safeguards, including assignment of legal and court costs?
4. Have you recently reviewed your collection plan?
   - Patient intake process
   - Patient education process
   - Payment arrangement process
   - Verification and preauthorization
   - Copayment collection procedures
   - Insurance billing procedures
   - Problem account detection procedures
   - Collection steps, sequencing, and timing
5. Do you have adequate collection control systems in place, and do *you* routinely examine them?
   - Aging analyses
   - Insurance aging analysis
   - Aging database
   - Collection database
6. Do you have collection performance standards for the collection administrator and others in the collection process?
7. Do you use the collection control systems and performance standards on a routine basis to:
   - supervise the collection administrator?
   - track collection trends?

tractors to gain sufficient staffpower to audit back accounts fast. Smart managers can use almost any employee to do some of the simpler tasks, such as calling insurance companies, searching remits for denials, pulling financial records, and the like. Find out the real size of your receivables.

- *Work smart.* Direct your personnel to "triage" the accounts. First, work those accounts with the greatest potential return. Write off truly uncollectable accounts and those not worth pursuing. If an account with an $80 balance would take four hours of a contractor's time at $10 per hour to audit and rebill, work it after resolving higher-value accounts.

- *Determine why your accounts have reached this state.* The reasons will become evident as the accounts are audited. Your collection personnel may have a self-interest in hiding the truth from you. If you suspect this to be the case, hire consultants, and have them report directly to you. The bottom line, however, is that if accounts are in disarray you will have to become personally involved for a period of time to understand the sources of the problem and be certain that it has been corrected.

- *Contain the problem now.* Once the sources of the problem are identified, your *highest* priority is to implement immediate corrections to the faulty process. It does you little good to resolve old accounts if you are creating additional new problems each day. Implement necessary policies and procedures. Discipline, terminate, or train ineffective staff. Do whatever is necessary *now.* This point is particularly important for building staff morale. There are few things more disconcerting than working hard to solve old cases, only to see another tidal wave approaching.

- *Set standards, and enforce them.* Most practices' receivables should not move into 90 days past current. If money does get into 90 days, someone should explain why to *you.* You should receive account aging reports at least monthly. Use the reports to set goals for and evaluate the performance of collection personnel.

As a physician manager, you should be actively involved in the management of your practice. This doesn't mean that you should be performing your subordinates' work for them. It does mean, however, that you cannot ignore your critical management role. Routinely reviewing aging reports and trends, looking for indications of potential problems, and determining and reviewing collection policies and standards are all appropriate activities for a physician manager. Your collection personnel should know that you are highly informed and very interested in the state of your practice's finances.

CONCLUSION

You should now be able to evaluate whether your practice has an effective, comprehensive collection plan. If it does not, you should be able to give your collection administrator or business manager guidance regarding the development of a collection plan and also be able to assess the results of his or her efforts. You should now be

familiar with the reasons why patients don't pay their bills and be able to implement procedures that reduce collection problems before they occur. In addition, you should now appreciate the diagnostic significance of receivables and be able to formulate a collections plan that will compartmentalize collection problems.

Finally, this chapter should have clarified your role in the collection process. As a physician manager, you will not be involved with the daily collection of fees. Your collection role, however, is crucial to your practice's financial security. Your *ultimate* responsibility for revenue collection is too important to delegate to a salaried employee. By reviewing financial reports and involving yourself in the design of your practice's collection plan, you will be able to ensure the collection effectiveness of your practice.

REFERENCES

1. "Improving collection performance: structuring the collection letter." With K. Locke. *Journal of Medical Practice Management*. 1994, January-February, 9 (4), 157–160.

2. A version of this section appeared in R. Solomon, Getting a Grip on Collections That Have Gone out of Control, *American Medical News*, 17 February, 1992, p. 34.

Sample Collection Plan (Partial)

(The following points are examples of the types of items that could be in a collection plan. Specific content will vary from practice to practice as a result of types of medical specialty, patient characteristics, and personal and ethical considerations.)

PATIENT INTAKE PROCESS

1. Patients will complete an intake form, which will provide sufficient biographical information to pursue collection should an account become delinquent.
2. The business manager will scan each intake form for obvious signs of financial hardship. If a patient is likely to be a hardship case, the business manager will advise the physician of this possibility, so that the physician can make an informed decision if long-term treatment is necessary.
3. The intake form will provide for authorization to bill the patient's insurance company.
4. The intake form will unequivocally state that the patient is ultimately responsible for settlement of the account.
5. New referrals that have been scheduled more than one day in advance will be reconfirmed the day before the scheduled appointment.

PATIENT EDUCATION PROCESS

1. A sign will be posted at the receptionist's window stating that payment is expected at the time of service.

2. When new referrals are taken over the telephone, the receptionist will inform the patient that payment or copayment is expected at the time of service. If the referral has any questions, the call will be immediately forwarded to the business manager.
3. Each new patient will be provided with a copy of the new patient pamphlet.
4. Patients who will be undergoing continuing treatment will be scheduled for a brief meeting with the business manager. During this meeting the business manager will review the patient's insurance coverage and copayment arrangements and answer any financial questions.

VERIFICATIONS AND PREAUTHORIZATIONS

1. Insurance information will be obtained from referrals at the time they schedule the initial office visit. All patients with CHAMPUS, Key Advantage, OPTIMA, or any other plans requiring preauthorization will be informed of their preauthorization responsibilities at this time.
2. All patients with a preauthorization responsibility will be flagged in the appointment book by the receptionist taking the referral.
3. Upon flagged patients' arrival for the initial office visit, the receptionist will verify that they have in fact received preauthorization.

4. If a patient has not been preauthorized, the receptionist will immediately inform the business manager, who will determine the best way to handle the situation.
5. Treatment authorizations will be placed in the patient's clinical chart. The need for additional authorizations will be monitored by the physician. The physician will inform the business manager when additional authorization is required, and the business manager will be responsible for obtaining the authorization or informing the physician of a denial.

COPAYMENT COLLECTION PROCEDURES

1. The receptionist is responsible for all initial payment, copayment, and deductible collections.
2. The receptionist is responsible for maintaining a current and accurate listing of any patients with copayments.
3. The receptionist is responsible for one collection attempt at the time of service. If the attempt is not made, the receptionist is responsible for contacting the patient that day and requesting payment by mail.
4. The business manager is responsible for ensuring that the receptionist is effectively performing these collection activities. This responsibility includes developing collection methods for when patients cannot or will not pay, employee collection training, and guidelines for when to refer the patient to the business manager.

INSURANCE BILLING PROCEDURES

1. The business manager is responsible for the accurate collection and transmission of all information necessary to receive insurance payment.
2. All procedures will be entered into the computer each day, and insurance claims will be generated and mailed at least three times each week. The objective, however, is daily insurance billing.

3. The business manager will maintain a file of all changes in billing procedures or notices received from insurance companies.

PROBLEM ACCOUNT DETECTION

1. Any denied insurance claim will be of the highest priority. The business manager will immediately investigate the denial, resolve the situation, do any rebilling necessary, and correct any problems with practice procedures, software, and the like.
2. The business manager will immediately inform the managing physician whenever there are any insurance billing problems that are related to computer software or have larger insurance billing implications.
3. The business manager will generate both aging and write-off reports each week. These will be forwarded to the managing physician.
4. The business manager is responsible for maintaining aging balances at acceptable levels as determined by the managing physician.
5. All accounts that have money in 90 days past current will be reviewed at least monthly by the business manager. The patient will be billed for personal fees. Insurance fees will be pursued either with a tracer or by resubmission of a claim.

COLLECTION STEPS AND SEQUENCING

1. Patients will be informed within one day that a missed copayment must be paid by the time of the next visit or within seven days. They will also be reminded that copayments must be paid at the time of service.
2. If a patient misses two consecutive copayments, the business manager will inform the physician, and, with the concurrence of the physician, appointments

will be suspended until the fees have been paid. The collection sequence will begin.

3. Patient fees that move into 90 days past current will enter the collection sequence.

4. The collection sequence is as follows: A detailed bill is sent with notice to pay in 21 days. On day 22, a first collection letter is sent with notice to pay in 14 days. On day 15, a second collection letter is sent with notice to pay in 10 days. Simultaneously, the business manager makes two attempts to contact the patient by telephone. On day 11, the account is sent to the collection attorney.

CHAPTER 9

Marketing

Chapter Objectives

This chapter will help you develop basic marketing skills. It begins by differentiating marketing from selling and progresses to the marketing planning process, which permits you to develop medical services and products that meet your customers' needs. You will learn how to evaluate your organization's internal competitive strengths and weaknesses and to identify and analyze potential problems and opportunities in your environment.

This chapter emphasizes thinking about your market in terms of market segments and targeting these segments with specific medical products and services. Finally, this chapter will also help you develop promotional skills. Promotion is the process of communicating what your health care organization can provide to its customers. Promotion skills are relevant to physician managers who are practice based as well as to those working in large health care systems. Promotion methods that will be discussed include:

- personal contacts
- using the media for both paid and unpaid ads
- using data, such as from clinical and management information systems, to describe quality and cost factors to referring organizations, such as primary care and specialist physicians, employers, and insurers.

The brief introduction to marketing in Chapter 1 emphasized the distinction between marketing and selling. To reiterate, physicians who market their services first identify their customers' needs. They then provide the products and services that their customers want in a form, at a price, and in a location that is attractive to customers (patients). In contrast, a selling philosophy begins with the products and services that the physician wishes to offer. Subsequent efforts are aimed at convincing customers (patient, employer, or health maintenance organization [HMO]) why they should acquire the health care provider's service. The differences, therefore, between marketing and selling are quite distinct.

Many physicians believe that *marketing* and *advertising* are simply two different words to describe the same process. This is not true, and therein lies a fundamental misconception about marketing. Marketing, in fact, affects the quality and characteristics of the products or services being offered. One outcome from marketing should be that your products and services will be changed so that they are more useful to your customers. When an organization markets its services, it recognizes that no matter how excellent they are, they are incomplete if customers fail to use them because:

239

- they are less useful than some other provider's services
- they are unaware of them
- they are offered at an inconvenient time or place or in an inconvenient manner
- they are not affordable or viewed as fairly priced

Marketing professionals have traditionally talked about four types of decisions that must be made regarding the marketing of a product or service. Often referred to as the four Ps, these decisions concern:

1. *product* or service characteristics
2. *place* or distribution of the product or service
3. *promotion* of the product or service so that customers will be aware of it
4. *price* of the product or service

The *marketing mix* is the specific combination of the four Ps that you develop for your organization as a whole or for particular services, such as oncology, cardiac services, outpatient services, and so forth.

Product decisions concern the specific products and services you intend to offer. To make these decisions, you need to identify groups of potential customers (e.g., patients, employers, and insurers), learn how they can be best served, and determine which products and services will attract them. The service that you offer might well include more than clinical outcomes. For example, it might include satisfaction, a sense of respect, and patient involvement. Patient-focused units and maternity centers are examples of how medical services can be modified to better encompass patient (customer) desires. Similarly, coronary artery bypass graft critical paths that can discharge some patients from the hospital sooner, thereby reducing cost, represent an expanded product definition that better satisfies employers' and insurers' needs.

Place (distribution) decisions concern where and when to offer services. Location and office hours are choices that can contribute to success. Using satellite, storefront, and shopping center locations and offering staggered and extended office hours are distribution options. In addition, convenient parking, easy access, and proximity to existing or desired patient bases are place considerations.

Promotion can include various forms of paid advertising, speeches, seminars to probable patient referral sources, free or low-cost blood pressure or cholesterol checks, and any number of activities that will familiarize the public with the organization, its physicians, and its services. This category also includes television infomercials on topics such as stroke, weight loss, and heart disease that are designed to familiarize potential patients with a health care system's physicians and facilities.

Pricing decisions concern the cost of services. This includes decisions related to participating with an insurance company and accepting its fee structure, participating with preferred provider organizations (PPOs) and HMOs, and agreeing to capitated contracts. Physicians and other health care providers can adopt conscious pricing strategies to undercut, match, or lead the market. Each pricing strategy can be appropriate if it fits into a coherent strategy to attract market segments.

Undercutting the market is a strategy to use in mature markets to gain market share. If you are a low-cost producer, it can be an effective approach. Matching the market generally makes pricing a nonissue. Adopting this approach emphasizes competing for patients on the basis of product or service characteristics, distribution, or promotion. Leading the market can be effective if your services are in great demand. Generally, consumers perceive higher-priced services and products to be of superior quality, so a price leader position can be consistent with introducing state-of-the-art procedures.

An effective marketing mix—the specific combination of product, place, promotion, and pricing decisions—is the result of a carefully developed *marketing plan*. A formal, written marketing plan contains, therefore, a product plan, a distribution plan, a promotion plan, and a pricing plan. Marketing plans are developed as a result of a thorough analysis of internal organizational strengths and weaknesses and external opportunities and threats. This process is sometimes referred to as SWOT (strengths, weaknesses, opportunities, and threats) analysis.

Health care organizations do not operate in a vacuum. To some extent, product and service decisions are influenced by external factors, such as the number, quality, and pricing of competitors; local geography; local and national economies; changes in medical technology; standards of care; government regulation; and local ethics regarding acceptable forms of promotion. It is important to develop a marketing plan in the context of these external factors, so that the plan considers how these issues may create impediments to success as well as opportunities to exploit.

In addition, a marketing plan should take into account internal factors, such as your organization's financial resources, the medical and professional skills of physicians and others, equipment and facilities, and the organization's mission. A marketing plan, therefore, should also be developed to build on internal organizational strengths and to compensate for its weaknesses.

As illustrated in Exhibit 9–1, the process of collecting data on external and internal factors is called situational analysis and leads directly to SWOT analysis. The SWOT analysis, in turn, defines the boundaries for developing a marketing strategy and, ultimately, specific marketing plans. Exhibit 9–1 also indicates that it is important to develop a marketing strategy before you construct a marketing plan. A marketing strategy is concerned with the long-range goals and general market orientation of your organization. It provides a context within which to develop a marketing plan. By having a strategy and developing marketing plans consistent with a strategy, you help ensure that the plan is more than an immediate reaction to market events. Here are two summary statements describing two different strategies:

1. *Carriage trade strategy:* Our practice will seek middle- and upper-income pa-

tients. It will be based on patients who seek superior quality and personalized service. We will offer state-of-the-art services in very comfortable surroundings. We will seek managed care arrangements that emphasize patient choice. Our boundaries are the world.

2. *McDonald's strategy:* Our practice will be directed at lower-paying patients who may not have good health insurance but who are most in need of care. We will provide our services in a "no-frills" atmosphere, so that prices will be affordable, but we will still be able to operate at a profit. The practice will prosper by efficiently treating many patients at very competitive prices. We will seek managed care contracts that will cover a large number of lives.[1]

Once a marketing strategy is determined, a specific marketing plan will logically flow from it. Obviously, it would be counterproductive to develop a marketing plan with "McDonald's" product, place, promotion, and price characteristics if in fact your real intention is to be a carriage trade practice, and vice versa. If you do not precede the development of specific marketing plans with the identification of an overall market strategy, you may unintentionally back into a questionable strategy as a result of a desire to undertake specific marketing activities. For example, the carriage trade practice may win a managed care contract without sufficient protections for cost shifting from hospitals and primary care physicians. As a result, the practice receives a volume that is inconsistent with its strategy. Having a good understanding of its marketing strategy will allow the practice to negotiate managed care agreements with characteristics that are important to it.

The process of developing a marketing strategy is discussed in Chapter 10, Strategic Management. In addition, Chapter 10 provides a framework for developing a marketing strategy based on your own situational analysis and SWOT analysis. The current chapter is designed

Exhibit 9–1 The Marketing Planning Process

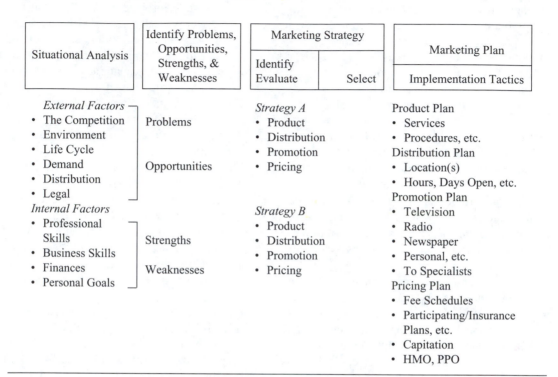

to place these planning processes in the larger marketing context. It is also designed to cover operational marketing skills that are used to put the marketing plan into operation, including promotion, segmentation, and marketing research.

CONDUCTING A SITUATIONAL ANALYSIS

The goal of conducting a situational analysis is to discover the external and internal factors that could affect your marketing plan. Factors to consider are outlined in Exhibit 9–1. These are a good starting point, but this list is certainly not exhaustive.

The Competition

To compete effectively, you must know who your competitors are and understand their competitive advantages and disadvantages. Questions to ask about your competitors include the following:

- How many competitors do you have? Are you, for example, the only urologist or hospital in town, or is the market divided among many competitors?
- Who are your competitors, and who are they likely to be in the future? Are they likely to be among the following:
  1. old, established practices/hospitals?
  2. new physicians or for-profit health systems moving into the market?
  3. alternative providers (e.g., HMOs and PPOs) or new types of organizations (e.g., management services organizations, Phycor, etc.)?
  4. specialists or primary care physicians who are broadening their spheres of practice?
  5. nonmedical competitors, such as chiropractors, psychologists, nurse practitioners, massage therapists, and health food stores?
  6. hospital emergency departments?
  7. emergency care centers?

- What are their competitive advantages and disadvantages? For example, do they have unique training, skills, cost structures, management skills, or equipment that set them apart? Do some have inside ties with hospitals and other potential referral sources? Do they have better or inferior locations? If you can understand the competitive advantages of your competition, then you may be able to:
  1. use similar strategies to your advantage
  2. avoid head-to-head competition that you cannot win
  3. devise tactics to circumvent your colleagues' competitive advantages
- What are their financial resources? Are they professionally well established?
- What promotional methods do they use, and how well do they appear to work?
- Do you think that your competitors will respond to your promotional efforts? That is, would they react in a retaliatory manner? Might they try to neutralize your efforts, or might they ignore you?

Environment

Environmental issues provide the scientific, professional, ethical, and social context for your market strategy and plans. Some environmental issues come and go, whereas others are more or less permanent. From a marketing perspective, it is important to understand where we are in the life cycle of an issue. For example, as I write this book it is impossible to open a magazine, turn on a radio or television, go to a movie, or have an extended conversation with a friend without some mention of the "drug crisis." Our social and political environment is saturated with this issue. A marketing plan that takes into account the public's intense interest in the drug problem may benefit your organization as well as lead you to provide a needed public service.

In contrast, eating disorders, such as anorexia and bulimia, are no less real now than they were a decade ago, but they no longer occupy the public spotlight. Does this mean that a health care system shouldn't develop programs to treat these disorders? Certainly not. The resources devoted to the problem and other marketing mix decisions, however, should take into account the current relative disinterest in the topic and the large number of medical and nonmedical providers that are now competing for this market. As a result of the changing social environment, a marketing plan that you would design today for an anorexia or bulimia treatment program would probably look very different from one that you would have designed 10 years ago. Similarly, the current controversy regarding silicon breast implants is an environmental factor that anyone performing this procedure should take into account before developing a marketing plan.

It is also important to take into account local environmental issues. For example, the Hampton Roads area in Virginia has a very large military population. This population is such a significant part of the market that it should be considered in the marketing plan of any local physician, hospital, or health care system. The implications of this market segment include the following:

- directing product/service decisions at young, low-income, temporary residents and providing services that might be highly utilized by this segment, such as obstetrics and children's disease, alcoholism, trauma, and drug abuse treatment programs (product)
- taking into account insurance coverage (CHAMPUS) and associated usual and customary rates (pricing)
- accessing the CHAMPUS system and other referral sources to reach this market segment selectively (promotion)
- selecting a location that coincides with areas of heavy military housing and commuter routes to the three major area naval bases and providing practice hours to harmonize with military base commuting schedules and routes (distribution)

Another environmental issue in the Hampton Roads area is the road system. The local highway system was poorly designed and does not have sufficient capacity. As a result, some parts of this area become virtually inaccessible between 7:00 A.M. and 9:00 A.M. and between 3:30 P.M. and 5:30 P.M. Some creative engineers have managed to link Norfolk to Portsmouth (two major urban areas) with a tunnel that opens onto a drawbridge. This means that at any given time a trip that normally takes a few minutes can take half an hour or longer. These transportation problems have created a certain mind set on the part of residents: They seek services in their immediate locality, they avoid certain areas and roads except during midday, and they plan commitments, such as medical appointments, to avoid the high traffic times whenever possible. These considerations affect product/service choices, including the number and location of hospitals, the feasible range of affiliation of physicians, and the location and hours of promotions, such as public presentations, blood pressure and cholesterol screenings, and the like.

Another important environmental issue to consider is local ethical standards regarding the use of promotion by health care organizations. For example, physicians in most parts of the country now feel comfortable placing a display ad in the daily newspaper describing their services. In addition, many physicians think that appearing on a local television talk show is an appropriate public service/promotional activity. How do physicians in your area feel, however, about combining the medium of television with the newspaper message? For example, what would the reaction be to a 30-second paid commercial extolling your skills and services? Many physicians would feel that this goes beyond the bounds of good taste or is even unethical. What would the consequences be if you were one of the first in your area to use this promotional approach? How would your peers react to you, and might there be some form of subtle or not-so-subtle retaliation?

Another area of environmental concern is changing technology. For example, what new types of equipment or diagnostic procedures are becoming available? This issue, which obviously has educational, technical, and financial implications, also has significant marketing implications. How would new equipment allow you to provide new or better services to your patients? How can you let patients or referring professionals know about your organization's capability to provide new services? To what extent will your colleagues follow suit, thereby limiting your competitive advantage to a window in time? Similarly, a technological change could be a major threat to your marketing plan if it eventually renders one of your services obsolete.

Life Cycle

Another external consideration is the life cycle of each service or procedure you offer. It is easy to understand that a product such as a computer or a car can have a life cycle. It is introduced into the market, demand for it grows, the market eventually becomes mature and stabilizes, then the demand for the product declines as tastes change or as competing products enter the market, and finally there is little or no need for it.

Many medical services and procedures also go through a life cycle of birth, growth, maturity, decline, and death. In most cases, the underlying disease continues, but the services, procedures, and medications that physicians use to treat the disease go through a life cycle. The change from one life cycle stage to another can be due to changing technology, such as new equipment or drugs, or to changing public awareness and acceptance of the disease. For example, bulimia has reached maturity in terms of public interest, and the number of patients who seek services for this problem has leveled off. Most areas abound with a myriad of different types of treatment facilities and programs to deal with eating disorders. AIDS, on the other hand, is still in the growth phase, as is multidrug treatment for the disease. Table 9–1 illustrates life cycles for procedures in several specialties.

Marketing professionals have noted that products or services in a particular life cycle stage have characteristic attributes. For example, the introductory phase is characterized by low sales, technical and marketing problems, and high

Table 9–1 Life Cycles in Health Care

	Introduction	Developmental/ Early Growth	Growth/Late Growth	Maturity	Decline
Administration	Shared Governance Quality Measurement and Qualifications Standard Treatment Protocols PACS	Total Quality Management (TQM) Decision Support System (DSS) Value-Based Pricing	Management Information Systems (MIS) Product Line Management	Discount-Based Pricing	Management By Objectives Zero-Based Budgeting
Cardiovascular	Lasers Lipid Clinics Percutaneous Bypass Intravascular Ultrasound Filmless Cath Lab Atherectomy Cardiac MR	Transesophageal Echo SPECT AICD Ventricular Assist Devices Valvuloplasty ECG Signal Averaging Freestanding Cath Lab	PTCA Conventional Echo Electrophysiology Color Flow Doppler Echo Thrombolytic Agents Stress Echo Mobile Cath Lab	Holter Monitoring CABG Cardiac Rehabilitation Diagnostic Angiography	Vectorcardiography Phonocardiography Stress Test Systolic Time Intervals Cardiokymography Ballistocardiography
Diagnostic Imaging	CT Angiography 3-D Radiologic Reconstruction Cine CT MR Spectroscopy PET	SPECT Ultrasound MR Angiography	DSA Vascular Labs Mammography Conventional CT MRI Prostatic Ultrasound Transvaginal Ultrasound	Nuclear Medicine Radiography	Encephalography Thermography Cut Film Angiography Bone Scan Head Scanners

continues

Table 9–1 continued

	Introduction	Developmental/ Early Growth	Growth/Late Growth	Maturity	Decline
Neurosciences	Photo Dynamic Therapy Alzheimers Testing Genetic Markers Tissue Transplants Image-Linked Navigation Systems Magnetoencephalography	Neurosonology Stroke Intervention Sleep Disorder Labs 3-D CT/MR	Radiosurgery Evoked Potential EEG Transcranial Doppler Interventional Radiology Stereotactic Surgery	EEG EMG	Contrast Arteriography Myelography
Oncology	Remote Afterloading Autologous Bone Marrow Transplantation Drug Sensitivity Assays Cancer Risk Assessment Cell Growth Regulation Laser-based Photodynamic Therapy	Gamma Knife Bio-Technology Neoadjuvant Chemotherapy Tumor Markers Granulocyte-Macrophage Colony Stimulating Factors Erythropolietin Immunotherapy (Monoclonal Antibodies)	Combination Chemotherapy Hyperthermia Multi-Modality Therapies Adjuvant Chemotherapy Interferon Cyto-Reductive Surgery Interstitial Implants Stereotactic Radiosurgery	Linear Accelerators Chemotherapy Hormone Therapy	Cobalt-60 Radiation Therapy (External Beam)
Orthopaedics	Bone Growth Stimulators Percutaneous Laser Diskectomy Robotic Tools	Cotrel-Dubosset Implants Paralysis Preventing Drugs Bone Transplantation Orthopaedic Oncology	Hip/Knee Replacement Sports Medicine Trauma-Related Violence-Related Arthritis	Laminectomy Diskectomy Fusion	Myelography CPM (Continuous Positive Motion)

					"Open" Surgeries
Surgery	Cochlear Implants Open Fetal Surgery Tissue Welding Laparoscopic Surgery —Bowel Surgery —Lung Tumors —CABG	Lasers Anesthesia Monitoring Laparoscopic Surgery Appendectomy —Pyloromyotomy (Peptic Ulcers) —Hysterectomy	Laparoscopic Cholecystectomy Autologous Blood Laparoscopic Herniorraphy	Lithotripsy	"Open" Surgeries
Other Clinical Services	Bedside Terminals Urinary Lithotripsy Biliary Lithotripsy Vascular Rehab	Fertility Clinics Patient-Controlled Analgesia Home Therapy Continuous Arterio- venous Hemofiltration	Peripheral Angioplasty Endoscopic Lasers Cataract Surgery Interocular Lens Implants Oximetry, Pulsed Oximetry Capnography	Autotransfusion Renal Dialysis Clinical Laborato- ries Pharmacy Radial Kerato- tomy Hyperalimentation	Therapeutic Phle- botomy

Source: Reprinted with permission from *Hospital Technology Scanner*, p. 5, © 1993, American Hospital Association.

costs in relation to revenues. These characteristics are due to the start-up costs and the costs of initial marketing. Physicians who decide to provide a service or procedure that is in the introductory stage should be future oriented and willing to assume some risk. Laser keratotomy, for example, is presently in this stage. Ophthalmologists who have invested their time and capital in acquiring the ability and equipment to perform this procedure face risks in terms of both its long-range effectiveness and the possibility that newer technologies may supersede it.

The growth phase is characterized by rapidly increasing demand for services by patients. Generally, the physicians who benefit most from the growth stage of a new service or procedure are those who first introduce it to an area. In the growth stage, it is not unusual for demand to exceed the ability to supply the service. The high revenues associated with the growth phase can also lead to a failure to control costs and may create the temptation to overextend. Overextension can be manifested as risky growth, such as buying new equipment or acquiring new facilities that will only pay for themselves if the growth continues. It can also be manifested as overwork. In short, the euphoria associated with the growth phase has inherent dangers.

The beginning of the mature phase is characterized by slowing growth. Eventually a peak is reached and patient demand flattens and may begin to decline. Most medical services and procedures will be in the mature stage, and some will remain there for many years. Health care organizations that are well entrenched and well managed will prosper even when providing mainly mature services and procedures. Because growth is no longer occurring as a result of increased demand from patients, it must occur by increasing market share. This means taking business away from competitors. Generally, this results in price competition. Therefore, controlling costs and differentiating yourself from your peers are particularly important in this stage.

The decline stage of a procedure or service is characterized by a decrease in the use of a proce-

dure or a decline in patient demand for it. This can be a slow and steady decline, such as would be characterized by changing social factors that might affect, for example, specific elective plastic surgery procedures. Declines resulting from technological change can, on the other hand, be precipitous. Other implications of product life cycle are discussed in Chapter 10, Strategic Management.

Demand

Demand is the extent to which current consumers seek the services or procedures you offer or intend to offer. To understand the demand for a given service or procedure, you must understand how potential patients currently buy similar services or procedures. Scott and colleagues list a number of considerations related to the nature of patient demand for medical services[2]:

- the number of physicians whom patients consider when seeking medical care
- the extent to which patients seek information before selecting a physician
- the loyalty that patients have to physicians used in the past or to referral sources, such as hospitals and other health care professionals
- the sources of information used by patients, such as the Yellow Pages, physician referral services, other health care professionals, and friends
- who makes the physician selection decision, and who influences the decision (e.g., the husband, wife, father, or mother)
- the degree of patient interest in the physician selection process (is the decision more like a decision to purchase hairpins or an automobile?)
- the perceived risk involved in making a bad physician selection decision
- attitudes regarding whether the illness or procedure is viewed as a necessity or a luxury (is the purchase of the medical service more like the purchase of food or a cocktail dress?)

- the length of the anticipated time involvement with the physician (is the time involvement with the consequences of the purchase decision analogous to that of buying gum or dining room furniture?)

The objective of asking these and other questions is to uncover implications for your services and procedures. By determining the answers, you may be able to design more effective services or communicate them more effectively.

Another issue related to demand is the concept of market segmentation. Market segments are groups of people who will respond in a similar manner to the marketing mix. By understanding the different demands associated with the segments of your market, you can more precisely direct your marketing efforts. If, for example, a plastic surgeon determines that a significant number of his or her rhinoplasty patients are women, are between the ages of 25 and 35 years, and reside disproportionately in two of the seven local counties, then he or she can use this information to design a more effective marketing plan. Similarly, if the decision about where to take a child with a cold for treatment is made by the mother in 75 percent of families, then this should influence promotion decisions.

Professional and Business Skills

To develop an effective marketing plan, it is important to assess your organization's professional and business skills. It makes no sense to market a service that cannot be delivered either clinically or managerially, to undersell a valuable or rare service, or to take on a well-entrenched competitor with little hope for success. Self-deception is self-defeating; you are obviously dependent upon a realistic determination of the relative quality of your professional skills.

The business end of your organization provides the support necessary for the delivery of professional services. If your business operations have weaknesses or strengths, then these must be understood, compensated for, taken advantage of, or changed. It is not advisable, however, simply to wish around weaknesses in office operations or to fail to take advantage of a strength.

An assessment of your organization's business strengths and weaknesses is very important because an effective marketing plan will put additional pressures on business operations. First, the marketing plan will, one hopes, result in an increase in patients treated, procedures performed, and so on. This, of course, will result in an increase in associated support work, such as laboratory testing, insurance filing, chart management, report writing, and so forth.

At the practice level, for example, marketing activities may include writing news releases and speeches and arranging appointments with referral sources, all of which take time and energy. Do you have an employee with enough skills to write a news release? Are your secretaries going to be able to take the additional load if you decide to produce a training and nutrition manual for the local Little League? Do your staff have the skill to approach local employers to negotiate covering lives for a capitated fee?

Finally, you should evaluate your own promotional skills and those of your colleagues. If you are terrified by the thought of standing before an audience to give a lecture, or if you are just not very good at it, then it is critical for you to acknowledge this. You may choose to work on your fear, develop your skills, or avoid this type of promotion. All are acceptable choices. What is not acceptable, however, is basing a marketing plan on something that you cannot or will not undertake.

Finances

Any strategic marketing plan will have financial implications. Developing new services and locations as well as promoting them cost money. Developing a pro forma budget can be a helpful exercise. Some promotional methods may cost little or nothing; many others can be quite expensive. It is important to be realistic about the funds that are available for product and service development as well as the cost of promoting them.

Personal Goals

For physicians in private practice, this is arguably the single most important internal environmental issue. What do you and your partners *want* to do? What do you want your practice to be like? What kinds of patients (defined any way you like) do you want to treat, and what type of clinical work do you really want to undertake? There is nothing so frustrating as working hard to achieve success only to realize that what you accomplished was not what you really wanted.

Consider more than just your clinical work when defining your goals. If, for example, it is important for you to have significant amounts of time with your family, then this should be taken into account in your marketing plan. For example, a plan, that, if successful, would result in your conducting 50 clinical hours per week, not to mention marketing and administration duties, is obviously inconsistent with a significant home life. Other issues, such as your status in the community or your ability to help ameliorate social problems, may be important to you. You will be happier and certainly more successful if your personal goals are reflected in how you run your practice. For example, the carriage trade practice and the McDonald's practice that were described above will have different degrees of attractiveness to different physicians. There is nothing inherently right or wrong with developing either type of practice. The important point is for you to be honest with yourself regarding what you want your practice to be so that you can develop a marketing strategy and plan that will help you get there.

Health care organizations similarly should pay attention to life goals, but in this context we usually use the term *organizational mission*. A for-profit health care system should develop a marketing strategy and specific plans that are consistent with its for-profit mission. Similarly, not-for-profit health care systems often have significant parts of their missions defined in terms of returning service to the community. Once again, the strategy and plans should derive from these goals.

SWOT ANALYSIS

A SWOT analysis involves taking the situation analysis information and determining your organization's strengths, weaknesses, opportunities, and threats.

Threats are external factors that result in an organization performing at lower levels than it would otherwise. Threats might include the following:

- numerous competitors in your specialty
- insurance carriers that have adopted less realistic usual and customary rates and require that more "hoops" be jumped through as prerequisites for payment
- a new emergency care facility that has opened two blocks from your hospital, skimming "cream" cases and revenue from your emergency department
- a downturn in the local economy that makes preventive health care generally less affordable
- physicians who have formed a management services organization with a major competing hospital and who also are on your staff

Opportunities are openings in the external environment of which you could take advantage. Here are some examples:

- The local school system decides to contract with a physician to provide medical examinations for all students in its athletic programs.
- An older physician with a successful practice is retiring and is interested in working out an arrangement for the care of her patients.
- A major commuting route passes your office, which allows you to provide treatment during commuting hours.
- Physicians, concerned about external threats, are willing to align with the hospital to form a management services organization that is closely integrated with the hospital and creates the potential for cost savings.

Weaknesses are internal factors that limit your organization's ability to compete for patients or provide them with services. Weaknesses might include the following:

- a patient reception area that is too small to support practice growth
- front office staff who are having difficulty coping with the current volume of patients
- a dislike on your part of talking before large groups
- a secretary who does not come to you with work problems but instead takes them out on other employees
- undeveloped management information systems, so that your hospital has poor cost data and, as a result, has difficulty making knowledgeable bids on managed care contracts

Strengths are internal factors that provide you with a competitive advantage over other organizations. The following are some examples:

- physician managers in affiliated health care practices who have been educated in business issues, who understand the need for hospital cost control, and who actively pursue total quality management thinking to improve hospital processes
- a thoroughly developed artificial hip critical path along with integrated financial and medical management information systems
- financial reserves that will allow you to deal with growth or any unforeseen circumstances expeditiously

Once you have completed a SWOT analysis, you will then use the information to develop a marketing strategy, which is the next step in the marketing planning process. Once again, this process is covered in detail in Chapter 10.

MARKETING PLAN

The marketing plan contains the operational details of how you will implement your marketing strategy. If the marketing strategy is somewhat analogous to the statement "We will open a second front in France in 1944," then the marketing plan will indicate which divisions will land where, what their objectives are, and what equipment and supplies they will need. The four elements of the marketing plan (product, place, price, and promotion) must fit together into a synergistic whole, and there must be a logical tie back to the marketing strategy. The marketing plan should provide concrete guidance regarding products and services, distribution, promotion, and pricing, and it must be consistent with and reflect the knowledge obtained in the preceding phases of the marketing planning process. Exhibit 9–2 provides an example of a marketing plan for a psychiatrist.

A marketing plan is subject to constant revision. For example, suppose that the first of the quarterly workshops referred to in Exhibit 9–2 is a great success. Many people attend, and within a week several have become patients. This would certainly suggest that the psychiatrist should consider revising his plans and should also try to determine exactly what happened at the workshop to attract the patients. Similarly, if the paid display ads are producing no noticeable results after six weeks, he should evaluate the ad content as well as the appropriateness of the medium.

PROMOTION

Promotion is probably what first comes to most people's minds whenever they hear the term marketing. Promotion is the process of presenting your services to prospective customers, such as patients, employers, insurers, and so forth. Promotional activities are often the most visible part of an organization's marketing activities to those outside the organization. The object of this section is to acquaint you with a number of specific promotional activities and indicate how and when to use them.

Personal Contact

Personal contact is one of the most effective ways of promoting a health care organization.

Exhibit 9–2 Sample Marketing Plan

Marketing Plan for a Psychiatrist

Product Plan

My objective is to spend 60 percent of my time doing medication work and hospital rounds. I do not want to be involved in much short-term psychotherapy, so I will select my psychotherapy cases to be longer-term, more chronic cases. I will seek to refer out short-term psychotherapy cases while retaining the medical component of the case.

I want to develop an eating disorders program. Once again, however, my primary interest is the medication and hospitalization components. I will try to find a psychology practice to develop and market this program jointly. That practice will handle the psychotherapy, and I will handle the medical component. If I can't find the "right" psychology practice, I will consider hiring a psychologist or clinical social worker and expanding my facilities, so that I can provide these services.

Distribution Plan

My practice is currently well situated to serve my patients. I will not expand my hours. The eating disorders program will have to be based in the "allied" practice. This practice must be in the eastern part of town, no more than 5 minutes or so from an expressway exit and no more than 15 minutes from my practice.

Promotion Plan

Paid Display Advertising

I will plan to spend $13,500 in paid print advertising. Based on market research provided to me by the publishers, I will spend $6,500 on biweekly display ads in the local entertainment newspaper and an additional $7,000 on a smaller weekly display ad in the daily newspaper. The ads will stress:

- the personalized nature of my services
- the comprehensiveness of psychiatry as opposed to the more limited skills of competitors, such as psychologists

I am willing to devote an additional $5,000 to the eating disorder program and would expect that the "allied" practice would contribute an equal amount. The specific nature of these ads will be determined with the "allied" practice, but it is necessary that the ads reflect a high-quality, scientific (as opposed to "pop psychology"), professional image.

Referral Source Development

1. I will refer out a significant proportion of psychotherapy patients to well-qualified and professionally competent allied providers, such as psychologists and clinical social workers, with the objective of receiving medication referrals. Once a provider has begun to supply me with his or her medication referrals, I will continue to supply him or her with psychotherapy referrals.
2. I will hold a one-day training program for family practice physicians to acquaint them with ways of determining when child behavior problems should be referred to a psychiatrist.

Television and Radio

I will have my secretary obtain a list of the names and addresses of all local talk show hosts. I will write each one a letter describing timely topics that I can talk about on his or her show. In addition, I will mail each one a press release on a specific issue at least once every two months.

---

continues

Exhibit 9–2 Sample Marketing Plan

Free Media

1. I will write at least one news release each month. These will be on the latest developments in mental health. Sources of information will be my professional journals. The news releases will be mailed to reporters and to local television and radio news departments.
2. I will conduct four free 1.5-hour workshops/seminars each year, which will be held in a nearby church auditorium. These will cover such issues as smoking, eating disorders, phobias, problem children, and the like. The workshops will emphasize the unique role of psychiatry in treating these disorders.
3. Six weeks before each free workshop, I will distribute a press release about it to all local newspapers and other media for inclusion in community announcements as well as to local churches and civic groups for inclusion in their newsletters.
4. I will try to find some source of free, recurring media exposure, such as a weekly mental health segment on a television news program or a weekly or monthly newspaper column.

Pricing Plan

I will participate with Blue Cross/Blue Shield until I feel that my patients are no longer particularly sensitive to the usual and customary rate or until I have more patients than I can personally treat. I will not participate with CHAMPUS. I will set my fees at about what my peers charge, but if I am off, I will be on the high side. My fees for the eating disorder program with not be different from my regular fees.

Personal contact means talking to large or small groups of people. It also includes one-on-one contact with another person. In either case, the target of personal contact can be potential patients or referral sources. One reason that this form of promotion can be so effective is that it is often not perceived as promotion. Another reason is that potential patients and referral sources get to know you and begin to see you as a person, not merely as a name or a title.

Let's first discuss how to promote yourself to groups of potential patients or referral sources. It is important to draw a distinction between making one or two presentations to groups and developing an ongoing personal contact strategy. The former is dabbling, the latter is promotion, and the distinction between the two is important. A real promotional effort requires commitment. In particular, it requires time and energy spent developing good presentations and a willingness to make presentations over an extended period of time. Hospital systems, for example, often have speaker series that are designed to familiarize potential patients with affiliated physicians and hospital facilities through the means of education.

Any form of promotion, to be effective, requires repetition, and personal contact is no exception. Physicians using this approach need ways to consistently develop interesting presentation materials. How do you do this? You create a special niche for yourself. Think about your specialty and interests. Select two or three treatment or disorder areas about which you are particularly knowledgeable or would like to be. Don't necessarily limit yourself to areas of current expertise. Be willing to expand your knowledge base when that is necessary or personally desirable. For example, if an employee assistance program will be conducting a seminar on drug testing, give it a shot even if you aren't an expert on the subject. A few hours of paid library work on the part of a student, coupled with a computer search, will give you the specialized knowledge that, in combination with your experience and medical education, will allow you to make an informative and effective presentation. Remember, you don't have to present yourself as an expert on a subject or procedure to make an interesting and effective presentation. You do have to present yourself, however, as one who knows what is current regarding a subject or procedure.

Remember also that the value of the personal contact lies largely in the quality of communication between you and your audience. The very fact that you are there has promotional value. Develop your presentation so that, whenever possible, it involves your audience. Asking your audience questions and giving them plenty of opportunities to ask you questions will help you establish a two-way dialogue. The presentation should allow your audience to sample your behavior. If your objective is to let the audience know that you are competent, concerned, and approachable, then conduct your presentation in this way. Give them facts, but also show them the type of person you are. Conduct the presentation so they understand that you care about their problems and are willing to listen to them. "But I don't have the time to do all that preparation," you say. If you really don't have the time, then you probably don't need to do the promotion in the first place!

Once you have defined a few presentation subjects, the next problem is finding someone who will listen. Begin by asking yourself "Who else works in these areas?" For example, suppose that you feel that you could make an effective presentation on sexual abuse. You might want to contact family service agencies, rape hotlines, ministries, women's groups, police departments, and others that come into contact with sexually abused individuals. There are a number of ways that you can make these contacts, including these:

- You can send a letter outlining the services that you can provide or your willingness to talk about a relevant subject.
- You can make a phone call. This can be particularly effective if you are not certain whom to talk to at an agency.
- A personal visit after a letter or phone call can be very effective in getting a commitment from groups to let you talk to them.
- You can make a call or send a letter in which *you* ask for advice. For example, state that you are looking for services that your patients might need, such as legal assistance or counseling.

Personal contact can also take place at the individual level. One of the most effective ways to conduct one-on-one promotion is over lunch. Meeting a referral source over lunch is advantageous in that neither of you "wastes" an hour (unless, of course, you normally don't eat during the day). Also, it allows you to develop a series of similar time-limited promotional opportunities that can be easily arranged by you or your secretary. If you make it a point to hold three luncheon meetings a week for a month, you will have captured approximately 12 hours of referral development time at virtually no cost in clinical hours.

Paid Ads

Table 9–2 contains an evaluation of the strengths and weaknesses of various major media. Many physicians use newspaper display ads in which they state their names and the services that they offer. If newspaper ads are to work, they require repetition; given the high cost of space in daily newspapers, this will invariably result in a large initial outlay of money before results are seen. If you are considering placing a display ad in a newspaper, be certain to ask yourself what will differentiate you from other physicians running similar display ads.

You should also consider the geographical area from which you draw patients. Although a newspaper may be read by hundreds of thousands of readers, most of this exposure may be of little value if your patients largely come from within a few miles of your practice. For example, a family practice located near residential neighborhoods may draw 90 percent of its patients from within a 10-mile radius. An advertisement in a widely distributed daily newspaper may be largely a waste of money; most readers will not travel long distances because there will be many competitors who are located nearer and because patients generally seek treatment close to home for illnesses perceived to be less serious. On the other hand, a specialist in cosmetic plastic surgery or a cardiologist may have a regional clientele, in which case the wide circula-

Table 9–2 Media Strengths and Weaknesses

Source	Advantages	Disadvantages
Newspapers	Good coverage in local markets Short time commitment Easy availability Tangible and believable	Low demographic selectivity Relatively short life Low reproduction quality
Television	Combines sight and sound High attention Conveys "big league" image Entertaining, energetic, and forceful	Low demographic selectivity Very short message life High production and presentation costs Commercial clutter
Radio	Low production and presentation costs High demographic selectivity Reaches mass markets	Less attention getting than visual messages Very short message life Commercial clutter
Billboards and signs	High repetition Low cost Visual	No demographic selectivity Very limited message
Magazines	High message permanence High demographic selectivity High reproduction quality	Long purchase lead time No guarantee of position
Direct mail	Demographic selectivity Personalized No competition surrounding your message	High cost per number of exposures Junk mail image

Source: Adapted with permission from S. Fajen, More for Your Money from the Media, *Harvard Business Review*, Sept.–Oct., © 1978, Harvard Business Review.

tion of the daily newspaper could be useful for reaching potential patients.

An alternative to advertising in the daily newspaper is to use smaller newspapers and newsletters. These can be especially effective if the publication targets an audience that is more likely to want your services than the general population. In addition, the lower advertising rates will allow you to achieve greater repetition. For example, a display ad in a Norfolk, Virginia gay and lesbian newspaper, which publishes monthly, can be run for a year for a lower cost than a single display ad in the daily newspaper. The gay newspaper could be a very good place for a practice to advertise if the gay and lesbian population would be particularly interested in the practice's services. If gays and lesbians would not be more interested than the general population, then it would in fact be a very expensive advertising outlet because its circulation is much smaller than that of the daily newspaper.

For example, if an ad in the daily newspaper costs $400 and is seen by 500,000 readers, then each dollar of advertising translates into 1,250 readers. By placing a similarly sized ad costing $30 in the 10,000-circulation gay and lesbian newspaper, you reach 333.33 readers for each advertising dollar. Advertising in the gay newspaper would be reasonable if you had a service or a message that would result in a response rate from the gay newspaper ad that was 3.75 times greater than the response rate from the ad in the daily newspaper. Promoting AIDS services or advertising the fact that you have special skills associated with helping gay and lesbian patients might produce a favorable return.

Whenever you advertise in a specialty newspaper or bulletin, you should consider designing your ad to speak *directly* to the publication's audience. Customizing the ad may cost a little more, but it will allow you to convey your message in a manner that might be particularly attractive to that market. Another benefit of utilizing smaller newspapers and newsletters is that some organization within the specialty audience may ask you to present a workshop or give a presentation, thereby providing additional exposure.

Another place to advertise is the Yellow Pages. An ad in the Yellow Pages is a relatively passive form of advertising because it does not increase demand for your services. A newspaper or television commercial can educate potential patients regarding the symptoms of a problem or the need for preventive care, thereby increasing demand. If prospective patients are to find you in the Yellow Pages, they must already know that they need your services. If they already know you and simply wish to find your telephone number, they will probably use the White Pages.

Many Yellow Pages referrals are price shopping. The Yellow Pages also represent one of the last places that people look for health care services. Yellow Pages shoppers often have exhausted other potential referral sources, such as friends and health care professionals. As a result, Yellow Pages referrals are less likely to show up for the initial appointment. One practice reported an overall first appointment show rate of 74 percent, whereas the rate for Yellow Pages referrals was 51 percent.

Yellow Pages ad copy should be designed for the consumer who does not know you. The top line should stress the services that you provide, not your name (an exception is when the practice name is descriptive of the services provided,

such as "Ear, Nose, and Throat Specialists, P.C."). Listing the most common symptoms you work with and a few of the most common disorders you encounter will also help Yellow Pages readers determine whether you can help. Other Yellow Pages ad design pointers are as follows:

- Use a large black border around your ad. A ¼-inch border will set your ad off from others.
- Color is not cost effective. In addition, as more advertisers resort to color, the color ad's ability to catch the eye is lost. Finally, many color ads look gaudy and do not promote a quality image.
- Strive to get the ad placed near the alphabetical listing. This will result in increased readership. The "dollar bill"–size ad has a greater chance of being placed near the alphabetical listing. An alternative is to create a small display ad in the alphabetical listing by purchasing several lines.
- Being toward the beginning of the listing is not that important. Many readers will fan through the book from back to front and will therefore search the listing in reverse order.
- Copy should use upper- and lower-case letters to increase legibility. Put your name near the telephone number. Don't use a map. It will waste space, and your ad may be torn out of the book. A short quotation in parentheses will attract attention.
- If you have been practicing for a while, note that in your ad. A group practice may be able to state, for example, "Over 40 Years of Professional Experience."

Finally, Yellow Pages spending should be a carefully assessed part of your overall advertising budget. By tracking how referrals are generated, you can determine the cost per referral, and comparisons can be made with other forms of promotion. The Yellow Pages budget can then be increased or decreased depending on the relative effectiveness of your Yellow Pages advertising.

Television and radio can also be used for advertising. Both media present messages that are very transitory. A daily newspaper may sit on a table for a day, and a monthly newspaper or newsletter may have exposure for several weeks. A 30-second television or radio ad is gone in 30 seconds. These media, however, can be exceedingly effective. The question is whether they are appropriate for your organization.

Radio and television ads require significant repetition if they are to have a significant impact. A rule of thumb is that the ad has to be seen or heard at least three times before the viewer or listener will fully comprehend the message and be able to recall the advertiser's name. In addition, the development, design, and production of the ad are critical because you have such a short period of time to make your point, and of course this costs money.

Production and air time costs will vary greatly depending on the market. In the Norfolk–Virginia Beach market (ranked 31st nationally), a simple 30-second television commercial can be produced and taped for about $2,000. The cost of air time will vary based on the ratings of programs on which the ad appears. For example, the local 6:00 P.M. news in this market costs about $800 for a 30-second ad. On the other hand, 30 seconds on David Letterman is currently selling for $200. If you have a $10,000 ad budget, the 6:00 P.M. news will not provide the repetition you need to have a good chance of success, but Letterman might. Production costs for radio are substantially lower than for television. Some radio stations will produce ads at no cost in return for the purchase of advertising time.

Larger health care providers are making effective use of television. With their greater financial resources, they can achieve the needed repetition. In addition, they can use alternative formats. Large health care systems have developed public service programming that includes several half-hour or hour long infomercials that appear in prime time spread over the course of a year. This is supplemented by 30-second spot commercials promoting the longer infomercials. The focus of the programming is to create public awareness of health care problems, such as stroke, heart disease, prenatal care, and so forth, that can be addressed at the system's facilities or by its physicians.

An understanding of patient characteristics is critical to using the electronic media effectively. For example, suppose that you are promoting a service that will be used primarily by women, such as cosmetic surgery. There are specific hours and programs that attract a disproportionate number of female viewers. Often, the rates will be lower for hours or programs that are most attractive to a particular market segment because *overall* viewership may be lower. A well-designed media plan for running an ad during hours and on programs where lower viewership is coupled with disproportionate viewing by your target market segment can make the cost-effectiveness formula for television and radio very favorable.

Television and radio stations have considerable amounts of data on ratings for various programs and time periods. Radio can be a particularly effective medium for targeting specific market segments because each station has a well-defined format that appeals to a different segment of the population. For example, talk radio stations tend to attract higher-income, better educated listeners, and rock stations have a high proportion of teenage and young adult listeners.

When talking to a station's advertising personnel, you should remember that their job is to sell advertising. Advertising that works is going to be in their long-term interest because you will continue to run ads if they generate patients. As with any purchase, however, you must be aware of the unscrupulous salesperson or the salesperson with a short-term profit orientation. According to one television executive, "A ratings book is like the Bible. You can find whatever you are looking for in it. An ad salesman will know what to show you to tell his story."

Given the 30- to 60-second length of electronic media ads, your ad must be well designed if it is going to be effective. This is one area in which you should rely heavily on professional advice. Television and radio professionals know how to take your ideas and convert them into visual and audio effects that will attract viewer attention and communicate your message. You should be involved in the ad development process, but you also should recognize your limitations. Concentrate on communicating to the professionals the visual and audio message that you want to convey, along with some thoughts on advertisement characteristics. For example, you might outline the content of the ad and ask whether the message should be presented by actors in dialogue, by one actor, or by you talking directly into the camera. If the professionals suggest an alternative approach and can give you a reasonable argument for proceeding differently, you should defer to their judgment.

You should also involve yourself in the selection of actors, graphic displays, and other decisions that will affect the appearance and placement of the message. You should rely very heavily on professional advice in these areas, however. Defer to professional judgment regarding specific use of language and technical production considerations, such as lighting, background, music, camera angles, dress, and make-up.

An alternative to this level of personal involvement is to hire a media consultant to act as an intermediary between you and the advertisement production personnel and the television or radio stations. The media consultant will also be able to tell you which programs on the local stations will provide the best mix of viewers and listeners to meet your marketing objectives. If you use a media consultant, it is critical to spend enough time together, so that you can make known your objectives and the image you wish to present.

If you decide to use paid advertising, you must be especially cognizant of the local ethics regarding this issue. If you get too far out in front of your colleagues, you may be subject to retribution ranging in form from mild ostracism or criticism to official censure. On the other hand, being out in front of your colleagues can be a very valuable competitive advantage.

Finally, if you determine that your practice might benefit from paid advertising, it might be worthwhile to read about some of the approaches used by successful advertising executives. This may give you some ideas for developing your own ads and ad copy and also may help you judge the ideas proposed by marketing and media consultants. For example, David Ogilvy, who has developed a number of successful advertising campaigns, has described his formula for print layout.[3] He concludes that the most effective way to lay out a print ad is to:

- place an illustration at the top of the page with a caption below it
- print the copy in a serif typeface
- set the copy in three columns 35–45 characters wide
- start the copy with drop initials
- print the copy in black ink on white paper

One particularly effective modification of Ogilvy's formula was used by Washington Hospital Center (Figure 9–1). This display ad uses color and paradox (luxury and cuisine in the context of a hospital ad) to attract the reader. The ad clearly is targeted at a market segment. In addition, the ad was run in *Washingtonian Magazine*, whose readership demographics are consistent with the ad's message. Of additional interest is the contrarian market strategy that the ad implies. At a time when everyone is trying to obtain managed care contracts, this organization has targeted a self-pay segment as at least one element in its customer mix. Ads of this type for a hospital hardly raise an eyebrow these days. Where hospitals and other health care providers pioneer, physicians often follow. The physician who is first in a market with aggressive ad copy may obtain a real competitive advantage, as well as the envy and criticism of peers.

Roman and Maas have written a guide that concisely describes what they believe works best in print, direct mail, radio, and television.[4] In the case of television, they recommend attracting the viewer's attention in the first five seconds by presenting a single-minded, uncomplicated, short, dramatic message featuring people instead of objects. In the case of radio, they suggest stretching the listener's imagination, presenting a memorable sound (e.g., an unusual voice), stating your name and your promise early, and target marketing by choosing

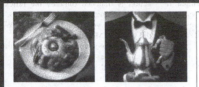

Gourmet food prepared to order. A waiter in bow tie and tails. Definitely not what you're used to in a hospital.

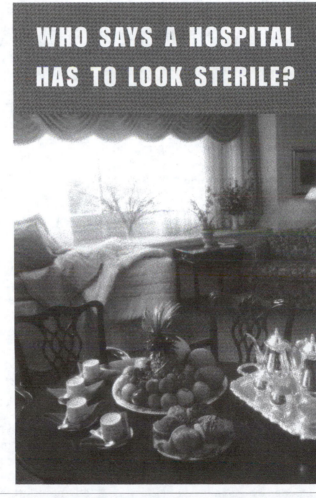

WHO SAYS A HOSPITAL HAS TO LOOK STERILE?

Luxurious. Comforting. Tranquil. Warm. If these are the last four adjectives you'd ever associate with the word "hospital," you'll know why we're announcing The Pavilion at Washington Hospital Center. An entire wing of deluxe, private hospital suites doing its very best impersonation of a luxury hotel. There's soft, incandescent light that flows from delicate, crystal fixtures. Carpeting so thick it makes your shoes feel more expensive. And a complete, gourmet menu prepared by The Pavilion's own chef, in The Pavilion's own kitchen.

In your suite there's fine art, fine furniture and fine linens. A spacious, tiled bathroom with marble vanities and heated towel racks. There are complete concierge and business services. And perhaps the best feature of all, utter quiet. In other words, the list of amenities goes on and on.

Even after you leave, your VIP treatment can continue, thanks to the personalized attention offered by the VNA Integrated Home Care System.

To determine if your doctor is affiliated with Washington Hospital Center, or to receive more information about deluxe suites at The Pavilion, call 202-877-DOCS. Washington Hospital Center. The area's most experienced hospital.

The Pavilion
WASHINGTON HOSPITAL CENTER
CenterLine (202) 877-DOCS
MEDLANTIC

Figure 9–1 Segment Directed Display Ad Using Modified Ogilvy Format. Courtesy of Washington Hospital Center.

stations and time slots to reach specific segments, such as teenagers or young adults.

Unpaid Ads

Some of the most effective promotions come in the form of free advertising. There are countless ways of getting free advertising, including the following:

- writing letters to the editor
- placing announcements in community bulletins about new services that you offer or workshops that you can or will conduct
- sending announcements to the local newspaper of honors that you have received or new associates who have joined your practice
- sending announcements to the local newspaper or appropriate community or church newsletters of open houses, talks, blood pressure clinics, cholesterol clinics, and so on
- volunteering to write a column for a local newspaper or newsletter
- distributing a news release on a newsworthy subject
- appearing on a local television or radio program or obtaining your own program[5,6]

A few of these strategies deserve particular comment because of the exposure they can provide. News releases are a particular favorite in the free ad category. As you might imagine, television ads during prime time can be very expensive. How much do you think that a two-minute advertisement would cost on the local 6:00 news? Writing effective news releases can get you the equivalent of several two-minute television ads per year as well as newspaper coverage that is equivalent to a large display ad.

The key to writing an effective news release is to remember for whom you are writing it. Your target is a reporter who is in need of a story. A news release must tell the reporter that he or she can get an interesting, timely story by calling you. The format of a news release is important. It should cover the five Ws of newspaper reporting (who, when, what, where, and why) and do this in a concise, clearly worded manner.

Exhibit 9–3 contains a news release. The *who*, of course, is you, but you want to indicate this in a clear and, if possible, visually exciting way. Next, you want to indicate the *when*, or the date of release. The *what* should be summarized in your headline. The headline needs to be enticing, but it should not be sensationalistic. Reporters are bombarded with news releases, and if they sense that you are trying to overstate your case, you will quickly be filed in the wastepaper basket. The *why* should be in the body of the news release. You must demonstrate the validity of your release. Why should the reporter care? Why should his or her readers, listeners, or viewers care? Generally, a good tactic is to point out the personal importance of the information to the reporter's audience. If appropriate, state how it can affect their lives. Finally, you want to end the news release with a clear statement of *where* the reporter can go to get additional information. This can be a paper or workshop that you are presenting, your name and office telephone number, or both.

News releases must be short and clearly written, and ideally they should include some numbers or catchy facts. You don't have to be a national expert to distribute a news release. The only requirements are that you be knowledgeable about the subject and possess a minimal amount of audacity.

Once you have developed a news release, the next task is to get it to the right people. Look in the local newspaper for reporters who are writing local articles. Don't limit yourself to the health, fitness, and science reporters. Your objective should be to assemble gradually a mailing list of local newspaper, television, and radio reporters. By reading the newspaper each day and by noting television and radio talk show hosts, you can establish a mailing list with virtually no effort. The same task can be given to your secretary or another employee.

Another tactic is to target a media outlet for concentrated attention. Because newspaper, television, and radio reporters receive dozens of

Exhibit 9–3 Sample News Release

NEWS RELEASE FROM THE OFFICE OF
DR. ROBERT BROWN

JULY 18, 1990
FOR IMMEDIATE RELEASE

Driver Training Students Tour Bayview Hospital Emergency Room

Students in Riverside High School's Driver Education Program are being given a tour of Bayside's emergency room in an effort to educate them on the perils of reckless and drunk driving. Emergency room personnel familiarize the students with the typical injuries suffered by accident victims and the necessary medical procedures.

Dr. Robert Brown, who initiated the program, stated "I hope that seeing the possible consequences of reckless behavior will act as a deterrent."

The program has been in effect for three weeks, and 47 students have toured the emergency room.

FOR ADDITIONAL INFORMATION CONTACT:
Robert Brown, M.D.
555-7639
or
5673 Anderson Dr., Virginia Beach, VA 23453

---

news releases each day, 95 percent of them are thrown out immediately after or even before they are read. To be effective, you have to get enough distribution of your news release within the newspaper or station to overcome the natural propensity to throw it out. This can be accomplished by targeting a cross-section of the organization. For example, you might target a television station by mailing releases to several reporters, the program director, the assignment director, and the public affairs director as well as the host and producer of each of the locally produced programs. A reporter may throw the release out, but perhaps it will appeal to the assignment director, who may then instruct a reporter to see whether there is an interesting story there.

In television, early morning news crews, noon news crews, and especially weekend news crews are often looking for program material. Be certain that your press releases get to these personnel. How do you obtain all these names? Have your secretary call your targeted media outlets and ask for names and job titles. It is that simple.

Getting a mention in a newspaper article or television story is often a function of timing. If you want to develop this aspect of marketing your practice, then you must be responsive to the needs of reporters. When a reporter calls, you must talk to him or her then or call back *very shortly* thereafter. Remember, reporters work under tight deadlines, and they need answers quickly. A print reporter probably will be in the process of writing the story at the time he or she telephones you. If you are not immediately available, the reporter will call the next physician down the list. The reporter will pass you by even if it was *your* news release that provided the initial idea for the story!

Another advantage of consistently responding quickly to reporters is that they will come to rely on you for medical information. Reporters will begin to call you and quote you in stories that they generate. For example, if there is testimony in a trial regarding a prescription drug, a reporter may contact you for information regarding the possible side effects of the drug. You may then be mentioned in the story: "Dr. Fred Wilson noted that the drug could cause the side effects claimed by the defense but that these side effects are rare." Another example of this type of promotion is presented in Exhibit 9–4. In this article, several local physicians give their opinions about a national news item.

Don't overlook distributing news releases to appropriate church, community, and specialty newsletters. Although their readership may be small, your chances of scoring a hit may be significantly greater. Also, a church or community newsletter may give you exposure to a relatively high proportion of potential patients. Once again, sending your news release to multiple targets within each organization will increase your chances of scoring a hit.

A personal appearance on a local radio or television program is another favorite in the free media ad category. You need a "hook" to get on a program, and a news release is a good start. Another alternative is to call the talk show host and explain what you would like to talk about on the program. The reaction you will get to this approach will vary, with the probability of success being greater in smaller markets.

How should you conduct yourself when you appear on a local television or radio talk program? It is important to remember that, to communicate effectively with the typical television audience, you must use a style of presentation appropriate for about an eighth-grade level. This means that you should use simple, direct language. If you use a technical term, you should immediately define it or explain it. Being very specific and using examples will also increase your communication effectiveness. Keep your discussion at the level of greatest general interest. Viewers will be less interested in your topic than your patients would be. Patients care about

their bodies, so they tend to be interested in what you have to say. If a viewer does not feel that your discussion is directly pertinent, he or she will probably not care, and with remote control and 50 cable alternatives readily available, you may be quickly "deselected."

Finally, a word of caution. No matter what you say or how clearly you state it, reporters will make mistakes. You will be frustrated because they will miss a major point you were trying to make, misquote you, or present only part of the total picture. All this "goes with the territory." As an example, take the story of a physician who was trying to persuade the city council in a rural Virginia community to allocate more money for emergency treatment services. She told a local newspaper that the cost of 24-hour-a-day emergency services was about $1.50 per year for each county resident. In an attempt to put the cost of these services in perspective, she lightly dropped the comment that services were cheaper than a six-pack of beer. The next day a newspaper headline proclaimed "Montgomery Emergency Services—Cheaper Than a Six-Pack!" To top it off, Montgomery was a dry county. Despite such possible pitfalls, it is important to remember that all exposure is valuable. Paraphrasing P.T. Barnum's adage: Short of overtly negative statements, don't be concerned with what the media say about you as long as they spell your name correctly.

A letter to the editor is another useful variety of unpaid ad. Writing a letter to the editor will increase the chance that potential patients will hear your name or learn something about you. A good strategy for getting a letter published is to expand on an issue or topic already covered by an article printed in the newspaper. A sample letter to the editor is shown in Exhibit 9–5.

What Promotions Work?

At this point, you may well be asking "But what works? What will give me the most promotional effect for my time and money?" All the ideas discussed can and do work *if you use them effectively and if you use them long enough.* A cornerstone of most successful medical promo-

Exhibit 9–4 News Story with Local Physicians

Henson's pneumonia treatable if diagnosed

Antibiotics could have saved him

By April Witt
Staff writer

The virulent strain of pneumonia that reportedly killed Muppets creator Jim Henson is common and usually curable if treated quickly with antibiotics, local doctors say.

"The streptococcus pneumonia is the most common kind of pneumonia to occur at home," Dr. William Edmondson, a Norfolk internist, said Thursday.

"It hits hard and once you have it you usually get sick enough to get help," he said. "It's something that drives you to the doctor quickly. It is the rare patient that toughs it out and does not get help."

Dr. Oscar E. Edwards, a Norfolk internist said: "Streptococcus pneumonia is tragic to die of. It is the most eminently treatable of them all. If he'd have just come in sooner, with a little bit of penicillin, and he'd probably have been well."

Henson, the creator of Kermit the Frog, Miss Piggy and a host of other beloved Muppets, died Wednesday in a New York Hospital of what his doctor said was "a massive bacterial infection, more specifically known as streptococcus pneumonia."

Dr. David M. Gelmont, director of intensive care at New York Hospital-Cornell Medical Center in New York, said the 53-year-old was healthy until coming down with flu-like symptoms Friday.

Asked why Henson failed to seek more aggressive treatment for his illness, Susan Berry, a spokeswoman for Jim Henson Productions, said: "My guess is he's totally absorbed. He couldn't be bothered. He was very cavalier with his health."

Henson worsened, returned to New York on Monday and checked into the hospital the next day. But by then the infection had spread through his body, damaging vital organs so severely that it could not be controlled by antibiotics, the usual treatment, Gelmont said.

Pneumonia, which strikes about 2 million Americans annually, is an inflammation of the lungs. Although a variety of bacteria and viruses can cause pneumonia, it is most commonly caused by streptococcus, the bacteria that reportedly killed Henson.

Once known as the "captain of the men of death," pneumonia has been much more easily treatable since the invention of antibiotics.

But pneumonia still kills more than 40,000 Americans annually. Most of those who do not survive pneumonia are either very young, elderly or debilitated by a serious disease such as cancer.

Among those at especially high risk of dying are people whose immune systems have been weakened by diseases such as AIDS or who are taking immune-suppressing medicines.

Asked Thursday whether Henson had AIDS, his doctor said: "Categorically, he did not have AIDS."

Dr. Scott A. Miller of Norfolk said no one needs to invoke AIDS to explain a pneumonia death in 1990. "If you get someone who comes in too late with this, you can't save them," said Miller, a Norfolk internist who specializes in infectious diseases. "It's upsetting, but it's the way of the world.

"A few years ago I took care of a 24-year-old woman — healthy, no AIDS — who came in with a little pneumonia and was dead in 24 hours. We don't have to invoke AIDS and we don't have to invoke alternative lifestyles to explain it. Mother Nature can do all of those things."

Streptococcal pneumonia is caused by a common bacteria. "Some people carry it in their mouths and are not affected by it," said Dr. Ignacia Ripoll of Norfolk, a specialist in pulmonary medicine.

People typically contract streptococcal pneumonia when "they have a little cold or a little virus," Ripoll said. "Then their body becomes more susceptible to this infection.

"Once they have this infection, they get sick very fast. Within a matter of hours, people are having chills and a fever and they feel quite ill."

Given a small dose of penicillin or another antibiotic, patients typically improve within 24 hours, Ripoll said.

Untreated, the infection can spread into the blood and damage vital organs, he said.

"We can still reverse it, but these people typically spend weeks in intensive care," he said. "When people develop multi-organ failure, 70 percent of them will die regardless of what you do."

tion is personal contact with potential referral sources and patients, including one-on-one meetings, lunches, community services, and community presentations. Paid media can be useful if you can adequately finance the projects. The expression "It takes money to make money" is particularly apt when it comes to advertising. Paid advertising, irrespective of the media, is

Exhibit 9–5 Letter to the Editor

December 17, 1990

Editor
The Virginian Pilot
150 W. Brambleton Ave.
Norfolk, VA 23510

Dear Editor:

I am writing in response to William Raspberry's article "The Horrors of Child Abuse" (Dec. 8, 1990).

As a practicing psychiatrist, I can testify that the horrors of physical and sexual abuse do not stop with the child and the child's parents. The scars and the pain follow the child into adulthood. As an adult, feelings of guilt, anger, and fear persist. The individual feels different, and he or she struggles to trust others. Sexual problems are common. Alcoholism, compulsive eating, and violence also are frequent companions of the adult who was abused as a child.

Recently, the media have given much attention to the sexually abused child. We must not ignore the adult who carries his or her own pain into adult life and who may need help and encouragement in dealing with the wounds.

Respectfully,

George Gravely, M.D.

---

most effective with repetition, and that costs money.

In general, the best way to generate referrals through the media is to get something to appear in print. People tend to cut out your name or announcement or an article that you wrote or in which you are quoted. They will often keep the clipping for weeks or months, and when they finally do need medical services, they will seek you out. In many ways, the ad, announcement, or article is like a business card with your name on it.

Television gives you outstanding visibility and name recognition. The fleeting nature of the medium, however, is a limitation, and you should not have great expectations based on a single appearance on a talk program. The cost of radio is substantially less than the cost of television. Once again, however, a few sporadic appearances will not constitute an effective radio campaign. Unless you devote substantial funds to advertising, the importance of these media lies in the part that they can play in your overall promotional effort, and this part should not be underestimated.

The final selection of a physician is often the result of many events that occurred over an extended period of time. It may result from name recognition gained over months or years of published letters to the editor, appearances on radio and television programs, quotations in the newspaper, and a few personal encounters. Slowly, a prospective patient or referral source becomes familiar with you and comes to believe that you are someone who may be able to help. When the prospective patient finally needs medical services, he or she is likely to call you because, in a sense, he or she has "known" you for an extended period of time. It should be clear from this that promotion is a long-term activity that must never cease but may change in nature as your practice develops and matures.

Patients can come from anywhere, and virtually anyone can become a referral source. If you are cognizant of this essential truth, then any interpersonal contact has promotional potential. Whether you are visiting your dentist or lawyer, getting your car repaired or your plumbing fixed, or simply mingling at a party, you should always be open to the possibility that you are talking to a potential patient or referral source. When appropriate, manage to work a few comments into the discussion about your profession. The key word here is *appropriate*. Remember, if you do this in a clumsy manner or in a way that is inappropriate given the context of the conversation, you may be doing more harm than good. It is far better to state your profession unobtrusively and then illustrate your good qualities by being an attentive listener and making appropriate additions to the conversation.

Finally, your own patients can be among your best referral sources. John Ernhardt, M.D., has offered several excellent suggestions for marketing to your own patients, including these[7]:

- Show regard for patients' time. This involves being punctual for your appointments and devoting sufficient time to each patient.
- Provide extra time for each patient who is hospitalized, and also make it a quality visit. Try to reduce the patient's anxiety. Also make courtesy calls, at no charge, to those of your patients who are under the care of another physician.
- Be available to talk on the telephone. In nonemergency situations, this could include having a staff person tell patients that you will return calls during a specified half-hour period.
- Provide patients with drug samples, thereby medicating them more quickly and relieving them of an expense if they cannot tolerate a new medication.
- Take the time to send appropriate letters and documents. This includes responding to patients who sent you greeting cards, forwarding medical records and test results to other physicians in a timely manner, and sending letters to family members of deceased patients.

It is important to approach these tasks with the proper mental attitude. They should not be undertaken as a way of manipulating patients. They should be done sincerely and considerately and should demonstrate that you are a professional who is concerned about your patients' welfare. If they are done with sincerity, then they will create patient goodwill and will also set an example of appropriateness and courtesy for your staff to follow.

PROMOTING UNDER MANAGED CARE

The discussion of promotion to this point assumes that the patient or a family member is the decision maker when it comes to selecting a physician, hospital, or health care provider. Managed care is changing that scenario. Increasingly, patients are being funneled through managed care organizations directly to contracting physicians and hospital systems. Under these circumstances, effective promotion becomes even more important because each referral source is more significant.

The content of the promotion becomes more critical and must be directed toward the needs of the referring physician or organization. Understanding the nature of the service that the referrer desires is critical both to design the appropriate service and to present the appropriate message. For example, what do primary care physicians desire when making referrals to specialists? Appropriate clinical care is a necessary but probably insufficient condition. Quick appointments, timely feedback, and clear and timely charting may be three additional issues. Given these considerations, how can specialists promote to primary care physicians?

Clinical outcome data represent one source of information that specialists can use to educate primary care physicians. Average length of hospital stay, infection rates, rework rates, mortality rates, and prescription medication costs are all examples of clinical data that specialists can use to promote their practice to primary care referring physicians. In addition, average time to initial office visit and average time for charting and feedback are also powerful messages to give to these physicians. In these instances, the promotion message cannot be provided without appropriate information systems to supply the data. Information systems, therefore, provide outcome data that can be used for more than assessing physician performance.

Similarly, primary care physicians in networks and multispecialty practices can use their referring specialists' cost data as well as their own when promoting their practices and networks to employers and other patient sources. Providing data per se tells employers that the physician provider or network is interested in cost control and has the tools to accomplish this goal. Outcome data, therefore, represent a very powerful promotion message in a managed care environment.

TARGET MARKETING AND MARKET SEGMENTATION

Market segments are groups of people who tend to behave in a similar manner or who have similar characteristics. Different market segments may have special needs and preferences, and this may justify developing special programs and marketing plans. For example, if people with homes in a particular ZIP code are especially likely to come to your practice, then they are behaving differently as a result of their geographical location. You may be able to use this information to direct your marketing efforts toward segments (geographical areas) that are more likely to be responsive to your practice. Similarly, if you know that an important component of your practice consists of patients with hypertension, then you can develop programs

and promotional efforts that will be particularly appealing to this market segment.

Identifying market segments is part of a marketing strategy called target marketing. Target marketing involves identifying one or more market segments and directing marketing efforts toward them. When physicians or health care organizations adopt a target marketing strategy, they do four things:

1. identify important market segments
2. systematically evaluate the attractiveness of each of the segments
3. select one or more of the segments for special attention
4. position the organization by developing a specific marketing mix to establish a competitive advantage in each of the selected segments

It is important to understand that identifying useful market segments is one part of an overall marketing strategy. The other essential elements are evaluating the value of these segments and designing services and communications to tap into them. It is also important to note that, although you may identify one or a few market segments deserving of special attention, your practice may still be largely composed of patients drawn from outside these particular segments.

Developing Market Segments

The first phase of target marketing is to identify potential market segments. Obviously, it would not be worthwhile to customize your services to meet the needs of every possible type of patient. You may find, however, that patients can be divided into a few broad categories on the basis of their needs. If that is the case, then it may be worthwhile to try to make use of these differences.

The potential bases of segments are only limited by your creativity. Kotler has listed a number of commonly used segmentation variables, which are shown in Table 9–3.[8] These segmentation variables can be classified as geographical,

Table 9–3 Segmentation Variables and Typical Breakdowns

Variable	Typical Breakdowns
Geographical	
Region	Pacific, Mountain, West North Central, West South Central, East North Central, East South Central, South Atlantic, Middle Atlantic, New England
County Size	A, B, C, D
City or SMSA size	Under 5,000; 5,000–20,000; 20,000–50,000; 50,000–100,000; 100,000–250,000; 250,000–500,000; 500,000–1,000,000; 1,000,000–4,000,000; 4,000,000 or over
Density	Urban, suburban, rural
Climate	Northern, southern
Demographic	
Age	Under 6, 6–11, 12–19, 20–34, 35–49, 50–64, 65+
Sex	Male, female
Family size	1–2, 3–4, 5+
Family life cycle	Young, single; young, married, no children; young, married, youngest child under 6; young, married, youngest child 6 or over; older, married, with children; older, married, no children under 18; older, single; other
Income	Under $5,000; $5,000–$10,000; $10,000–$15,000; $15,000–$20,000; $20,000–$25,000; $25,000–$30,000; $30,000–$50,000; $50,000 and over
Occupation	Professional and technical; managers, officials, and proprietors; clerical, sales; craftsmen, foremen; operatives; farmers; retired; students; housewives; unemployed
Education	Grade school or less; some high school; high school graduate; some college; college graduate
Religion	Catholic, Protestant, Jewish, other
Race	White, Black, Oriental
Nationality	American, British, French, German, Scandinavian, Italian, Latin American, Middle Eastern, Japanese
Psychographic	
Social class	Lower lowers, upper lowers, working class, middle class, upper middles, lower uppers, upper uppers
Life style	Straights, swingers, longhairs
Personality	Compulsive, gregarious, authoritarian, ambitious
Behavioral	
Occasions	Regular occasion, special occasion
Benefits	Quality, service, economy
User status	Nonuser, ex-user, potential user, first-time user, regular user
Usage rate	Light user, medium user, heavy user
Loyalty status	None, medium, strong, absolute
Readiness stage	Unaware, aware, informed, interested, desirous, intending to buy
Attitude toward product	Enthusiastic, positive, indifferent, negative, hostile

Source: MARKETING MANAGEMENT, 9/E by Kotler, © 1988. Reprinted by permission of Prentice-Hall, Inc., Upper Saddle River, NJ.

demographic, psychographic, and behavioral variables. Geographical variables divide a market on the basis of location. Even though you may draw all your patients from one city, you may be able to divide this area into useful smaller units, such as ZIP codes or districts. If the practice or hospital is obtaining a disproportionate number of patients from particular ZIP code areas, then this may be a useful segmentation variable because it could indicate where to direct marketing. If a health care provider has more than one location, then understanding which patients go to each location may allow you to determine more precisely the services and promotion activities that are best suited for each location.

Demographic variables divide the market on the basis of patients' personal characteristics, such as age, sex, and insurer. Demographic variables are the most commonly used basis for defining market segments. This is because patient desires, attitudes, needs, and utilization rates often correlate with demographic variables. Segmentation on a demographic basis is commonly used in the marketing of consumer goods. By understanding the demographic characteristics of market segments, it is possible for you to utilize marketing messages and media that directly address the most promising segments. For example, it is much more likely that Mercedes-Benz ads will appear in *Architectural Digest* and *Vogue* than in *Wooden Boat Magazine* or *Easy Rider* because the demographic characteristics of *Architectural Digest* and *Vogue* readers are more similar to the demographic characteristics of Mercedes-Benz buyers. The ad in Figure 9–1 illustrates an appeal to a demographic segment.

Demographic variables can be important segmentation variables for a health care organization. Age, sex, family income, occupation, education, and race can be important because patient service needs vary across the segments defined by these variables. Women, for example, have a different distribution of diseases and procedures than men. In addition, women probably have more decision-making power in regard to the treatment of children. Lower-income groups may be less able to afford elective procedures, such as annual examinations, contact lenses, and cosmetic surgery. They may also need a different mix of services, such as dialysis and treatment for diabetes and hypertension.

Better educated groups may be more receptive to messages delivered through informa-

tional seminars and may be more willing to use preventive services, whereas groups with less education may be more responsive to Yellow Pages ads. It is important to understand that using demographic variables to define market segments does not mean that you need to neglect men, for example, or low-income and low-education groups. If in fact you want to attract these groups, then you will simply have to offer a different mix of services, which your segmentation research will help you identify.

Age is another useful demographic variable. For example, the medical problems associated with sports differ among various age groups. Middle-age athletes experience different types of injuries and have different medical needs than teenagers. Members of these two segments can also be attracted to a practice in different ways. Middle-age athletes may be accessed through athletic and golf clubs and softball leagues, whereas teenage athletes can be accessed through schools, parents, and coaches. Each segment also will be responsive to different messages and media.

Perhaps the most obvious and important demographic variable is disease or health problem. Not every disease, however, has to be taken as defining a separate market segment. The issue is whether you can develop additional specific services for or ways of communicating with a group defined by a disease or health problem.

For example, developing a program to help the families of terminally ill patients deal with the eventual loss of their loved one would be a service that you could provide to this segment. The particular causes of death would not have to be taken into account. An ophthalmologist might consider all patients who require sight correction as a segment irrespective of whether correction is through the use of glasses, corrective surgery, or contact lenses.

Examining market segments defined by diseases or treatments can suggest new services to provide or new ways to communicate with potential patients. Exhibit 9–6 contains some diagnostic market segments arranged by medical specialty. Each of these diagnostic segments can

Exhibit 9–6 Diagnostic Market Segments

Cardiology
- Post–myocardial infarction
- Coronary artery bypass graft
- Dysrhythmias
- Chronic congestive heart failure

Dermatology
- Chronic dermatitis
- Skin cancer
- Allergic dermatitis

Family Practice
- Hypertensives
- Diabetics
- Sick children
- Upper respiratory infection
- Psychosomatic illnesses

Pediatrics
- Well babies

- Chronic ear infections
- Allergic children
- Orthopaedic problems

Psychiatry
- Depression
- Anxiety/phobias
- Sexual dysfunction
- Obsessive compulsive disorder
- Rape/sexual assault
- Separation and divorce

Pulmonary
- Chronic obstructive pulmonary disease
- Asthmatics
- Industrial lung diseases
- Pulmonary fibrosis

Source: Adapted with permission from S. Brown and A. Morley, *Marketing Strategies for Physicians*, pp. 181–182, © 1987, Practice Management Information Corporation.

be divided into smaller segments. For example, a dermatologist may choose to focus on the adolescent chronic dermatitis segment, whereas an orthopaedist may market to adult sports medicine patients.

Psychographic segmentation divides patients on the basis of social class, life style, or personality. Social class is strongly associated with preferences for consumer goods, habits, clothing, and so forth. There clearly are social class differences in the kinds of medical treatment desired and needed. People lower on the socioeconomic scale have more chronic health problems and have less sophisticated medical knowledge. This implies that the services you offer and the way you promote them will vary based on the social class of your present patients and of the potential patients you wish to attract.

Personality assessment, as we saw in Chapter 3, involves time-consuming assessment procedures. You can certainly make guesses about a patient's personality, but it is obvious that these guesses are going to be less accurate than your assessment of the patient's age, geographical residence, and sex. The marketing research literature is ambivalent about the real-world usefulness of personality segmentation. You may be able to devise some reasonable hypotheses, however, regarding personality segments. For example, if you have an oncology practice, you may well have a disproportionate number of situationally depressed patients. This would be a patient segment that could benefit from treatment for this problem and might be very responsive to a practice that communicates a recognition of this problem.

Behavioral segmentation is based on attitudes toward, use of, or response to medical services. One important behavioral segmentation variable is benefits. This means constructing groups based on what the patients seek from treatment, that is, the benefits that they desire. Kotler and

Clarke state that most health care consumers can be grouped into the following four benefit-seeking segments[9]:

1. *Quality buyers* want the best product and are unconcerned about cost.
2. *Service buyers* are primarily concerned with acquiring the most caring and personal service.
3. *Value buyers* examine the price–quality trade-off. A value buyer would go to a physician who had a "reasonable" reputation and who had "reasonable" fees.
4. *Economy buyers* are most interested in the least expensive alternative.

You may find that your patients are homogeneous with respect to the benefits that they seek. If that is the case, then you are probably conveying a message to prospective patients about the benefits that you provide. This may or may not be desirable. For example, if you are trying to provide family practice services to a broad spectrum of the community, yet your patients are mostly quality buyers, then you may be excluding a significant number of potential patients. If that is the case, you would do well to consider the nature of your practice's reputation. For example, are you conveying an unintended message that dissuades service or value buyers?

Multiple Segments

It is often possible to find more than one basis upon which to segment your practice. For example, you may find that young women with children, older patients, and professionals either are or should be important practice segments. On occasion, you may find it useful to combine two segments. For example, Woodside and colleagues examined how demographic variables interact with benefit segments in the selection of a hospital.[10] They found that benefit segments are closely associated with unique demographic profiles. Because demographic variables are easily determined, their findings could be used

by hospitals to develop new products and marketing strategies for promoting products and services to specific demographic segments.

Evaluating and Choosing Market Segments

The second and third components of target marketing involve evaluating and choosing segments. Larger health care providers, such as hospitals and nursing homes, determine the usefulness of various market segments through marketing research. The research process typically involves many in-depth interviews and focus groups composed of patients and potential patients. The data are then evaluated, and a profile is developed of a potential patient's demographic, psychographic, geographical, and behavioral characteristics and media consumption habits. This obviously can be a time-consuming and expensive process. An alternative approach is to look at current patients and search for prominent segmentation patterns. Concentrate on large, obvious groups defined geographically, demographically, or behaviorally, such as residence location, sex, occupation, age, or disease. Don't try to create a myriad of narrow, multivariable segments because each segment will be too small to market to effectively. Large homogeneous segments will allow you to make marketing decisions that will affect a substantial number of patients.

When evaluating whether a segment will be useful for target marketing, consider the size and growth potential of the segment, its attractiveness, and your practice's objectives and resources. The size of a segment is important because you do not want to put time, effort, and resources into a segment that is too small to obtain a reward commensurate with your efforts. Growth potential is important because successfully marketing to a growing segment will result in practice growth. Remember, however, that a growing segment will tend to attract attention, which translates into competition. Good examples of growth potential leading to increased competition include coronary artery bypass graft and excimer RK surgery in the 1990s, and overeating-bulimia-anorexia in the 1980s.

Another aspect of segment attractiveness is the degree of existing competition. If there are already a number of other medical practices competing for a segment, you should ask yourself the following: Is this market segment large enough to support another provider? Do I have a competitive advantage such that I will be able to do better in this segment than my peers?

Evaluation of the current attractiveness of a segment can be particularly important if you will be competing against nonmedical organizations or hospitals. Nonmedical competitors may be used to lower fees, and this may foreshadow an erosion of a market's profit potential. Nonmedical competition may be encountered in problem segments such as smoking, weight loss, anxiety, pain management, eye care, and foot care. Hospitals can be tough competitors because their enormous resources allow them to undertake expensive promotional campaigns that saturate a market with highly visible television, radio, and newspaper ads. They also can offer a service at a loss or a break-even price as a way of attracting patients, who will then turn to them for other services at a later date. Segments that have attracted the serious attention of hospitals must be approached with caution.

For practice-based physicians, perhaps the most important consideration when evaluating the desirability of a segment is the degree to which it is consistent with their own personal and practice goals. For example, if you derive little or no satisfaction from working with children, then you should give careful consideration before targeting this segment, even if you are likely to reap financial rewards.

Ultimately, the selection of segments is a qualitative, subjective decision. It may be based either on objective data from marketing research or on intuitions derived from personal knowledge of your patients coupled with a healthy dose of speculation. In the final analysis, it is a management decision, and it should take into account the benefit that you can add to your patients. Going back to the four Ps, can you provide some benefit in terms of product (service), place (location), promotion (communications), or price that will give you a competitive advantage? If you cannot provide something of special value to patients in a given segment, then you should probably not select it for special attention.

POSITIONING YOUR ORGANIZATION

The final phase of target marketing is to position yourself so that you will market to the previously identified target segment or segments. Segmenting is the difficult task. Once good segments have been identified, positioning is relatively easy. The positioning should be determined by your evaluation of the particular competitive advantages that you have vis-à-vis the segments. This should then be reflected in the specific marketing plan you construct. Dr. Smith, a psychiatrist, for example, might identify the "upscale, higher-income, better educated" segment as deserving of special attention. She determines that her competitive advantages are as follows:

- She is a physician, not a psychologist or clinical social worker.
- She can prescribe medication, unlike many of her competitors.
- She can diagnose physiological problems, unlike many of her nonmedical competitors.
- She has more years of postgraduate training than competitors with other kinds of degrees.
- She is a psychoanalyst, unlike many of her medical colleagues.
- All major insurance carriers will cover her services, unlike competitors in other professions, who are only covered by some carriers.
- Because she employs a psychologist, she can provide a complete range of mental health services, unlike many of her com-

petitors, who can only provide some of these services.

After talking with several of her patients who are in the upscale, higher-income, better educated segment, Dr. Smith determines that they are largely quality buyers. Her marketing strategy, therefore, is to approach this segment by appealing to the desire to obtain the best services from the most qualified provider. Her marketing plan for this segment is different only in regard to the promotion component. The services that she will provide are the same as those offered to all her other patients. She is not providing additional services (product), offering different hours or locations (place), or charging different fees (price) to attract this segment. She places print ads emphasizing her superior position in the provider "pecking order," including her ability to diagnose physiological causes of mental disorders, and uses this to emphasize the superior quality of her services. She places television and radio ads on talk programs with demographics that are heavily biased toward the better educated and upper-income segments. Finally, she makes presentations before business groups and employers with more highly educated workforces, where she emphasizes the medical aspects of mental health and the overall superiority of psychiatry among mental health care professions.

MARKETING RESEARCH

Marketing research is a tool you can use to better understand the external and internal environmental factors that confront your organization. For example, you can use marketing research to evaluate your competition, the feasibility of various locations, patient demand for particular services, and patient perceptions regarding your services and your organization. You can also use marketing research to test alternative marketing strategies and plans before you put proposed strategies and plans into operation.

The process of actually conducting marketing research can be broken into five phases:

1. defining the problem
2. designing the research study
3. collecting data
4. analyzing the data
5. interpreting the data

Beyond the very simplest of patient attitude surveys, marketing research should be conducted by professionals trained in the field.[11] Larger health care systems may have qualified personnel on staff, but many health care organizations will have to hire a consultant. Knowing how marketing research is conducted will help you understand and evaluate the work that the consultant will be performing for you.

Creating a clear definition of the problem you intend to investigate is essential if the end product is to be meaningful. For example, suppose that you decide that you want to learn why your patients select and continue to use your practice or hospital. This question could be examined in a number of different ways. The answer could involve referral sources, advertising or other forms of promotion, location, patient satisfaction with previous treatment, fee schedules, and so on. If you have not clarified in your own mind what you really want to learn, then you might easily design a study in which you waste time and effort collecting data that are not relevant to your real concern.

Designing the study is the next step in the process. At this point, a decision must be made regarding how to collect the information. For example, will you use quantitative methods, such as a questionnaire, or qualitative methods, such as a focus group? If you are primarily interested in understanding concepts and issues, then a qualitative method will probably be appropriate. On the other hand, if you need statistical insight to answer your questions, then you will probably have to use a quantitative method. For example, if you want to know what the major patient satisfaction and dissatisfaction issues are regarding billing, then you can obtain this information with qualitative methods. If you want to know what proportion of patients are satisfied and what proportion are dissatisfied, then you will have to use a quantitative method.

The next stage involves collecting the data. Sometimes practice or hospital staff will be used to collect the data because they are the ones in contact with patients. This will raise a number of practical difficulties that, if not properly addressed, can result in invalid marketing research. For example, secretaries may not get questionnaires to patients because of ringing telephones or other job demands, patients may not respond because they don't have time, and sampling will be compromised when a questionnaire was given to Mrs. Smith instead of Mr. Jones because that was easier.

The next phase of marketing research is the analysis and interpretation of the data. Data analysis methods include examining simple descriptive statistics, such as means, standard deviations, percentages, and frequencies. The relationship between two or more variables can be assessed by a number of methods including correlation, regression, factor analysis, and cross-tabulation. Qualitative data must be analyzed by looking for common themes and ideas in subjects' responses. The final interpretation, however, should never be totally left to a consultant. The study results are only useful to you if they directly pertain to the specifics of your organization. A consultant cannot know your organization as well as you do. It is essential, therefore, for you to subject any consultant's research conclusions to a thorough logical analysis based on what you know about your practice or health care organization.

Sometimes it is not necessary to collect new research data to answer a marketing question. For example, your medical office management software almost certainly contains important marketing research information, such as patient demographics, referral sources, procedures conducted, diagnoses, and so on. These internal sources of marketing data can be particularly attractive because you know something about

their existence, thereby avoiding long, involved research. You also know something about their accuracy. You probably know, for example, if your secretary does a good job of determining referral sources before entering them into the computer.

External secondary sources of marketing research include the published research literature. Probably the easiest way to access this literature is via the Internet. Searching key words in medical databases such as MEDLINE, specific journals such as the *New England Journal of Medicine* and the *Journal of the American Medical Association*, and nonmedical sources is a very time-effective way of finding research results that may pertain to your problem.

Other sources of marketing research findings include national and state professional associations; the American Marketing Association; the American Medical Association; state or regional offices on aging, adolescence, and so on; school boards; state hospital associations; state and regional economic development agencies; university bureaus of business research; and local chambers of commerce. Many of these groups publish marketing reports or studies containing data that can be used to evaluate various market segments. For example, the American Medical Association's Council on Long-Range Planning and Development has assessed the changing demographics of internists' patient populations. It concluded that the increasing number of elderly patients will affect the nature of illnesses treated by internists. It also predicted that there will be increasing competition among subspecialties within internal medicine.

The primary advantage of using secondary marketing data is that you can obtain information without having to collect it yourself. As a result, you may be able to answer market research questions without using your time or a consultant's time to construct a questionnaire, interview patients, and so on. Assuming that there is nothing unusual about your market or your practice (i.e., nothing that would make the study results inapplicable to your circumstances), use of published findings can be very cost and time effective. At a minimum, secondary source data will help you define more precisely your research questions given the experiences of other researchers.

Survey Research

Survey research data can be collected by telephone, by mail, or in person. The questionnaire must be designed so that the questions clearly pertain to the research question, are unambiguous, and have appropriate response scales. In addition, a thorough understanding of the statistical methods that will be used to analyze the data must be applied to developing the questionnaire. Otherwise, it is possible to develop a questionnaire that is not statistically interpretable. Use of professional assistance is critical when you are using questionnaire because it is very easy to bias or invalidate the results through inadequate question and questionnaire design.

Survey questionnaires are particularly appropriate for assessing proportions of respondents who hold particular opinions or have certain attitudes. Exhibit 9–7 contains a survey used at Hartford Hospital to assess patient satisfaction. Questionnaires of this type also can be used longitudinally to determine whether attitudes are changing over time.

Focus Groups

A focus group is a qualitative marketing research method in which a group of 5 to 15 people or so is assembled for an open-ended discussion regarding one or several issues or topics. The object is to obtain qualitative information from the subjects. The discussion should be led by a professionally trained moderator, and you may be present as an observer if you wish. One advantage of a focus group is that the group "process," or the interaction among group members, can often disclose more about a topic than would be revealed by conducting one-on-one, in-depth interviews or quantitative research. A focus

group contains a small sample of nonrandomly selected participants, so they may well not represent the population of patients or referral sources. If a focus group is properly conducted, however, and if you are aware of its inherent weaknesses, the weaknesses need not interfere with its usefulness to you.

Focus groups can be used for a number of different purposes. They are excellent for stimulating your own thinking regarding your organization and how your practice or hospital is perceived by your patients. Ideas generated by this exploratory approach may or may not then be tested using quantitative research. Focus groups can also be used to obtain information that is not accessible through quantitative methods. For example, information obtained from a focus group regarding the difficulties of scheduling a first appointment to address the problem of rectal bleeding would be very difficult, if not impossible, to obtain using an anonymous patient survey. It simply is too personal a matter to be explored in depth in a questionnaire. Focus groups can provide an opportunity to explore patients' decision-making processes. Why do patients decide to return? What are the aspects of your practice, hospital, or health care system that first attracted them? What issues do patients consider when they evaluate the quality of care, level of information provided, and the like?

Focus groups can also help determine how patients and prospective patients will respond to a new service or advertisement. Axelrod graphically described a further reason for using a qualitative approach, such as a focus group, when he stated:

> [It is] a chance to "experience" a "flesh and blood" consumer [patient]. It is the opportunity for the client [physician] to put himself in the position of the consumer [patient] and to be able to look at his product and his category from her vantage point.[12(p.6)]

To put it another way, a focus group can let you "hear your patients talk." As Donald J. Messmer, president of Mid-Atlantic Research

Exhibit 9–7 Hartford Hospital Patient Survey

Today's Date: ___/___/___	Please fill in the circle like this: ●
	Form Completed by: ○ Patient ○ Other

Diagnosis Specifics (For Office Use Only.)
○ ○
○ ○
○ ○ Other

Your opinions are very important. They will help us plan for improving the quality of our care.

	Always	Usually	Sometimes	Seldom	Never
1. The staff treated me with respect and courtesy.	○	○	○	○	○
2. The staff treated my family and visitors with respect and courtesy.	○	○	○	○	○
3. The staff introduced themselves and explained their role in my care.	○	○	○	○	○
4. The staff responded to my questions in a professional manner.	○	○	○	○	○
5. I received a clear explanation of the treatments or tests to be done (purpose, benefits, risks).	○	○	○	○	○
6. I received a clear explanation of the results of these treatments or tests.	○	○	○	○	○
7. Those close to me were informed of my condition and needs. (Leave blank, if doesn't apply).	○	○	○	○	○
8. When I needed help, I received it within a reasonable time (i.e., eating, bathing, or getting to the bathroom).	○	○	○	○	○
9. When I used my call button, I was answered promptly.	○	○	○	○	○
10. My pain was relieved. (If no pain, leave blank.)	○	○	○	○	○
11. If I had a concern or complaint, someone listened and responded.	○	○	○	○	○
12. My hospital room was clean.	○	○	○	○	○
13. The doctors were caring.	○	○	○	○	○
14. The nurses were caring.	○	○	○	○	○
15. I participated in decisions about my health care.	○	○	○	○	○

16. The staff adequately prepared me for discharge.   ○ Yes   ○ No
17. Parking was reasonably priced.   ○ Yes   ○ No
18. Parking was both safe and accessible.   ○ Yes   ○ No
19. My overall impression of the health care I received is:
     ○ Excellent   ○ Very Good   ○ Good   ○ Fair   ○ Poor

20. I would recommend Hartford Hospital to my family and friends.
     ○ Definitely Would   ○ Probably Would   ○ Probably Would Not   ○ Definitely Would Not

My age group is: ○ Under 21 ○ 21-34 ○ 35-50 ○ 51-64 ○ 65-74 ○ 75 or Over	
Sex: ○ Male ○ Female	
Overall, I would say my health is: ○ Excellent ○ Very Good ○ Good ○ Fair ○ Poor	

Some companies have expressed an interest in knowing their customer group's level of satisfaction with Harford Hospital. Your current insurance carrier is:

○ Aetna   ○ Blue Cross/Blue Shield   ○ CT Care   ○ Kaiser   ○ Other HMO   ○ Medicare   ○ Medicaid   ○ Other

We welcome your comments. Please turn this page over to complete the survey.

Courtesy of Hartford Hospital, 1995, Hartford, Connecticut.

and a professor at the College of William & Mary, stated:

> Clients will often say "This is the first time that I have actually heard my customers talk about my product or service." You can't wipe that image of their comments away. It can be a powerful tool to get management's attention—It can be a revelation.

Keown has suggested a framework for organizing a focus group.[13] The first step in the process is to hire a consultant to conduct the focus group research for you. This assumes that you don't have appropriately trained personnel on staff. The consultant will arrange for an appropriate meeting place, possibly find group subjects, and provide the group moderator. An effective focus group moderator must be trained and experienced in using a focus group to be able to stimulate a group process from people who are total strangers. To do this, the moderator must be able to determine the conscious and unconscious causes of behavior and use the group process to obtain information that is more insightful than normally could be obtained through simple discussions.

A focus group moderator can be retained through a marketing consulting firm or by contacting the business school at a local university. You should personally meet the moderator and be certain that he or she understands the objectives of your research. If you are not comfortable with the moderator, then select another one. If you are working with a consulting firm and it will not or cannot replace the moderator, then go to another firm.

The moderator is under considerable pressure during a focus group session. If the moderator does not perform effectively during the few hours of the session, then you will have wasted this opportunity. The moderator must be able to respond to totally unpredictable events as they occur. This includes being adept at dealing with quiet, passive groups or group members; overly excited groups or group members; outspoken group members; the "wise guy"; inconsistencies that develop in the group discussion; and groups that go off on a tangent.

To be effective, the moderator will have to do some homework. He or she must understand the characteristics of your patients and choose clothing and a communication style that will allow group members to work together effectively. The moderator will require spontaneity, humor, self-awareness of personal biases, and the ability to express thoughts clearly. In addition, the moderator should construct a moderator guide, which is an outline used to ensure that all the relevant topics are covered. An effective moderator will use this guide as an initial agenda but will let a conversation develop if it appears to be relevant.

After you select a consultant, you must define your research questions. The consultant should help you with this process. Research questions involving more complex and personal issues will be most suited to examination through the focus group method. As the group session proceeds, participants will tend to explore the reasons for their actions, and they will probably develop a greater level of comfort in discussing them because there will be others present who have been in similar situations or have experienced similar feelings. In a sense, there has to be something that is complex enough or debatable enough over which to develop a group process.

Next, you must decide who should be in the focus group. For example, should it be current patients or people who are potential patients? Often, the research questions will help you identify the appropriate group participants. For example, if you are investigating questions related to patient satisfaction, you would obviously have to use current patients. On the other hand, if you are trying to assess the impact of a proposed television commercial or newspaper display ad on people who are choosing health care providers, then a group composed of potential purchasers will provide you with better information.

Because people generally feel more comfortable talking to others who are similar, several focus groups with different participants in each may be necessary. For example, one group might be composed of mothers with children, another group might be composed of working white-collar men, and a third might include working women with no children. Nonpatient groups can be recruited from church, social, and civic groups as well as through notices in community newsletters and daily newspapers. Obviously, when you are using a patient group, confidentiality must be a primary concern. All patients whom you ask to participate should sign a written release stating that they will be voluntarily participating in the project and that they understand that their status as one of your patients will be revealed to others.

The number of participants will depend on the preferences of the moderator, what you hope to obtain from the group, the meeting place, the length of the focus group agenda (longer agendas call for fewer participants), and your budget. The number of groups is a function of the number of market segments and the size of your budget. Generally, you should organize at least one focus group for each distinct market segment. On occasion, a focus group will contain participants from more than one segment. For example, an emergency department might organize a focus group around heart attack patients and trauma victims, with the goal of exploring whether the segments react differently to the issues raised in the group. Whether this is a feasible strategy depends on the complexity of the issues being discussed and the ability of the moderator to facilitate a group process in which the participants of neither segment inhibit the participants of the other segment.

To derive the most benefit from focus groups, they must meet in an appropriate facility. Groups can be run either in an office or in a facility designed for the purpose. Generally, a commercial focus group facility will give superior results. This is because group members will respond in a more typical fashion if they are on "neutral turf." This is especially true if you are using patient groups because feelings connected with being a patient, including being in a subordinate, dependent position, will be associated with your facility. These feelings may interfere

with the development of a group process and with the honest expression of opinions. In addition, commercial facilities have equipment that will help you obtain the most information. This equipment typically includes the following:

- a one-way mirror, so that you or several other observers can unobtrusively observe the group process (group members must always be informed if they will be observed or taped)
- taping equipment (video or audio), so that you can record the session for future reference and interpretation
- overhead projectors, flip charts, and other aids to help the moderator work with the group

It is particularly important for you to observe the focus group, either by using a one-way mirror or by viewing a videotape. This will help you interpret the moderator's findings. You may also have an opinion about the conduct and composition of future groups based on your observations of the content and intensity of participants' comments. Finally, your insight regarding your own organization and the issues raised in the focus group will help the moderator provide you with the most useful conclusions.

Because focus groups are not composed of participants randomly drawn from the population of patients or potential patients, it is inappropriate to categorize comments quantitatively or interpret them statistically. A participant's statement could be idiosyncratic, or it could reflect the views of many other patients or potential patients. What is essential is to understand the reasons behind the participants' statements. A good moderator will be able to comment on the reasons behind the statements.

CONCLUSION

Success may provide the luxury of not having to market. If you are in a specialty that is in high demand, or if there are relatively few competitors in your area, you may be able to limit your marketing activities to announcing your presence, affiliating with a hospital, and associating with colleagues. If you are the only hospital in town, you may be able to get away with little more than putting your name on the front of your building, until someone else comes to town or your market dynamics change so that selling beds is not as successful a formula. Apart from these circumstances, however, marketing should be a regularly occurring function. The question then becomes whether you will do it well or poorly.

Physicians, practices, and health care organizations that must market their services to prosper or even survive should undertake the complete process, including performing a thorough situational analysis and SWOT analysis, developing a marketing strategy, and writing specific marketing plans. These then evolve into operational marketing decisions, such as seeking to serve selected market segments, pricing, location decisions, and the like.

The purpose of this chapter is to familiarize you with the marketing concept and to demonstrate how the various marketing components fit together. This chapter provides the foundation for developing a marketing strategy and marketing plans, which are discussed in detail in Chapter 10.

REFERENCES AND NOTES

1. See, for example, J. Norman, Can a Practice Serving the Poor Avoid Financial Quicksand?, *Medical Economics*, 5 February 1990, pp. 79–87.

2. J. Scott, M. Warshaw, and J. Taylor, *Introduction to Marketing Management*, 5th ed. (Homewood, Ill.: Irwin, 1985), 11–12.

3. D. Ogilvy, *Ogilvy on Advertising* (New York, N.Y.: Vintage Books, 1985). Ogilvy devised the slogan for Rolls-Royce: "At 60 miles an hour, the loudest noise in the new Rolls-Royce comes from the electric clock." He also developed campaigns for Volkswagen, Dove soap, Hathaway shirts, and Marlboro cigarettes.

4. K. Roman and J. Maas, *How To Advertise* (New York, N.Y.: St. Martin's Press, 1975).

5. For an example of how a physician took advantage of serendipity to obtain a radio talk program, see D. van Amerongen, I Was Chicago's Answer to Dr. Ruth, *Medical Economics,* 19 March 1990, pp. 101–105.

6. Some radio and television stations will charge you for hosting a program, others will pay a salary for your services, and still others will neither pay a salary nor assess a fee. Generally, cable stations will charge a fee. Commercial stations may be more inclined to pay a salary. Some commercial stations may give you a program and pay you a salary if you advertise with them.

7. J. Ernhardt, Marketing? My Patients Do It for Me, *Medical Economics*, 2 October 1989, pp. 58–64.

8. P. Kotler, *Marketing Management: Analysis, Planning, Implementation, and Control*, 6th ed. (Englewood Cliffs, N.J.: Prentice-Hall, 1988).

9. P. Kotler and R. Clarke, *Marketing for Health Care Organizations* (Englewood Cliffs, N.J.: Prentice-Hall, 1987), 244.

10. A.G. Woodside, et al., Preference Segmentation of Health Care Services: The Old-Fashioneds, Value Conscious, Affluents, and Professional Want-It-Alls, *Journal of Health Care Marketing* 8 (1988): 14–24.

11. For an example of attitude survey research conducted in a practice, see R. Solomon, Using a Patient Survey To Market Your Practice, *Journal of Medical Practice Management* 6, no. 1 (1990): 51–55.

12. M.D. Axelrod, Marketers Get an Eyeful When Focus Groups Expose Products, Ideas, Images, Ad Copy, etc., to Consumers, *Marketing News*, 28 February 1975, pp. 6–7.

13. C. Keown, Focus Group Research: Tool for the Retailer, *Journal of Small Business Management*, April 1983, pp. 59–65.

CHAPTER 10

Strategic Management

Chapter Objectives

This chapter provides physician managers with a paradigm for thinking about strategy in a rapidly changing health care market. This paradigm, called the pentagon and triangle, links marketing concepts (e.g., product/service, price, place, promotion, and staffing considerations) with management issues (e.g., performance appraisal, employment systems, organizational integration, and management information systems) to produce an outcome called strategic management.

This chapter describes how to develop a strategic plan based on internal organizational and external market considerations. Generic strategies are discussed and placed in the larger context of strategic planning. These are standard strategic approaches that are generally appropriate for a given market challenge or organizational objective. Finally, a series of worksheets are provided to guide physician managers through the strategic planning process.

Strategic management is the process of having managers, physicians, and other key personnel, perhaps with the assistance of consultants, examine and evaluate options for the future of your organization. The strategic management process, sometimes called strategic planning, and the resulting strategic plan can be contrasted with operational planning, which focuses on immediate or near-term objectives. Strategic plans and operational plans should be consistent with each other. Strategic management addresses questions such as these:

- What do I want this practice, hospital, or health care system to be like in the future?
- What changes are occurring in health care, the community, patients, competitors, and

so on that may affect the way we provide services in the future?
- What things must I begin to do *now or in the near future* to ensure that we will be competitive in the medical environment a few years hence?

In a sense, strategic management is an extension of the marketing process. It was emphasized in Chapter 9 that marketing decisions should be based on a thorough evaluation of an organization's strengths and weaknesses and the environment's opportunities and threats (SWOT analysis). As part of the marketing process, you were asked to consider your long-range vision for your organization. This *strategic* thinking was then translated into a marketing plan—an *operational* plan—describing immediate and near-term tactical goals and courses of action. Developing your marketing plan, therefore, is intimately associated with the strategic process.

Strategic *management* can also be contrasted with strategic *planning*. Strategic management means continuously managing as well as thinking in strategic terms. Physician managers who manage strategically are continuously considering the long-term implications of daily events or emerging trends. Strategic management is an ongoing process. Changes in the health care environment, technology, your personal goals, local demographics, insurance, government regulation, and the competitive environment should all generate continuous, evolving strategic thought. Strategically managing any health care organization is characterized by a state of mind in which managers, physicians, and physician managers at all levels are continually evaluating events in terms of their long-range implications. It is closely related to the mind set associated with total quality management (Chapter 12), in which there is an emphasis on seeking what could be, as opposed to being satisfied with what is, and then translating what could be into concrete process changes to bring about that future.

Strategic planning without strategic management is an older paradigm for addressing the long-term planning process. It localizes the strategic planning and thinking to a point in time and usually is undertaken by a limited group of employees whose mission is to plan for the organization. Here, strategic planning is separated from line managers and physicians, and planning is viewed as the territory of experts, who at a given time undertake mapping out the organization's future. Often, this process is conducted by consultants or with the aid of consultants, who may specialize in health care. In larger organizations, strategic planning may be the territory of a strategic planning staff. The executive summary may well fill a thick three-ring binder, with the actual plan filling several additional volumes.

The problem with this approach is that the planners may be isolated from real customers (patients, insurers, referring physicians, employers, etc.) or unfamiliar with the day-to-day operational issues of a particular hospital, practice, or health care system. In addition, because the strategic planning process takes place at a point in time, it can be unresponsive to the changing health care environment. Finally, all strategic plans are implemented by operational personnel, including managers, physicians, physician managers, and other health care professionals. A strategic planning process that is insulated from key operational players runs the danger of not having patrons who really understand it and are committed to its success.

A STRATEGIC MODEL: THE PENTAGON AND TRIANGLE

Larry Ring, a colleague of mine at the College of William & Mary, and Douglas Tigert of Babson College have developed a model or way of thinking about marketing and strategy that summarizes how a physician, group, or health care organization can think strategically. Their model helps identify where you can add value to your medical product or service by incorporating marketing, management, and strategic planning processes to provide a comprehensive approach to strategic management. Their approach is composed of two components: the pentagon and the triangle (Figure 10–1).

The pentagon describes your relationship to your customer. It is composed of the four Ps of marketing with some minor modifications. The pentagon points are product/service, place, value (price), communication (promotion), and an additional P: people. The key to a successful strategy is to win on at least one point of the pentagon, or to have a better mix on the pentagon than your competition, so that your overall strategy creates a favorable marketplace niche.

The triangle issues provide the infrastructure to compete successfully on the pentagon. An organization's logistics, systems, and suppliers are central to determining the nature of the pentagon points. For example, a hospital with a superior clinical information system will have thorough knowledge about its procedures, physicians, programs, outcomes, and costs. It can then use this information to compete more effectively on the value and product/service pentagon points.

The Pentagon

Product/Service

Product or service includes all elements related to the nature of the service that you offer. For a physician, this would include procedures, diseases, the quality of patient relations, the ambiance of your office or outpatient diagnostic area, and so forth. A plastic surgeon, for example, who decides to orient his or her practice more toward reconstructive procedures than cosmetic is making a product/service decision. Major categories for hospitals might include inpatient, outpatient, diagnostic services, and emergency care. Health care systems would consider mixes across a

broader range of themes, such as hospital services, outpatient, insurance, hospice, dialysis, mental health, physical therapy, health maintenance organization (HMO) products, preferred provider organization (PPO) products, and the like.

Thinking about the product/service in the context of market needs and your competition is central to strategic management. The SWOT analysis process that was described in Chapter 9 is a fundamental tool that you will use to identify product/service strategic considerations.

Place

Place includes all the issues related to your location and your size. This could include neighborhood characteristics, proximity of competition and patient base, number of locations, their placement, and so on. Determining whether to have multiple locations, including a hospital location, is a place decision often made by special-

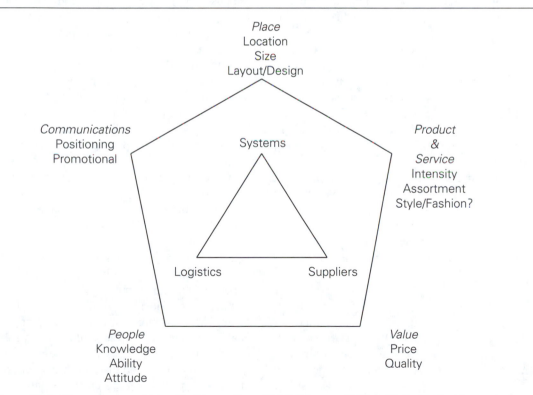

Figure 10–1 The pentagon and triangle. *Source:* Copyright © Lawrence J. Ring, Ph.D., used with permission.

ists. Hospital systems often make place decisions to have access to a patient base with desirable characteristics.

Recently, one Virginia hospital acquired an inner city hospital to have access to its Medicare patient base. At the same time, it opened a new tertiary care facility as a joint venture with a competitor in a wealthy suburb to position itself in front of expected population trends. Similarly, a hospital in South Carolina opened a satellite location between a wealthy suburb and a competing hospital. As a result, many emergency cases with desirable socioeconomic characteristics, including insurance, stop at this hospital's satellite instead of its competitor's main location.

As with all points on the pentagon, decisions about place should be made with the customer in mind. A hospital operating a dialysis center needs to locate that center for the convenience of its patients, not its staff. On the other hand, sometimes place problems can be solved by redefining the nature of the product/service. For example, kidney dialysis is often associated with lower income and alcohol and substance abuse. A hospital dialysis center that is being underutilized because of poor proximity to user groups can provide transportation, thereby effectively relocating itself by redefining the nature of its service. Similarly, new technology that permits easier home dialysis, and using slower dialysis during sleeping hours are additional examples of rethinking the place issue.

Centers of excellence with potential capacity and attractiveness beyond a given locality can market their services regionally or nationally by overcoming the location problem through competitive package pricing that includes transportation.

Value

Previously we discussed the issue of price as a marketing consideration. We must offer a product or service at a price that our customers will perceive as appropriate. Value takes the notion of price a step further and factors in the issue of quality. Conceptually, value is the product of price times quality. Quality, of course, is a major consideration for all health care organizations. Many of the challenges faced by health care organizations these days often revolve around defining quality.

One of the fears about managed care is that low price will be the determining factor in all decision making. Employers, insurers, and physicians may talk quality, but when coverage and treatment decisions are finally made, cost may be the real determining basis. When thinking about this issue, we need to make a distinction between the customer and the purchaser and between short- and long-term effects. Often, in health care, the customer and the purchaser are not the same. For example, one customer is the patient. The purchaser, however, for this customer is likely to be the customer's employer or the government. In the short run, the employer may make a decision based on price alone. Let's play out this example a little further, however. Suppose that the customer has a bad experience. Perhaps the atmosphere that we must have to deliver primary care services at the lowest possible price is a little too much like a "cattle car." Dissatisfied customers will, over time and as an aggregate, comment to their human resources administrators, and over time this should result in more serious consideration of the trade-off between price and quality. Often, this is expressed by giving employees more choices of insurers, networks, and providers.

Will every purchaser respond this way? Certainly not, and that is the point. In our society there are lots of choices. It is very likely that a variety of needs will develop on the value point, and that will create many opportunities for health care organizations to compete on the value equation. The display ad in Figure 9–1 (Chapter 9) is one example.

You may consider this discussion naive, but it is not. Markets are continually evolving. A health care organization that builds its only strategy around the lowest possible price and is insensitive to quality, and therefore value, considerations may find that a significant part of its market has shifted and that its products no longer coincide with purchasers' needs as modified by customers' needs.

Alternatively, parts of your product/service may well be defined almost exclusively by price, such as some HMO products and very expensive but competitive procedures such as coronary artery bypass graft. Here, however, quality is an understood necessary but insufficient condition for customer and ultimately purchaser satisfaction. Providing high quality is viewed simply as the entry ticket into the ball park. For example, let's look at grocery stores to gain some perspective on this issue. If you ask people why they buy their groceries at a particular store, they will typically give you one of three reasons. About 50 percent of the people will say that they choose their grocery store based on location. They go to the grocery that is most convenient to their home or commuting route. About 25 percent choose the store with the lowest perceived prices. The remaining 25 percent will state that they shop where they can get the best assortment, superior quality, or some other aspect of service. Implied, however, in all these choices is that quality is acceptable, and acceptable is operationally defined at a very high level.

Quality quickly becomes of paramount importance when it is perceived as unacceptable. For example, a few years ago Food Lion, a mid-Atlantic region grocery chain, was accused of washing its meat in bleach to extend shelf life. The allegation made national news, and quality immediately became the salient issue when people were considering whether to shop at this chain. Sales plummeted, and the chain's reputation as the low-price leader became irrelevant to consumers almost overnight.

In health care, implicit quality should always be assumed to be the customer's primary concern. It may not surface as a choice or satisfaction issue until it is perceived as unacceptable. Once it does surface, however, it will be of paramount importance. Value, then, implies an acceptable trade-off between price and quality. This may mean, for example, controlling price by redefining the product/service so that value is improved by reducing cost, but in ways that don't affect patient perceptions of quality. For example, reducing surgeons' choices of sutures, valves, and joints can reduce cost, which reduces price and improves value without affecting customer satisfaction. Similarly, one hospital saved $26,707 per year by eliminating asparagus from the mix of vegetables served to patients.[1]

People

The people component looks at winning through the interaction with customers. Once you have defined the nature of the product or service, you should consider who can offer them to the customer, so that the customer will be most satisfied. Obviously, this means that employees must be technically proficient. As with quality, customers often assume that this will be the case, unless an employee demonstrates incompetence, at which point it becomes an issue. Generally, therefore, gaining a competitive advantage on the people point of the pentagon means staffing so that your employees have personal characteristics and abilities that go beyond technical proficiency.

For example, nurses working with patients in chronic situations such as hospice, a dialysis center, or physical therapy, whose inclination is to be more patient focused than procedure focused, would create more customer satisfaction. A dialysis nurse who naturally thinks in terms of asking patients whether they need an aspirin or a blanket, or who is naturally inclined to ask how the grandchildren are doing, could provide a competitive advantage on the people point. Similarly, employees who are less inclined to need interpersonal interaction may be a better fit in laboratory technician positions, where the work is more solitary and where employees who like a lot of interpersonal interaction may distract coworkers.

As with many pentagon issues, the key to achieving success may be in an underlying triangle or support system that provides the organization with a competitive advantage. For example, obtaining employees who most advance the idea of meeting customer needs can result from using more effective employment methods (see Chapter 3). A second key to success on the people point is to use performance appraisal and reward systems that are congruent with employees' improving customer satisfaction (see Chapter 2). Finally, using a TQM philosophy (see Chapter 12), in which employees are encouraged to look creatively at the organization–customer interface, identify problems, and find solutions, is an additional example of a triangle system that facilitates winning on the people point.

Communications

This issue includes all ways in which you communicate with patients, employers, insurers, and others. We can think of this in the form of traditional promotion methods, which are discussed in Chapter 9, such as newspaper and Yellow Pages advertising. The communication, however, that is becoming most important in health care is increasingly being aimed at decision makers, who often are not patients. For example, outcome data, such as cost, rework rate, infection rate, and time to schedule an appointment, are often of paramount importance when primary care physicians make referrals to specialists. Specialists who communicate these types of data to primary care physicians to obtain referrals are trying to win on the communications point.

Similarly, health care systems that can communicate outcome measures to insurers and employers are trying to win on the communications point. For example, favorable rates of vaginal births after Cesarean section compared with a normative sample could give a health care system a chance to win on the communications point. Once again, this can't be done effectively unless the triangle systems that are needed to obtain and report the data, and to use the data to affect medical decision making, are in place. The need, however, for the triangle system might not be fully recognized unless the organization has a strategy of winning on communications and thereby the need for outcomes assessment.

We can also talk about communication within an organization. For example, when nursing, medicine, pharmacy, and housekeeping staffs are effectively integrated so that they release patients on average three hours earlier than a competing hospital, that hospital has a cost advantage and also an outcome measure to communicate. Internal communications, therefore, can also be a point on the pentagon where a health care provider can obtain a competitive advantage. Once again, underlying infrastructure (triangle) systems can create the ability to win on the communications pentagon point. In this case, the systems would be those that affect integration, such as organizational structure, performance appraisal, and compensation and reward plans. It also would work best when the staff know that the goal is to act integratively and to develop internal systems to improve communications.

The Triangle

The triangle is composed of the organization's infrastructure. Specifically, it includes systems, logistics, and suppliers. Systems are the procedures and processes by which the organization operates. Often, systems collect data and are used for decision making on issues such as cost, quality, and production. Other important systems, however, include the employment and performance appraisal systems that are necessary to hire the right employees and physicians and to motivate them so that there is a self-interest to satisfy patient, customer, or organizational needs.

Systems that improve pentagon competitiveness can be manifested in a number of ways. One particularly effective example is the development of care paths or critical pathways. These spell out in fine detail how patients who meet entrance criteria for the pathway will proceed through a course of treatment. A critical path is generally developed through consensus involving all constituencies who have a role in the pathway. A critical pathway team for coronary artery bypass graft might include cardiac surgeons, cardiologists, nurses (operating room and unit care), management information system specialists, and administration (billing, discharge, and medical records). In addition, critical path content including specific procedures, medications, and length of stay, is generally based on current research, when available, as opposed to anecdote or past practice in isolation. Finally, critical pathway systems are evolutionary. Based on experience and new research, the pathway will be modified to improve quality. This whole process of system development is, therefore, very closely aligned with the notion of TQM and continuous improvement. Exhibit 10–1 and Figure 10–2 present a critical pathway and a flowchart, respectively, for a total hip arthroplasty.

Logistics are the specialized systems that bring the right resources in appropriate amounts to the point where they make a difference. Why stock 10 artificial hips if 2 will generally do? Why have operating teams scheduled for late morning surgeries waiting because of procedural variance unrelated to quality of outcome that is occurring in earlier surgeries? Information systems can provide data on the financial and quality effects of different alternatives and make logistical improvements predictable and feasible.

Finally, suppliers are a part of the infrastructure that is taking on new importance to health care providers. In recent years, manufacturers of industrial products, such as automobiles and computers, have used suppliers to relieve themselves of having to carry an expensive, space-consuming inventory. This is possible if suppliers work closely with users, who can specify the qualities and characteristics of a limited number of items and provide accurate information about exactly when they will be needed.

Limiting the number of choices allows health care organizations to make larger-volume purchases and get a lower price so that the per unit costs go down. Specifying when units will be needed means that all parts of the supply chain can produce the units when needed, and inventory costs for everyone in the production process are reduced. Once again, information systems that provide the needed data to the right people "just in time" are critical. In one documented instance, a hospital achieved a one-time savings of $1.3 million in inventory reduction and reclaimed 11,000 square feet of space through better inventory control.[2]

Information systems are expensive to develop and maintain. Developing cost and productivity information systems requires skills that most medical practices don't possess and a level of medical knowledge that most hospital administrators don't possess. Some large practices and hospitals are developing cost-based management systems so that they will know what it costs to provide a service or procedure (see Chapter 6). Practices that provide hospital-based services, such as cardiac surgery and radiology, are partnering with hospitals to develop the needed information systems that can mutually benefit both in making the pentagon decisions. Developing alliances and partnering on limited, problem-focused projects that develop the information and operating systems that allow physicians and medical care organizations to perform more effectively may define the way these parts of the health care system will interact in the future.

STRATEGIC MANAGEMENT: TOOLS AND TECHNIQUES

The strategic planning process described below takes the pentagon and triangle and uses them to plan for the future. Strategic planning can be applied to any unit of analysis. For example, the strategic plan could be developed for an organization, such as a health care system composed of hospital, medical, and insurance components, or for any one of these components. Similarly, it could be developed for a practice or for a new product or service that a health care system, practice, or solo physician is planning to introduce.

Exhibit 10–1 Critical Pathway Excerpt: Total Hip Arthroplasty

DRG #209 Total Knee	CARE PATH—TOTAL KNEE ARTHROPLASTY			
	PRE-ADMIT/PRE-OP	DAY OF SURGERY	POST OP DAY 1	POST OP DAY 2
FLOOR:	Ortho/Neuro Unit	Ortho/Neuro Unit	Ortho/Neuro Unit	Ortho/Neuro Unit
CONSULTS/VISITS: Physical Therapy, Social Service Discharge Planning	Financial Coordinator Educator Discharge Planner Visit to gym area 8 East (On unit PAT and registration). Notify diabetic clinical specialist of diabetic admission.	8 East prepares pt/family for OR *PT*-CPM as ordered Place in PACU	*PT*—at bedside in AM Review precautions Wt. bearing per MD order Chair in AM Ambulate in PM Stand and transfer Instruct isometrics Quads, hamstrings, gluteals, ankle pumps *CPM* advance per protocol. *OT*—evaluation of ADL function *Social Service* referral	*PT* BID (Reinforce Day 1) Ambulates 10–20 ft with assist. *OT* continues with ADI *Discharge Plan* Reassess patient and family needs. Confirm discharge disposition with patient/family. Activate discharge plan. *CPM* advance per protocol.
TESTS:	AP/Lat. Chest X-ray. EKG, UA, CBC, Chem Profile, PTT, PT, Platelets, Electrolytes, Type/Cross/Screen	X-Ray PACU H & H @ 1800 P.T. if on Coumadin	H & H @ 0600 P.T. if on Coumadin	H & H @ 0600 P.T. if on Coumadin
NUTRITION/HYDRATION:	As at home: NPO after MN	Clear liquids to DAT. IV 2000/24 hr Auto/Constavac blood per protocol	Diet as tolerated IV—decrease to KVO if on PCA INT if tolerating PO.	Diet as tolerated. INT IV if PO intake adequate. May D/C INT if Hgb > 8

continues

	PRE-ADMIT/PRE-OP	DAY OF SURGERY	POST OP DAY 1	POST OP DAY 2
FLOOR:	Ortho/Neuro Unit	Ortho/Neuro Unit	Ortho/Neuro Unit	Ortho/Neuro Unit
ACTIVITY:	Up ad lib	Bedrest turn with pillow to side q4–6h. Elevate affected calf on pillow—not under the knee. HOB up 45 degrees. Up to bedside commode/ stand to void PRN with assist.	Chair × 2, walk with therapist. Out of bed (2–4 hrs total per day). Weight bear per MD order. Bedside commode to void.	Weight bear per MD order. Walk with PT—increase ambulation, chair BID, BSC, walker with assist. Out of bed 4–6 hrs total per day.
INTERVENTIONS:	Begin nursing admission assessment. Assessment of at home meds. Nurse calls MD of any lab/ X-ray/or EKG deviation	VS Q ½ hr × 3, then VS q4h. Neurovascular checks q2h prn. I & O q8h prn. Head to toe assessment. Assess skin condition. Knee drsg & drain (empty q8h). Assess bladder elimination.____ Assess bowel elimination. TED hose reapplied BID. CPM machine as ordered. Ankle exercise q1h w/a. Biox—begin to wean as per protocol. IS per order. Goal____.	VS q4h. I & O q8h. Neurovascular checks q4h. Head to toe assessment q8h. Change knee drsg per protocol. Assess skin condition. Assess bladder elimination.____ Assess bowel elimination. D/C drain per protocol. IS per order. Goal____ CPM machine as ordered. Ankle exercise q1h w/a.	Change wound drsg. IS per order. Goal____ CPM machine as ordered. Ankle exercises q1h w/a. Reinforce exercises.

Exhibit 10-1 continued

MEDICATION:	Instruct pt. regarding use of NSAIDS or anticoagulant treatment at home. Instruct to bring in specific meds from home (i.e., inhaler). PT to obtain from medical MD any meds he/she should take on day of OR.	Ancef 1 gram IV q8h *Analgesia* PCA Epidural IM Coumadin or ASA, Lovenox. Resume at home meds as ordered.	Ancef 1 gram IV q8h *Analgesia* PCA Epidural IM Coumadin, ASA or Lovenox. Colace 100 mg BID MOM 30 cc prn HS PO	Analgesia IM or PO (PCA or Epidural D/C) Coumadin, ASA or Lovenox MOM 30 cc prn hs PO Colace 100 mg po BID
KEY ACTIVITIES/ TEACHING PLANNING:	General Pre-op and Post-op teaching. TKR teaching. Review list of what to bring. Review equipment needs. Instruct on use of IS. Instruct on use of PT exercises.	Review pre-op teaching before surgery. Orient to room. Review post-op teaching after surgery.	Reinforce PT instructions. *Anticoagulant* instructions. (Coumadin, ASA, Lovenox) *PT exercise:* quad sets × 20 Bid Straight leg raises × 20 Bid Heel slides × 20 Bid Sitting knee flex/extend × 20 Short arc quads × 20	Reinforce PT instruction. Reinforce anticoagulant instruction. Coumadin video/teaching. Lovenox video/teaching.
KEY PATIENT ACTIVITIES/OUTCOMES:	Verbalizes understanding of teaching. Demonstrates use of IS. Demonstrates PT exercise. Verbalizes understanding of discharge process. Verbalizes discharge needs.	Hemodynamically stable Demonstrates correct turning techniques with help. Demonstrates correct use of call light. Pain level is < or = 4 on 0-10 scale. Demonstrates use of IS. Demonstrates use of PCA. Biox > 90 on room air. Biox < 90 per protocol. Tolerates CPM if ordered.	Demonstrates correct way to transfer from bed to chair WA. Up to commode/jeep with assist. Does ½ of bath in bed. Feeds self. Tolerates PT. Tolerates CPM. Pain level is < or = 4 on 0-10 scale. Biox > 90.	Transfers from bed to chair with min assist. Transfers from chair to walker with min assist. Walks to BR with walker. Had BM or flatus. Does ½ of bath at bedside. Tolerates PT. Tolerates CPM. Verbalizes bleeding precautions. Begins self inj. if on Lovenox. Pain level is < or = 4 on 0-10 scale.

Courtesy of Memorial Health System, South Bend, Illinois.

Figure 10–2 Critical pathway flowchart. Courtesy of Memorial Health System, South Bend, Indiana.

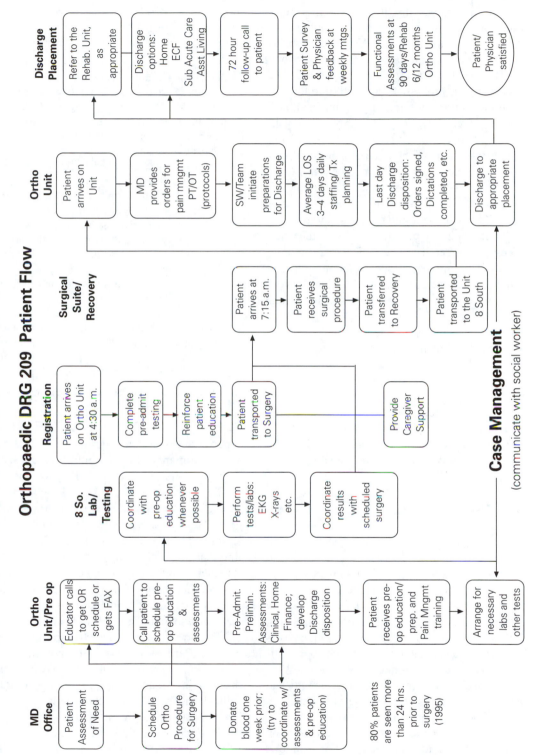

Orthopaedic DRG 209 Patient Flow

To think strategically, it is important to separate yourself emotionally and psychologically from present circumstances. You need to break from the present and be able to look at events unaffected by the compulsions of the moment. The planning process begins with defining the customer service mission of your medical business, product, or service, not simply restating the training that you received in medical school or the services that your practice or hospital currently provides. This distinction goes back to the definition of marketing, which is to define the product/service in terms of customer needs as opposed to what you find convenient to provide.

When exploring the idea of new medical services, remember that the technical medical product may be only one aspect of your mission. Other aspects to consider could relate to your own personal strategic plan and might include the following:

- self-fulfillment and personal satisfaction
- developing collegial relationships
- product/service positioning relative to managed care, such as the possibility of developing products and services with a high proportion of self-pay patients
- working with state-of-the-art techniques
- fulfilling various social responsibilities

The Mission Statement

Defining a mission is important because it will provide you with guidance when responding to daily events. Exhibit 10–2 contains a mission statement for a health care system. At the smaller health care organization level, defining a mission should not take days or weeks of introspection, long meetings with partners, or hours of exploration with a consultant. Be honest with yourself. If you have partners, be sincere with them. What are you trying to achieve both professionally and personally? By answering these questions, you can define the essence of your mission.

A mission statement can provide guidance on fundamental strategic direction. For example,

Exhibit 10–2   Fort Sanders Health System Mission Statement

We are an alliance of people and organizations with a common dedication to serve the people of East Tennessee as the area's preeminent health care system. We are committed to lead, minister, and manage effectively, seeking opportunities to enrich the health and quality of life in our communities.

- with values anchored in Christian teachings
- with programs and services of highest quality and lowest practical cost
- with progressiveness and innovation
- with fervent commitment to the principles of local ownership and voluntary governance
- with a supportive atmosphere in which to work and grow
- with sensitivity and caring

We are a united team, pledged to a common vision of leadership in the health care community and uncompromising service to God through service to our fellow men and women.

Source: Used by Fort Sanders Health System from 1990–1996. Reprinted with permission.

suppose that you conclude that a particular response to managed care would be inconsistent with your mission statement. Perhaps cosmetic plastic surgery offers a financial niche but the essence of your practice is reconstructive surgery. This conflict would suggest that you at least reevaluate your practice mission. You may find that you are willing to modify the mission statement and thereby make new alternatives accessible that you previously would not have considered. On the other hand, you may conclude that a cosmetic niche needs to be a very limited offering so as not to deflect you from your core mission. Perhaps its role is to subsidize other, less profitable areas. Finally, you may determine that this is a road that you just choose not to walk. Either way, your mission statement will have precipitated an internal discussion that needs to take place if you are to take control over your destiny.

Don't, however, view a mission statement as an inflexible constraint. Instead, it should be a constant reminder of what you are about and why your organization exists. Operational policies that are inconsistent with this mission should be examined very carefully. For example, a large, affluent, suburban health care system with a religious affiliation recently purchased an inner city hospital with a very different set of demographics. One reason—certainly not the only one, but still a significant one—was this hospital's mission to serve the community and those who are less affluent. Acquiring a failing inner city hospital and ensuring continuing services to its clientele were consistent with this hospital's mission statement and were not inconsistent with other aspects of the decision, including a realistic financial evaluation. The point is that the hospital's mission statement pointed it in a direction that resulted in it asking questions and looking for opportunities that it might not otherwise have explored.

An organization that routinely violates its mission statement runs the risk of becoming fragmented and uncoordinated in its actions. An organization that will not modify its mission in the face of continuing messages from its various customer constituencies (patients, colleagues, employees, employers, insurers, etc.) runs the risk of becoming irrelevant.

The next objective is to translate the mission statement into a strategic plan. To ensure relevance and subsequent strategic management of the plan, those who will have to put the plan into operation should be involved in developing the plan. Professional strategic planning assistance may come in the form of corporate staff in larger health care organizations. Smaller health care organizations may contract with a consultant to facilitate the strategic planning process. In either case, it is critical for administrators, physician managers, and line personnel representing all major organizational constituencies to participate in the strategic design process, so that a broad range of information is accessed and buy-in from the eventual implementors is obtained. Inclusion of these groups forms the bridge from strategic planning to strategic management.

The Strategic Planning Process

An outline to guide you through the strategic planning process is found in Appendix 10–A. This outline will allow you to develop a strategic plan in significant detail. This approach is an adaptation of one developed by Ring and Tigert.[3] It will guide you through three major questions:

1. What is the current situation?
2. Where do we want the organization to go?
3. What is the path that we should use to get there?

Each worksheet in Appendix 10–A is designed to help you explore a specific part of the planning process in detail. In preparation for completing the worksheets, you will find it helpful to think about the issues that they raise. The following section and its associated figures will be helpful in preparing you to think about the issues raised by the Appendix 10–A worksheets and the data that may be helpful for completing those worksheets.

Competitive Analysis

The purpose of a competitive analysis is to identify those features of your organization's internal and external environment that will govern the feasibility of attaining goals and adopting strategies for achieving them. Figure 10–3 presents a competitive analysis model. You can use this model to organize your thoughts regarding market competitive issues and your organization's specific circumstances. The resulting data will then allow you to evaluate strategy options and complete the A worksheets in Appendix 10–A. Consider the following:

- The economic characteristics of your market
  1. Is your market growing?
  2. Who are your rivals?
  3. What is the pace of technological change?

4. What is the geographical range of your competition: local, regional, or national?

- The driving forces
  1. Who is the service purchaser?
  2. What is the relationship between the service purchaser and the customer/patient?
  3. How are advances in technology or medical knowledge affecting the type and price of services you provide or that others in your field provide?[4]
  4. How are innovations in marketing, such as promotional methods and changing standards, affecting the communication of information to patients, purchasers, and providers?
  5. What changes are occurring in cost and efficiency?
  6. Are there regulatory and governmental changes that may affect your services?
  7. Is society changing its attitudes toward your services?

- The competition
  1. Who are your rivals, and what things can you do to gain a competitive edge?[5]
  2. What is the potential for new competition?
  3. What is the potential for alternative health care fields to provide substitute services?
  4. How much power do buyers have? Will individual consumers, PPOs, HMOs, employers, and others affect pricing?
  5. What market strategies are used by your competition?

Key Success Factors

Key success factors are those things that a health care organization must do well to succeed. As we have seen, the pentagon (people, place, value, communication, and product/service) and triangle (logistics, supplier, and systems) are respectively the bases for a competitive marketing mix and the infrastructure that is necessary to provide that mix. Consider your

ability to compete effectively on at least one pentagon point or to deliver a service that is competitive across a mix of the points. In addition, what is the triangle infrastructure that will be necessary to attain this competitive mix?

The second part of a competitive analysis consists of a review of your organization's specific situation. You can analyze your own competitive situation by examining your current strategy.

Your current strategy can be evaluated using a number of criteria, including income relative to competitors, financial reserves for future growth, and professional reputation.

- Are there parts of your current strategy that aren't working?
- Are there parts of your strategy that are particularly effective?
- If you don't have a formal strategy, identify the strategy that has evolved.

SWOT Analysis

As mentioned earlier, SWOT is an acronym for strengths, weaknesses, opportunities, and threats. A strength is something that your organization does well. A weakness is something that your organization lacks or doesn't do well. An opportunity is an opening in the market that you may be able to exploit. Threats are environmental issues that may negatively affect your organization. Exhibit 10–3 lists some considerations to look for when you are performing a SWOT analysis. An effective strategy will do some or all of the following:

- It will build upon strengths.
- It will compensate for weaknesses.
- It will take advantage of opportunities.[6]
- It will provide defenses against threats.

Strategic Options

A successful strategy will be consistent with both the external and internal findings of your competitive analysis. Table 10–1 outlines some generic strategies and summarizes some of the internal and external issues to consider when

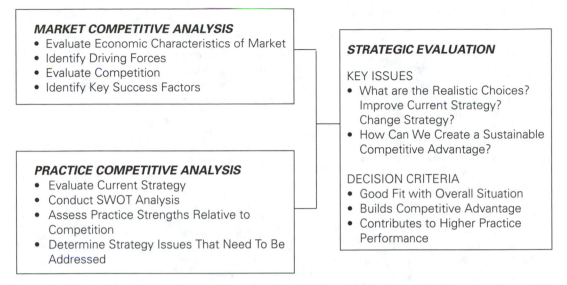

MARKET COMPETITIVE ANALYSIS
- Evaluate Economic Characteristics of Market
- Identify Driving Forces
- Evaluate Competition
- Identify Key Success Factors

STRATEGIC EVALUATION

KEY ISSUES
- What are the Realistic Choices? Improve Current Strategy? Change Strategy?
- How Can We Create a Sustainable Competitive Advantage?

DECISION CRITERIA
- Good Fit with Overall Situation
- Builds Competitive Advantage
- Contributes to Higher Practice Performance

PRACTICE COMPETITIVE ANALYSIS
- Evaluate Current Strategy
- Conduct SWOT Analysis
- Assess Practice Strengths Relative to Competition
- Determine Strategy Issues That Need To Be Addressed

Figure 10–3 Competitive analysis model. *Source:* Adapted with permission from A.A. Thompson, Jr., and A.J. Strickland, III, *Strategic Management Concepts and Cases*, 5th Edition, p. 58, © 1990, Irwin Publishers.

you are evaluating strategies. When you are evaluating strategy alternatives, it is important to keep the following considerations in mind:

- Realistically evaluate whether your personnel have the skills, time, and motivation to follow through on a strategy. An overly ambitious plan may create internal problems and put strains on your resources and personnel. In addition, a strategic change may not be consistent with the personal objectives of some employees or partners. People work to achieve their own objectives. A change in strategy may result in turnover, hostility, and perhaps sabotage if it is perceived as inconsistent with an individual employee's objectives. This should not deter you from pursuing strategic change, but you should take into account potential resistance to change and plan to deal with it (see Chapter II).
- A strategy that is a radical departure from your current course can be very risky. Such a strategy should only be undertaken after considerable analysis and thought.
- Avoid a strategy that can work only if everything goes smoothly. There will always

be surprises, and few things in life go exactly as planned. You should assume that most, if not all, surprises will be bad ones.
- Prepare for the responses of your competitors. If the strategy works, how will your competitors react? Are there any defensive strategies that you might implement along the way so that you can retain your newly gained competitive advantage?

GENERIC STRATEGIES

Although specific strategies only make sense given the particular details of your situation, there are generic strategies to consider. Use them as a jumping-off point. They are intended to stimulate your thinking, not to be a formula answer to a strategic challenge.

The Low-Cost Producer

This strategy may be relevant when you are trying to attract groups of patients from a large employer, a group of employers, or a managed health care system or when you are targeting certain types of patients.[7] The strategy is to cut

Exhibit 10–3 SWOT Analysis: What To Look for

Potential Strengths
1. A distinctive competence
2. Financial resources
3. Interpersonal skills
4. Medical skills
5. Respect of peers
6. Economies of scale/volume
7. Insulated from competitive pressures
8. Proprietary or exclusive technology/skills
9. Cost advantage
10. Marketing skills
11. Management skills
12. Referral sources
13. Strong position on any of the 5 Ps
14. Strong position on any of the three triangle issues

Potential Weaknesses
1. No clear strategic direction
2. Obsolete facilities
3. Subpar profitability because . . .
4. Management skills
5. Marketing skills
6. Narrow scope of services
7. Poor position on any of the five Ps
8. Weak position on any of the three triangle issues

9. Financial resources
10. Cost position
11. Dissention between partners or organizational parts

Potential Opportunities
1. Identify additional market segments
2. Broaden or redefine services to meet customer needs
3. Diversify into related services
4. Enter new geographical regions
5. Complacency among rivals
6. Growth market
7. Form alliances and partnerships

Potential Threats
1. Entry of more competitors
2. Entry of alternative health care providers such as chiropractors, nurse practitioners, psychologists, etc.
3. New forms of health care delivery: PPO, HMO, integrated hospital delivery systems
4. Changing technology
5. Slow market growth
6. Changing patient tastes and needs
7. Adverse demographic changes

costs to the bone, so that you can offer lower prices and thereby gain market share. Profit is achieved by high volume that is leveraged to create low costs.

Offering low prices relative to competitors means that the organization must be cost conscious in every aspect of business. Tight budgeting, elimination of waste, frugal design of office space, and thin personnel staffing are intrinsic to this strategy. Developing effective triangle systems and pursuing and growing at the maximum digestible rate during the growth phase of the market/product/service life cycle are two methods to become the low-cost producer.

Differentiation

A differentiation strategy is based on identifying purchasers or patients with different sets of needs. One or more of these needs form the basis for a strategy. Medical services can be differentiated on each of the five pentagon points. A sole provider of a service in an area has achieved differentiation. Structuring a practice or center around a unique service can provide a strong competitive advantage. For example, excimer retinokeratotomy surgery has formed the basis for national and international practices. Currently, European providers are advertising laser procedures that are not yet available in the United States, thereby differentiating themselves from U.S. competitors.

Differentiation can also be based on providing superior quality or superior perceived quality of service. For example, the orthopaedic surgeon who can offer hip replacement patients a complete in-house package of radiographic examination, surgery, and physical therapy may have a

Table 10–1 Generic Strategic Options

Medical Environments	Organizational Positions	Situational Considerations	Market Share Options	Strategy Options
Rapid growth	Dominant leader	External	Grow and build	Competitive approach
Consolidating to a smaller group of competitors	Leader	Driving forces	Capture bigger market share and grow faster than competitors	Low cost
Mature/slow growth	Aggressive challenger	Competitive pressures		Differentiated services, locations, hours, skills, technology
Aging/declining	Content follower	Anticipated moves of key rivals	Invest heavily	
Fragmented	Weak/distressed candidate for turn-around/exit	Key success factors	Fortify and defend	Offensive initiatives
Rapid change	No clear strategy or market image	Internal	Protect market share	Attack, end run, guerrilla warfare
Increasing high technology		Current performance	Grow as fast as medical market	Defensive initiatives
		Strengths/weaknesses	Retrench and retreat	Fortify/protect
		Threats/opportunities	Surrender weakly held positions when forced	Retaliatory
		Cost position		Harvest
		Competitive strength	Fight hard for core markets	Turnaround
		Strategic issues and problems	Maximize short-term cash flow	Revamp strategy
			Minimize reinvestment of capital	Operational changes: reduce cost, increase revenues, sell assets, etc.
			Overhaul and reposition	
			Try to turn around	
			Abandon/liquidate	
			Sell out	
			Close down	

Source: Adapted from A.A. Thompson, Jr. and A.J. Strickland III, *Strategic Management Concepts and Cases*, 5th ed., p. 158, © 1990, Irwin Publishers.

competitive advantage. Similarly, centers with reputations for excellence, such as the Texas Heart Institute, the Jones Reproductive Clinic, and the Cleveland Clinic, have managed to differentiate themselves on perceived, if not actual, quality. Interestingly enough, as we have seen, this can also allow them to be the low-cost provider. The perceived high quality allows many centers of excellence to compete for regional and national contracts, which results in higher volume. This, in turn, results in better utilization of fixed costs, and it also allows them to negotiate lower costs on supplies, both of which result in a lower cost structure. High quality and low price is obviously a very powerful combination.

Differentiation, however, can also fail in the following situations:

- The differentiation is based on something that doesn't really lower the price or isn't perceived as really increasing the customer's or patient's well-being.
- The price is set too high.
- The value is not perceived by the patient or customer even though it is real.

Attacking

Generally, it is not acceptable in medicine to attack your competitors directly. You can, however, attack your competitors' strengths and weaknesses. Opening satellite locations, using image advertising, and using price reductions to obtain managed care contracts are all legitimate forms of attack. Similarly, providing something that competitors can't can be used as an attack. For example, quick access to high-quality medical care is being used in an attack fashion by U.S. providers to obtain foreign customers/patients who can pay for services in cash.

Guerrilla Warfare

Guerrilla warfare is characterized by attacks directed at the weak points of carefully selected competitors, who often are much more power-

ful. It can be a very effective strategy for a smaller health care organization in a market with mature, larger, well-entrenched competitors. This strategy also can be useful for new practitioners in a no-growth or slow-growth market.

Guerrilla attacks focus on a market segment or service that is weakly defended. For example, hospital systems may be vulnerable to attacks on selected surgical procedures that can be performed in physicians' offices. Surgeons who selectively seek contracts by offering insurers better rates for practice-based procedures that formerly were hospital based are conducting guerrilla warfare.

Fortifying and Protecting

This is a defensive strategy designed to block the advances of adversaries. Generally, service businesses use a fortifying and defending strategy to protect referral sources. Obtaining written contracts, wining and dining, acknowledging referrals, and providing quality service make it difficult for challengers to divert referrals. Some health care systems have been purchasing primary care practices as a defense against the entry of large outside managed care organizations. By buying up the available sources of primary care, they make it very difficult or very expensive for outside players to enter the market.

Harvesting

Harvesting is a strategy for orderly withdrawal from a market while at the same time collecting a harvest of cash.[8-10] Harvesting is accomplished by cutting budgets to a minimum, reducing advertising expenses, reducing quality in those areas where it will not show, eliminating nonessential services, reducing or eliminating equipment maintenance, subletting or selling excess office space, and so on.

Harvesting is appropriate when an organization is in an undesirable position and the goal is to restructure the organization totally or kill it off. Harvesting also is appropriate for services where demand is flat or declining *and* you have a small market share. Harvesting can create the capital necessary to finance a turnaround, or it can precede liquidation. In any event, it is a strategy that can buy time for a final decision.

Consider the following case example. Ralph Early did not enjoy his solo private practice. He found the experience to be lonely, he did not enjoy cultivating referral sources, and he did not find managing the day-to-day affairs of a small practice to be rewarding. In addition, his financial position had been in a long, steady decline because the economics of solo practice were no longer favorable in a market that was 40 percent managed care. His lease expired in six months, and he decided that he would prefer working for a large hospital doing clinical, educational, and administrative work.

While negotiating an agreement to work for a hospital, Dr. Early began a harvesting strategy. He eliminated a part-time clerical position, a nursing position, and a telephone line and reduced his supply inventory to a minimum. He also accelerated into his remaining months of private practice any legally appropriate personal expenses that he thought his future employer might not compensate him for, such as buying a new cellular phone. Finally, he limited the time each day that his business manager would take patient calls so that she could work back accounts and maximize account collection.

Boston Consulting Group Strategies

The Boston Consulting Group has developed generic strategies that integrate the issues of market share and product life cycle. Table 9–1 illustrates product life cycles for some medical services. Dichotomizing both growth rate and market share into high and low, it is possible to assemble a 2-by-2 table. Low share of a high growth market often characterizes the introductory life cycle phase. Generic strategies in this cell are either to invest to gain market share while the competition is fragmented and margins are large, or get out (harvest), and reinvest capital, effort, time, etcetera, in other products/

services/procedures. Growing market share generally will result in both negative cash flow and income statement net income because of the need to reinvest gains. This phase is called the "Question Mark," because of the uncertainty of the procedure's future and which strategy to pursue. Table 9–1 demonstrates that not all Question Marks succeed.

If you and the procedure/service are successful, the result will be a high share of a high growth market. High share creates economies of scale and lower costs, and results in a very competitive position. The generic strategy in this cell is to grow at the maximum digestible rate. As Satchel Page said, "Don't look back because someone may be gaining on you!" This phase is called the "Star." The goal is to retain or even gain more market share. Investment of net income continues, and Stars often are cash and net income neutral.

As with all markets, products, and services, eventually the growth rate declines. Generally, price competition breaks out in this phase as competitors try to increase volume, and gain associated cost advantages in a flat market. If you have high market share in a low growth market you can choose to undercut the competition on price, or match them on price and gain substantial net income and cash. This is the "Cash Cow" phase. Here, the generic strategy is to milk the cow, take cash and profits, but not kill it. Simultaneously, you should reinvest some net income in Question Marks, because they will be your future.

The final cell, a low share of a low growth market is referred to as a "Dog." Generally, you get into this cell by never gaining market share during the growth phase. You simply drop from a low share of a high growth market to a low share of a low growth market. The generic strategy here is to divest. The problem is that Dogs are often pets; a pet hospital, clinic, program, procedure, service, etcetera, and it is often difficult to kill off a pet.

This approach may be helpful if market share and growth convey competitive advantages Some products and services, however, are not sensitive to these issues. Lexus, Mercedes-Benz, and American health care organizations that cater to overseas cash patients and patients desiring upscale service for cosmetic or choice procedures (see Figure 9–1) are examples that run counter to this model.

Turnaround

A turnaround strategy is appropriate when an organization is in crisis and is worth saving but the current strategy has led to very serious financial or management problems. The first task in a turnaround strategy is diagnosis. A misdiagnosis can be fatal because the organization by definition is already in a weakened state. It is essential at this point to determine whether the crisis has been caused by poor implementation of an effective strategy or an ineffective strategy. Common problems that can precipitate the need for a turnaround strategy include the following:

- buying market share with low fees while underestimating the actual cost of delivering the services; this can be a real danger of capitation and some HMO and PPO arrangements
- excessive fixed costs associated with underutilized office space, equipment, or personnel
- never gaining, or even losing, market share as a result of competitors' actions
- overreliance on a new procedure or technological innovation that does not generate the expected revenues

Attempting a turnaround can be very risky. Hall studied 64 companies that had attempted a turnaround and none of them succeeded.[11] The turnaround attempts failed because the firms either waited too long to begin or had insufficient cash or managerial talent to recover in slow-growth industries. Here are five generic approaches to undertaking a turnaround[12]:

1. *Revamp the existing strategy.* If the cause of the problem is strategic as opposed to operational, then this approach is appropriate. Strategic problems are essentially flaws in the approach to the market. Operational problems usually result from incompetent execution of the strategy. Revamping can be undertaken with any of the strategies noted above.

2. *Increase revenues.* This approach is necessary when there is no way to cut expenses. The strategy for approaching the market remains the same, but operational changes are made to increase revenues. Revenues can be increased through better utilization of physician time, using more physician extenders, offering additional services, adding office hours, coding more thoroughly, and so on. If demand is inelastic and you are a nonparticipating physician with an insurance plan, you can raise your fees. If demand is elastic, raising your fees may result in driving patients to your competition, thereby reducing your revenues.

3. *Reduce costs.* Once again, the strategy for approaching the market remains the same. Operational plans, however, stress cost reductions in all organizational aspects. Reducing costs will only work if the items associated with the costs do not generate revenue or if their associated costs can be reduced at a greater rate than their associated revenues. To use this tactic, cost inefficiencies must be identifiable, and the cost-volume-profit relationship must be understood (see Chapter 6). Costs can be reduced by eliminating unneeded or underemployed positions, eliminating underutilized services, making better utilization of automation (e.g., electronic claims), using flexible budgets to manage expenditures, and undertaking a general belt tightening.

4. *Sell assets.* Big-ticket capital items (e.g., radiology equipment, computers, and laboratory equipment) that are not being efficiently utilized can be sold. The cash generated can then be used to finance

other revenue-generating programs and services.

5. *Use a combination of approaches.* A turnaround need not be elegant. Use any and all of the approaches that seem relevant. A change of strategy can be coupled with the other approaches, or these approaches can be used with the current strategy. Generally, the more serious the problem, the more likely it is that you will have to consider a broad, rapid attack on the problem.

Implementing the Strategic Plan

After you identify a strategy, the next step is to implement it. The object is to achieve the tightest possible fit between the strategy and how your organization operationalizes it in each of the functional areas covered in this book. Everything this book may have taught you regarding staffing, performance evaluation, leadership, motivation, organizational structure, budgeting, marketing, and revenue collection should be reevaluated in the context of your changed strategy.

Employee rewards must act as a link between employees' perceptions of their own personal objectives and the implementation of the strategy. As noted in Chapter 5, people don't work for you, they work for themselves. If you properly structure the situation, people will work *with* you to achieve your goals because of the mutually desirable consequences. This is what occurs when an organization successfully implements team-building concepts, TQM, and an empowerment philosophy. Successful application of all these management concepts results in an alignment of personal and organizational rewards.

A financial assessment is critical to any planned change in strategy. A budget is the financial planning part of your strategic plan. Therefore, creating a pro forma budget for your plan will help ensure that it is realistic.

Computer hardware and software and information systems must be examined to ensure their ability to contribute to achieving your objectives by way of the specified strategy. For example, a strategy that is based on cost control and alignment of physician and health care system incentives will be greatly enhanced by an information system that assesses comorbid conditions and adjusts physician production statistics accordingly (Chapter 15). Similarly, developing activity-based cost systems for procedures critical to success may also be important to the success of the strategy (Chapter 6).

Supporting all this should be shared values and shared ethical standards. If employees or partners don't truly believe in the mission and the means of achieving that mission, then they will not have the commitment to follow through on the strategic plan.

Finally, the physician manager's role in this process is to orchestrate the implementation of the strategy. Possible leadership styles range from directive to delegative, and the physician may choose to pursue strategic imperatives quickly or slowly. The decisions regarding leadership style and pace must be based on the appropriateness of the different leadership strategies (see Chapter 5) and any anticipated resistance to change (see Chapter 11). Consultation with others spreads the ownership of an idea, thereby creating motivation on the part of others to make the idea work. If, on the other hand, the organization's existence is being threatened, it may be necessary to use a more directive approach because the changes may have to be put in place sooner.

It is also appropriate to personalize the strategic planning and management concepts. Residents, for example, should think in terms of a personal strategic plan. Similarly, physicians should periodically reevaluate their personal strategic options. As the world in which you are practicing medicine or managing a health care organization changes, the considerations that were important to you several years ago may well have changed. For example, you may be practicing in a small group. Strategically, you may have concluded that you need to get larger to compete effectively and provide appropriate medical care. In terms of your personal strategy, you should be considering what this means to you. Is this your vision of what you consider professionally desirable? As you evaluate the impact on your job description, does this sound like a positive career change? If not, what can you do now to redirect your future toward a more desirable outcome?

A physician who is entering private practice has the opportunity to define a personal strategy. The new physician can easily be faced with too many strategic options, however, and not enough time or information to make an informed decision. There are no easy solutions to this problem.

Perhaps the best tactic is to approach strategic planning with some degree of humility. Admitting that you don't know and asking for opinions and advice is a far better tactic than acting with bravado on the basis of rudimentary information. Consulting with peers, colleagues, and mentors and judiciously using consultants can give you a perspective on how best to put your strategic plan into effect.

CASE EXAMPLE

Dr. Fred Stanley was the founder of a group psychiatric practice. He had been dissatisfied working for other physicians, so he decided to develop his own practice. He envisioned a practice composed of two or three other owners that would provide a very high standard of care in a well-appointed, upscale office suite. He was looking for a relaxed team atmosphere in which he could work with respected, cooperative colleagues. Consistent with this strategy, he rented an office suite in a class A office building and proceeded to decorate the waiting room with Chippendale reproductions and his own office with art deco furnishings highlighted by a large black marble desk. He had five other treatment offices, and by the time he opened his doors he had hired three other providers.

During the practice's first year, Dr. Stanley hired George Michael, Ph.D., to fill one of the two open offices. Dr. Michael had a full caseload, but his patients required considerable front office attention. They tended to be more remiss in paying their copayments and generally had less desirable insurance coverage. In addition, Dr. Michael was very demanding of the office staff. He was abrupt, often interrupted conversations between the office staff and others, and was almost always running too late to be courteous. In addition, he required far more typing, transcription, and scheduling support than any other provider. All this created tension within the practice. Nevertheless, Dr. Michael generated substantial revenue for the practice, so Dr. Stanley tolerated, and to some degree tried to manage, his behavior. Dr. Stanley discussed these problems on several occasions with Dr. Michael, and on more than one occasion the discussion degenerated into a confrontation.

Toward the end of the practice's first year, the building owners contacted Dr. Stanley regarding his first right of refusal on the unrented office space adjoining his suite. An attorney had offered to rent the space, so Dr. Stanley either had to rent the space now or be precluded from expanding during the four years remaining on his lease. A month before Dr. Stanley had been notified about the office space, Lionel Filbert, M.D., had contacted him about joining his practice. Dr. Stanley at first rejected the idea, although he did not immediately communicate this to Dr. Filbert. Dr. Filbert's caseload was almost entirely composed of chemically dependent families and adolescents. Because of the nature of their problems, these patients tended to be irresponsible. They often canceled or did not show for appointments, avoided their financial responsibilities, and came up with many creative ways of not paying their bills. In addition, Dr. Filbert had a reputation for being demanding of office staff, having unrealistic expectations, and responding emotionally to everyday problems. On the other hand, Dr. Filbert treated in excess of 45 patients each week plus hospital rounds, and his reputation with this patient population was excellent.

In light of the office space option, Dr. Stanley reconsidered his decision regarding Dr. Filbert. Using a break-even analysis, Dr. Stanley calculated that Dr. Filbert's contribution margin would cover the additional monthly rental. The added office space could provide room for five additional providers. Dr. Stanley calculated that, if he could fill several of the other offices, he would have a very profitable practice. In addition, Dr. Filbert would be brought in with the expectation of partnership, and he would bring new referral sources and insurer alignments. Balanced against this was the knowledge that his present office suite was still not filled and that, in the event that he was not able to recruit additional providers, he could have a serious financial problem if Dr. Filbert decided to leave or partnership did not materialize. In addition, he anticipated that it would be difficult to work with Dr. Filbert.

Dr. Stanley, tempted by the opportunity to have a larger practice, retained Dr. Filbert with a partnership option and leased the additional office space. The next year and a half was very difficult for him. He had numerous problems with Dr. Filbert's patients, hired three secretaries for Dr. Filbert (none of whom Dr. Filbert considered adequate), and received a fairly steady stream of "emergency" calls from him on weekends and evenings regarding "office problems." In addition, Dr. Filbert and Dr. Michael formed an "alliance of misery." Staff meetings were largely consumed with responding to their complaints, and from Dr. Stanley's perspective they never had anything positive to say or to contribute to the practice atmosphere. Finally, other producers were becoming dissatisfied because the "squeaky wheels" in the practice did get oiled. The secretaries and the business manager attended first to the needs of Drs. Filbert and Michael.

During this period of time, Dr. Stanley was able to hire two additional producers. The office morale, however, was very low. Dr. Stanley became concerned that two other producers, whom he eventually wanted to become partners, would become so dissatisfied that they would leave. In addition, Dr. Stanley was becoming very frustrated with his practice, as indicated by these comments:

> In hindsight, I can see what happened. I lost sight of what was really important to me and where I wanted to go. Dr. Filbert didn't fit with the practice strategy. Unfortunately, I wasn't thinking *strategy* when I hired him. I knew what it would be like to work with him, but I only saw that as a daily inconvenience. I didn't understand that, in combination with Dr. Michael, I would be inadvertently changing the fundamental philosophy and reason for being of this practice. We went from a low-volume, high-quality, calm practice to a high-volume, frantic crisis center. Our location, our rent, our furnishings, our marketing, our strategy, and our mission are all based on my original mission statement. These are all wasted on our current clientele. I could just as easily attract them in a strip shopping center office space with crate furniture at 50 percent less rent. In addition, the office chaos and animosity have given us a reputation as a bad place to work. I now find it very difficult to attract additional producers.

> Dr. Filbert and Dr. Michael are not bad people. They simply don't belong here. To make them belong here, I would have to adjust our mission—to include their approach to practice. It's not a question of right or wrong, good or bad. It's simply an issue of fit. Right now we don't have a fit, and life is difficult for everyone.

Beyond the satisfaction issues, Dr. Stanley anticipated some additional long-term consequences as a result of the lack of fit. Dr. Michael would probably leave in six months when his contract expired. Dr. Filbert might well leave when his contract expired in eight months, simply because he was always dissatisfied about everything! In addition, the continuing presence of both Drs. Michael and Filbert for the next several months might drive away Dr. Stanley's other producers. Dr. Stanley saw the prospect of having a large office suite to himself in eight months. He stated:

> I have to go back to my initial strategy. This will be very difficult and dangerous. I could choose to continue going in the direction in which my practice has evolved, but I can see now that it would mean developing a very different practice, and I don't *want* to do that. I will have to terminate both Dr. Michael and Dr. Filbert. In addition, I must do it soon, so that the others will see that I intend to change the direction of this practice.

> A break-even analysis shows that we should be able to scrape by if we are really careful about costs, sublet the added office space, and cut our nonessential spending to the bone. Hopefully, over time, the reputation of the practice will improve so that I will be able to recruit other producers and fill my original office space.

FORESIGHT

The strategic planning/strategic management process that has been described in this chapter can be a helpful guide to developing a competitive strategy for a physician, practice, hospital, or health care system. To have its greatest impact, however, it must be used in the context of foresight. It is all too easy to abandon creativity to the dictates of a customer-led strategy. The health care industry is rapidly redefining itself. Hospitals are acquiring physicians and become insurers. Physicians, similarly, are repositioning themselves. Pharmaceutical companies are getting into the outpatient services business. Where are the boundaries?

If health care providers are to excel beyond simply gaining a larger share of yesterday's market definition, then they must break the limitations of being customer led. Hamel and Prahalad propose that customers often lack foresight.[13] Fifteen years ago, customers did not know that

they wanted cellular phones, faxes, personal computers, Internet access, CD players, and the like. These authors' position has a grain of truth to it in that customers did not know that they wanted these specific products. Customers, however, *did* know that they wanted the problems solved or the opportunities created by these products, and herein lies the role of foresight.

Developing a strategic plan around the nature of things as perceived by customers today may limit your ability to outflank competitors in the future. Leading with new conceptualizations of health care service that satisfy customers' needs, even if customers don't realize that they have the need yet, and then educating and communicating with customers can result in a redefinition of the organization and the business. Hal Sperlich, who created the minivan for Chrysler after Ford rejected the idea, states:

> [Ford] lacked the confidence that a market existed, because the product didn't exist. The auto industry places great value on historical studies of market segments. Well, we couldn't prove that there was a market for the minivan because there was no historical segment to cite.

> In Detroit most product development dollars are spent on modest improvements to existing products, and most market research money is spent on studying what customers like among available products. In 10 years of developing the minivan, we never once got a letter from a housewife asking us to invent one. To the skeptics, that proved there wasn't a market out there.[14(p.92)]

In an industry in which the nature of service delivery and the underlying financial relationships are fundamentally changing, it may be important to get beyond a customer-led strategy. By this I don't mean losing sight of your customers' needs, but I do mean going beyond their current perceptions of how those needs are best fulfilled. Ideally, strategic planning should explore the "white space," those areas between and beyond the currently conceived boxes (product, service, provider definition, etc.) or the current definitions of the five pentagon points.

USING APPENDIX 10–A

Once you have reached this point, you are ready to complete the worksheets in Appendix 10–A. These worksheets provide a self-guided basis to begin the strategic planning process. Use the worksheets as a guide to explore internal and external issues, the competition, and strategic alternatives and to indicate where you may need to collect additional information.

After you complete the worksheets, consider the following issues:

- Is your proposed strategy likely to succeed given the information at hand?
- How well does your strategy fit with current key success factors and organizational strategies?
- How robust is your strategy to changes in response to future external threats and internal weaknesses?
- What aggressive moves could be made to take advantage of opportunities, make your plan more competitive, reduce costs, and deter or block threats?

Next, *realistically* examine the choices that are available to you. Is it possible to improve on your proposed strategy? Modifying a current strategy will generally be less disruptive and risky than going off in a totally new direction. What things, if any, can you do to create a sustainable competitive advantage?

CONCLUSION

Having a clear strategy will help you make operational decisions that are consistent with organization objectives. In the absence of a strategy, decisions may be made that have very significant unintended consequences. This chapter should have made you aware of why you should think in strategic terms and encouraged you to undertake strategic planning and conduct strategic management on a routine basis.

There are a number of tools that can help you organize your strategic thinking. There are also a number of generic strategies that you can use as points of departure when evaluating strategic options. The discussion of these tools and options, as well as case examples of physicians who had to contend with the consequences of implicit and explicit strategic choices, should provide you with the means and the motivation to evaluate strategic choices and put your strategic plan into effect.

REFERENCES AND NOTES

1. VHA, Inc., *Utilization: A Guide to Reducing Variations To Improve Outcomes* (Irving, Tex.: VHA, 1994).

2. VHA, Inc., *Electronic Data Interchange: Using EDI To Reduce Total Delivered Cost* (Irving, Tex.: VHA, 1994).

3. Personal communication with L.J. Lawrence and D.J. Tigert.

4. There appears to be a trend in general internal medicine toward providing more care in the office and less in the hospital. In addition, the nature of office care seems to be changing, with an increased emphasis on preventive care and health maintenance. As a result, internists now devote more of their time to talking to and educating their patients. These trends may have implications for office staffing and design. See S. Wartman, Internal Medicine, *JAMA* 263 (1990): 2649–2651.

5. You can answer this question by examining the local market as well as national trends. For example, a report by the American Medical Association's Council on Long-Range Planning and Development stated that the primary source of competition for internists in coming years will be subspecialty internists and that some subspecialties may expand their range of services to obtain a larger and more secure patient base. See The Future of General Internal Medicine, *JAMA* 262 (1989): 2097–2100.

6. For example, the American Academy of Family Physicians found that only 40 percent of its members provided some level of obstetrical care and that an additional 40 percent had discontinued obstetrical services. The risk of malpractice litigation was cited as the reason for this trend. At the same time, the decrease in the availability of obstetrical services may create an opportunity

for less faint-hearted family practice physicians. See R. Bredfledt, J. Colliver, and R. Wesley, Present Status of Obstetrics in Family Practice and the Effects of Malpractice Issues, *Journal of Family Practice* 28 (1989): 294–297.

7. For an example in which low cost was an inherent part of a practice strategy, see J. Norman, Can a Practice Serving the Poor Avoid Financial Quicksand?, *Medical Economics*, 5 February 1990, pp. 79–87.

8. P. Kotler, Harvesting Strategies for Weak Products, *Business Horizons* 21, no. 5 (1978): 17–18.

9. P. Kotler and R. Clarke, *Marketing for Health Care Organizations* (Englewood Cliffs, N.J.: Prentice-Hall, 1987), 98, 342.

10. F. Paine and C. Anderson, *Strategic Management* (Hinsdale, Ill.: Dryden Press, 1983), 246–247.

11. W.K. Hall, Survival Strategies in a Hostile Environment, *Harvard Business Review* 58, no. 5 (1980): 75–85.

12. C.W. Hofer, Turnaround Strategies, *Journal of Business Strategy* 1 (Summer 1980): 19–31.

13. G. Hamel and C.K. Prahalad, *Competing for the Future* (Cambridge, Mass.: Harvard Business School Press, 1994).

14. H. Sperlich, quoted in G. Hamel and C. K. Prahalad, *Competing for the Future* (Cambridge, Mass.: Harvard Business School Press, 1994).

Strategic Management Planning Worksheets

Use these Worksheets as a template. If you find that you need more rows or columns, for example, simply add them to a rendition of the worksheet in a spreadsheet or on a ruled piece of paper.

Worksheet A-1 Product/Service Definition

Define the nature of the product or service that you wish to supply. This could be on the basis of diagnosis, procedure, service, patient characteristics, or the like.

Worksheet A-2 Market Profile

1. What is the size of the market? State in any relevant terms (patients, fees, geographical area, etc.).

2. What is your current market share?

3. What market share do you seek?

4. What market growth trends do you anticipate?

5. What life cycle stage is the market in (question, star, cash cow, dog, uncertain)?

6. Who are your biggest competitors, and what is their market share?

Source: Copyright © Lawrence J. Ring, Ph.D., used with permission.

Worksheet A-3 Segmentation: Identifying Important Market Segments

---

Now that you have described the total relevant market, how can it be subdivided into useful groups or segments? Look for major differences in the market. If the service is provided to a group of people, look for segments within the group or in treatment method. If the product is a treatment or procedure, look for subpopulations of customers.

Are there factors that might result in different levels of attractiveness across parts of the market? Examples might include demographics (age, sex, income, etc.), location (near, far, suburban), behavioral (benefits sought, usage rate, loyalty, etc.). Refer to the text for a discussion of segmentation.

Criteria for successful segmentation include the following:

- What segments are reachable?
- Are there segments that are differentially responsive to the pentagon marketing mix?
- Are there differential costs associated with reaching different segments?
- Is your segmentation exhaustive? Does your segmentation encompass the whole market?
- Are excluded segments ones that you don't care about or would prefer not to treat?
- How well do your market segments fit with how you currently provide service?
- How does segmentation fit with your mission statement?

What are some differences across the total market?

Worksheet A-4 Segmentation

Customer Benefits Sought	Segment A	Segment B	Segment C	Segment D	Segment E

Rank order benefits sought within each segment.

Source: Copyright © Lawrence J. Ring, Ph.D., used with permission.

Worksheet A-5 Decision Making

	Segment A	Segment B	Segment C	Segment D	Segment E
Who makes decisions?					
What is the decision-making process?					

Source: Copyright © Lawrence J. Ring, Ph.D., used with permission.

Worksheet A-6 Segment Profiles: Where Are We Now?

	Total	*Segment A*	*Segment B*	*Segment C*	*Segment D*	*Segment E*
Size ($, units)						
Your current share						
Share sought						
Expected growth						
Life cycle stage						
Largest competitor today						
Largest future competitor						

Source: Copyright © Lawrence J. Ring, Ph.D., used with permission.

Worksheet A-7 Environmental Analysis

1. What are current market trends?

2. Describe what competitors are doing in this market. What are the critical elements of their strategy?

Worksheet A-8 Competitive Analysis by Benefits

Use customer benefits identified in Worksheet A-4

Major Competitors	Benefit 1	Benefit 2	Benefit 3	Benefit 4

Source: Copyright © Lawrence J. Ring, Ph.D., used with permission.

+ = We are better
– = They are better
/ = We are about the same
? = Uncertain

Worksheet A-9 Evaluating Your Competition by Segment

Major Competitors	Segment A	Segment B	Segment C	Segment D	Segment E

Source: Copyright © Lawrence J. Ring, Ph.D., used with permission.

+ = We are better
− = They are better
/ = We are about the same
? = Not certain

Worksheet A-10 Situational Analysis (SWOT)

Evaluate strengths, weaknesses, opportunities, and threats by the overall market and by segments.

Refer to Chapter 9 for a discussion of SWOT analysis.

	Strengths	Weaknesses	Opportunities	Threats
Overall Market				
Segment A				
Segment B				
Segment C				
Segment D				
Segment E				

Source: Copyright © Lawrence J. Ring, Ph.D., used with permission.

Worksheet B-1 Marketing Strategy and Objectives

1. *Strategic Statement*: What is the overall plan of action that you have for approaching the market? Are there any elements of generic strategies that are relevant? Consider market segments.

Worksheet B-2 Risk Analysis

Event	Probability of Occurrence	Potential Impact	Contingency

Source: Copyright © Lawrence J. Ring, Ph.D., used with permission.

Worksheet C-1 Building the Pentagon and Triangle for Your Strategy

	Segment A Current Position	Segment A Plan	Segment B Current Position	Segment B Plan	Segment C Current Position	Segment C Plan	Segment D Current Position	Segment E Plan
Pentagon implications								
Product								
Place								
Value								
Communication								
People								
Triangle implications								
Systems								
Logistics								
Suppliers								

Source: Copyright © Lawrence J. Ring, Ph.D., used with permission.

CHAPTER 11

Organizational Integration

Chapter Objectives

The goal of this chapter is to help you get the parts of your health care organization to work together as an integrated whole. Integration is an outcome that can be improved by choosing or modifying the organization's structure. Organizational structure, therefore, is discussed as a tool for improving organizational integration.

Some people will resist change because they are afraid or feel that they will lose something as a consequence. This chapter presents strategies that the physician manager can use to overcome resistance to structural changes and other sources of change as well.

Integration is the process of getting the parts of an organization to perform in a coordinated, synergistic manner. Integration is important to health care organizations because it is a strategy for reducing costs and improving quality. If, for example, a hospital's nurses, medical staff, laboratories, pharmacy, housekeeping, and billing work more effectively with each other, so that patients on average are discharged four hours sooner than a competitor across town can achieve, this provides a competitive advantage. If, in addition, this integrated performance across jobs, departments, and professions results in patients, for instance, not waiting two hours in the radiology department or three hours for their physician to discharge them, then improved patient satisfaction will also occur.

The examples cited above make it sound as though employees and departments want inefficiencies to occur. Far from it. Generally, these inefficiencies occur as a result of employees,

groups, or departments trying to do what they do exceedingly well. They do it so well, in fact, that it is done to the exclusion of any other person's or group's needs, including perhaps the patient's!

For integration to occur, the achievement of employee, departmental, and professional goals must be subordinated to the larger organizational need. When this doesn't happen, and organizational units such as pharmacy, radiology, and respiratory therapy go off on their own, this is called suboptimization. As a perverse consequence of the organization's parts trying to excel in achieving their own narrow objectives, overall organization productivity is reduced.

As the size and diversity of an organization's product and service offerings increase, integration becomes more difficult to achieve. Diversified health care organizations have the most to gain from achieving integration. Consider a diversified health care system that provides tertiary level hospital services, outpatient surgery, outpatient primary and specialty care, nursing home services, and insurance, including indemnity, preferred provider organization (PPO), and health maintenance organization (HMO) products. Each of the products and services is contained in a separate part of this health care system, such as shown in Figure 11–1. Now, consider all the ways in which each part can perform that will make it look good but at the same time hurt the performance of the total organization.

Primary care physicians may shift costs to specialists by referring to them for procedures that they themselves could conduct. Similarly, specialists may choose to use the hospital's surgical facilities as opposed to their own if, as a result, they can shift costs to the hospital. The insurance company may be going after market share through low rates and as a result is flooding the system with more patients than the primary care physicians can handle.

If integration is the process of getting the parts of a health care organization to function together more effectively, then we will have to understand in detail the nature of the organization's parts, including their missions and incentives. Organizations are composed of parts. In the smallest organizations, each part is a separate job description. For example, in a solo private practice, the front office staff may comprise one person who performs all front office functions, such as answering the telephones, scheduling, insurance billing, and so forth. In this instance, it is relatively easy to achieve front office integration because it occurs in the brain of the office manager. In this type of organization structure, the challenge will be to integrate the roles of the office manager and the physician.

As organizations get larger, the size and degree of organizational unit specialization increase. The front office of a large, multispecialty practice might be divided into several functions, such as clerical, scheduling, collection, billing, insurance, and the like, each of which is part of the job description of the business manager in the solo practice. Each of these functions might well have a supervisor, and several persons may be employed within each function. In addition, the large, multispecialty practice probably has front office functions that the solo practice does not have, such as managed care contracting and information systems management.

STRUCTURE

The manner in which the parts of the organization are pieced together is called the organization's structure. An organization's structure should help it solve problems. If the organization's internal or external environments change, the structure often must change in response. Perhaps one of the most dramatic examples of this has been the decline in the number of solo practitioners and the growth of ever larger single specialty and multispecialty practices. Fundamental changes in the economics of medicine that place a premium on better utilization of fixed costs and competition for managed care contracts have resulted in practices changing their structure.

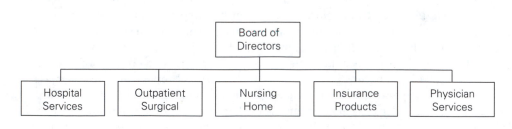

Figure 11–1 Diversified divisional health care organization.

Understanding the way in which the parts of the health care organization are assembled, or its structure, helps you answer the following questions:

- *Where do we draw the boundaries that define the specialized parts of the organization?* These lines are the boxes that appear on an organization chart. The boxes represent the grouping of human resources. In effect, these boxes or boundaries determine who works closely with whom.
- *What type of measurement and reward systems will be needed?* As we have seen in Chapter 5, employees ultimately do what is in their self-interest. Similarly, they will work in the aggregate toward those goals that they believe are in their group's, unit's, function's, or division's self-interest. By creating boundaries, we also create the need to think about the rewards that we have created for these organizational units. For example, if we reward a finance department for keeping costs under control, we should not be surprised when it limits resources to a pathology laboratory that is exceeding its expense budget. Unfortunately, this may occur even though the laboratory also is exceeding its net income goal by an even larger amount! If departments, and consequently their employees, are given goals and rewarded for keeping costs down and not for encouraging growth in net income, then we shouldn't be surprised by the wayward consequences.
- *How do we integrate the parts of the organization so that their individual contributions combine to achieve the organization's overall goals?* This objective can be achieved if we think carefully about how we draw the subunit boundaries, how we measure performance, and how we structure the rewards that define the relationship among employees, groups, and the organization.

We will begin discussing how to answer these questions by exploring the boundary choices that are available. There are three fundamental strategies for organizing all organizations, including those in health care: functional structure, divisional structure, and matrix structure. Each structure has strengths with some types of integration challenges and weaknesses with others.

A functional structure arranges the human resources by their function, or what they do. Figure 11–2 illustrates a hospital that is functionally organized. How is it determined where to draw the organizational boxes? Ultimately, this is a subjective judgment, but there are certain logical groupings. All the medical services are grouped together and report to one vice president. Similarly, marketing, nursing, and medical support services each have their own "boxes," so that people who work in these functional areas are grouped, work, and led together. As we descend deeper into the organization structure, we can see that functions may be broken into smaller subareas. Medical support, for example, has three major groupings within it: laboratory, radiology, and pharmacy. Medical is broken into orthopedic, cardiology, oncology, and emergency units.

Figure 11–3 illustrates the functional structure of a multispecialty practice. Once again, the basis for grouping people together is what they do. Notice that on occasion different aspects of the same process may be organizationally divided, such as the marketing groups under business administration and internal medical planning committees. In this case, the marketing professionals and physicians on the marketing committee are doing different aspects of the marketing function. Clearly, however, the two groups need to be coordinated, and this would be one important integration challenge and objective for this practice.

The organization chart also indicates the specific jobs that would have primary integration responsibility. The director of medical administration is responsible for integrating across the medical specialties (functions) of primary care, orthopedics, cardiology, oncology, gastrointestinal, and nursing. The directors of the internal planning committee and the external planning

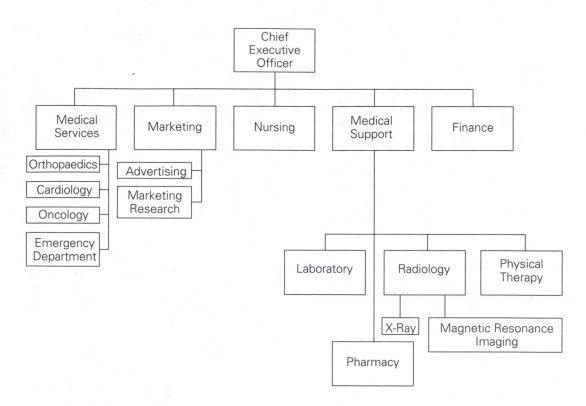

Figure 11–2 Functional hospital organization structure.

committee are responsible for integrating across committees that they supervise. The chief executive officer (CEO) is responsible for integrating across business administration, medical administration, internal medical planning committees, and external medical planning committees. Often, integration at this level will be supported by meetings chaired by the CEO and staffed by the functional heads.

Functional designs have the following potential advantages:

- *Economies of scale and high efficiency are possible*. Because all those performing a function are grouped together, they can work closely with each other, and the fewest number of employees will be needed.
- *Similar employees will develop collegiality*. Similar backgrounds, education, and training, coupled with common department goals, develop group cohesiveness. Employees who work together all the time

know each other's strengths and weaknesses and can compensate and adjust accordingly.

- *Performance standards are easy to set*. Everyone in a department is working toward the same goal, and the goals of the department are defined by the homogeneous function. Marketing is evaluated on marketing performance. All of the cardiologists work together and can set their own internal quality and cost standards, and so on.
- *Decision making and lines of authority are simple and clear*. If, for example, the director of information systems has a question about cardiology services, it is clear where he or she can go for an answer.

When a functional design is being used, the goal is to achieve these advantages while not incurring some of the potential disadvantages of this structure. The potential disadvantages include the following:

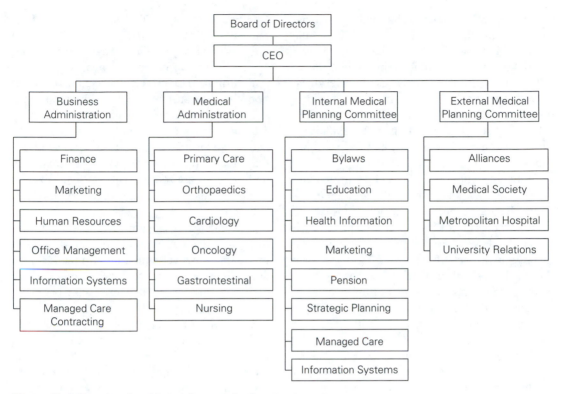

Figure 11–3 Functional multispecialty organization structure.

- *The functions may maximize (suboptimize) at the expense of the organization.* For example, if the information systems group develops information systems that meet its own needs regarding capital acquisition cost, maintenance budget, software budget, staffing, and functionality but don't fully meet the needs of users, such as the oncology group, then this would be suboptimization.

- *Members within a function can become insulated from the rest of the organization.* The horizon within a functional group is the function. Cardiologists will have a tendency to look at the practice from that perspective, and human resource professionals will have their own functional perspective on the practice. This within-group perspective can lead to narrow thinking, poor communication, and ultimately suboptimization.

- *There may be a tendency for "buckpassing."* Because no single function is responsible for a complete product, failure often results in everyone pointing a finger at another function. Oncology's failure to meet performance criteria may result in this department blaming information systems for producing misleading or incomplete outcome data reports and managed care contracting for contracting with the local asbestos factory. No one is willing to take responsibility because no one really has responsibility for the overall product.

In a functional structure, the ability of the CEO to integrate across functions and the willingness of the functional unit heads to think and act beyond their functions become critical to organizational success.

When the product mix or geographical dispersion of an organization create too many integration problems in a functional design, a divisional design is an alternative. Figure 11–4 shows the organization chart for the General Hospital System. We can refer to some of the components of General Hospital, such as Senior Services, HealthNet, and Professional Insurance Products as companies, because they have a complete functional structure within them, as denoted by the marketing (M), sales (S), and finance functions (F).

Why not combine all of General Hospital into one health care company? Selling hospital services, insurance products, senior services, and primary care services are so different from each other that they require a degree of specialization in order to do each of them well. There also may be regulatory and professional reasons to keep some of the companies, such as Professional Insurance Products and HealthNet Primary Care as separate distinct organizations with their own functional structures.

To illustrate this point further, consider the archetype of divisional organizations: General Motors Corporation. Why have a Chevrolet Division, Cadillac Division, Saturn Division, and so on? Consider the marketing problem for a moment. It certainly would be possible to have marketing people working back and forth across Cadillac, Chevrolet, and Saturn marketing projects. If I want to get really good at marketing Cadillacs, however, I probably need to spend a lot of time understanding the Cadillac product and the Cadillac customer. The Cadillac customer is different from the Chevrolet customer, and, as we have seen, the key to successful marketing (product, place, price, promotion, and people) is knowing your customer. If I really want to get good at marketing Cadillacs, given the complexity and expense of marketing cars, I probably have to specialize in this product line. Repeating the functions across different product or geographical companies allows an organization with a complex customer mix to match that complexity in its product mix. Because a whole product line or region is now an organizational unit, the lines of responsibility are also clearly established. If corporate is dissatisfied with Cadillac's productivity, it is clear where to look. Cadillac can't blame Chevrolet or Saturn. This structure, therefore, makes "buckpassing" more difficult because a unit has clear responsibility across all functions for a product or geographical area.

Returning to Figure 11–1, we see an organization chart for an integrated health care system that uses a divisional structure. Why have separate divisions for hospital services, nursing home, and insurance products? Just as with General Motors, the products and services that each unit provides are so different that specialization in marketing, finance, and service delivery is necessary.

The potential disadvantage of this structure is that, once again, suboptimization may occur. In this case, however, the suboptimization may arise out of the divisions. Divisions may achieve their objectives at the expense of the organization. In the early 1980s, Cadillac tried to increase its sales by developing a "low-end" product. The Cimmaron was a restyled Chevrolet Cavalier that sold for substantially less than other Cadillacs but about $4,000 more than the Cavalier. Not only was the Cimmaron a poor product in terms of quality and design, but it achieved some of its sales at the expense of Oldsmobile and Buick products. When one division's success is achieved at the expense of another division as opposed to external competitors, this is called cannibalization. When the outpatient services division opens an outpatient surgicenter that competes with the hospital services division's outpatient surgical services, that also is cannibalization.

Finally, a divisional structure has a lot of potential for unneeded personnel and resources. If all the marketing personnel and their support equipment and systems across the several General Motors divisions were consolidated into one huge marketing function, it is likely that fewer positions, computers, secretaries, and water coolers would be needed. It is likely, however, that the marketing product would suffer greatly as a result of the lack of specialization and the unwieldy size of the homogeneous marketing unit. The goal, of course, is to achieve the specialization that divisionalization can achieve without too much inefficiency.

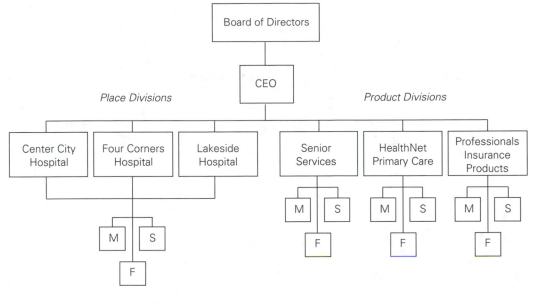

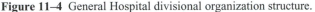

Figure 11–4 General Hospital divisional organization structure.

The role of top management in a divisional structure is to coordinate the roles of the different divisions. Top management sets overall divisional goals, helps define product and service parameters, provides financial resources, and allocates them to the divisions. All this is done with the objective of minimizing both suboptimization and unnecessary duplication.

Some organizations have developed a structure that combines aspects of both functional and divisional structures into a matrix. Figure 11–5 illustrates a matrix structure for an aircraft manufacturer. The columns contain the traditional functions of manufacturing, marketing, engineering, research and development, maintenance, and human resources, and each is headed by a functional director. The rows represent the different aircraft projects that are underway, such as the 727, 737, 747 projects. Each project is led by a project director. Inside the matrix is the 2-boss manager, who reports to a functional director on a career basis and a project director on an operational basis.

Each project director is responsible for a complete project across all functions. Similarly, each functional director is responsible for a function across all projects. Both the functional directors

and the project directors are at the same organizational level. Neither side of the matrix is superior or subordinate to the other. This means that, for the organization to be successful, both sides must cooperate.

For example, suppose a sales agent returns from southeast Asia with the news that there is an opportunity to make a new sale of 737s. He or she needs some additional sales and marketing assistance to put together a proposal. The 737 project director, who is responsible for all aspects of the 737 project, including sales, does not have the line authority to move marketing and sales personnel across projects. This must be coordinated with the functional, marketing, and sales directors as well as with the other affected project directors.

In a well-run matrix organization, top management is totally outside the matrix. Top managers should not resolve issues between the two sides of the matrix. To do so would remove the need for discussion, negotiation, and ultimately integration across the two sides of the matrix. If top management provides the solutions, then the name of the game is "get to top management first." Instead, top management's role is to provide strategic direction and financial resources.

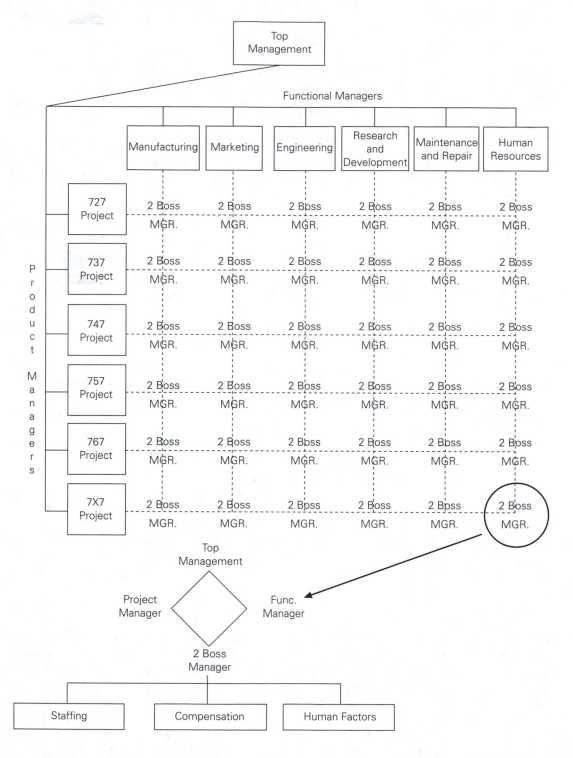

Figure 11–5 Matrix organization structure.

Working in this type of environment requires considerable interpersonal skill. Communication and negotiation skills, seeing the problem from other groups' perspectives, and understanding organizational goals are all absolutely essential in this type of structure. Matrix organizations require a high level of integration. Why create a structure that is so highly dependent on successful integration? The answer lies in the types of industries where matrixes have emerged. Generally, these industries utilize sophisticated, expensive technology that is in a constant state of change. To succeed, they must be constantly changing and successfully reallocating their expensive resources and personnel to where they are most urgently needed. Aircraft manufacturing (Boeing), shipbuilding (Newport News Shipbuilding), and space exploration (the National Aeronautics and Space Administration) are three industries that have successfully applied matrix structure concepts.

The matrix structure also is applicable to some health care organizations. For example, many integrated health care systems need to pay close attention to operational efficiency, which can be best managed functionally. Clinical and business information systems, for example, need to be effectively managed across the entire organization. Human resources costs need to be controlled, and personnel need to be assigned to where they are most needed. Financial controls need to be applied across all programs and departments to create a level financial playing field. At the same time, rapid changes in medical technology, managed care, and the desires of patients create value in closely managing critical product and service lines. For example, coronary surgery, emergency department, oncology, maternity, insurance products, primary and hospitals care may be product lines that are critical to a health care system's success in the marketplace. Someone needs to be paying undivided attention to each of these "profit centers." After all, patients and employers (i.e., customers) have no intrinsic interest in the underlying functional support systems. Their concern is with the service.

Figure 11–6 illustrates a hospital matrix in which support services, cardiac services, and information systems cut across the major "product lines" of the organization's hospitals and outpatient physician services. Patients come to this organization for the services offered by the product lines, and the product line directors are therefore patient-focused. They are interested in providing the most efficient highest quality services possible. If they were left to their own devices, however, they might create organizationwide inefficiencies, such as redundant cardiac service facilities and standalone information systems that only met local needs. The "row" directors are concerned with producing the most effective and efficient systems from a total organization perspective. This may result, for example, in a common information system that attends to all provider needs, but does this in a coordinated *organizational* fashion. Similarly, cardiac surgery services may be limited to one hospital. If the heads of both sides of the matrix can work together, then the needs of each side of the matrix can be balanced. The reward, measurement, and support systems will be critical to the success of this matrix. The matrix will have to be staffed with people that understand this integrated mission and who are committed to it. Selection and employee development become critical so that the right people with the right mindset staff the matrix.

Figure 11–7 contains a matrix for the Department of Nursing at Abbott Northwestern Hospital. Notice, once again, that each side of the matrix is attending to a different need. The columns are patient-focused and the rows are system-focused. Notice also, that this chart tells us nothing about the rest of Abbott Northwestern's structure. Different parts of a larger organization can have a local structure that meets local needs. Matrix units, for example, can exist in an organization that is otherwise departmental, functional, or matrix.

If the health care organization is structured functionally, there may be little coordinated emphasis on realizing the potential of each service line. Information systems may tend to be de-

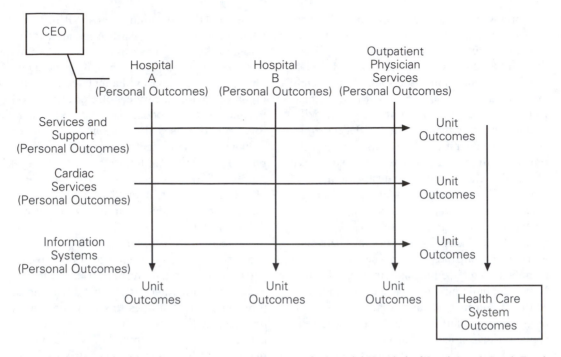

Figure 11–6 Matrix health care system structure. Courtesy of Memorial Hospital of South Bend, South Bend, Indiana.

signed with the needs of the information systems, people (function) foremost. Alternatively, organizing only around products and services could easily result in overspending on resources and suboptimization across product and service lines as each one tries to maximize its position in the organization. For example, why should oncology use the hospital's information system or electronic medical record if oncology can develop its own that will best serve oncology's needs? Without the control of a functional constituency, no one will say "Hold it! We need to talk about this. Perhaps I can make it work better for you!"

Under these circumstances, a matrix structure could offer some obvious strengths by simultaneously attending to both the functional and the product/service axes. This situation points out, however, that a matrix structure must be more than a drawing on a piece of paper. Critical to a matrix's success is that those on the matrix's sides and in the matrix must truly behave in an appropriate manner. Communication, negotia-

tion, cooperation, a desire to achieve organizational goals (i.e., to act in an integrated manner) become essential. The key to achieving these behaviors are measurement and reward systems that create personal incentives to act in appropriate ways. Failure to act in these ways can lead to the bane of matrix organizations: too many meetings, too much talk, and not enough action.

In summarizing all three structures, we can see that integration becomes a central concern for each one. What needs to be integrated varies with each structure. In a functional organization, integrating across functions is the challenge; in a divisional organization, the challenge is to integrate across products and locations. The challenge in a matrix organization is to integrate within and among functions and products/services. Understanding the type of structure that you have will help you identify where you need to develop organizational integration. Finally, given the integration issues that you identify, you may want to consider changing the organizational structure to one that more directly

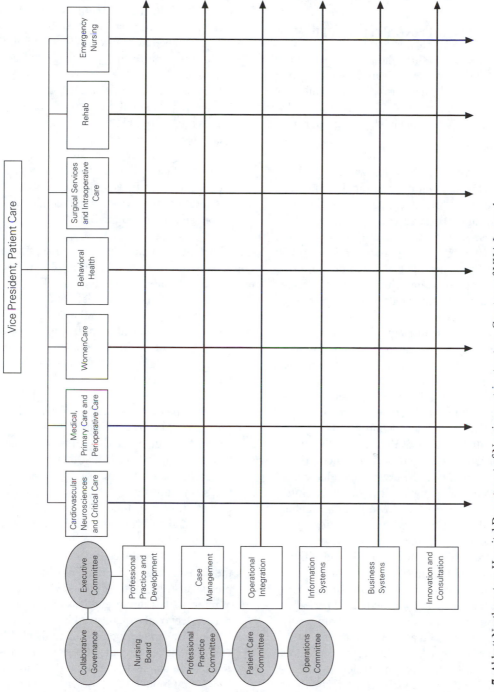

Figure 11–7 Abbott Northwestern Hospital Department of Nursing matrix structure. Courtesy of VHA Inc. and Abbott Northwestern Hospital.

complements the nature of your products and services.

FACTORS INHIBITING INTEGRATION

We have seen that the nature of the organization's boundaries can either help or hinder integration. There also are other sources of inadequate integration. At a generic level, four additional factors that inhibit integration are as follows:

1. *Complexity*. This occurs when there is a large volume of information that must be exchanged for integration to occur, but the support systems are not adequate. Because of the inadequate information exchange, two or more parts of the organization cannot optimally coordinate their actions. An example would be the coordination required to reduce waits for testing and special services in the hospital. Each unit, such as radiology, has its own schedule, as does the attending physician and the patients, based on where they are in their respective treatment protocols. Coordinating all this activity to reduce average patient waiting time is a complex data exchange and scheduling problem. As a result, it often doesn't happen effectively.

2. *Differentiation*. This occurs when different subunits in the organization have different values, attitudes, and behaviors. Differentiation can arise from a number of differences, including education, professional orientation, and goals. Historically, differentiated groups include physicians, administration, and nursing.

3. *Poor informal relations*. When differentiation goes on for an extended period of time, a history of distrust and animosity can build, so that it takes on a life of its own. In some hospitals, for example, this has occurred between physicians and administration. Administrators assume that physicians just don't understand their perspective on decision making, never will understand, and have no interest in

understanding. As a result, physicians are viewed as adversaries and often are not brought into the decision-making process. Similarly pessimistic attitudes can be developed by physicians about administrators. The result is unintegrated actions.

4. *Physical size and distance*. Size and distance can also inhibit the coordination of activities. Obvious examples include a hospital system with facilities and personnel spread across an area. Similarly, within a facility the physical distances between patient beds, physician offices, laboratory, physical therapy, administration, and so on can inhibit integration.

The electronic revolution has great potential to reduce size and distance barriers. Electronic medical records, integrated clinical and financial databases, e-mail, local area networks of personal computers, personal digital assistants, image digitizing and transmission, faxing, and the like all serve to reduce this integration problem.

Barriers to integration that are specific to health care organizations include the following:

- *Embryonic development of most clinical information systems*. Clinical information systems are difficult to maintain and develop. One difficulty is that they are intrusive. Clinicians who are trying to treat patients find it difficult to record clinical data because this takes time. In addition, unless the clinical information system can take into account the illness burden of a physician's or health care system's patients, the data can be misleading. For example, if physician A has a higher than average system mortality rate or readmission rate, this may reflect on the quality of his or her care. It may also simply indicate that this physician has sicker patients. Information systems, such as the Johns Hopkins Ambulatory Care Group (ACG) system, attempt to adjust for illness burden. These systems, however, are relatively recent and are only partially successful.

- *Separate, unintegrated financial and clinical information systems*. Health care organizations developed financial information systems first because of the need to bill accounts. Clinical information systems evolved out of the financial systems because the financial systems did capture some clinical information. Overall, however, the financial information systems were inadequate for making clinical decisions, such as evaluating treatment protocols and physician outcomes. The financial information systems did not capture the right pieces of clinical information, and they did not adjust for the sickness of patients. Until the financial and clinical information systems become integrated, each alone may create incentives for its respective users that send them off in different directions. For example, in an unintegrated setting, financial data may indicate that building a new cancer treatment center may not be justifiable. Similarly, physicians may look at clinical outcomes and argue that care could be improved, cost reduced, and market share gained. If the financial and clinical systems are not working on the same basis and using the same data, then it is impossible to resolve the divergent conclusions.
- *Nonalignment of goals among parts of the health care organization*. Employed physicians working for a health care system with no productivity incentives often reduce their productivity to levels below those before their contracts were purchased, and they often stop looking for ways to improve efficiency and reduce costs. The physicians' gain is the hospital's loss. Similarly, primary care physicians working under capitation may be able to reduce their costs by overreferring to specialists to the detriment of total system cost.

INTEGRATION MECHANISMS

How do we overcome these barriers to integration? There are a number of standard approaches to this problem that are applicable to health care organizations. These are summarized in Table 11–1.

Probably the most basic approach to integration is to establish a management hierarchy. In effect, we create a job whose responsibility is to create integration. For example, the position of medical support director in Figure 11–2 has responsibility for coordinating across laboratory, pharmacy, radiology, and physical therapy. This approach of adding organizational layers is in contrast to an empowered approach to managing, which goes in the direction of pushing decision making down to lower levels.

When the amount of work that managers must do to integrate becomes too great, they can be "extended" by adding staff positions. The staff's role is to work with the organization units, gather information, report back to the integrating manager, and help each unit coordinate with the others.

Rules and procedures are an effective integration strategy when integration is required around routine matters. We can establish a rule, for example, that says "Whenever X-ray film inventory reaches 35 percent of nominal, contact purchasing to order more" or "Whenever an account goes into 90 days past current, audit it and take some action within two business days."

Figure 10–2 illustrates a patient flow process for diagnosis-related group (DRG) 209 that integrates the functions that need to be coordinated if the DRG is to be treated in an efficient and effective manner. Similarly, critical pathways can be thought of as sophisticated integration methods. Exhibit 10–1 contains part of a critical pathway for total hip arthroplasty. The columns contain the time standards, the rows the activities, and the cells specify what should happen for integration to occur. These diagrams illustrate how triangle systems can serve as a source of integration.

Goals and plans are another integration tool. A hospital system's management services organization (MSO) sets a goal of improving its managed care competitiveness in eight months. The MSO's management concurs that some of the things that must occur include:

- training physicians to understand how they affect financial outcomes,

Table 11–1 Comparison of Integration Methods

Integrating Methods	Advantages	Disadvantages
Management Hierarchy	Links together all the organization's functional parts.	Cumbersome and can break down.
Staff	Can supplement hierarchy.	Can create its own integration problems.
Rules and procedures	Economical way to create integration around routine matters.	Limited to repeatable issues.
Plans and goals	Can handle nonroutine matters.	Cost in terms of time, effort, and physician involvement.
Committees and task forces	Can handle a large number of unpredictable problems.	Costly. Team members need group skills.
Integrating roles	Can handle a large number of unpredictable problems.	Difficult to find the person with the right skills and characteristics.
Measurement and reward systems	Can use motivation to obtain integration.	Unmeasured activities or outcomes can be ignored or undermined. Can produce dysfunctional behavior.
Selection and development systems	Acquire and improve skills needed for integration.	Expensive and can take a long time to achieve.
Organizational boundaries		
Functional	Integrates within functions.	Does not facilitate integration across functions.
Product/geographical	Integrates within a product, service, or geographical lines.	Does not promote integration among product, service, or geographical lines.
Matrix	Promotes integration among and across functions and products.	Expensive, complex, can generate tension and conflict.

Source: Adapted with permission from P.F. Schlesinger et al., *Organization: Text, Cases, and Readings on the Management of Organizational Design and Change*, p. 119, © 1992, Irwin.

- training reception staff to send triage patient calls to appropriate levels,
- acquiring managed care projection software,
- training employees and physicians in the use of the software and the assumptions that it makes, and
- developing a patient education process, so that patients will understand when to call, thereby eliminating many unneeded office visits.

The goal, as a result, has increased integration. For instance, physicians who understand the business aspects of their medical decisions are more likely to practice in a manner consistent with the assumptions being made in the managed care projection software. Similarly, those working with the software will be more likely to make reasonable assumptions if they work with business-knowledgeable physicians during the model building phase. By establishing these integrated goals, the physician services office begins training physicians in the business aspects of medicine. Simultaneously, the information systems unit begins evaluating managed care decision support software.

Committees and task forces can be effective ways of using current staff to make integrated decisions. By drawing physicians and administrators from various medical specialties and management functions across the health care organization to staff a committee, we can bring a wide range of perspectives to the table. Figure 11–3 illustrates a multispecialty practice that uses committees as part of its standard structure.

Committees and task forces also provide flexibility because, by their nature, they are temporary structures. A task force is a temporary grouping of personnel who are given a specific goal to achieve. After the goal has been reached, the task force is dissolved. Sometimes task forces are referred to as project teams. Once again, this is a temporary unit that will be dissolved after the mission has been accomplished. They can expand and contract in size, add members to bring in additional relevant constituencies, and even go away if the need for them no longer exists. Often, physicians feel that committee work is frustrating and inefficient. When contrasted with the alternative, however, which is to create full-time positions to do the work of the committee, it can be an efficient, low-cost option.

Integrating roles are usually used when integration is difficult to achieve but is nevertheless very important. Generally, integrating roles have no direct authority over the areas to be integrated. This prevents "railroading." Instead, integration is achieved through personal influence and leadership skills. Often, the physician staff office in a hospital system performs this function.

Another approach to using integrating roles is to create a project manager position to integrate services across a product line. An oncology project manager could, for example, integrate all inpatient and outpatient oncology services across a health care system. This position's perspective would cut across professions, specialties, and organizational units with the goal of improving the cost and quality of oncology services. If this approach becomes common in a health care system, then the structure has evolved into a matrix.

Measurement and reward systems are two of the most powerful integration tools. The goal is to assess personnel and subunits based on their cooperation and achievement of joint goals. Giving employed physicians incentives that are congruent with health care system goals for lower costs and improved clinical outcomes is one example of how a reward system can integrate two parts of the organization.

It is important to remember that the reward system must support integration and not work against it. Providing rewards without thinking about the system effects can foster suboptimization. Independently rewarding physicians based on outcomes, laboratories on reduced turnaround time, and administrators on lowered costs without considering how these measurement and reward systems may interact can create a suboptimizing outcome.

Selection and development systems are long-term approaches to improving integration. Managers and physicians can be selected based in part on whether they have the interpersonal skills and attitude necessary to work cooperatively. Similarly, providing team development and employee development training can improve current employees' integration skills. Promotion across functional lines and systematic job rotation across functional or divisional lines are two commonly used ways to develop employees' abilities to think in integrated terms. Physicians, nurses, pharmacists, and others with clinical experience who acquire management skills can make excellent managers because they can see both sides of a problem.

Finally, we can modify organizational boundaries to include interdependencies. Patient-centered units in which diagnostic and treatment facilities are located under unit control can increase the integrated delivery of services. Moving from a functional structure to a divisional structure based on medical services, such as illustrated in Figure 11–1, will increase the integration around the service. Often, the move from a functional to a divisional structure is a result of increased size and the need to specialize in the delivery of services. As health care systems grow in size and diversity of products and services, the evolution into a divisional structure is an appropriate response. For health care systems

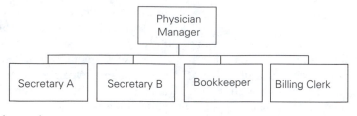

Figure 11–8 Simple practice structure.

that have particularly important integration issues across both function and product/service line, adopting a matrix structure may be an appropriate response.

SMALL PRACTICE STRUCTURES

The challenge of integration also applies to small practices. The structural choices available to small health care providers, however, are different. Small providers generally adopt a simple structure (Figure 11–8). This structure is often so simple that none of the participants may perceive that there is any structure at all! In a simple structure, everyone reports to the physician manager. As a result, the physician manager becomes the focus of all the upward and downward practice communication. If Joanne, a secretary, has a problem that she can't resolve herself, Dr. Smith, the physician manager, is the one she will tell. Dr. Smith will then have to do something about it, even if it is nothing more than telling Joanne to work it out with one of the other secretaries. This type of structure can provide the physician manager with a lot of information about daily practice operations, especially if the physician manager is willing to listen to employees and they feel that the physician manager is responsive to reasonable requests.

One of the primary responsibilities of the physician manager in the simple structure is integration. The physician manager becomes personally responsible for making certain that each employee's contributions fit together, so that the totality of employees' efforts results in a smooth-running, coordinated, and productive team effort. The problem with this scenario is that it takes too much physician time. An alternative is the office manager structure (Figure

11–9). In this structure, the office manager takes over some of the management responsibilities that were previously assumed by the physician manager, and performs the front line management tasks. In effect, this is the simplest of functional organizations. The office manager directs the daily activities of office staff, sets priorities, implements standard office policies, and coordinates the efforts of the front office to produce integrated, effective group performance. The physician manager's management role is to supervise the office manager, focus on long-term planning, and assist the office manager in problem solving and procedure revision on more significant front office issues.

Effective communication between the physician manager and the office manager is essential to the success of this structure. Weekly meetings often form the basis for vertical integration between the physician manager and the office manager. For example, if the accounting reports indicate that expenditures for supplies seem to be rising, the physician manager would ask the office manager to determine the reasons why and propose solutions. The office manager would be responsible for implementing changes and keeping the physician manager informed of progress made in controlling these expenditures.

A potential disadvantage of this structure is that the physician manager is removed from day-to-day operations and is dependent upon the skill and ability of the office manager. If the office manager is not capable of making decisions that are generally consistent with your management philosophy, you will find yourself micromanaging and constantly reviewing your office manager's daily decisions. You will effectively be operating as though there were no office man-

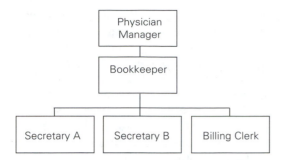

Figure 11–9 Office manager structure.

ager, yet you will be paying a salary for one! In addition, the office manager will come to resent the micromanagement, and the office manager's subordinates will realize that he or she is a figurehead. All this will tend to create dissension and dissatisfaction. This scenario points out the need for employees to have the right personal characteristics to operate with the level of independence required by the structure.

If you find yourself in the position of reviewing all of an office manager's decisions, you should ask yourself some hard questions, such as these:

- Are you perhaps too perfectionistic?
- Are you able to recognize that there may be more than one effective solution to a problem?
- Is it possible that the office manager's solutions to problems could be as effective as your solutions?

If, after sincerely considering these questions, you conclude that the problem lies with the office manager, then you need a new office manager. Unfortunately, with this type of practice structure, you may not notice that the details are going unattended until a major problem develops. The delegation of power and authority through an office manager structure can provide you with great power because it effectively multiplies your presence. Unfortunately, delegation is a double-edged sword that can wound you seriously if your office manager is inadequate.

The office manager structure suffices for most private practices. Larger practices, however,

may find it necessary to evolve additional structural elements to deal with the complexity and quantity of information in such functional areas as marketing, information systems, collection, billing, and human resources. In effect, they evolve into fully developed functional structures.

As functional structures in practices grow, partners often take responsibility for supervising one or more functions. One physician might take on quality management, another assumes responsibility for human resources, another supervises financial issues, and so forth. By dividing the management responsibilities in this manner, the partners achieve two objectives: they reduce the amount of time that each partner devotes to practice management, so that no one is unduly burdened, and each partner develops a relative degree of expertise in one or two functional areas, with the result that the practice as a whole acquires more total management expertise.

When physicians functionally specialize, it is important for them to integrate across functions. On occasion, the partners should meet with the objective of achieving integration. Each partner should familiarize the others with what is happening in his or her functional area of responsibility. These meetings also should focus on integrated goal setting for the functional areas. Often, one physician will act as a managing partner, making daily business decisions and chairing the cross-functional partner meetings.

CHANGE

Physicians have always had to adjust to a changing clinical environment as science has developed new procedures, medications, and equipment. The health care business environment, however, has been characterized by stability. That is no longer the case. There are a number of forces generating change in health care organizations. Technology is a major source of change. Clinical and financial information systems that produce data that physicians can be evaluated on, such as clinical outcomes, cost, and patient satisfaction are changing the nature of how physicians practice. Some physicians adapt while others resist these changes.

Another source of change is social trends. In 1993, everyone thought that fundamental health care change would occur as a result of government regulation. Fundamental change did occur, but it came from an unexpected direction: the private sector. In reaction to the rising cost of health care, physicians, commercial insurance companies, and for-profit and not-for-profit health care systems have made significant changes in both the clinical and the business parts of health care.

Competition is a major source of change. Providers are reacting to and in anticipation of change. Reducing inpatient beds, purchasing physicians' practices, reorganizing hospitals, and developing MSOs, PPOs, and HMOs all force the competition either to change or to risk being uncompetitive and irrelevant.

The natural evolution of product/service life cycles can also be a source of change. Table 9–1 contains life cycles for a number of specialties as of 1993. The dynamic nature of medicine has resulted in many of the procedures already shifting from one life cycle stage to another.

Finally, new ways of thinking about health care are also a source of change. Physician managers with management and financial skills who can apply total quality management (TQM) methods and understand the relevance of developing an activity-based cost management system, among other abilities, are changing their organizations. It is hoped that the readers of this book will be a source of change in their organizations.

All these forces are resulting in the need for physician managers and others working in health care to change the way they are organized and how they deliver and practice medicine. Unfortunately, many resist change. Resistance can arise for a number of reasons. Some people realize that they will lose power and political control. For example, you decide that your practice has grown to such an extent that it is necessary to move from a simple practice structure to an office manager structure. As a result, a secretary who previously reported directly to you and was allowed considerable autonomy sees that she will lose the status of reporting directly to you, be more closely supervised by an office man-

ager, and have less discretion regarding the utilization of her time. As a result, she resists the change instead of embracing it as necessary given the changed circumstance. Others resist because they don't really understand the nature of the change. Some resistance is a result of informed, honest disagreement. Finally, some resistance occurs because of individual differences, such as having a personality with a high need for control.

Often, underlying all these reasons is a simple and basic motivation for resisting: fear. When people are afraid of something, they will create all sorts of rationalizations and justifications within which to wrap their resistance. Fears that they may not be able to adjust, that they perhaps don't have the necessary skills, or that they won't be able to learn the new skills are all motivations for resistance to change.

It is important to recognize, however, that not all resistance to change is bad. Resistance creates a hurdle, so that ideas are scrutinized and modified if necessary to make them work. Having too low a hurdle for change can result in organizational chaos and bad decisions. An example of this problem occurred during the mid-1980s. This physician saw the potential of personal computer–based office automation and decided that he was going to automate all aspects of his small group practice, including billing, account management, collection, scheduling, and word processing. He tried to do this using a computer with 128 kB of RAM and a 20-MB hard drive. In addition, the medical office management software was inadequate to the task, and the database software was "buggy" and lost several mailing lists. To make a long story short, after six months of frustrating effort on the part of his staff, the computer system found its appropriate place as a dust collector in an unused back office. In this case, the hurdle for change was too low. The physician's partners did not sufficiently challenge him to justify why the whole business operation should be automated, whether it could be, and why that should occur at this time and on such a broad basis. The outcome was disastrous and eventually was an element that led to the dissolving of the practice.

The type of resistance that I am concerned about is resistance that is not based in rational thought and occurs after a thorough analysis still indicates that change is necessary. What can you do to reduce or eliminate this type of resistance to change? Over the years, a number of tactics have been devised to introduce change in ways that will lower or overcome resistance. These strategies vary in terms of how quickly they implement change, the amount of planning required, and how much others are involved in the change process. Following is a number of change strategies proposed by Schlesinger and colleagues that are summarized in Table 11–2.[1]

Education and Communication

This tactic relies on familiarizing potential resisters with the reasons behind the change. This tactic is particularly effective when resistance is based on erroneous or insufficient information. Relying on education and communication to reduce resistance can take time. It also means that potential resisters must trust you. If they do not, they will simply dismiss the information as propaganda.

A classic example of resistance at the practice level resulted from the personal computer revolution in the 1980s that brought widespread office automation to private practices. Many office managers resisted this trend. Using education and communication involved discussing the reasons why automation was needed. Pointing out the increased ability to manage the collection process, generate more accurate and timely insurance billing, and so forth fits into this category.

In the 1990s, the development of critical pathways is generating physician resistance in large hospital systems. Education and information focusing on how critical pathways help physicians improve quality and lower cost are fundamental strategies for addressing this issue.

Participation

In this approach, potential resisters are allowed to participate in the design and implementation of the change. If you don't have all the information that you need to design the change, participation allows you to obtain additional information from others. Participation also creates ownership, and owners are more likely to want the change to succeed. There are some risks to using participation. Participation can lead to changes that you didn't anticipate or that don't meet your needs. In addition, the participation process can absorb large amounts of time. Perhaps one of the most destructive decisions that a manager can make is to use "false participation." This occurs when managers tell others that they will participate in the decision-making process, but if a solution is produced that management disagrees with, the participation is then withdrawn. This teaches others to distrust management.

Returning to our office automation example, including the office manager in the selection of hardware and software would have helped lower fear, gain access to the best information about what really would have worked in the office, and created a sense of ownership on the part of the person who was most critical to the project's success. Similarly, including physicians who will be critical to implementing critical paths on the teams that develop them not only provides access to information necessary for developing high-quality pathways, but also creates commitment to using the pathways.

Facilitation and Support

This approach to diffusing resistance to change involves providing training and support for employees, so that they will be able to adjust to the new circumstances. For example, in the office automation instance, effective facilitation and support would have included extensive software training as opposed to throwing employees in a room with the training manuals and saying, "Okay, go to it!" The 1990s analog is providing physicians with training in the use of an electronic medical record.

Negotiation

Negotiation amounts to buying out the opposition. In effect, you give the resisters something they want in exchange for something you want.

Table 11–2 Change Strategies

Tactic	Best for	Advantages	Disadvantages
Education/ Communica- tion	Resistance based on lack of information or inaccurate information and analysis.	Once persuaded, people will often help with the implementation of the change.	Can be time consuming if large numbers of people are involved.
Participation	Situations in which initiators do not have all the information needed to design the change and others have considerable power to resist.	People who participate will be committed to implementing change, and any relevant information they have will be integrated into the change plan.	Can be time consum- ing. Participants could design an inappropriate change.
Facilitation and Support	Dealing with people who are resisting because of adjustment problems.	No other tactic works as well with adjustment problems.	Can be time consuming and expensive and still fail.
Negotiation	Situations where someone or some group will clearly lose out in a change and where they have consid- erable power to resist.	Sometimes this is a relatively easy way to avoid major resistance.	Can be too expensive in many cases. Can alert others to negotiate for compliance.
Co-optation	Very specific situations where the other tactics are too expensive or not feasible.	Can help generate support for implement- ing a change (but less than participation).	Can create problems if people recognize the cooptation.
Manipulation	Situations where other tactics will not work or are too expensive.	Can be a relatively quick and inexpensive solution to resistance problems.	Costs initiators some of their credibility. Can lead to future problems.
Coercion	Situations when speed is essential and the change initiators possess considerable power.	Speedy. Can overcome any kind of resistance.	Risky. Can leave people angry with the initiators.

Source: Adapted with permission from P.F. Schlesinger et al., *Organization: Text, Cases, and Readings on the Management of Organizational Design and Change,* p. 119, © 1992, Irwin.

This, of course, implies that you have some bar- gaining chips. Negotiation can be effective when it is obvious that the change is going to result in an employee losing something of value, but you have something to offer that will mitigate this loss. Remember, however, that negotiation sets a precedent that you will "pay" for resistance to

change. In the future, others may choose to resist with the hope that they too will be able to extract a price for their cooperation.

Co-optation

When you co-opt someone, you make him or her part of the change process by giving him or her a desirable or visible role in the change process. Co-optation can be a quick, effective way to overcome resistance because it ties the resister's fate to the fate of the change.

There are two dangers associated with co-optation. First, if an employee is intent on doing employment suicide just to spite you or just to demonstrate to everyone that you were wrong, everyone will go down in flames. Second, as with negotiation, you will teach others that they can benefit by resisting. This may result in encouraging future resistance.

Manipulation

Manipulation is defined as attempting to influence behavior covertly. It often involves selectively revealing information. You tell others only enough to obtain their cooperation. Manipulation can also include telling half-truths and even outright deception and lying. The downside of this strategy is that it can eventually result in reprisals. You may find yourself justifying its use by thinking "I have to get this change implemented now. I'll worry about the consequences later." If you don't have the power to coerce and you need to get something done quickly, manipulation can be an effective strategy. The downside of manipulation is that, almost always, people eventually learn that they have been manipulated or misled. Once this occurs, there will be a price to pay. Manipulation often leads to reprisals in a similarly indirect manner, such as passive-aggressive behavior.

Coercion

When you use coercion, you try to force employees to accept the change by telling them that, if they don't like it, they can quit, be fired, lose additional benefits or power, or be passed over for promotions or pay raises. The advantage of using coercion is that it is fast. If you must put a plan in place tomorrow, then coercion will allow you to quickly overcome immediate resistance. This is a risky way to introduce change, however, because people resent being coerced. Once again, as with manipulation, you will engender retaliation at a time and in a place of the other's choosing.

Summary

Most health care organizations should gravitate toward using "top of the list" strategies. By this I mean that, because of the nature of health care organizations, they should generally rely on education and communication, participation, facilitation, and support. They should rely to a lesser degree on cooptation and negotiation. Manipulation and coercion are generally not appropriate in most health care settings and situations. There are a number of reasons for this. Most health care organizations have found value in a TQM philosophy of management. Education, participation, and facilitation fit well with the idea of creating an organization climate in which employees are motivated to find problems as opposed to hiding them, and are rewarded for fixing them as opposed to continuing to do things in the same way. In addition, integration is much easier to achieve when all understand why they must integrate and how their actions affect others. Once again, this is not likely to occur in an organization characterized by manipulation, coercion, and the fear and distrust that these tactics can engender.

Here are some pointers regarding choice of change strategies[2]:

- The greater the anticipated resistance, the more consideration should be given to using slow change methods. Greater levels of resistance are more difficult to overcome. Low levels of resistance can be blitzkrieged.
- The greater your power, the better your relationship with employees and peers, and the more they accept the legitimacy of your acting unilaterally, the easier and more productive it is to use fast change methods. If your position is weak relative to the potential resisters, such as relative to your peers in an equal partnership, then you should use slower methods.

- The more you will need others to help you design or implement the change, the more you should rely on slow change methods. For example, if you know that you need to develop a local area network across several primary care practice locations, then including physicians from each location in the selection of the system would be important. This will take more time than unilaterally selecting a system. You would do best to employ one or several slow change methods that directly include system users.
- The greater the immediate threat to organizational survival, the more you may have to rely on fast change methods. If the immediate stakes are not high or if the negative effects of postponing change will not occur for some time, then you may be able to afford to use slower methods.

The final step in the change process is planning it. Think seriously about the significance of the problem. There are few situations in life in which an opportunity is irrevocably lost if it is not immediately grasped. Many of us have inclinations to act quickly and decisively. This tendency needs to be tempered by considering whether this speed will be gained at the cost of resistance, and for no material gain in competitive advantage.

Next, thoroughly analyze the sources of potential resistance. Who might resist and why? Think about who has the necessary information and whose cooperation is essential. Consider your level of power relative to potential resisters. Finally, construct a change plan. How will you go about working with those who are likely to resist? What change methods will you use? What will be the timing and sequence? As you implement your plan, retain some flexibility. As unforeseen events arise or as new information surfaces, be flexible enough to change your tactics to fit the developing situation.

CASE APPLICATION: UNITED FAMILY PRACTICES, LTD.

As Fred Anderson, M.D., signed the final document creating United Family Practices,

Ltd., he wondered whether he and his colleagues really knew what they were getting into. The financial logic behind the joining of seven previously independent practices and 25 family practice physicians was compelling.

Currently, about 15 percent of local patients were under some form of managed care. Most of Anderson's colleagues believed, however, that within three years 50 percent of local patients would be under some form of managed care. The practices brought with them a patient base that Anderson estimated to be 15 percent managed care, most of which belonged to a large PPO run by the state Blue Cross company.

As a group, United Family Practices would constitute a significant percentage of local family practice physicians and would have to be reckoned with by any managed care organizations in the area or entering the area. Its purchasing power should result in obtaining the best possible prices for medical and business supplies and capital items. Over time, the partners planned to consolidate their locations, thereby reducing fixed costs for rent, personnel, and capital equipment. By controlling these costs, they could compete effectively for managed care contracts. Finally, as members of a large group, they hoped to have the resources to invest in the best technology and personnel and thereby be able to provide the highest-quality care.

No, Anderson wasn't worried about the finances. After all, an assemblage of accountants and consultants had assured everyone that this was a sound financial and strategic decision. What Anderson was worried about was how to manage 25 physicians and an initial support staff of 94.

The plan that Anderson, the other physicians, and consultants developed to organize United Family Practices seemed to make sense. One physician from each of the seven founding practices would serve on a board of directors. The board would elect from its members a managing physician as the CEO, who would be appropriately compensated for this work. In addition to his or her clinical practice, the CEO would make most daily decisions needing physician concurrence, such as final approval of advertising and promotions, small managed care contracting decisions, and routine supply purchases. The CEO would seek board concurrence for decisions with major financial or long-term implications, such as making a job offer to a physician, accepting HMO and other managed care contract proposals, and developing a practice strategic plan.

The CEO and the board hired an administrator, Pete Reynolds, who had an MBA and four years of practice administration experience working as an internal consultant to the physicians of a large integrated health care system. His responsibility was to handle day-to-day practice management. His duties included supervising the billing/receivable process, developing internal practice policies and personnel procedures, assisting the CEO, making sure that costs in all parts of the practice were being controlled, and coordinating all aspects of daily practice operation.

Anderson felt confident about the CEO's and the administrator's job descriptions. He was uncertain, however, about the structure below the administrator. The seven founding practices were spread across nine different locations. To keep things simple and retain some semblance of normalcy for the physicians, the new practice would retain most of the old physician–staff reporting relationships.

The former office managers of each practice would still be responsible for the operation of their locations, and they would report to Reynolds. Billing would remain decentralized, but each office manager would send Reynolds daily paper reports, such as work completed, cash receipts, insurance billings, insurance collections, and aging analyses. In addition, physicians would retain their previous staff relationships with nurses and secretaries. Purchasing of supplies, however, would be centralized through Reynolds.

Anderson and most of the other physicians strongly supported this organization structure because they retained significant local control, which made the whole experience less frightening. For example, if a secretary or a nurse had performance problems, the affected physician

and local manager could quickly handle it. Hiring would be handled locally also, with the needs of the local physicians being of paramount importance.

A feeling of local control was especially important for location A, which primarily had an inner-city, Medicaid patient base, and location F, which was positioned in the two most affluent suburban counties and still had a high proportion of indemnity insurance patients. Physicians in these locations felt that their needs and their patients' needs were somewhat different from the group's other locations, and it was important to them to be able to practice accordingly.

A minority of physicians had some reservations about the practice's structure. One of the physicians commented:

> One reason for forming a large group practice was to operate more efficiently. The way we have organized, however, doesn't do much to help us act as *one* practice. We need to encourage interdependent, coordinated behavior, but our organization structure appears to work against this. The days of 25 or even 7 Lone Rangers, each charging off in their own direction, are over or will be soon. But how do we integrate the parts of United Family Practices, Ltd., so that as a group we are better than we were as seven competing practices?

This case illustrates the importance of structure and change to a practice that is adjusting to the challenges of managed care. The current structure creates all sorts of integration problems. Other than purchasing, there is virtually no integration. Billing, contracting, human resources, office procedures, information systems, and treatment protocols are all separate and uncoordinated across the locations. In its current state, United Family Practices possesses none of the advantages of a large group practice.

Why is it this way? This may have been the price of admission. Probably what we see here is the most that all the physicians were willing to give up to come together under one roof. The structure, even with all its faults, at least allows them to affiliate. It gives them the opportunity to reshape themselves so they can compete as an integrated organization in a managed care environment. In a sense, perhaps the very fact that they exist as a practice is an indicator of successful integrative negotiating. If, however, this is the level of integration that exists a year from now, United Family Practices will not be realizing its potential.

This case also points out the importance of anticipating resistance to change and then effectively managing it. Duplication in some positions, such as the former office managers, ensures that there will be a lot of fear and suspicion surrounding any proposed changes. United Family Practices does not need seven office managers. In addition, the practice needs some positions that currently do not exist, such as positions to direct and coordinate information systems, human resources, and managed care contracting. Some of the office managers may be capable of performing or being trained to perform these jobs. Some of the current office managers may have to be terminated. Similarly, many of the office staff will be changing duties and reporting relationships, and some will no longer be employable. In this environment, the CEO and the administrator will have to anticipate resistance and effectively address it.

Physicians will also be a source of resistance. Reward systems, reporting relationships, adoption of treatment protocols, referral standards, taking personal responsibility for managing costs, and implementing clinical quality control (including peer evaluation) on a routine basis are some of the challenges that United Family Practice's physicians will face if they are to compete successfully in a managed care environment. Once again, the task facing all the physicians and the administrator will be to identify the needed changes and put them into operation in spite of the fears and resistance that will arise.

To overcome, or at least lessen, the level of resistance, extensive use of education and communication, participation, and facilitation and support will be essential for the practice to put the changes in place that will be needed. It should be obvious that any reliance on manipulation or coercion in as fragile an environment as exists at United Family Practices would be a certain prescription for disaster.

CONCLUSION

Physician managers need to be aware of how to use structure and change to improve organization integration. Structure should help the health care organization deal with internal and external challenges. As the challenges change, the structure may need to adapt in reaction to or in anticipation of these changes.

Resistance to change is a natural response to fear engendered by the unknown. Resistance that is not addressed can result in failure to implement needed changes. Currently, a common source of resistance in many parts of the country is to managed care. Some physicians still feel that it will never arrive in their community or that it can be worked around. Expressed in this manner, this is hope, not the result of careful, considered thought and certainly not the outcome of a plan. They may be correct, but if they are then they will be lucky. If they are wrong, then their resistance may result in delaying actions on their part that could further their survival.

REFERENCES

1. P.F. Schlesinger, et al., *Organization: Text, Cases, and Readings on the Management of Organizational Design and Change* (Homewood, Ill: Irwin, 1992), 352.

2. J. Lorsch, "Managing Change," in *Organizational Behavior and Administration*, ed. P. Lawrence, L. Barney, and J. Lorsch (Homewood, Ill.: Irwin, 1976), 676–678.

CHAPTER 12

Total Quality Management

Chapter Objectives

Total quality management (TQM) is an important force in the evolving health care system. You will learn the fundamentals of the TQM management philosophy and why processes, employee participation, and a TQM organization culture can be critical to the success of both large and small health care organizations as they adjust to the changes being generated by managed care. In addition, you will become familiar with TQM tools and their uses, such as run charts, Pareto charts, fishbone diagrams, and statistical analysis. Finally, you will understand where your role as a physician manager fits into the TQM process.

Quality is a concern that has become an expressed preoccupation of U.S. business. It is difficult to pick up a copy of the *Wall Street Journal*, *Business Week*, or *Fortune*, or for that matter *The Journal of the American Medical Association* or *American Medical News* without seeing an article on or reference to the importance of quality or a story documenting an organization's attempts to improve its quality. Historically, quality has been of paramount concern to physicians. The life and death nature of health care services, coupled with their complexity, results in quality being an obvious element in the success of any health care organization. The question, however, is: How can health care organizations achieve quality, and at what cost?

Total quality management (TQM) is a term that has been applied to the most highly developed, all-encompassing management strategy for obtaining quality. TQM principles are applicable in varying degrees to all levels of health care organizations, ranging from solo private practices to hospitals and managed care companies, and go by a number of other names: quality improvement (QI), continuous quality improvement (CQI), and so forth. The benefits in terms of patient, customer, and employee satisfaction as well as quality of service delivered, reduced costs, increased profitability, and productivity can be substantial. TQM, however, is not without its costs. TQM requires major investments in changing the organization's culture, developing ways of assessing performance, and inventing new ways of providing services. Just as there have been well-documented TQM success stories, there have also been notable failures. TQM, when put into operation as a quick fix, an impulsive response to competition, an advertising gimmick to attract customers (patients, employers, or insurers), or a fad to utilize because that is what sophisticated organizations are "supposed" to do at the millennium, is likely to fail. With it will go the substantial psychological capital invested by managers and employees as well as time and financial cost.

Physician managers need to understand the implications of instituting TQM so that they can make an informed choice about whether this approach to managing will be helpful to their organization. Physician managers normally don't have technical TQM skills, just as they don't have technical skills in accounting, finance, business law, and marketing. As a result, physician managers typically will not apply technical TQM tools, such as statistical analyses, Pareto charts, and run charts, just as they would not identify a specific personality test to use in employment or assemble an income statement. Instead, their role will focus on determining the need and the targets for TQM, setting direction, and marshaling resources: in effect, managing the process. To do this, physician managers need to be familiar with TQM concepts and methodology. Physician managers in clinical roles will be important participants in improving clinical processes, so they reflect both medical and management considerations.

THE ROOTS OF TQM

The fundamental nature of TQM was defined during the 1920s and 1930s by two employees of the Hawthorne Works of Western Electric, the manufacturing arm of AT&T. AT&T, and the Hawthorne Works in particular, had a long history of industrial engineering and management research. Walter A. Shewart, an engineer on a team investigating quality and control problems, discovered the significance of understanding, measuring, and displaying variability. Figure 12–1, for example, contains a control chart that displays the variability in a hospital's business chart error rate. It reports the percentage of a sample of a hospital's charts containing one or more errors. An error, for example, might include a missing signature, incomplete insurance verification information, illegibility, or the like. The UCL line is the upper control limit. The UCL can be statistically defined. A standard, for example, can be set at two standard deviations

around the mean. Variability above or below the UCL is considered out of tolerance.

The importance of variability is that it can be used to identify the sources of quality problems. For example, what happened in months 2, 4, and 18? Were these months in which new employees were working? Was there a volume increase, or were new management procedures implemented? Once variance is identified, then causes can be sought, problems identified, and variance reduced. If, for example, the variance in Figure 12–1 is associated with new employees, then the cause might be inadequate training or ineffective employment methods. Changing the training or employment processes should result in increased quality.

This example illustrates that work is performed through processes. In this case, the process defines when and by whom charts are completed. Generally, quality problems occur because the work process has been poorly designed or not designed at all. By studying variation and changing the process through which work is performed, one can dramatically improve quality. Focusing on the process as opposed to the individual is central to TQM.

The control chart in Figure 12–1 illustrates one of the tools that TQM practitioners use to display variability and describe quality. This is one of the TQM tools that Sashkin and Kiser have referred to as the seven old tools; the other six are charts, fishbone diagrams, run charts, histograms, scatter diagrams, and flowcharts.[1] Each of these tools is discussed below. In each case, an example is provided in the context of receivables collection.

Figure 12–2 illustrates a Pareto chart, named for Vilfredo Pareto, an economist who first noted that most wealth is controlled by a few individuals. A Pareto chart displays the number of quality problems by their source. Figure 12–2 displays a practice's out-of-tolerance receivables (90+ days) by various causes. One widely noted observation is that most problems are attributable to a limited number of causes or sources. Pareto charts, therefore, can be helpful to determine where your effort can have the greatest payoff. In this case, understanding why practice policies are

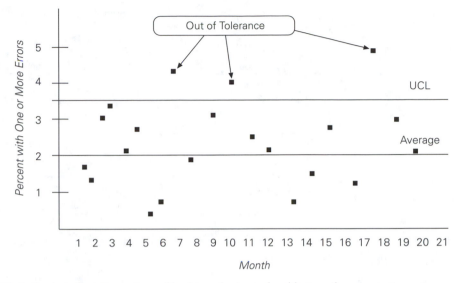

Figure 12–1 Control chart: Percentage of business chart sample with more than one error.

not being enforced and fixing that problem appear to be the first places to direct effort.

Figure 12–3 contains a fishbone diagram, also called a cause-and-effect diagram. The diagram represents hypotheses regarding the major sources of the effect noted at the end of the diagram. Constructing a fishbone diagram helps stimulate thinking about a problem. Because it is difficult to represent the interaction among various causes (bones), fishbone charts should not be taken too literally. Displaying information this way can be useful, however, to summarize the results of brainstorming and to express logical thinking about a problem.[2]

A run chart shows quality trends over time. Figure 12–4 contains a run chart for the receivables in 90+ days. A run chart can be particularly helpful in collection management because it will allow you to detect when a change has occurred. The physician manager can then inquire and di-

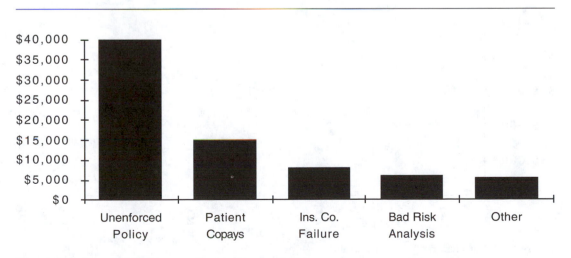

Figure 12–2 Pareto chart: Sources of receivables in 90+ days.

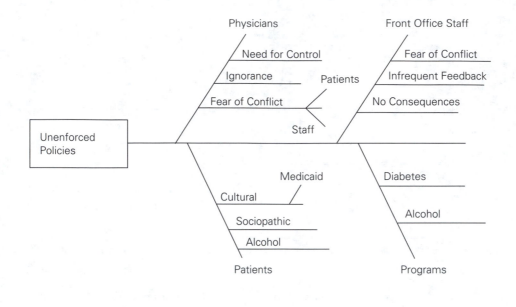

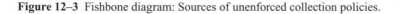

Figure 12–3 Fishbone diagram: Sources of unenforced collection policies.

rect corrective action. For example, the chart shows that something happened in July. The control level at approximately $10,000 was exceeded in that month, and a steady climb in receivables ensued. If the practice regularly utilized a run chart, this would probably have been noticeable in July and certainly by August.

A histogram can be useful for displaying the relative frequency of data by categories. Figure 12–5 displays a practice's receivables by aging categories. Histograms or bar charts are helpful for showing a static display of the relative size of different categories. They can, however, hide trends that are occurring over time. For example,

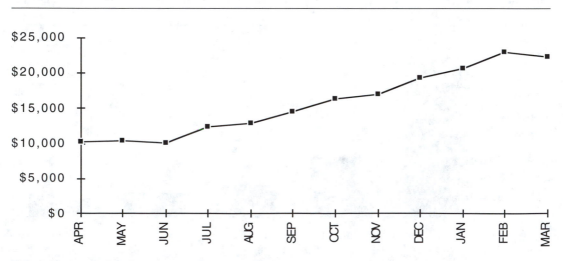

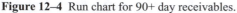

Figure 12–4 Run chart for 90+ day receivables.

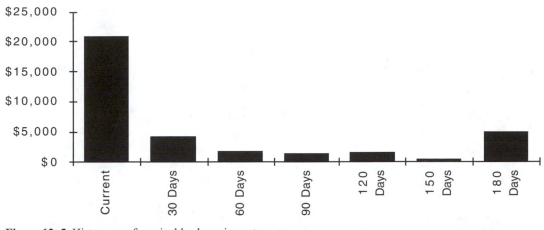

Figure 12–5 Histogram of receivables by aging category.

if most of the values in the 180 days category have recently entered it, the meaning would be different than if most of the entries had entered the category three months ago.

A scattergram displays data for two variables and can indicate the relationship between them. Figure 12–6 shows a scattergram illustrating the relationship between number of procedures per month and new patient receivables (0 to 30 days old). The general slope of the relationship from lower left to upper right indicates that the two variables covary: As procedures increase, the size of new receivables also increases. This *may* be due to cause and effect, but scattergram data are correlational and do not prove cause and effect. For example, suppose that a hospital acquires an inner-city outpatient dialysis program. This program could be expected to attract low-income patients with a higher incidence of alcohol and drug problems that are causal to their disease process. Social, economic, and cultural issues, not volume per se, are the drivers, and the scattergram data in themselves do not directly point us to these causes.

Shewart's work centered on developing statistical methods for identifying and displaying variability in the manufacturing process. W. Edwards Deming, also at Western Electric at that time, extended Shewart's work into a general theory of management. Deming was instrumental in developing statistical tools and display methods, and he trained a generation of engineers and managers in their use. He observed, however, that the ability to use these tools did not ensure that quality would necessarily improve. Deming, who became the personification of the TQM philosophy, recognized that control charts, statistical analyses, and exhortations to improve quality don't solve quality problems. Improvements in quality only occur when managers and employees are willing as well as able to use the information to change the production process.

As he examined his successes and failures, Deming concluded that the management and organizational contexts within which the TQM tools were used were critical to quality improvement. He summarized the management characteristics that he felt were necessary for quality to flourish as his 14 Points.[1] They define the parameters of the TQM management philosophy and provide insight into the physician manager's TQM role.

1. *Create constancy of purpose for improvement of product and service.* Deming stresses that quality should be the primary goal, not profit. Profit is a by-product that will flow from quality. Although this may sound naive, it can be expressed in an-

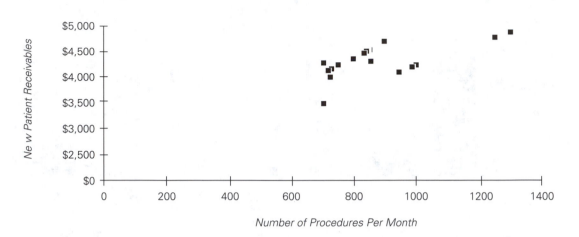

Figure 12–6 Scattergram of new patient receivables in 0 to 30 days and number of procedures per month.

other way: Quality is a less direct but more certain route to obtain profits.

2. *The whole organization must adopt the new philosophy.* The central importance of quality must be accepted by all employees, not just selected pockets, levels, or work teams. It must permeate the organization from the highest level down to the bottom. If this doesn't occur, TQM can result in limited successes on the more easily defined quality problems. There will not be the opportunity, however, to improve in unexpected areas where quality problems are not obvious to the initiated or to improve beyond what is now considered acceptable.

3. *Understand the purpose of inspection.* Mass inspection assumes that quality can be added on at the end by correcting errors. Errors are wasteful because it is much more expensive to fix a mistake than to build the product right or provide the service correctly to begin with. The most important purpose of inspection, therefore, is to identify the reasons for poor quality. Generally, this can be achieved much more easily and effectively by sampling than by inspecting all output.

4. *End the practice of awarding business on price alone.* The primary criteria to use when selecting suppliers should be their willingness to meet customers' needs and their willingness to work toward improving quality. Price should be considered, but only as a secondary issue. Many health care organizations are wrestling with this issue. In a sense, short-term, immediate cost savings may be incompatible with long-term quality improvements, which ultimately may be more frugal *and* effective.

5. *Constantly improve, and continue to improve production and service systems forever.* Quality improvement must be an ongoing process. It never ends, and there is no improvement level beyond which quality is considered excessive.

6. *Institute training.* Deming recognizes the need to train workers in statistical control methods and the use of quality control tools. He also states that all workers must be fully trained in the technical skills needed to perform their jobs. Finally, he notes that it is necessary for managers to have training in management and organizational skills because these are essential to create a climate in which TQM can flourish.

7. *Teach and institute leadership.* This means developing managers' skills to set a vision, gather the necessary resources,

obtain the cooperation of others, and design management systems, including TQM. It means creating a culture in the organization that truly values quality.

8. *Drive out fear*. For quality to flourish, employees at all levels must feel secure. They must know that making or finding errors will not lead to retribution. Telling the truth, pointing out a problem, and thinking of new ways to do the job will not occur if employees believe that they will be punished overtly or covertly as a result of their acts. Deming views regular performance appraisals as fear inducing and detrimental to quality because they focus on and tie compensation to short-term job performance. Deming's position in this regard is at odds with ideas expressed in Chapter 2 of this book. This contradiction will be discussed in more detail below.

9. *Break down organizational barriers*. Often, work groups, teams, departments, divisions, and so forth will compete with each other. This can be over budgets, personnel, reputation, or power. When this happens, the organization as a whole loses because the parts of the organization won't work together with an undivided interest to satisfy the customer's needs. Organizational barriers, therefore, turn coworkers and colleagues into competitors. These barriers will prevent the integrated delivery of health care services. They must be removed. Strategies for improving integration were discussed in Chapter 11.

10. *Eliminate exhortations and slogans*. Quality cannot arise from short-term motivational and inspirational "highs." If workers want to do better but don't have the tools to do it or are working in an organizational culture that punishes it, then exhortations to improve are viewed as hypocritical. If, on the other hand, employees are motivated to improve quality and work in a climate in which this is rewarded and not punished, exhortations and slogans will be viewed as superfluous if not demeaning.

11. *Eliminate numerical production quotas*. When production goals become the primary goal, quality will suffer even if quality standards are met. Production quotas will replace the emphasis on stretching quality beyond the current standard. Instead, the emphasis will be stretching production statistics beyond the current standard while producing standard quality.

12. *Remove barriers to developing pride of skill*. Providing adequate training, high-quality materials and tools, and an organizational culture that encourages developing skills and producing a high-quality product will enable employees to develop pride in their product or service. Employees who take pride in their work will have a built-in incentive to improve quality because it will increase their pride and personal satisfaction.

13. *Encourage education and self-improvement*. Beyond using the tools and methods of quality control, Deming believed that employees need to learn how to work together as a team. They need to learn new behaviors and ways of interacting. Behavioral science skills, such as team building, leadership, and change management can help employees develop these skills.

14. *Take action to accomplish the transformation*. Top management must put these ideas into action. Managers cannot leave it up to lower level employees because the key to improving quality is to involve the whole organization in a culture of quality improvement. Only top management has the stature and resources to animate the whole organization toward a common quality objective.

In Deming's view, TQM does not exist until these 14 points are endemic to the organization. This goes beyond platitudes and grand statements by top level management. These policies must be truly incorporated into every employee's way of thinking about his or her job. Deming's approach to quality goes far beyond the use of statistical tools and control procedures, which are necessary but insufficient in themselves for quality to flourish.

Implementing variance charting and other quality tools is the easiest part of instituting TQM. The most difficult part is to develop the organizational culture in which quality is central. It should be no surprise, therefore, that some organizations limit their operationalization of quality to the tools of TQM, the mechanical instruments. The success of this approach is generally limited because employees at a fundamental level do not have a reason truly to excel toward quality.

Our discussion of quality to this point describes a process to achieve it. There is another element to add, however, that focuses on the purpose of quality. Deming proposed that the purpose of quality is to produce a product or service that "meets the demands of the market."[3(p.41)] In other words, *the purpose of quality is to obtain customer satisfaction.*

Defining quality by focusing on the customer's needs should sound familiar. This is consistent with our definition of marketing. A marketing approach starts with customers' needs. Products and services are then developed around these needs, and they are then priced, placed (distributed), and promoted and the organization is staffed so that they meet customers' needs. This contrasts with a selling approach, in which a product or service is developed because it meets *your* needs, with the subsequent goal being to convince the customer why he or she needs to buy it.

Joseph Juran further developed Deming's idea of satisfying customers' needs as the focus for quality through what he calls the Juran Trilogy. The Juran Trilogy comprises quality planning, quality control, and quality improvement. The idea behind quality planning is to build quality into the product or service at the outset as opposed to plating it on by catching mistakes before they reach the customer. Figure 12–7 il-

lustrates the impact of quality planning. In this example, the current level of quality planning has built in a 20 percent operating deficiency. Examples could include procedures that build in wasted operating room time, physician time, X-ray film, payroll dollars, and the like.

The quality control process focuses on "fire fighting," such as identifying and fixing the sporadic spike, sometimes referred to as special variance. Special variance is due to intermittent causes. For example, why does the success rate at a fertility clinic suddenly "spike down" by 50 percent over a three-month period? Once the spike has been detected, the search for personnel, material, and procedural causes can proceed. Notice, however, that this says nothing about, nor does it address, the adequacy of a clinic's "normal" in vitro fertilization success rate.

Some waste, however, is chronic because of the way the activity was planned from the very beginning. This doesn't imply bad motives on the part of the planning personnel. Instead, the planned-in waste may be due to lack of thought or failure to consider some issues. The quality improvement process (Figure 12–7) focuses on driving down the overall level of waste by changing the basic process, as opposed to simply catching the spikes and special variances.

Using Juran's Trilogy, it becomes clear that the greatest and least costly opportunity to improve quality is in the initial quality planning. It should not be surprising, therefore, to note that Juran discusses marketing research as intrinsic to successful quality planning. Specifically, marketing research is a process for identifying the quality needs of customers. It is a method of finding out what features are important and how your product or service compares with those of your competitors[4]. It allows you to build in the quality from the customer's perspective, as opposed to finding out after the fact that your service does not fit the customer's needs or wants.

Juran describes a road map for quality planning that focuses squarely on meeting customer needs[5]:

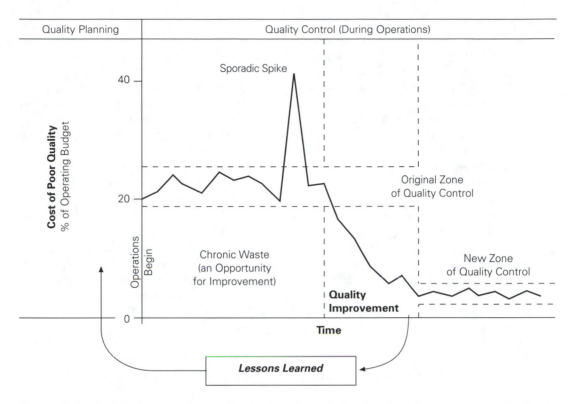

Figure 12–7 The Juran Trilogy. *Source:* Reprinted with permission from J.M. Juran, *Juran on Planning for Quality*, p. 12, © 1988, The Free Press.

- *Identify the customers*. Customers are those who will be affected by your efforts. For a health care organization, there could be a wide variety of customers. As noted in Chapter 9, the definition of customer in the 1990s is complex and may include patients, patient families, insurers, employers, government, and primary care physicians. A patient's primary care physician is the cardiologist's customer. Similarly, the cardiologist may be a customer of a hospital's billing staff, critical care nurses, and laboratory. Not all constituencies are equally important, but all are relevant. This intertwined customer list lends additional importance to Deming's observation that quality must be endemic to the whole organization. Customers are *everywhere*. Pa-

tient customers will be affected by several processes, such as admitting, scheduling, billing, and discharge, which in turn may be reciprocal customers to each other. If we define quality as meeting customer needs, then we must also consider the needs of these internal customers.

- *Determine customers' needs*. Do this in *their* language, so that they can communicate effectively with you. As a physician manager conversant in business thinking and language, you should be able to solicit this information from business customers, such as insurers, finance, marketing, and management administrators, and others. Your medical background will also allow you to solicit the needs of medical customers, such as referring physicians, staff physicians, pharmacy, personnel, nurses, and so forth. This ability to communicate across both sides of what previously was a fence is a unique strength of the physician manager.

- *Translate those needs into your language.* Here, the role of the physician manager becomes particularly important. As a physician who understands the language of business and the perspective of management, you can be a particularly skilled translator because you also understand the issues from a medical perspective.
- *Develop a product (service) that can respond to those needs.* Physician managers need to be able to work with other health care professionals to develop services that meet internal and external customer needs. As the professional with the optimal management and medical perspectives, the physician manager has a critical role.
- *Optimize product or service features so that they meet your needs as well as the external customers' needs.* Here, Juran is talking about balancing the needs of the various constituencies. Physician managers, once again, are uniquely qualified to balance the medical and business considerations of a problem.
- *Develop a process that is able to produce the product or service.* Remember, improving faulty processes, not personnel, is at the heart of quality improvement. A practice, hospital, or health care system can develop treatment protocols and a process for revising them based on clinical outcomes, cost outcomes, and research. Similarly, it could conduct patient attitude surveys, focus groups, and brainstorming to assess systematically patient and physician perceptions, and it could use these findings to develop the treatment protocol further.
- *Optimize the process, don't suboptimize it.* Just because customer needs can be identified does not mean that all employees will work toward their achievement. Suboptimization (see Chapter 11) occurs when various constituencies deviate from the organization's goals to meet their own needs. The surgeon, for example, who insists on stocking a lens that is not demonstrably superior and the management information services department that insists that all computer consultants be under its direct supervision may both be suboptimizing. Joint planning, avoiding subunit goals, evaluating managers on organization success and customer satisfaction instead of department goals, and obtaining participation from all constituencies are ways to avoid suboptimization.
- *Prove that the product works under operating conditions.* For example, put the treatment protocol into effect. Observe clinical, cost, and patient satisfaction outcomes. Are they as expected? If they are not, study the problem again. If they are, then:
- *Transfer the process to the operating forces.* Put the changed process into operation, and use it according to the operating plan. The plan should also have feedback mechanisms so that, as conditions change and as the definition of quality evolves, quality can be continuously improved.

Envisioning quality as encompassing internal and external customers and variability assessment tools leads to the possibility of intervening in the quality process at several points. These checkpoints are places where quality can be assessed and inserted into the process. These are described in Figure 12–8, where they have been related to the pentagon issues of infrastructure (discussed in Chapter 10) that are so critical to delivering integrated care. Because quality is first defined by the customer, quality checkpoint 1 (QC1) is the opportunity to assess customer satisfaction. Examples of QC1 assessments include patient surveys, interviews, and focus groups. Because parts of the organization are the customers of other organizational parts, these same methods are appropriate for internal use. In a hospital, for example, a QC1 assessment might

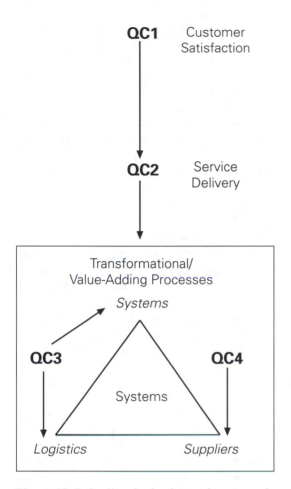

QC1   Customer
Satisfaction

QC2   Service
Delivery

Transformational/
Value-Adding Processes

Systems

QC3   **QC4**

Systems

Logistics   *Suppliers*

Figure 12–8 Quality checkpoints and pentagon issues.

include a critical care staff focus group of physicians, nurses, and respiratory therapists. Similarly, patient data that incorporate quality of life measures would constitute a QC1 assessment. Organizational climate surveys are another form of QC1 data. QC1 data are a particularly important quality issue for medical procedures with aversive side effects, such as bone marrow transplantation.[6,7] Understanding patient perceptions of quality and then using these data to improve quality not only provides a better patient outcome but also makes the provider more competitive.

QC2 is located at the point of service delivery. Control tools such as Pareto charts, run charts, and other ways of describing clinical and cost outcomes and their variability focus on this checkpoint. Many organizations concentrate all their quality efforts at QC2 without appreciating that performance at this point is an input to QC3 and an outcome of QC1. Reinfection, mortality, morbidity, time, number of procedures, and an almost limitless number of financial variables are all ways of assessing QC2 quality.

QC3 is located at the point where materials come into the organization. These materials can be physical, such as antibiotics, syringes, and magnetic resonance imaging machines, but they also can be human. For example, using effective employment methods (see Chapter 3) to hire the best staff can pay substantial dividends at QC2 and QC1. Consider the costs of using work samples, simulations, role plays, and tests for hiring administrative and professional personnel. Think of all the ways that a higher caliber of employee manifests itself downstream in higher quality at QC2 and QC1. Imagine now the value that can be added by using work samples and other truly effective selection procedures to improve medical and administrative performance. Other QC3 examples are logistical and purchasing systems that ensure that specifications are appropriate and supplies are acquired in a timely manner.

QC4 moves the quality process back one more step to the supplier. For example, Japanese auto manufacturers work closely with vendors and suppliers, to the degree that they help them design parts and develop their management systems. In the United States, auto manufacturers are doing the same thing. Currently, Ford has greatly reduced the number of engineers designing engine seals and gaskets by moving the design work back to the parts supplier. The Ford engineers then assume the role of coordinators, integrators, and project leaders. Developing this close relationship with the supplier pays off in better-fitting parts that are more reliable and are delivered reliably when they are needed, not before and not late.

Working with suppliers that are willing to consider designing their product to satisfy their customer's (i.e., the health care organization's) needs is the basis for Deming's admonition to end the awarding of contracts on price alone. Because the cost of rework increases at each successive step, quality that can be designed in before your organization acquires the product or service is the least expensive way to add value. For example, a supplier that studies a hospital's utilization patterns and packages sutures and heart valves in more useful quantities may be a better choice than the low-cost vendor. Similarly, health care organizations that work with internship programs and universities to develop physicians with management skills as well as medical skills may produce higher-quality physician managers than health care systems that try to train physicians in management skills in midcareer.

TEAMWORK: THE CORE OF TQM AND ORGANIZATION INTEGRATION

In a hospital or medical practice, internal customers reside in different functional parts of the organization. The challenge is to integrate these different parts. As we have seen in the discussion of organization structure (Chapter 11), different parts of an organization have different perspectives, goals, and incentives. This can result in suboptimization, or the achievement of local goals at the expense of the organization's goals. Complex processes, such as medical treatments, cut across many different organizational groups. How, then, do you integrate these diverse groups, which have different immediate goals, perspectives, and even languages?

A fundamental TQM concept for addressing this integration problem is the idea of a quality team. Quality teams are assembled to cut across organizational boundaries. They include members from all groups that contribute to or affect a process. Because even processes in fairly small practices cut across organizational boundaries, teams become important because no one can see the whole process. In this way, differing per-

spectives can be focused on a problem or process. Often, quality teams are assembled to tackle a specific problem. In this case, their members should include all constituencies that are affected by the problem.

For teams to function effectively, they must develop a culture that is consistent with long-term objectives. Why would an employee want to contribute to solving a problem if he or she knew that the solution would result in a lower personal performance evaluation? Obviously, the employee wouldn't. Why would a team member want to contribute ideas that might be viewed as counterproductive back in "the shop"? Once again, he or she wouldn't. To make TQM teams effective, therefore, it is important to develop an organizational culture and environment that focus on solving problems as opposed to assigning blame and on achieving integration among organizational parts as opposed to protecting turf. This issue of individual responsibility for job performance is one in which the TQM culture may be at odds with some traditional management thinking.

Traditional management thinking says that employees must be responsible for their personal behavior and that there should be consequences as a result. Traditionally, managers used the performance appraisal process to evaluate and document job performance and then, as a consequence, to make compensation and promotion decisions. Traditional management thinking is more short-term focused; TQM is more long-term focused. Traditional management thinking assumes that, if there are no short-term evaluation consequences, employees will lose focus and not excel. TQM, on the other hand, assumes that relieving employees of short-term performance requirements will free them to look at their jobs in a larger and longer-term perspective. The discussion of empowerment in Chapter 5 may be helpful for thinking about this problem.

Empowerment, or pushing decision making and involvement down to lower levels, is essential for team-based TQM to succeed. As Bowers and Lawler discussed, empowerment is appropriate under some circumstances and not others.[8] One of the variables that they used to determine the appropriateness of the situation for empowerment was type of person. Employees with high growth needs (high need for achievement, recognition, responsibility, etc.) who are flexible and adaptable and have or desire to possess strong interpersonal skills are good candidates for empowered jobs. These also are the characteristics of employees who can flourish under TQM. Employees who seek achievement for achievement's sake and an internal sense of satisfaction do not need the regimentation of a short-term focused appraisal system to structure their performance. In contrast, some employees obtain little or no satisfaction from the work itself. They are rigid and set in their ways, have limited interpersonal skills, and do not wish to develop the range and depth of their talents. These employees will be frustrated by empowered jobs and will have great difficulty adapting to the fluidity of a TQM environment. In addition, they may take advantage of a system that does not pay close attention to short-term performance through regular performance evaluations.

In a larger sense, there is no conflict between a TQM culture and traditional management thought. The link between the two lies in the employment process. If employees are being selected whose personal characteristics and work ethics are inconsistent with the TQM culture, then this is a process problem that is located in the selection process. The wrong people are being hired. The selection process needs to be changed, so that the organization will be more likely to select those employees who will thrive in a TQM culture. Work samples, personality testing, simulations, and other sophisticated employment methods that were discussed in Chapter 3 need to be utilized to solve this process problem.

What is the role, then, of performance appraisal in a TQM environment? Performance appraisal must become more oriented toward goal setting and employee coaching than an after-the-fact accounting of past performance. Similarly, the performance evaluation system should be changed to emphasize and evaluate teamwork, contribution of ideas, and problem identification, so that it is consistent with the TQM management philosophy. For this to occur, one must first hire employees who want to work in this type of environment.

What is necessary, then, for a TQM culture to flourish is a synergy of management systems. For teams to function effectively, employment methods must first select employees with the interpersonal skills, independence, and need for achievement required in a TQM system. Training must be supplied so that employees develop the communication and management skills, including TQM skills, necessary to work effectively in groups. Finally, management systems, such as performance appraisal and compensation systems, must complement the long-term perspective that is an inherent part of TQM. The eventual goal is to blur the line between improving quality and the definition of an employee's job. Both should be viewed as one and the same.

A final element of the culture that is necessary for successful TQM teams to develop is to use the scientific method for problem-solving. Problems are identified, data are collected and displayed using the TQM tools described above, hypotheses are formed, processes are adjusted in response to the data and hypotheses, effects are observed, and processes are adjusted again if necessary. Finally, conclusions are reached, and the process of hypothesis generation, testing, and system implementation continues—*forever*. This is a process that health care professionals generally feel comfortable with because it is the basis for the sciences of their professional disciplines.

CASE ANALYSIS: HIGHER QUALITY AND LOWER COSTS IN DIALYSIS*

Recognizing the potential to save lives, the Joint Commission on Accreditation of Health-

---

Source: Reprinted with permission of Higher Quality, Lower Cost, *American Medical News*, May 13, © 1996.

care Organizations now requires hospitals to set up quality improvement programs.[9] Only a handful, however, have implemented the measurement systems, developed the protocols, and fostered the teamwork needed to make it work. More often, attempts bog down in endless meetings and fractious infighting. Even rarer is the small medical practice that can muster the vision, resources, expertise, and commitment to adopt a rigorous continuous quality improvement (CQI) program. For those that do, however, the payoff can be huge. Just ask Ernie Rutherford, M.D.

Five years ago, Dr. Rutherford set out to improve performance at five dialysis centers that he owns and operates with partners Joan Blondin, M.D., and Herschel Harter, M.D., in and around Monroe, Louisiana. A Deming devotee with no formal business training, Dr. Rutherford was convinced that statistical process control and CQI could work the same wonders for medicine that it has for industry. Four years into the program, the results have far exceeded Dr. Rutherford's expectations. Mortality rates have dropped from about 23 percent (close to the national average) to 11 percent. Hospitalizations are down 40 percent. Patients report feeling better than they have in years. At the same time, marginal costs per dialysis treatment have fallen 35 percent, netting an additional $500,000 this year for the dialysis centers.

Dr. Rutherford believes that his approach is significant for other reasons as well. As physicians are being asked to take more and more risk, statistical process control gives them a powerful tool for understanding and controlling risk. It will help physicians who master it retain control of medicine. "If you can get rid of variation [in a process], you can predict how it will perform. If you can predict, you can take risk. We can't wait for capitation," he says.

Others are interested in Dr. Rutherford's approach. He has presented his results to meetings of the Renal Physicians Association and is working with a local hospital to develop treatment algorithms for congestive heart failure. Representatives from other dialysis centers and the Health Care Financing Administration's (HCFA's) renal network have visited Dr. Rutherford's centers to find ways to improve quality. Even the Institute of Medicine has taken a look.

The key is to focus on quality, not cost, Dr. Rutherford says. "If you focus on cutting costs, quality will go down. If you focus on improving quality, costs will eventually go down." That's largely because improving quality through process control also means eliminating waste and duplication of effort to fix mistakes. Implementing quality improvement with strict process controls is not a simple task, however. Dr. Rutherford and his colleagues had to overcome both technical and cultural hurdles that have halted CQI programs at other facilities.

The Scientific Method

Dr. Blondin describes CQI as "just the scientific method applied to business." CQI proposes that products, in this case the health and functioning of patients with end-stage renal disease, are the result of processes. For the product to improve, the process must change. That's where the scientific method comes in. First, the process is defined. This step is analogous to generating a hypothesis and designing an experiment. At the North Louisiana Dialysis Center, teams of physicians, nurses, nutritionists, and technicians develop algorithms, or detailed flowcharts, of standard treatment procedures for processes ranging from controlling blood chemistry to treating malnutrition. These algorithms are then tested on groups of patients.

Second, the capabilities of the process are measured. Quality indicators, including hospitalizations, complications, adverse drug events, and blood chemistries, are monitored. Once a process is standardized, over time normal variation in its outcomes can be established. These data track the results of the experiment and function as control charts. They are collected in a computerized patient record system.

Third, the process can be changed. Results quickly become evident on the control chart. They may move an indicator up or down, or they may reduce or increase the normal variation of the process. Likewise, monitoring of control charts can alert physicians and staff that a change has crept into a process.

If data points leave the normal variation range or establish a trend above or below the median, it's time to look for the cause. "What we're doing now is practicing evidence-based medicine," Dr. Rutherford says. "We don't have to guess anymore. We have the data. Dialysis lends itself well to process control because the same procedure is done over and over, allowing opportunity to measure outcomes and improve processes." He believes, however, that it can work with other types of medical practice, particularly managing chronic diseases.

Physician Leadership

One element that is missing from many hospital CQI programs is strong physician involvement, according to Dr. Rutherford. Often, administrators are the first to be trained, and physicians are the last to be brought in. That's a mistake because physicians control 80 percent of the resources and are positioned to make the greatest impact. They often catch on to CQI quicker than others because they have scientific training, Dr. Rutherford adds.

Physician leadership proved critical at the North Louisiana clinics. To train staff in CQI basics, Dr. Rutherford brought in the training team from Hospital Corporation of America. Physicians and key staff were flown to seminars for advanced training, one of which was taught by Deming himself.

The total training cost exceeded $70,000, which represents a large investment for a small practice. Because CQI is predicated on teamwork, however, everyone must be trained, physicians especially. "At first I thought that if we had one or two people trained they could tell us what

to do," Dr. Harter says. "But everyone at the top has to know it. If you don't understand the system, you can't critique the process."

Once implementation began, leadership played an even bigger role. Typically, the transition to CQI means an initial drop in productivity as the charting process and the need to come up with measurement criteria are piled on top of regular duties. For the North Louisiana clinics, this lasted about 18 months, says Jennifer Bennet, R.N., who directs the program. The first set of algorithms took six months to complete. The process required bringing five physicians to consensus with input from all staff involved.

By all accounts, Dr. Rutherford's vision pulled the clinics through. "There was more than one occasion when I dropped into a chair in his office and said 'I quit,'" Bennet says. Dr. Rutherford was steadfast in his faith that the system would work.

After several months, it became clear that recording and properly interpreting data were problems. Dr. Rutherford brought in statistician Ray Carrey, Ph.D., for advice. One problem was that the clinics chose some complex processes to chart as they launched the program. Biological processes in homeostasis proved particularly difficult to chart and measure. "If we had it to do over, we would start with some simpler processes," Dr. Rutherford says.

Learning to use software to produce algorithms, which are flowcharts of every step in a given process, and to generate control charts was also a challenge. The clinics began with one big advantage, however: They were already using computerized patient records. Without them, retrieving data for control charts from paper patient records would have been impossible. "You couldn't hire enough monks to do it," Dr. Rutherford says.

Once the technical hurdles were cleared, the program began to show results. Results inspired confidence, and now enthusiasm for the program is palpable. Dr. Bennet commented, "Everyone is excited. They're saying, 'What are we going to do next?'"

Drive out Fear

As significant as teaching the technical end of CQI was, fundamental changes had to be made to make the process work. The first was changing the working relationships among staff and physicians. In place of hierarchical arrangements, where nurses and technicians exercised little judgment and always deferred to physicians' orders (even when they knew the order was wrong), Dr. Rutherford fostered a culture of cooperation. "Free input from all parties is needed to understand and get control of every part of the process," he noted.

"Staff have to know they won't be punished for speaking up. Drive out fear—that's the most important thing in the beginning." It's crucial for two reasons. First, for CQI to work, the collective knowledge of everyone on the team must be tapped and codified. When quality teams meet to develop algorithms, everyone has an equal say. Of course, once an algorithm is developed, it must be approved by consensus of all physicians on staff.

Second, staff must feel comfortable defending the algorithm once it is in place because success depends on keeping processes regular. The CQI method of looking at patient treatment as a process with normal statistical variation has become so ingrained that nurses will ask physicians "Are you sure you want to make a decision based on just one data point?"

The algorithms don't take authority from physicians. Rather, they represent a consensus on the best current method for dealing with a problem. Physicians can override them. The algorithms are subject to constant review and update. In practice, they free physicians from making many routine adjustments by spelling out how staff should deal with problems. "They've cut down a lot on phone calls, and the calls I get now are usually the ones I really need to get," Dr. Harter says.

Dr. Blondin concurs: "It is one of the most effective ways of extending physician practice that I have seen. It allows me to concentrate on the problems that really require a physician's atten-

tion." Ironically, removing physicians from constant interaction with patients has improved results in some ways. Before CQI, physicians saw patients every time they were dialyzed, usually three or four times a week. Generally, they'd write prescriptions based on the patient's vital signs that day.

"We thought we were practicing high-quality medicine, but what we were really doing was tampering with the system," Dr. Rutherford says. "One day blood pressure would be high, and a doctor would write a prescription for that. The next day it would be low, and a different doctor would write a prescription for that. Before you knew it, the patient was on three different blood pressure medications when he or she didn't really need any."

The HCFA now requires physicians to see patients at least once a week. "We see them, but we leave our prescription pads behind." Dr. Rutherford's goal is to leave day-to-day operations to staff as much as possible, reducing direct physician intervention to quarterly meetings with care teams. "I'd like to meet with them and say 'Great work, people, you did well.' We're not there yet, but we're getting closer."

Break down Barriers

Some of the most spectacular results have been the direct result of breaking down traditional barriers between departments and completely rethinking how care is delivered. For example, malnutrition was known to be a significant factor in hospitalizations and mortality, so the North Louisiana centers shifted the focus of care toward nutrition services.

All staff are more aware of patients' nutrition needs. The centers now employ one nutritionist for every 100 patients, about twice the usual ratio. "What's different is that physicians and nurses believe in nutrition," says nutritionist Kathy Baker. Most important, an algorithm has been developed to spot malnutrition early, determine causes, and aggressively treat it with everything from diet to treatment for depression to parenteral feeding. The centers' high use of parenteral feeding drew attention from the HCFA at first, but the centers were able to demonstrate that it lowered costs by preventing hospitalizations.

Another improvement was an increase in the average length of time on dialysis by 30 to 40 minutes per session. Often, dialysis centers try to save money by shortening sessions. Dr. Rutherford and his colleagues, however, found that longer sessions improved patients' health and quality of life and saved money by reducing hospital stays.

The centers can afford longer dialyses because they have cut overhead. Here again, knocking down traditional barriers between departments played a major part. For example, reuse of artificial kidney filters jumped when the reconditioning department started working with the dialysis units to get the filters into reprocessing within 3 to 5 minutes after use instead of 30 to 45 minutes. It became easier to clean them, and reuse leaped from 8 to 45 times per filter. The centers also cut costs by settling on one supplier for nonbiocompatible filters and one for biocompatible filters. That eliminated inventory costs and emergency shipping costs for overnight delivery of out-of-stock filers.

CQI not only has improved quality but also has brought the staff together around the centers' central mission: saving lives. "The most exciting thing has been the involvement and participation of staff and patients," Dr. Blondin says. Dr. Rutherford adds "It's been gratifying both professionally and personally."

CONCLUSION

The physician manager's TQM role is both managerial and operational. The managerial role involves creating an organization culture where TQM can develop throughout the practice, hospital, or health care system. There is no magic to doing this. Skillfully applying your knowledge about organization structure, employee motivation, leadership, performance evaluation, and compensation and reward systems and having a vision of what a TQM-managed organization looks like are essential. Your role as a manager will then involve working with these issues in the context of the problems and opportunities confronting your organization.

In addition, your role as a manager will involve acquiring the TQM expertise for your organization by providing training in TQM skills, including the tools, such as variance analysis and charting, communication, team building, and so forth. This does not mean that you should be the one in the trenches providing TQM training. On the contrary, your role as a manager will involve acquiring this training for your organization by creating positions for staff experts (if you are in a large health care organization) or by bringing in consultants or using training programs (if you are in a smaller organization).

Your operational TQM role will involve applying TQM to both clinical and management work. On the clinical side, you should be constantly looking for ways to improve your organization's clinical processes. This will involve a constant vigil to improve clinical outcomes and reduce costs. Operationalize this by working with your staff in an atmosphere where they can contribute ideas. This will involve actually doing TQM, including holding quality team meetings, conducting variance analysis, using TQM tools, and applying the scientific method to observe the effects of changes. In this regard, you may need to call on consultants or staff to create the statistics and charts.

Finally, the physician manager's role involves using TQM to improve the management process, such as by altering organization structure, performance appraisal methods, or employment processes. The unique contribution that a physician manager can make is that he or she is more likely to understand how changes in the management system can affect medical outcomes and how medical personnel are likely to react to these changes. As a participant in designing these changes, you can bring a unique perspective to the quality team discussion that will be essential to achieving integration across medical, other health care, and administrative constituencies.

REFERENCES

1. M. Sashkin and K.J. Kiser, *Putting Total Quality Management to Work* (San Francisco, Calif.: Berrett-Koehler Publishers, 1993).
2. G. Bounds, et al., *Beyond Total Quality Management* (New York, N.Y.: McGraw-Hill, 1994) 382.
3. W.E. Deming, Report to Management, *Quality Progress* (July 1972): 35–47.
4. Deming, Report to Management, 47.
5. J.M. Juran, *Juran on Planning for Quality* (New York, N.Y.: The Free Press, 1988) 14.
6. R.T. Skeel, Quality of Life Assessment in Cancer Clinical Trials—It's Time to Catch Up, *Journal of the National Cancer Institute* 81 (1989): 472–473.
7. C.M. Moinpour, et al., Quality of Life End Points in Cancer Clinical Trials: Review and Recommendations, *Journal of the National Cancer Institute* 81 (1989): 485–495.
8. D. Bowers and E.E. Lawler, The Empowerment of Service Workers: What, When, How, and Why, *Sloan Management Review* 33, (1992): 31–39.
9. Case analysis by H. Larkin, "Higher Quality, Lower Cost," *American Medical News* (13 May 1996): 9.

CHAPTER 13

Negotiation

Chapter Objectives

This chapter will tell you how to negotiate more effectively with peers, subordinates, superiors, and those outside your organization. It will give you strategies for understanding your own self-interest as well as those of your adversary. Understanding these interests is central to effective negotiation. It will also provide tactics to guide you in responding to an adversary's negotiation offer.

Negotiation is the art of settling disputes between two or more parties. For negotiation to be appropriate, there must be a dispute, there must be some uncertainty about the most appropriate solution, and there must be some willingness on the part of both parties to compromise. Physician managers are continually negotiating with those both inside and outside their own organizations. Inside medical practices, those negotiated with include physician partners, affiliated physicians, physician applicants, medical assistants/extenders, and senior level practice managers such as business managers. Common external negotiation adversaries include insurance and managed care organizations, hospitals, landlords, suppliers, and other practices. Physician managers working in managed care and hospital organizations often negotiate with subordinate employees, affiliated and employed physicians, other corporate executives, and a host of external agents, such as physician groups, suppliers, consultants, insurance companies, and hospitals. Finally, physicians continually find themselves negotiating with patients over compliance with treatment plans, referrals, and so forth.

It can be argued that most of what encompasses the skill of management must eventually be expressed or made operational through some form of negotiation. For example, the positive benefits of performance appraisal discussed in Chapter 2 depend upon obtaining employee acceptance of the appraisal and goal setting processes. Similarly, introducing change to an organization, such as activity-based costing of medical services, information technology, and use of clinical outcome measures are dependent upon obtaining the cooperation of those who will have to implement these methods. Obtaining this compliance is generally a negotiated process and usually cannot be implemented unilaterally.

Negotiation, as it is applied in real medical organizations, is an art, not a science. Although there are many scientific studies of the negotiation process, they are largely artificial and abstract investigations whose external validity is highly questionable given the necessary simplifying assumptions. Nevertheless, there have been some studies that take on significance because their findings validate the experiences of those who have described the art of negotiation. What I will next discuss are those ideas, many of which are subjective artistic negotiation conventions, that have developed over the years, some of which have been buttressed by experimental validation.

Many of the concepts that have become central to the art of negotiation appear at first to be self-evident. In hindsight, they are. The problem for the unskilled negotiator is utilizing the appropriate piece of "common sense" at the right time. Having a strategy, therefore, of how to approach the negotiation process can be a helpful way to make certain that you consider and incorporate your knowledge in a systematic manner.

THE ART OF NEGOTIATION: KEY CONCEPTS

Know Yourself

Understanding your own interests and goals is fundamental to any successful negotiation. You cannot protect your self-interest or achieve your objective if you don't have a clear idea of what you are trying to achieve from the negotiation. Understanding what you are trying to achieve requires, at a minimum, some honest introspection. Often, however, it requires collecting information or data, anticipating the business implications of various outcomes, and considering the personal and interpersonal implications of various negotiation outcomes. Generally, negotiation with another person, group, or organization is not a one-time event. Anticipating the relationship that you would like to have after the negotiation and the atmosphere that it will create for future interactions is a critical part of understanding what you wish to obtain from the negotiation process.

Many of the chapters in this book will give you the basis to determine what you are trying to

achieve from the negotiation. For example, your performance appraisal skills will help you set employee goals. Your financial management skills will help you identify managed care, compensation, and vendor agreement goals. Knowledge of organization change will help you identify sources of potential resistance and develop strategies to overcome this resistance. In each instance, the knowledge provides the context for negotiations with those whose cooperation will be essential for implementing change.

One of the most important considerations to identify before beginning to negotiate is your reservation price. This is the point beyond which you are willing to walk away from the negotiation. Sometimes, an estimate of your reservation price can be obtained directly by surveying the market. For example, if you are negotiating to lease office space, knowing that other suitable office space is leasing for $15.00 per square foot may help you determine that under no circumstance will you go beyond $17.50.

Sometimes the reservation price can be determined by examining your internal data. For example, given your space needs, perhaps you determine that you can't afford to pay more than $16.00 per square foot. Similarly, you may look at last year's revenue from a particular insurer who is converting to a capitated network. After considering the percentage of your patient base that will be involved, you conclude that you would rather not get the contract at a price, for example, of less than $0.70 per member per month. Sometimes, the reservation price can be a qualitative statement. For example, after evaluating Dr. Johnson's specialist utilization rate and cost data, you may determine that, to continue as a preferred provider organization (PPO) affiliate, Dr. Johnson must be willing to participate in additional utilization review training. If Dr. Johnson is not willing to accept this, you will not extend his PPO privileges.

Another concept that is critical to understanding yourself is determining your best alternative to a negotiated agreement (BATNA) before you begin to negotiate.[1] Your BATNA is what you will do if the negotiation fails. Knowing your

BATNA before you begin to negotiate with an adversary is important because it will place the negotiation in a larger perspective. Sometimes, negotiators may concede too much because they aren't aware of other relatively desirable alternatives. On other occasions, negotiators fail to reach agreement, not understanding that their best alternative is far less desirable than being somewhat more flexible in the current negotiation.

For example, your first choice for an office lease is in Sycamore Medical Arts building, which is adjacent to your primary admitting hospital. The offer is for $16.00 per square foot for a three-year corporate lease. Your BATNA is only $14.75 per square foot, but it is located eight miles farther away from the hospital, and the landlord is asking for a four-year, personally guaranteed lease. The BATNA provides a context for the ensuing negotiations. Knowing your BATNA might allow you to make some concessions on price to obtain the more desirable location and lease terms, which overall would be preferable.

Returning to Dr. Johnson, perhaps your BATNA is to do nothing. You may conclude that if you can't reach an agreement with him that ensures that he will get his consulting referrals and costs under control, then you would rather not have him on board. Perhaps you have plenty of other primary care physicians (PCPs), so that his patients will eventually have to switch over to your other PCPs, or they will lose coverage. Knowing your BATNA in this case will allow you to negotiate with Dr. Johnson with no second thoughts about compromising your goals or rescinding his plan privileges.

Know Your Adversary

Adversary is a charged word. Even so, the person with whom you are negotiating *is* an adversary. At the same time, it is important to understand that adversaries can share common interests. They can mutually benefit from cooperation, but fundamentally they remain adversaries.

Knowing your adversary is important to negotiating an agreement because it will help you determine where to begin the negotiating process. Think about the considerations that might be important to your adversary. Put yourself in his or her shoes. What would you want if your places were reversed? What issues would be most important to you? Which ones might be of lesser importance? Think about the probable limits of how far your adversary may be willing to go to compromise.

Begin the process of knowing your adversary by estimating his or her reservation price. What is the point beyond which he or she is likely to walk away from the negotiation? After all, you have a limit beyond which you won't go. Your adversary, similarly, has limits. How far would be too far for him or her to go on each identifiable issue? When thinking about this, consider what issues may influence the adversary's reservation price. Revisiting the lease example, you estimate that the owner's financing costs for the Sycamore Medical Arts Building are $10.00 per square foot and that insurance, taxes, and other overhead costs for the property are about $1.00 per foot. Next, you assume that the owner will probably want to make a 10 percent margin over expenses, which adds another $1.10 per square foot. Both these pieces of information were obtained from your helpful real estate agent. After preliminary plans are assembled, you determine that reconstruction and build-out costs for the suite will be about $1.30 per foot. An estimate of the owner's reservation price, therefore, would be about $13.40 per foot ($10.00 + $1.00 + $1.10 + $1.30).

Similarly, you may estimate Dr. Johnson's reservation price as public censure within the PPO network if he has to consult with a mentor to review referral standards. Based on your past dealings with Dr. Johnson, you feel that he is a proud person, and has a strong need for control. You estimate that holding him up to scrutiny by other network physicians would go beyond his "price." Your proposals, therefore, for additional training and supervision by another physician will have to be arranged so that they don't publicly disclose his current unacceptable performance.

Next, estimate your adversary's BATNA. If a negotiated agreement can't be reached, what is the adversary's probable next best choice? Evaluating the adversary's BATNA will provide information about how likely he or she is to be flexible. For example, perhaps the office leasing market is soft. If the owner does not reach an agreement with you, the BATNA may be vacant space and a loss of $11.00 per month of fixed costs for an indeterminate time. Obviously, this could have a profound effect on the owner's reservation price, your estimate of the reservation price, and both your subsequent actions.

Be Prepared To Dance

The term *negotiation dance* has been used by many to describe the give and take, maneuvering, and strategizing that take place between negotiating parties. Remember, there are no guarantees that an agreement will be reached. The negotiation dance determines whether an agreement will be reached as well as its final terms.

Now, let's change the circumstances a bit in the lease example. Assume that the office suite that you are trying to lease is currently occupied by Ms. Jones, the owner, who is planning to use your rental income to purchase an additional office suite, where she will move her business. You estimate her BATNA to be forgoing the purchase of the other office until she can find a suitable tenant for her current space. You perceive her to be a conservative businesswoman, not one to take undue risks, and therefore unlikely to impulse buy the other suite, acquire it under unfavorable financial circumstances, or purchase the other suite while risking a loss of $11.00 per square foot for an undetermined time or renting her current suite for less than her target net income.

Conceptually, the negotiation dance takes place between the reservation prices of the adversaries, which is referred to as the zone of agreement. Figure 13–1 illustrates the zone of agreement for the lease example in which the owner will not purchase a suite to move her business unless she first obtains a renter. In this example, the zone of agreement ranges between $13.50 and $16.00 per square foot. Naturally, the owner wants to move the final contract price above the $13.50 point, and the physician wants to move it below the $16.00 point. This area then becomes the turf for the negotiation dance. Normally, of course, neither side knows for certain the other's reservation price, so the dance involves both identifying those boundaries and trying to conceal one's own boundary.

Interests versus Positions

Conceptually, it is useful to separate a party's interests from his or her positions. Positions are the items placed on the bargaining table. They are specific goals or outcomes that you desire from the negotiation. "Rent of $15.50 per square foot," "Carve out pediatric patients from the capitation coverage," and "You agree not to practice within 25 miles of our location if for any reason you do not complete the term of this contract" are all examples of positions.

Interests reflect a side's needs, wants, fears, and so forth. They are the basis on which a negotiating position is formed. In effect, interests motivate the formation of positions. Interests may be based on fundamental issues, such as financial stability, fairness, or relationship. On occasion, parties will have clashing positions, but their underlying interests may not conflict. When this occurs, and one or both parties realize it, then there is an opportunity to move the negotiation toward agreement.

Dr. Johnson, to whom we have referred previously, is a PCP. His specialist utilization rate and cost data are significantly above those of others in the PPO's physician panel. Ms. Adams, the network administrator, has talked to him several times about this in the past. She has shared network referral data with him, but this hasn't changed his referral pattern. Figure 13–2 presents the interests and positions for both Dr. Johnson and Ms. Adams, the PPO network administrator.

Although their respective positions are in conflict, the same degree of disharmony is not found

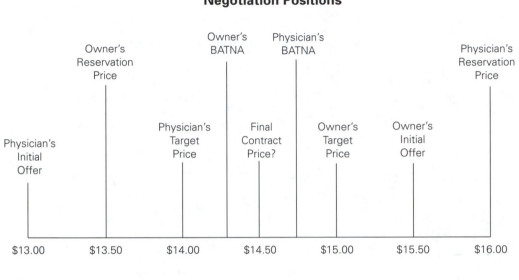

Figure 13–1 Office space negotiation.

in their respective underlying interests. Dr. Johnson wants to remain on the PPO panel, and Ms. Adams wants to keep him. Dr. Johnson is concerned about appropriate medical care, and so is Ms. Adams. It is apparent that the way each party is expressing its interests in terms of specific positions is really the major source of conflict. Perhaps Dr. Johnson views the PPO's referral guidelines as endangering him and his patients. As a result, additional training is irrelevant. His opposition to Dr. Argyle as a mentor could be founded in his interests of need for control and embarrassment avoidance.

Ms. Adams, on the other hand, has operationalized her interests in terms of two particular actions: providing Dr. Johnson with additional education, and mentoring him over an extended time period to be certain that the training "sticks." These are ideas that she generated to operationalize her interests. As an effective negotiator, she should be willing to modify her positions, so long as she does not sacrifice her interests. Similarly, if Dr. Johnson's interests can be protected while satisfying the PPO

administrator's interests, he may be willing to modify his positions. Examining the negotiation from this perspective creates room to maneuver and the potential to reach an agreement.

Thinking about the negotiation from the perspective of interests as opposed to positions may give each side the opportunity to modify its position without compromising what is dear or losing face. As a negotiator, then, one of your most fundamental tactics should be to recast the discussion away from positions and toward interests. We cannot, however, be a Pollyanna about this. There will be times when interests are so divergent that it makes the chance of identifying a mutually acceptable position unlikely. If that is the case, using interests as a lens to focus your thinking about the negotiation should allow you to determine this sooner as opposed to later. Ending a negotiation that has little or no possibility of being successfully concluded also is of value.

Next, try to focus the nature of the negotiation process away from a confrontation of personal wills and arbitrarily held positions and toward using objective criteria. Fisher and Ury refer to

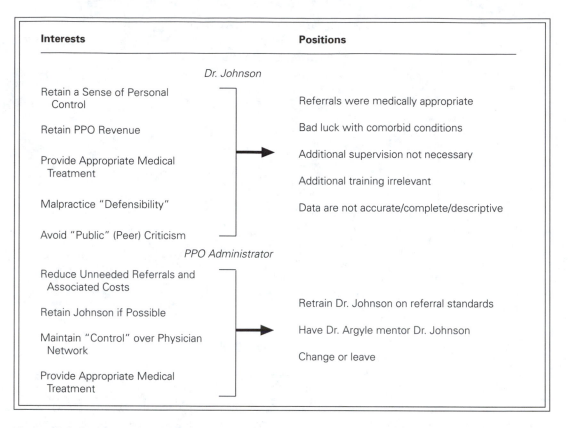

Figure 13–2 Interests and positions of two adversaries.

this approach as principled negotiation.[2] Examples of external objective standards that they propose include market value, precedent, scientific judgment, professional standards, efficiency, cost, law, moral standards, equal treatment, tradition, and reciprocity.[3] Using external standards to guide a negotiation reframes it into a more objective problem-solving process. This moves the focus of the negotiation toward a discussion of determining what would be an objective, fair basis to formulate an agreement and away from personal, arbitrary positions. It also provides a basis for each party to change its position without losing face or feeling foolish.

Returning to our real estate example, Ms. Jones, the owner, initially offered a rate of $15.50 per foot. Several days later, you respond as follows:

My agent has surveyed several other "Class A" office suites in this part of town that are either on the market now or that have rented in the past six months. The price has ranged between $13.00 and $14.00 per square foot. Please correct me if I'm wrong on this, but this seems to be the market range. Is there some reason, perhaps some characteristic of your suite, that would warrant going outside this range?

You have reframed the discussion into what is externally fair and away from a direct contest of wills. Ms. Jones is now in the position of having to do one of the following:

- produce alternative data that encompass her offering price of $15.50 (perhaps, for example, she believes that you and your agent are not being truthful or that your sample is not valid)

- identify an alternative objective standard, such as her internal costs, irrespective of what other real estate is renting for
- offer a justification for why her office suite may merit a higher rent
- state that she will not be governed by any standards; this simply is her price

If Ms. Jones chooses the last strategy, then the negotiation can be quickly concluded. You know that from the owner's perspective there is no basis to modify her position. You must choose between the offer at $15.50, which is lower than your reservation price, and your BATNA. On the other hand, any of the first three alternatives can provide a basis for you and Ms. Jones to modify your positions and reach a negotiated agreement.

Returning now to Dr. Johnson, the administrator made the following comments to him when she first proposed retraining and mentoring:

> There were 14 cases that you referred on to consultants that easily fit within our guidelines for nonreferral. These guidelines were initially developed by a national panel and then reviewed and modified by local board-certified PCPs. In addition, we have been modifying these standards over the last three years based on our local network experience. Our incidence of malpractice claims is well below national standards and lower than that of local PCPs outside our network. Finally, our clinical outcomes data show that our PCPs are providing excellent quality of care.

At this point, Dr. Johnson can debate the appropriateness or accuracy of the administrator's data. If his reaction is that the data are irrelevant, and he has no suggestions for either making them relevant or identifying another objective standard, then the administrator can quickly conclude the negotiation. If Dr. Johnson is unwilling to satisfy the administrator's interests, then they

will certainly have to part ways. Alternatively, if he accepts the data as appropriate and valid, then this can change the focus of the negotiation to how he can become skilled in using the referral guidelines while still protecting his interests. Correspondingly, if Dr. Johnson identifies some truly distorting aspects of the data, then Ms. Adams should be interested in his observations.

The negotiation dance can be affected by initial bargaining positions. An adversary's extreme initial offer can result in you negotiating in reaction to that position as opposed to an objective standard. If an adversary takes an extreme initial position, ask questions to understand why the position was taken. Essentially, ask the other party to state his or her interests. Next, choose one of the following based on your understanding of these interests:

- Ignore the adversary's initial position, and try to refocus the negotiation on the basis of some objective standard.
- Make a counteroffer that is equally extreme in the other direction. Remember, the median between the two offers is a natural focal point for future negotiations.[4,5] Determine your counteroffer, therefore, so that the midpoint between the two offers is well within your acceptable range.
- Break off negotiations until your adversary makes a more reasonable offer.

Utilizing these tactics not only retains a level playing field but also communicates a message to your adversary that you know the initial offer was extreme and that you will not agree to anything near it.

DISTRIBUTIVE NEGOTIATING

In its simplest form, negotiating is the process of distributing a fixed resource between two competing adversaries. For one side to win something, the other side must lose something. This circumstance is frequently referred to as a zero sum game because, for me to gain $50, you must lose $50, and the sum of the two is $0. This distributive or competitive approach to negotiation assumes that the size of the pie is fixed and that each side wants to maximize its gains. The goals, therefore, of the competing parties are in direct conflict. A distributive negotiating situation can arise when any of the following are present:

- There is a single issue to be negotiated.
- Resources *are* limited, each side truly *does* need more, and each side can only get it at the expense of the other.
- One or both sides envision negotiation as a confrontational, "macho" exercise (to many, the essence of negotiation is "I win, you lose").
- One or both sides don't take the time or are unwilling to expend the effort to see whether there is an alternative to this approach.

Integrative bargaining, which is discussed later in this chapter, occurs when two parties recognize that there are several issues to be negotiated and that, in total, it isn't necessarily true that each side can gain only at the other's expense. For integrative bargaining to be feasible, the parties must differentially weigh the importance of various issues. For example, both parties may view the contract price as being of paramount importance. An option to renew clause, however, may be more important to party A than to party B, whereas B attaches more significance than A to the length of the contract. Under these circumstances, it is possible to trade or "log roll" the price, renewal option, and contract length so that both parties gain what is most important to each.

Generally, it is best to begin negotiations using an integrative approach. Most negotiations, with the exception of buying a used car, will have some integrative characteristics. There will be occasions, however, when a distributive strategy is more appropriate as well as adversaries whose skills or preferences may be limited to that approach. It is necessary, therefore, to understand how to use both strategies.

To illustrate a distributive negotiation situation, let's return to the lease example. After determining a reservation price and a BATNA, the owner's next task is to choose a target price, or the price that she would prefer to get. You guess that her reservation price is $13.50 per square foot, so the target price will be above this point. Ms. Jones may determine a target price by examining her costs, thinking about the issue of profit, and then assessing the market and the adversary (you) to determine what she might be able to get. Next, she will formulate an initial offering price, which is her initial negotiation position. Because people expect give and take in the negotiation process, the initial offering price needs to be above her target price.

Selecting an initial offering price can have a profound impact on the subsequent negotiation. If the initial offer is perceived as totally unreasonable, the other party may immediately withdraw from the negotiation having concluded that no agreement will be possible and that continuing would be a waste of time. Lewicki and colleagues propose that extreme initial offers extend the negotiation process, thereby allowing more time to learn about the adversary's priorities and to influence him or her.[6] They also convey the message that the parties are far apart and that more concessions than originally anticipated may be needed.

It should be clear at this point that an important goal in distributive negotiating is to get a good estimate of the adversary's reservation and target prices and then perhaps to influence them. Data to help you evaluate this include:

- indications of time pressure that the adversary is under
- the cost to the adversary if the negotiations fail, including his or her probable BATNA
- the adversary's perception of how much you need to reach an agreement or value a particular negotiating point

Naturally, adversaries are hesitant to reveal critical information, so that often the data available will be problematic. An action you can take to affect your adversary's perceptions is selectively presenting information. For example, you could mention that your current lease rate is $12.00 per square foot without disclosing that the current renewal offer is $15.00 per square foot. Consciously choosing emotions, verbal language, and body language can also create an impression. Although it may be appropriate to provide less than full information and to consider carefully how you present information, it is not appropriate to lie.

As the negotiation proceeds, generally each side will make concessions. Concessions recognize the legitimacy of the other side's interests as represented in its positions. Concessions also affect the offerer's status and position. Making a concession conveys information. Generally, concessions that successively decline in size indicate that the side is nearing its target or reservation price. Effective negotiators will gauge the size of concessions relative to the initial offer. High initial offers create more negotiating room and hence are generally associated with larger concessions.

Sometimes, distributive negotiators can use "hardball tactics." These tactics attempt to force the adversary to do something that he or she doesn't want to do. They change the focus of the negotiation away from content and interests toward context and positions. Many people find these tactics to be offensive and perhaps unethical. At a minimum, they are dangerous to use because they can hurt your reputation, cause the adversary to break off negotiations, or create an incentive to get even. The following are some examples of hardball tactics:

- *Good guy/bad guy*—One negotiator takes a threatening, belligerent, and perhaps extreme bargaining position. He or she temporarily leaves the negotiation (e.g., for a previously arranged meeting). The good guy takes over, expresses sympathy for the opponent having to deal with the bad guy, and then proposes that they try to reach a quick agreement before the bad guy returns. This tactic is often transparent and can easily alienate the opponent.
- *Lowball/highball*— This involves making a very low (or high, whichever would be more favorable to you) initial offer that will not be honored. If the opponent accepts the offer, he or she is told that there are addi-

tional elements to the negotiation that had been "overlooked." Auto dealers use this tactic so that buyers will return before accepting another dealer's offer. This gives the first dealer another shot at the sale. This tactic creates hard feelings because the accepting party learns that the deal really isn't complete and that it will cost more. Sometimes this tactic becomes "bait and switch" when the buyer learns that the product really isn't available but a similar one with a few more bells and whistles (and a higher price) is ready for sale.

- *Nibbling, salami slicing, nickel and dime*— This involves asking for a small concession after one side thought an agreement had been reached. The classic example is a customer who asks for a free tie after the tailor has taken measurements and written up the ticket on a suit. The cost of the tie is small relative to the suit, so there is great pressure to comply. This tactic creates ill will for a small gain and may result in future retribution.
- *Chicken*—This is bluffing with a very threatening position. An important cardiac surgeon threatens to move his or her surgeries to another hospital unless some changes are made to the physicians' lounge. You may feel strongly that the surgeon is bluffing, but can you take the chance? The problem with this tactic is that the stakes are high and a bluff may be called. If the bluffer doesn't follow through, he or she will lose all credibility. Once again, future retribution is another possible outcome.
- *Intimidation*—This involves using threats, false anger, guilt, and the like. These tactics can be used to distract the opponent from the basis of negotiation by focusing on context.
- *Presenting false facts*—This should not be confused with less than full disclosure. This tactic is dangerous because there is no fallback position if your opponent challenges you to support your facts. If an opponent confronts you with data that affect your position, it is always appropriate to ask for

substantiation or time to collect your own data. Separate this from the "people" issue of trust by asserting that you always verify factual assertions.

Your response to a given hardball tactic will depend on the specific circumstances, including your BATNA. All responses, however, are dependent on you being able to recognize the tactic for what it is: an attempt to shift the focus from the content of the negotiation to contextual issues and thereby gain an advantage. Here are some specific ways to counter hardball strategies:

- Ignore them. Change the subject, or pretend it didn't happen. For example, responding in a calm manner can be disconcerting to an opponent who is ranting and raving. Responding to an extreme price offer by stating "The new food services management contractor must be ready to go by August 10" tells the opponent that his or her price position isn't even worth talking about.
- Recognize the hardball strategy for what it is, and confront your opponent with it. In effect, negotiate the negotiation process. Fisher and Ury give an example of doing this[7(p.130)]: "Say, Joe, I may be totally mistaken, but I'm getting the feeling that you and Ted here are playing a good guy/bad guy routine. If you two want a recess at any time to straighten out differences between you, just ask."
- Respond in kind. Once your adversary understands that you can be equally extreme or irrelevant, he or she may move on. For example, a janitorial service offered to clean a hospital's new outpatient clinic for $2.00 per square foot per year. The physician manager immediately responded "I was thinking more on the order of $0.10!" "Where did you get that number from?" the service negotiator replied. The physician manager then responded "Look, instead of just throwing numbers around, why don't we talk about this in terms of what it costs

us to provide this service with our current staff at our other locations?" Combining an equally extreme counteroffer with a quick proposal to change the *basis* of negotiation often results in moving the discussion away from unsubstantiated, arbitrary positions to one based on objective criteria: the hospital's current cost.

In summary, distributive bargaining is a win–lose approach in which negotiators try to reach agreement by influencing beliefs about what is possible while at the same time trying to obscure their own real interests as they attempt to ascertain their opponent's interests.

INTEGRATIVE NEGOTIATING

Integrative negotiation is characterized by a recognition that the parties will have to live together after the negotiation. The issues in integrative negotiations may first appear to be win–lose, but what separates this from a distributive process is how the opponents respond. The negotiation atmosphere is characterized by a sincere interest in trying to understand the adversary's real interests and objectives. This is not to say that the two sides are not advocates. They are, but both sides also recognize that they may be more successful through a mutual understanding of interests. Because each side has an interest in the other understanding its interests, there is a much freer flow of information between the two parties than in a distributive negotiation.

Lewicki and colleagues have identified four steps in the integrative negotiation process[8]:

1. identifying and defining the dimensions of the problem
2. bringing interests to the surface
3. generating alternative solutions
4. choosing specific solutions

Several points characterize an integrative strategy for defining the dimensions of a problem. First, there is an attempt to define the problem in terms that are mutually acceptable to both parties. For example, in negotiating a pharmaceutical supply contract, the dimensions may be cost, timeliness, quality, and service. Once both parties agree on the dimensions to be negotiated, then they can formulate positions on each dimension.

Second, the problem needs to be stated as a goal to be attained, as opposed to a statement of a solution. An example is "We view reducing inventory as a real opportunity to lower our costs" as opposed to fixing immediately on a proscriptive statement of *how* to do this.

Third, the problem identification needs to be depersonalized as much as possible. When one side or the other has ownership, it can become defensive. A personalized statement would be "Your pharmaceutical sales people are always pushing too much stock on us and overestimating order lead time." A depersonalized statement would be "There is a difference of opinion on necessary inventory and when orders need to be placed to have appropriate inventory levels."

Finally, separate problem identification from finding a solution. If the two occur at the same time, then negotiators may jump into problem solving before fully evaluating the nature of the dispute. Because integrative negotiating is characterized by exchanges between the parties, discussing solutions before all the problems are fully explored and stated is premature and may result in both parties having to revisit solutions that were reached prematurely.

Next, the integrative process focuses on interests. By examining the problem at this deeper level, we move behind positions, which are really particular attempts to satisfy underlying interests. Because there generally are several positions that can satisfy an interest, this increases the chance of reaching a solution. Fisher and Ury provide an excellent example of how moving beyond positions to interests can result in a solution that is better for both parties:[9(p.40)]

> Consider the story of two men quarreling in a library. One wants the window open and the other wants it closed. They bicker back and forth about how much to leave it open: a crack, halfway, three quarters of the way. No solution satisfies them both.
>
> Enter the librarian. She asks one why he wants the window open. "To get some fresh air." She asks the other why he wants it closed. "To avoid the draft." After thinking a minute, she opens wide a window in the next room, bringing in fresh air without a draft.

This example points out several advantages of redefining the problem in terms of interests. While the problem remained defined as positions, it was likely that neither side would be happy because any opening dissatisfied one party and even half-open dissatisfied the other party. The librarian's intervention was successful because she focused on the question of why. Why was each party unhappy? This refocused the dispute in terms of the underlying interests.

The third aspect of integrative bargaining is generating alternative solutions. Four methods of generating alternatives are expanding the pie, log rolling, cost cutting, and brainstorming.

Conflicts often arise because there simply are not enough resources available. By making the pie bigger (i.e., allocating more resources), conflict can be reduced. A hospital wishes to reduce the number of artificial hips that are used from 11 to 3. It estimates that this will save $1 million over three years. Surgeons, however, are resisting the change. Some initially will have longer operating times because they are beginning at the start of the learning curve. In addition, they will have to receive training on unfamiliar hips. Expanding the pie in this instance may mean that the hospital may provide training and return some of the cost savings to the surgeons.

Log rolling involves trading off issues so that both parties achieve success in the issues that are most important to them. To log roll, however, it is necessary for each party to have different priorities on several issues. In this instance, perhaps there are some favorable committee assignments and surgery times that could go along with the agreement.

Cost cutting involves understanding the costs to the opponent if your interests are met, and then providing appropriate compensation. Exhibit 13–1 contains some questions that can reveal integrative solutions using each of these strategies.

Finally, brainstorming is an idea generation strategy that has had widespread use and is helpful for creating "breakthrough" thinking about a problem. All too often, original ideas are prematurely rejected or never given full consideration. Brainstorming overcomes these problems by separating the generation of ideas from their evaluation. Brainstorming is generally a group idea generation process, but it can be done individually. The basic rules of brainstorming include the following[10]:

- No idea is too ridiculous to be stated. Everyone is encouraged to state any idea irrespective of how extreme, ridiculous, or outlandish.
- Each idea that is presented belongs to the group, not the person stating it. This allows members to build on the ideas of others without getting into issues of personal credit.
- No idea can be criticized. The purpose of the session is to generate ideas, not evaluate them.

Once the ideas have been generated, they are evaluated. Many of the ideas will be of no value. Some, however, may have an element that had not previously been considered. Others, when taken in combination, may provide the basis for a new way of looking at the negotiation.

The final stage in integrative negotiation is to evaluate the options that have been generated and to choose the best alternatives. This will involve evaluating the options in terms of both quality and acceptance. As noted above, using

Exhibit 13–1 Three Strategies and Questions To Expand Integrative Negotiation Alternatives

---

Expanding the Pie

1. How can both parties get what they are demanding?
2. Is there a resource shortage?
3. How can resources be expanded to meet the demands of both sides?

Log Rolling

1. What issues are of higher and lower priority to me?
2. What issues are of higher and lower priority to the other?
3. Are issues of high priority to me also low for the other, and vice versa?
4. Can I "unbundle" an issue, that is, make one larger issue into two or more smaller ones that can then be log rolled?
5. What are things that would be inexpensive for me to give and valuable for the other to get that might be used in log rolling?

Cost Cutting

1. What risks and costs do my positions create for the other?
2. What can I do to minimize the other's risks and costs so that he or she would be more willing to go along?

Source: Adapted with permission from R.J. Lewicki et al., *Negotiation*, 2nd Edition, p. 94, © 1994, Irwin Publishers.

objective criteria and external, mutually accepted standards to evaluate quality will depersonalize the process. Ideally, the basis for deciding among alternatives should be determined before the decision-making process begins. Pay particular attention to differences in the importance of interests, willingness to assume risk, and issues related to time. These can create opportunities to log roll solutions.

Let's apply some of these ideas to a negotiation between a hospital that wants to introduce an activity-based management control system into its breast cancer program. Some of the physicians oppose this because they believe that it would be intrusive, would create more paperwork, and could jeopardize their ability to make clinical decisions. If the physicians felt that one problem would be increased paperwork and time needed to develop the management systems, one solution would be for the hospital to provide more administrative and clinical support (expand the pie). Log rolling could involve the physicians agreeing to be part of the system development team if the hospital provides a new position in its grants office that would focus on oncology. Creating a committee in which oncologists are dominant and that would have oversight of the activity-based management project might reduce the fear (cost cutting) that administrators would be dictating clinical decisions through policy. Finally, a brainstorming session containing representatives of all interested parties (administration, oncologists, oncological surgeons, nursing, quality control, etc.) may generate some breakthrough ideas, such as restructuring the position of the breast cancer program in the hospital organization so that it prepares its own budget within hospital constraints and has departmental status. These two changes would allow the program to protect its own self-interest better.

CHOOSING A NEGOTIATION STRATEGY

Savage and colleagues propose choosing a negotiation strategy based on the importance of the substantive and relationship outcomes of the negotiation.[11] Substantive outcomes refer to protecting or obtaining your interests. Relationship outcomes deal with how the negotiation and its results will affect future relations with the adversary.

When you are only interested in substantive outcomes and you don't care about how maximizing the tangible benefit from this negotiation may affect future relations with your adversary, then a distributive strategy is generally appropriate. If you are interested in both achieving substantive outcomes and developing a positive, long-term relationship with your adversary, then an integrative strategy has the best chance of simultaneously achieving both goals.

If the real value to you in a negotiation is retaining or enhancing the relationship and the substantive outcome is of little or no value, then accommodation is most appropriate. For example, a new physician in town has an opportunity to bid on a school board contract to be a high school's team physician. The real value to the physician is in the relationship that can be developed with local community leaders, name recognition, and referrals. The immediate compensation as team physician is of relatively little value. As a result, the physician should undertake every part of the negotiation trying to maximize the relationship-building considerations.

If you are interested in neither substantive nor relational outcomes, then avoidance will be most appropriate. An avoidance strategy means that you don't negotiate. Negotiating takes time and consumes resources. There will be some parties who, because of reputation, past experience, qualifications, or some other issue, are simply not worth this investment. For example, a catering firm whose past performance in managing the hospital cafeteria was unacceptable wishes to bid on the contract again. You are not interested in continuing the relationship, nor are you interested in getting a low bid, because of your past experience. There are no substantive or relationship issues that need to be discussed. They are irrelevant to your plans, and you should not waste your time or the catering firm's in a negotiation. Similarly, the insurance company that has been hounding you for three months is offering a product that you don't need, and you could care less about a long-term relationship with this company. Under these circumstances, don't negotiate. Don't even meet.

THE PRISONER'S DILEMMA AS A METAPHOR

Suggestions have been provided for when integrative and distributive negotiation strategies may be most appropriate. There will be circumstances, already described, when one or another will be more appropriate. The dilemma that the negotiator faces when considering whether to approach a negotiation integratively is whether cooperation will be reciprocated or will be used as an opportunity for exploitation by the adversary. In effect, "If I see integrative possibilities and pursue that approach, but my adversary views the situation as distributive, will I be taken advantage of?" Similarly, there is the temptation to take advantage of an adversary who acts cooperatively.

This dilemma occurs in many real-life situations. For example, the members of a cartel all do well if all cooperate. If one member of the cartel defects, he or she does extremely well. If all behave this way, however, then all lose. Similarly, if everyone in my community recycles trash and I do not, then I experience the benefits of a cleaner community without the inconvenience of sorting my paper and glass. If everyone behaves this way, then all lose. Immunizations are another example. If everyone is immunized and I am not, then I am insulated from the disease without incurring the small but real probability that I will have an adverse reaction to the immunization. Once again, if everyone behaves this way, all will lose.

The Prisoner's Dilemma is a game that can be used to clarify some of the risks and opportunities associated with cooperation and noncooperation. In this game, each adversary has a choice of cooperating or defecting. Neither side can communicate with the other before a decision, and after a decision each side learns of the other's choice. The players don't know how many rounds there will be in the game. The reward matrix is presented in Figure 13–3. For example, if one party chooses to cooperate and the other also does, then both receive 3. If one chooses to cooperate and the other defects, then the defector is rewarded for giving in to the temptation and receives 5, and the other gets the "sucker's payoff" of –5. If both choose to defect, then both receive a modest loss of –2.

This reward system, in a general sense, describes many real-world situations. If you can "clean the other's clock" through deceit or manipulation, then in the short run you can win big. In effect, it pays to defect if you think that your adversary will cooperate *and* if you are not concerned about future relations. If as a result, however, you teach your opponent that he or she can't trust you to cooperate, then he or she won't cooperate in the future, and you will do less well than you would have if you had taught your adversary that you could be trusted to cooperate. The dilemma is that the act of defection, which could generate the greatest possible gain in the short run for each player, generates mediocre outcomes for all in the long run.

This game has formed the basis for a substantial game theory literature that has produced results that provide an interesting perspective on negotiating. Axelrod, for example, asked a number of experts in game theory and related disciplines to submit computer programs for a Prisoner's Dilemma tournament.[12] The tournament was structured as a round robin, so that each program was tested against every other one, with each game comprising 200 moves. Axelrod's goal was to see which strategies performed best. Fourteen programs were submitted. Some programs chose each move (cooperate or defect) randomly. Others used complex exploitative strategies that calculated an opponent's defection rate based on previous rounds and then defected just a little bit more frequently.

Axelrod noted several characteristics of the better programs. All of the eight top-ranked programs were "nice." That is, they started off cooperating. The best of the "mean" entries scored 401 points, and the lowest of the "nice" entries received 472 points. When nice entries played against other nice entries, they averaged almost 600 points, which suggests the premium that may be possible for mutual cooperation. Another common characteristic of the best programs was that they were provocable. They punished defection by defecting themselves. In other words, they were not martyrs. The best programs were also forgiving. They didn't hold grudges. Defection was not an irredeemable sin. They gave the opponent the opportunity to resume cooperation. Finally, the best programs gave clear messages. Obtaining continuing cooperation is tricky. Complex strategies can be difficult for the opponent to decipher and could result in unprofitable defections. The best programs signaled clearly when they would cooperate and when they would defect.

The program that achieved the most success was called *Tit for Tat*. This program cooperates in the first round and thereafter does whatever the opponent did on the preceding round. If the opponent defected on the previous round, then *Tit for Tat* defects on the next round. If the opponent cooperated on the previous round, then *Tit for Tat* cooperates on the next round. This strategy was nice, provocable, forgiving, and clear. Axelrod had a number of interesting comments about the programs, which sound all too much like the actions of real people in the heat of negotiation[13(p.40)]:

> . . . the entries were too competitive for their own good. In the first place, many of them defected early in the game without provocation, a characteristic which was very costly in the long run. . . . Even expert strategists from political science, sociology, economics, psychology, and mathematics made the systematic errors of being too competitive for their own good, not being forgiving enough, and being too pessimistic about the responsiveness of the other side.

Axelrod, encouraged by the success of the first tournament, held a second one. Entrants were given a report describing *Tit for Tat* as well as the conclusions regarding niceness, provocability, forgivingness, and clarity. Sixty-two entries were received from six countries. Once again, *Tit for Tat* proved to be the most successful program. Next, Axelrod tried to determine whether *Tit for Tat*'s success was due to its competitors' "knocking each other off." In other words was *Tit for Tat* robust? Could it do well in different, narrower environments? Axelrod constructed six hypothetical tournaments. *Tit for Tat* won five and finished second in the sixth. He commented[14(p.54)]:

> What accounts for *Tit for Tat*'s robust success is its combination of being nice, retaliatory, forgiving, and clear. Its niceness prevents it from getting into unnecessary trouble. Its retaliation discourages the other side from persisting whenever defection is tried. Its forgiveness helps restore mutual cooperation. And its clarity makes it intelligible to the other player, thereby eliciting long-term cooperation.

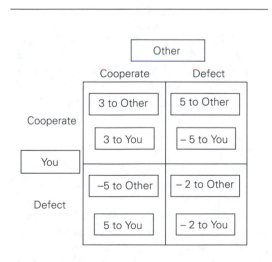

Figure 13–3 Prisoner's Dilemma payoff matrix.

Finally, Axelrod concluded, once again with comments, that if offered in the context of humans as opposed to computer programs provides much to ponder[15(p.54)]:

> ... *Tit for Tat* foregoes the possibility of exploiting other rules (programs). While such exploitation is occasionally fruitful, over a wide range of environments the problems with trying to exploit others are manifold. In the first place, if a rule defects to see what it can get away with, it risks retaliation from rules that are provocable. In the second place, once mutual recriminations set in, it can be difficult to extract oneself. And, finally, the attempt to identify and give up on unresponsive rules (such as *random*) or excessively uncooperative rules often mistakenly led to giving up on rules which were in fact salvageable by a more patient rule like *Tit for Tat*. *Being able to exploit the exploitable without paying too high a cost with the others is a task which was not successfully accomplished by any of the entries in round two of the tournament* [emphasis added].

Clearly the Prisoner's Dilemma has many characteristics that are problematic in real negotiations. To mention a few, each player knows with certainty whether the other has defected or cooperated in the previous round. In real life, you often don't know with certainty whether cooperation really is cooperation or artfully disguised defection. Reward contingencies in real negotiations will vary greatly from the ratios used in the game, and this obviously could have a major impact on behavior. Finally, negotiators in real life can talk to each other before they make or respond to an offer. They can express intentions, propose commitments, and threaten. All these considerations should give us pause about the generalizability of Axelrod's findings.

Nevertheless, there do seem to be some lessons that could be cautiously drawn and applied from this research:

- Unless you are given reason to believe otherwise, it may be beneficial to begin negotiations assuming that the adversary will be willing to be cooperative.
- Retaliation for a violation of expectations is a reasonable response. Don't, however, overreact. Be certain of your facts, and choose the degree of your reaction so that it is appropriately proportional to the violation.
- Don't hold a grudge. If it appears that your opponent is willing to move from confrontational to cooperative negotiations, be willing to respond accordingly.
- Clear communication is critical. Although the content of the negotiation may be complex, strive to communicate in direct, unambiguous language and signals. Don't give confounding messages, such as nonverbal cues that contradict written and verbal messages.
- Don't be greedy. Even if the immediate negotiation is limited and there is little chance that you will have future dealings with your adversary, think long and hard about being exploitive. Even if you don't believe in fate, karma, balance in the universe, or "what goes around comes around," your reputation will precede you.

CASE ANALYSIS: THE BLACK BOOK

Paul Grant, M.D., and Larry Jones, M.D., partners in Down East Internal Medicine, Ltd., were simultaneously facing a professional and business crisis. Two years ago they made their first foray into managed care by contracting with Portland Shipbuilding and Down East Dreadnoughts, both major local employers, to provide capitated primary care services. As a result of obtaining these contracts, they greatly expanded their practice. They hired three additional nurses, two secretaries, and two nurse practitioners and doubled their office space by acquiring an adjacent, vacant suite. Finally, they hired two physicians to work as employees. Fran Johnson, M.D., was fresh out of residency. Her career plan was to work for a while before making any permanent commitments. Bill Herald, M.D., was retiring from the Navy at age 51. He was looking to begin a new career, but he wasn't sure that he wanted to stay in Portland for his next career or, for that matter, to be in a small private practice.

Both physicians were only interested in an employment relationship, and both were happy to sign two-year employment contracts. Drs. Grant and Jones saw this as an opportunity to profit substantially while still paying Johnson and Herald equitable salaries. Grant commented "I figured that if one or both became successful, and we got along, we could work out a partnership arrangement later. If it didn't go well, I could hire someone else."

Eighteen months later, the effects of international peace struck. Portland Shipbuilding, a subsidiary of a major conglomerate, closed its doors as a result of the Navy canceling all its new construction contracts. Down East Dreadnoughts also lost all its new construction contracts and was barely staying alive doing ship repairs. As a result, Down East laid off 70 percent of its hourly employees. With the decline in employment, Drs. Grant and Jones saw an immediate and precipitous decline in cash flow from their managed care contracts as their per member per month covered lives declined. In addition, they noted that copayments were becoming more difficult to collect, indemnity insurance patients were increasingly reluctant to schedule annual physicals and preventive care, and receivables were increasing.

At about this time, Dr. Johnson decided that she didn't like the climate and was moving to the southwest. She gave six months notice.

Dr. Grant saw the handwriting on the wall. The first thing that he did was ask his business manager to run a breakeven analysis (see Chapter 6 for a discussion of breakeven analysis) to see how the projected loss in revenue would affect the practice's profit position. After he reviewed the analysis, he said:

> The results were sobering. If things continued the way we were projecting, we would be losing over $20,000 a month within six months. We had to make some immediate changes, so Larry and I sat down with the breakeven analysis to see what changes we could make to our expenses, with the goal of survival. We also saw the specter of bankruptcy in the background.

The first to go would be Dr. Herald, whose contract would not be renewed. Both physicians figured that they could absorb his declining case load. Next to go were the physician extenders and unneeded clerical support. Still, however, they had a projected annual loss of almost $165,000. This left two major areas to cut: their own salaries and rent. Currently, they were renting 6,000 square feet at $20 per square foot. They no longer needed this amount of space. In addition, with the decline of the local economy, the bottom had fallen out of commercial real estate rents. Office space that had rented for $20 per square foot could now be leased for $13 to $14 per square foot. Dr. Grant commented:

> We decided that we would try to renegotiate our lease. We would get the best deal that we could. Any remaining shortfall would have to be taken out of our salaries. We were both willing to take substantial salary hits to keep the practice going, but we also both agreed that at some point it wouldn't make sense and that we might have to choose other alternatives, such as Chapter 11 bankruptcy, or even Chapter 7, and move elsewhere. Chapter 11 provides a court defined "breathing space" for the organization to restructure its finances. Chapter 7 results in liquidation of the organization's assets.

> We felt that the building owner would be willing to work with us. We had been in the building for seven years, and they had always been cooperative in the past. Plus they were local, and all of us had this siege mentality that if we could stick together, we might all be able to weather the storm.

> Then the other shoe fell! We receive a certified letter telling us that the building was

in foreclosure. In hindsight, that shouldn't have been a surprise; this was a high-rise, first-class office building, but occupancy was only about 50 percent, and I knew that several occupants were really hurting financially. The new owners were Conglomerated Insurance Company of America (CICA), out of Los Angeles! How do you negotiate with an insurance company? What are their interests, and what do they want? We had this image of an administrative bureaucracy that would be difficult if not impossible to negotiate with. This was a real blow. We felt that we needed advice, some help in understanding how CICA would look at what we would propose, so we turned to our attorney.

Their attorney, Duncan Foster, suggested that CICA's goal was to position the property for sale. A property generating more revenue would support a higher selling price. This meant that CICA would try to increase occupancy, which of course would have to be accomplished at current market rates. Another element of value in commercial real estate was lease lengths. All other things being equal, a building with longer occupant leases was worth more than one with shorter leases. Foster commented "I think that your strategy of renegotiating the lease is viable. If we can come up with a plan that makes sense given *today's* real estate reality, CICA will probably listen. Yesterday's real estate circumstances are history."

"How do we do this?" asked Grant.

"Well, I would begin by constructing a black book," responded Foster.

"What's that?"

Foster continued:

A black book is something that we use in bankruptcy negotiations, and that is where you fellows are at. If your numbers are correct, you will go under unless CICA will work with you. A black book contains the alternatives that are available and spells out the financial implications for the other side given each alternative. For ex-

ample, what will CICA receive if they accept your proposal, and what will they receive if you go into Chapter 7? Then they can make an informed choice.

We need to provide a breakeven analysis incorporating your proposal to show that you will be a viable long-term tenant, that the plan you are proposing will result in a tenant that is financially stable. That's important because long-term leases are probably important to CICA. Next, we can show them how much revenue they will receive from you if they accept your proposal and what they are likely to get if you file for Chapter 7 bankruptcy. That's important because those are the choices that they will have.

Two days later, Jack Duggan, a senior vice president at Maple Leaf Realty Group, a regional commercial real estate firm, contacted Dr. Grant to inform him that his firm would be managing the property for CICA. Dr. Grant scheduled a meeting with him to tell him about the practice's financial problem. Dr. Grant stated:

My objective for the meeting was to tell Duggan about our financial problem and then to *listen*. I wanted to learn as much as possible about Duggan's and CICA's goals for the building and what might be their underlying interests. Duggan either played his cards close to his vest or simply didn't know much about CICA's plans for the building; I suspect more the latter than the former. I threw out some of Foster's hypotheses—that they would be interested in retaining tenants at current market rates and trying to fill the building as much as possible for a resale. Duggan said that filling the building and dealing with the reality of current market conditions made sense under any circumstances. The meeting concluded with my promise to have a proposal to him in one week.

Grant, Jones, and Foster then met to identify their interests and what they guessed would be CICA's interests (Exhibit 13–2). This would

Exhibit 13–2 Interests of Down East Internal Medicine, Ltd. and Assumed Interests of CICA

Interests of Down East Internal Medicine, Ltd. partners	*Assumed interests of CICA that could affect negotiations*
• Preserve the personal assets of Drs. Grant and Jones • Reduce operating costs • Achieve financial stability under projected financial conditions • Preserve the practice for Drs. Grant and Jones if possible • Conclude negotiations expeditiously, so that in the event that they fail, Drs. Grant and Jones can pursue other alternatives	Probable • Generate maximum rental income for property • Raise current building occupancy rate • Minimize concessions to Down East Internal Medicine, Ltd. Possible • Sell property in an expeditious manner; avoid a "fire sale"

form the basis of the proposal that they would make.

Appendix 13–A contains a copy of the black book that Foster and Dr. Grant assembled for Jack Duggan. In addition, Dr. Grant wrote a cover letter to Mr. Duggan describing the history of the practice, the impact of the local financial crisis on the practice, his desire to consider any alternative that makes financial sense, and the need to conclude the negotiation in 30 days.

Upon receipt of the proposal, Mr. Duggan called Dr. Grant and told him that he would pass the proposal on to his contact at CICA and that he hoped to be back to Dr. Grant in 1 week to 10 days. Two weeks elapsed with no word from Mr. Duggan. Dr. Grant called him, and after several unreturned phone calls over three days Duggan's secretary called and said that the proposal was still under consideration.

In the meantime, Dr. Grant, being aware of the importance of a BATNA, had contacted a real estate agent to begin a preliminary search for more affordable space. During these discussions, Dr. Grant learned that CICA also owned several other properties around town and that it had developed a reputation as an exceedingly slow decision maker. He also met with Mr. Foster again to position the practice for either Chapter 11 or Chapter 7 bankruptcy.

Twenty-eight days after Mr. Duggan received the black book proposal, he called Dr. Grant and told him that CICA was making a counterproposal. The next day the counterproposal arrived by express mail. The letter in Exhibit 13–3 contains CICA's counterproposal. Grant, Jones, and Foster then met to analyze it. Its content indicated that they had anticipated CICA's interests. All the terms related to the themes of living with current market rates, trying to fill the building, and cooperating with Down East in a financial workout that would be mutually advantageous.

The annual rent of $45,000, or $15 per square foot, was perhaps a little above market, but this only translated into $3,000 more per year than Down East's proposal. Dr. Grant commented, "I'm sure there is $3,000 worth of slop somewhere in our numbers. I just hope that it's slop in our favor! We can always take it out of our salaries. . . . We won't let this go over that small an amount."

CICA's counterproposal to be able to move the practice around in the building or perhaps even out of the building was obviously related to its desire to seek large tenants, who might take half a floor or a whole floor. Dr. Grant continued:

> This could be a problem. You just can't move a medical practice on that short a

Exhibit 13–3 CICA Counterproposal

February 3, 199X

Paul Grant, M.D.
Down East Family Practice, Ltd.
1100 Corporate Drive, Suite 705A
Portland

Dear Dr. Grant:

CICA management has evaluated your proposal and authorized me to make the following offer:

1. The annual rental shall be $45,000.
2. Down East Internal Medicine, Ltd. shall vacate suite 705B and relocate in suite 705A.
3. Down East Internal Medicine, Ltd. shall cover any building costs necessary to separate suites 705A and 705B.
4. Down East Internal Medicine, Ltd. agrees to be relocated elsewhere within the building at CICA's expense with 60 days notice during the remainder of the lease, should CICA find it desirable to do so. If no suitable space is available, CICA shall cover reasonable moving expenses. Build-out costs and other expenses associated with moving to another building would not be borne by CICA.
5. Down East Internal Medicine, Ltd. agrees to extend the length of its lease for an additional year with a 4% rent increase in this third year.

Please contact me if there are any other issues to resolve.

Very truly yours,
Jack Duggan
Sr. Vice President
Maple Leaf Realty Group

---

notice, especially if we had to find another building. On the other hand, flexibility would be very important to them, if one of their fundamental goals is to fill the building. Maybe they would provide more than 60 days notice; probably any move would be to another suite in the building. It would be in their self-interest to do that. Probably they will never ask us to move. Larry and I didn't like it, but we could live with it.

The year extension was no problem. Our breakeven showed that we could reach financial stability, so what's an additional year to us given what we gain? The net effect on the cost of the deal, however, makes their numbers look a lot better. Our proposal had a total value to them of $84,000 in rental payments over two years. We were on the hook for $240,000 over two years. Adding the third year along with the 4 percent escalation and the $15 per foot price brought the value of their counterproposal to $136,800.00. Finally, they *weren't* proposing any personal guarantees. They were willing to leave this as a corporate debt. That could have been a big stumbling block.

Dr. Grant called Mr. Duggan the next day and indicated that he would accept the proposal. He asked whether the move notification could be increased to 90 days. Duggan stated that he did not have personal authority to make that change and implied that it would be tortuous to reenter the CICA bureaucracy. He then stated:

> I doubt that we could get CICA's approval on a new tenant in less than 60 days. In all practicality you will probably get plenty of notice. If you don't have any other issues, then I will proceed to have this agreement drafted into an amendment to your current lease.

Dr. Grant agreed. It took CICA six weeks to get him the amendment and an additional three months before a fully endorsed copy sporting the signatures of three CICA vice-presidents was returned to him.

CASE ANALYSIS: PARAGON HEALTHCARE

Paragon Healthcare is a case that has been written to help you apply the concepts of negotiation to the common managed care challenge faced by many physician managers of negotiating a capitated contract. The case, which is presented in Appendix 13–B, is designed to stimulate thinking about positions versus interests, your BATNA and your adversary's BATNA, and your respective reservation prices on a number of issues.

The case involves responding to a managed care request for proposal. The practice's response illustrates how it tried to control risk, log roll, and cut the other's costs and at the same time propose a package that protected its own interests. The value of the case is in helping you think about the negotiation process in the context of managed care, not in the particular positions taken by this practice. Perhaps one of the most valuable lessons is not to accept the adversary's positions as stated in the request for proposal as a fait accompli but rather to consider the interests that they represent and to think creatively about a counterproposal that respects mutual interests. You can most effectively utilize this case by reading it carefully and then answering each set of questions that follow the case.

CONCLUSION

Physician managers constantly encounter situations that require effective negotiation skills. On occasion, negotiations can be distributive, and when that is the case distributive skills are appropriate. On many occasions, an integrative strategy will result in both sides achieving more than if they had adopted a win–lose approach.

Identifying your interests, as opposed to becoming fixated on positions, is a good place to begin any negotiation process. Identifying the interests of your opponent will help you move your opponent away from positions that serve neither of your interests. Being "nice," "provocable," "forgiving," and "clear" is a reasonable place to begin the negotiation process.

Negotiation is an art, not a science. A physician manager who wishes to succeed in this art must use common sense and an insightful understanding of the adversary to shape his or her negotiation positions. He or she also must use good judgment and humility to know when all that can be achieved has been achieved.

REFERENCES

1. R. Fisher and W. Ury, *Getting to Yes: Negotiating Agreement without Giving in*, 2d ed. (New York, N.Y.: Penguin Books, 1991).

2. Fisher and Ury, *Getting to Yes*, 83.

3. Fisher and Ury, *Getting to Yes*, 85.

4. L.R. Weingart, et al., Tactical Behaviors and Negotiation Outcomes, *International Journal of Conflict Management* 1 (1990):7–31.

5. D.G. Pruitt and H. Syna, Mismatching the Opponent's Offers in Negotiation, *Journal of Experimental and Social Psychology* 21 (1985):103–113.

6. R.J. Lewicki, et al., *Negotiation*, 2d ed. (Burr Ridge, Ill.: Irwin, 1994), 63.

7. Fisher and Ury, *Getting to Yes*.

8. Lewicki et al., *Negotiation*, 83–110.

9. Fisher and Ury, *Getting to Yes*.

10. J.L. Gibson, et al., *Organizations,* 8th ed. (Boston, Mass.: Irwin, 1994), 620–621.

11. G.T. Savage, et al., Consider Both Relationship and Substance When Negotiating Strategically, *Academy of Management Executives* (1989):37–48.

12. R. Axelrod, *The Evolution of Cooperation* (New York, N.Y.: Basic Books, 1984).

13. Axelrod, *Evolution of Cooperation*.

14. Axelrod, *Evolution of Cooperation*.

15. Axelrod, *Evolution of Cooperation*.

The Black Book Proposal

PROPOSAL FOR LEASE MODIFICATION

Down East Internal Medicine, Ltd. proposes to reduce the annual rent for the remaining two years on its lease with Conglomerated Insurance Company of America (CICA) to $42,000 per year, payable in 24 monthly installments of $3,500. This adjustment is being requested because of the effects of the local economic downturn on our practice's financial condition. To facilitate this proposed rent reduction, Down East Internal Medicine, Ltd. also proposes to vacate suite 705B and move all its operations into its original location in suite 705A. If this proposal is acceptable, then the proposed annual rent of $42,000 would represent a rate of $14 per square foot, which is representative of current market conditions. This would also provide CICA with the opportunity to lease suite 705B.

Under this proposal, we project that the landlord will receive at least $42,860.30 more than it would recover under Chapter 7 bankruptcy, as illustrated in Exhibit 13–A1.

Before making this proposal, Down East Internal Medicine, Ltd. has developed a plan to make severe reductions to its expenses, which will amount to approximately $621,000 over a 12-month period. This is illustrated in Table 13–A1. Of this amount, 12.56 percent would be due to the proposed lease modification. The largest reductions will come from eliminating salaried physician and medical professional positions as well as administrative salary reductions on the part of the two partners, Drs. Grant and Jones. The proposed rent reduction will be the final reduction to fixed costs, which will allow the practice to break even.

The alternative, which we have discussed with legal counsel, is Chapter 7 bankruptcy. If the fixed assets (Exhibit 13–A1) are liquidated, an optimistic recovery would be $9,258.80. If Down East Internal Medicine, Ltd. must proceed with bankruptcy, it is likely that the accounts receivable will suffer significantly as a result of the loss of a continuing practice to pursue collection. In addition, the legal and administrative costs of even a straightforward Chapter 7 corporate liquidation would be at least $5,000.

The practice under the proposed arrangement will be a viable, competitive entity, and it will be in a position to rebuild its patient base. It retains several strengths that will ensure that it will be able to meet the revised lease terms:

- an excellent clinical reputation
- two well-respected physicians with full case loads
- a managed care contract with a local shipyard, which may produce additional revenue as the shipyard recovers
- established referral sources
- an experienced business manager
- extremely efficient collection of receivables

Exhibit 13–A1 Financial Comparison of Proposal and Chapter 7 Bankruptcy

Landlord recovery under proposed lease arrangement:		
Rent: 2 years at $42,000	$84,000.00	
Total		$84,000.00
Landlord recovery under Chapter 7 bankruptcy:		
Value of fixed assets per 199X tax return	$23,147.00	
Adjustment for market value	($13,888.20)	
Market value of fixed assets	$9,258.80	
Accounts receivable	$52,687.00	
Adjustment for collection of receivables	($15,806.10)	
Net receivables	$36,880.90	
Projected legal and administrative costs under Chapter 7		($5,000.00)
Total		$41,139.70
Net gain for lease modification proposal		$42,860.30

- extensive marketing and promotion expertise and practice visibility
- an excellent location for attracting patients throughout the greater metropolitan area
- no debt other than to the partners

In conclusion, the proposed annual rent of $42,000 will result in the landlord receiving substantially more financial benefit than would be received under the bankruptcy alternative. The partners are committed to staying in practice if that is financially feasible. We have developed a plan that, with your cooperation, will make this feasible.

To proceed with the necessary restructuring, it is essential that we know as soon as possible whether you will accept this proposal. I propose that we determine whether we can reach an agreement within 30 days. If the negotiations extend much beyond this time, we will begin to incur losses that will be unacceptable, and we will have to consider other alternatives.

Table 13–A1 Projected Expense Reductions

Operating Expenses	Projected Next 12 Months	Prior 12 Months	Reduction
Advertising—Marketing	$2,065.00	$2,065.00	$0.00
Advertising—Yellow Pages	$1,048.93	$1,048.93	$0.00
Credit card discounts	$1,475.00	$1,475.00	$0.00
Bank service charges	$395.70	$395.70	$0.00
Interest expense	$471.80	$471.80	$0.00
Travel—Business related	$1,000.00	$6,894.00	($5,894.00)
Licenses—Professional	$600.00	$600.00	$0.00
Licenses—Business	$3,385.41	$5,924.47	($2,539.06)
Other taxes and licenses	$2,000.00	$2,554.87	($554.87)
Business meals	$2,876.00	$4,578.00	($1,702.00)
Food/entertainment—Marketing	$1,000.00	$5,498.00	($4,498.00)
Legal expenses	$2,578.00	$2,578.00	$0.00
Accounting expenses	$500.00	$500.00	$0.00
Other professional expenses	$2,487.00	$6,500.00	($4,013.00)
Rent—Office space	$42,000.00	$120,000.00	($78,000.00)
Rent—Equipment	$4,000.00	$7,500.00	($3,500.00)
Office supplies	$6,895.00	$10,598.00	($3,703.00)
Medical supplies	$26,597.00	$35,895.00	($9,298.00)
General overhead	$3,548.00	$3,548.00	$0.00
Computer repair/Maintenance	$1,123.50	$1,123.50	$0.00
General repair and maintenance	$1,206.25	$1,206.25	$0.00
Payroll taxes—Employer total	$10,370.00	$20,740.00	($10,370.00)
Postage	$2,275.75	$2,730.90	($455.15)
Health insurance	$6,000.00	$12,000.00	($6,000.00)
Professional liability insurance	$16,000.00	$26,000.00	($10,000.00)
Insurance—Other	$972.00	$972.00	$0.00
Salaries—Medical	$300,000.00	$700,000.00	($400,000.00)
Salaries—Physician management	$0.00	$50,000.00	($50,000.00)
Salaries—Front office staff	$93,000.00	$123,000.00	($30,000.00)
Telephone	$4,259.00	$4,684.90	($425.90)
Total	$540,129.34	$1,161,082.31	($620,952.98)
Net income	$24,105.67		

Percentage expense reduction due to lease proposal 12.56%

Paragon Healthcare

Prepared By
Irving M. Pike, M.D.
Gastroenterology Consultants, Ltd.
Virginia Beach, Virginia
and
Robert J. Solomon, Ph.D.
Graduate School of Business
The College of William & Mary
Williamsburg, Virginia

PARAGON HEALTHCARE

843 Powhatan Place
Hampton Roads, VA 23455

February 1, 1996

Dear Dr.
Enclosed is a package of information concerning Paragon's Request for Proposals (RFP) for a Gastroenterology Capitation Program. We are inviting proposals for a capitated network from all currently participating gastroenterology (GI) practices in the area. It is Paragon's intention to select a reconfigured network of GI practices, and to put the GI Capitation Program into effect on July 1, 1996.

We strongly urge you to carefully read all of the enclosed material. We have enclosed a copy of the GI Database Report for 1995. The Market Share information in this report is important, as it will become your initial Market Share for this Capitation Program.

We must receive a final copy of your proposal by April 1, 1996 in order for you to be considered for our new network.

If you have any questions, or require additional information to prepare your proposal, please contact Janice Smith, Provider Relations Supervisor at 555-2345, or my direct line at 555-4567. We are eager to meet with you and discuss your proposal. We stand ready to assist you in thoroughly understanding this program, and in preparing a proposal for our new GI Capitation Program.

Sincerely,

Andrew Carey, M.D., M.B.A.
Medical Director

PARAGON HEALTHCARE REQUEST FOR PROPOSALS: GASTROENTEROLOGY NETWORK CAPITATION PROGRAM

General Requirements

Paragon Healthcare is seeking proposals from all participating gastroenterology (GI) practices for in-network adult and pediatric services rendered under our HMO and related managed care programs in the Four Corners area.

There are three separate factors which are multiplied together to determine your monthly capitation payment. The first factor is your practice's Market Share. We have enclosed a report documenting your market share as of January 1, 1996. We will update the market share data for 1996 when the final data have been compiled prior to determination of the initial capitation payment in July. We will recalculate Market Shares once every six months during the course of this contract.

The Market Share is determined by each practice's percentage of the total number of unique referred patients and the practice's percentage of relative value units of service submitted in encounters as compared to all practices in the GI network in the same service area. These two factors are equally weighted to determine each practice's Market Share. Paragon will adjust practice Market Shares semi-annually based upon encounters submitted by all GI practices in your Service Area.

The second factor used to determine your overall reimbursement level is the total number of eligible Members in your Service Area. The Service Area for this capitation program is defined as the Four Corners area. As of December 31, 1995, there were approximately 77,000 members in this Service Area. The actual number of eligible members will vary from month to month. No minimum or maximum number of members are guaranteed in this program, but will depend entirely upon how well we are able to market our HMO and related Point of Service products in this community.

The third and final factor used to determine capitation payments is the Capitation Rate, for which you must submit a competitive bid. Your proposal must specify a Capitation Rate expressed in per member per month (PMPM) terms that your practice is willing to accept as one of the three basic factors used in the formula for reimbursement under this program. Each GI practice's monthly capitation payment will be determined by multiplying the practice's Capitation Rate by the practice's Market Share, and then multiplying that product times the total number of eligible Paragon members in your Service Area.

Only those practices whose proposals are accepted by Paragon will be admitted into our new GI network effective July 1, 1996. Over the last several years there has been steady growth in this service area. However, Paragon does not guarantee any minimum level of membership in the service area during the term of the contract.

Paragon Healthcare reserves the right to accept or reject any or all proposals submitted, and to use competitive negotiations during the final selection process. The final selection criteria will be based not only upon the specific financial terms proposed, including any proposed financial incentives, but also upon the mixture of services provided, hospitals and geographic areas served, board certification status, and all quality of care and cost effectiveness data which Paragon maintains in its own files on physicians. Finally, Paragon will interview each group practice to assess who will partner the most effectively with us to meet our medical management goals and objectives.

Paragon is not obligated to accept the lowest bid submitted in this process, but will weight all the above factors to select a capitated GI network which in its sole judgment provides the best overall value in terms of quality of care, service to our participants and primary care physicians, and medical cost effectiveness. Paragon expects that the total number of GI practices and physicians participating in our network will be reduced from current levels after the final selection has been made.

Incentive Programs

Paragon believes that GI services represent a major opportunity for medical cost containment in the Four Corners area. The first critical cost factor for GI disease is the cost for professional services associated with your specialty. Your capitation rate proposal will directly address this cost factor. The capitation rate will include all professional services rendered by you in your office, the emergency room, in-patient and out-patient areas of the hospital.

Our studies have shown that over the last three years the average cost for GI professional services across all of our providers in the Four Corners area have averaged $0.82 PMPM. Comparative national costs for GI capitation contracts range from $0.42 to $0.59 PMPM. (50th and 70th percentile capitation rates as reported in a national survey covering 132 different capitation rates.)

For comparison, our Hudson Valley region has a very similar population with a similar age and sex distribution. The cost in Hudson Valley is $0.64 PMPM for this same time period, using the same fee schedule used to reimburse the Four Corners area. The data clearly point to extremely high GI costs in the Four Corners market. Your capitation proposal must reduce the excess costs in the Four Corners service area for this cost factor.

In order to make the GI capitation program successful, we need a significant reduction in total medical costs associated with GI services and diseases. There are three other major cost factors in treating GI diseases. Paragon believes that a properly structured incentive program for our capitated physicians is an important tool to assist both parties in achieving our objectives in reducing these other three factors. All of Paragon's incentive programs are designed to support one or more of the three medical management objectives which guide our health care program:

1. Improve patient access, service and satisfaction
2. Improve quality of care
3. Keep total medical costs as low as possible

The other three areas of potential cost savings are:

1. Reduce inpatient hospital costs by reducing hospital length of stays associated with GI admissions; converting some very short admissions into medical observation stays (23-hour short stay), preventing low acuity admissions through the aggressive use of home health services;
2. Reduce the frequency and cost of endoscopy services;
3. Reduce the cost of GI prescription medications.

Paragon maintains databases appropriate to each of the above three GI cost factors. For example, our studies have shown that the cost of H2-antagonists and other GI drugs averaged $2.06 PMPM in Four Corners in 1995, as compared to the Paragon national average based on 44 HMOs throughout the US of $1.15 PMPM. Thus, the cost for GI prescription drugs in Four Corners is 88 percent higher than our national average as measured on a PMPM basis. This suggests a dramatic opportunity to reduce costs to levels closer to the national averages. We believe that a properly structured incentive could be the catalyst for encouraging such an improvement.

We have also found that a very large percentage of total medical costs associated with GI results from elective endoscopy procedures performed in the outpatient suites of our participating hospitals. The rate of endoscopy services has historically been 2.1 procedures per 1,000 members. Our comparative information suggests to us that such services could be reduced by at least 20 percent through the use of careful clinical protocols. There are many cases where the use of acceptable alternative diagnostic or therapeutic protocols could reduce the number of elective endoscopy procedures without affecting the outcome or quality of care given to the patient. We believe that a capitation program coupled with appropriate incentives again could reduce this very important factor.

See Table 13–B1 for the *GI Hospital Medical DRGs Database*, which contains data on those hospitalizations that are primarily controlled by your specialty. This indicates the current number and rate of admissions, total bed days, and length of stays as well as the expected performance targets in a well managed health care system for each of these parameters.

The data show that in the first six months of 1995 in the Four Corners Area, the number of GI admissions per 1,000 members of 2.33 was close to the performance target of 2.15, which calls for an improvement of approximately 8 percent in the GI admission rate to meet the target. The actual average length of stay at 3.62 days is a full day longer than the performance target of 2.6 days. Likewise, the total number of bed days per 1,000 members is 8.31 compared to the performance target of 5.76, which indicates that an improvement of 44 percent is possible in a well managed integrated health care system. We have already developed an incentive program for our Cardiology Capitation Program based upon an equivalent table for Cardiovascular DRGs. Similarly, we believe that a structured incentive program would be effective in reducing GI hospital admissions and bed days.

All of these studies demonstrate that costs for GI services in this community are extremely high. We must reduce the total GI medical costs to a level that is closer to national norms. In order to achieve this important goal, a major determinant of our final GI network physician selection decisions will be on the basis of those practices that can demonstrate to our satisfaction the best overall plan to reduce total medical costs for all four GI cost factors, and who can work with us in a collaborative manner in developing the best combination of capitation and financial incentives to achieve such goals.

The details of an incentive program to accomplish this will need to be developed and clearly understood by all parties before we can make our final network selections. Your proposal should address how you would work in partnership with Paragon to reduce the total cost associated with each of the GI cost factors noted above

through the use of a properly structured capitation program coupled with an incentive program. Please feel free to discuss your ideas with us for a GI incentive program prior to submitting your proposal.

COMMONLY ASKED QUESTIONS

1. *What is capitation?*

   Capitation is a method of paying physicians on the basis of the total number of patients for whom they are responsible for providing specialty services, rather than on the basis of a set fee for each individual service performed. Paragon uses a specialty prepaid capitation budget which is divided according to the Market Share of each practice participating in the network.

2. *How does the market share capitation method work?*

   Each month each participating specialty practice receives a fixed rate of payment per member. This is called the capitation payment. For example, the practice might be responsible for specialty services for 75,000 members. If the agreed upon capitation rate was $0.50 PMPM, the total specialty budget would be $37,500 each month for the entire population in the given service area. If more than one practice was responsible for this group of patients, each practice would receive a pro rated Market Share of this total specialty budget.

3. *What is the advantage of capitation to the specialist?*

   It assures the practice a financially sound and growing patient base. It also decreases the administrative burden of collection, and makes cash flow more predictable and reliable. Well run specialty practices will immediately recognize a positive cash flow advantage. It positions the practice to compete more effectively by increasing its Market Share, because

Table 13–B1 GI Hospital Medical DRGs Database—Four Corners Area

January 1, 1995–June 30, 1995

DRG	Description	Admits	Total Bed Days	AVG. LOS	Actual Admits/ 1,000	Actual Bed Days/ 1,000	Expected Days	Expected AVG. LOS	Expected Admits/ 1,000	Expected Bed Days/ 1,000
172	GI Malig. w CC	6	66	11.00	0.08	0.83	23	3.77	0.05	0.18
173	GI Malig. w/o CC	1	1	1.00	0.01	0.01	4	3.77	0.05	0.18
174	GI Bleed w CC	15	79	5.27	0.19	1.00	45	3.03	0.11	0.34
175	GI Bleed w/o CC	4	7	1.75	0.05	0.09	12	3.03	0.11	0.34
176	Compl. Peptic Ulcer	2	4	2.00	0.04	0.05	6	3.03	0.11	0.34
177	Unc. Peptic Ulcer w CC	2	15	7.50	0.03	0.19	6	3.03	0.11	0.34
178	Unc. Peptic Ulcer w/o CC	5	17	3.40	0.06	0.21	15	3.03	0.12	0.34
179	Inflam. Bowel Dis.	7	50	7.14	0.09	0.63	26	3.77	0.05	0.18
180	GI Obstruct. w CC	7	26	3.71	0.10	0.33	26	3.77	0.06	0.18
181	GI Obstruct. w/o CC	5	18	3.60	0.06	0.23	19	3.77	0.05	0.18
182	Esophagitis, Gas, >17 w CC	39	153	3.92	0.49	1.93	90	2.31	0.37	0.86
183	Esophagitis, Gas, >17 w/o CC	53	121	2.28	0.67	1.52	122	2.31	0.37	0.86
184	Esophagitis, Gas, age 0-17	31	81	2.61	0.39	1.02	72	2.31	0.39	0.87
188	Other GI Dx, >17 w CC	0	0	0.00	0.00	0.00	0	1.19	0.06	0.19
189	Other GI Dx, >17 w/o CC	3	19	6.33	0.04	0.24	4	1.19	0.07	0.19
190	Other GI Dx, age 0-17	2	2	1.00	0.03	0.03	2	1.19	0.07	0.19
	Total	182	659	3.62	2.33	8.31	472	2.60	2.15	5.76

Expected LOS, admits/1,000, bed days/1,000 performance targets are based on national statistics.

Source: Copyright © Robert J. Solomon, Ph.D., Irving M. Pike, M.D., and Sentara Health System, used with permission.

the number of practices accepted into the specialty capitation network is limited.

4. *What is the advantage of capitation to the health plan?*

Capitation has the potential to improve referral interactions between specialty and primary care physicians. There is a strong financial incentive to create common referral protocols and patient management guidelines between primary and specialty providers. Ineffective or unnecessary consultations, treatments, and procedures usually decrease when the presence of fee for service financial incentives are removed. Experience in numerous areas suggest that specialty driven utilization will typically decrease 20 percent under capitation.

It creates the opportunity to work more closely with a limited number of high quality, cost effective specialty practices. It allows the health plan to more accurately predict medical costs from year to year. Administrative costs for claim processing will decrease.

5. *Will patients have unlimited access to specialists?*

No, the health plan will continue to use primary care physicians as gatekeepers to initiate all specialty referrals, except in an emergency.

6. *What is included in capitation?*

Reimbursement for all professional services provided by your specialty to all eligible participants is included. This includes all office and hospital based professional services, as well as any diagnostic testing, laboratory and radiology procedures performed in your office. Payment for facility costs, such as hospitals and surgicenters, is not included in the professional capitation given to specialists. But all of your professional services rendered by your practice and provided in your office, and any hospital surgicenter, or emergency room treatment provided by you are included in the capitation payment. Paragon participants are responsible for a copayment due at the time of office service which adds to the total compensation of the capitation package.

Out of area emergency care and patient self-referred elective care is not included in the capitation. Care rendered to participants in our PPO program is not included in the capitation, and will be paid with our PPO fee schedule.

7. *Does this mean that I won't be paid a separate tray fee?* (The tray fee covers the variable costs [consumables] associated with a colonoscopy, EGD, flexible sigmoidoscopy, etc. It includes costs for such items as Betadine, disposable instruments, alcohol, swabs, etc.)

Yes. The tray fee is covered in your PMPM price. There is no extra payment for a tray fee.

8. *How can I communicate with the health plan about participants?*

In the near future we will link key practices to the health plan electronically, which will provide immediate eligibility information. Next, it will allow the practice to record referrals, encounters, procedures, and hospitalizations electronically. PCP referrals can be confirmed instantly without a call.

9. *What will happen to practices that do not become part of the capitation plan?*

Paragon will transition care of patients from terminated practices and transfer the care of these patients back to their primary care physicians or to those specialty care practices who are in the program. This will have the effect of increasing the Market Share over time of those practices selected to participate in the Specialty Capitation Program. We generally expect such transitions to be completed within 90 to 180 days of implementation of the network.

10. *Are there incentives or bonuses available in the capitation program?*

Paragon typically provides an incentive program for capitated physicians above the capitated rate for meeting specified performance targets involving quality, access, patient satisfaction, and/or reduction of total medical expenses. A formula for reducing total medical expenses might include inpatient and outpatient hospital costs, diagnostic costs, laboratory, and/or pharmaceutical charges. The exact formula and timing for distribution for the incentive program is determined by agreement with the Paragon Medical Director.

11. *How are the specialty capitation rates determined?*

Paragon maintains a claims database for all care in your specialty, and uses that information as a starting point to determine costs in your specialty on a PMPM basis. The claims experience will be shared with you so that you can understand some of the areas of inefficiency and opportunities for improvement. We also review national sources of capitation rates, such as the Warren Survey.

Paragon has also determined a historical Market Share of each specialty practice that participates with us. The overall specialty capitated budget will then be divided according to the Market Share of each practice. Ultimately, the final capitation rate agreed upon will be negotiated based upon these parameters.

12. *How often will Paragon adjust the Market Share for each practice?*

We will adjust this semi-annually during the first two years of the program to account for those practices which are no longer participating with us, and the resulting shift in referral patterns. After the first two years, we will adjust the Market Share annually.

13. *Are we at risk to lose market share if we become more efficient, but other practices in the specialty capitation network don't evolve to more efficient methods of utilization?*

This is a theoretical risk, but one which can be controlled. First, remember that one of our criteria is to select practices with demonstrated ability to control unnecessary utilization. Second, we will be sharing utilization data on all groups through a Specialty Advisory Committee composed of your peers. If it appears that one practice is acting inappropriately, we will request input from the Specialty Advisory Committee on how to deal with this situation. In essence, we will ask each of you to monitor the performance of your peers in the program.

14. *How should I determine what capitation rate to put in my proposal?*

You have two sources of data: (1) the historic costs for your specialty within your service area; (2) national sources of specialty capitation rates, such as those determined by the Warren Survey.

15. *What criteria will Paragon use to select specialty practices?*

We will consider the following:
- the geographic area and hospitals at which each practice provides services;
- a statistical review of historical patterns of care and costs for each practice;
- a review of the unique procedures and services performed by each practice;
- measures of quality of care, clinical outcomes, complaints, compliance with health plan policy and procedures, board certification;
- the monthly capitation rate proposed by the practice;
- the general attitude of the physicians in the practice, their contributions to our managed care program, and the ease with which we have been able to work with the practice historically;
- any creative ideas which you may propose to lower total medical costs, as well as improve service access or quality of care to our members.

16. *If I'm not selected for the specialty capitation network, what will happen to my patients?*

Paragon will assist you in transferring the care of your patients back to their primary care physicians. In most cases the transfer will take place between 30 and 90 days of the implementation of the Specialty Capitation Program.

17. *Will our total reimbursement be more or less under the Specialty Capitation Program?*

That depends upon a number of factors. Clearly, one will be the Capitation Rate that you submit in your proposal. In addition, physicians who practice a conservative, efficient utilization style of practice are more likely to see an improvement in cash flow on a per patient basis.

We expect to have fewer specialists within our network after the program is fully implemented, and those physicians selected to remain in the program should see an increase in total referrals, and hence Market Share. This should lead to an increase in overall cash flow.

The prepaid nature of capitation provides cash flow significantly faster than the traditional method of submitting claims and awaiting payment. A typical wait for traditional claims processing is 45 to 90 days. Instead, you will receive your capitation check no later than the 20th day of each month. In addition, there are no denied claims because you receive prepayment.

18. *What about copayments?*

This can be a significant source of cash. Member copayments add about 3 percent to 5 percent of additional reimbursement.

19. *How should our practice divide the monthly capitation revenue to individual physicians?*

This is an important question, and it should be thoroughly discussed with members of your practice. There are several methods, and all involve developing a formula and implementing the accounting methodology on a monthly basis. One method is to divide the revenue based upon relative value units of service provided by each physician. Other groups have chosen to split capitated revenue on the basis of the number of patients seen. Third, you could choose to share the revenue using the Market Share methodology and equations that we have developed to administer this program. A final method is to split the capitation revenue according to the percentage of billings for each physician.

MARKET SHARE FORMULA

The Market Share for each practice is the percentage that each practice has of its designated service area. The formula adjusts both for the number of patients seen, as well as the intensity of care that must be rendered to each patient. The Market Share for each practice is calculated using the following formula:

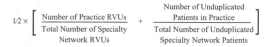

$$\frac{1}{2} \times \left[\frac{\text{Number of Practice RVUs}}{\text{Total Number of Specialty Network RVUs}} + \frac{\text{Number of Unduplicated Patients in Practice}}{\text{Total Number of Unduplicated Specialty Network Patients}} \right]$$

Monthly Capitation Payment

The Monthly Capitation Payment for each practice is calculated using the following formula:

Specialty Capitation Rate × Practice's Market Share × Total number of members in the Service Area

Example

Practice XYZ is a GI practice with three physicians. Over the last year it treated a total of 100 unique unduplicated Paragon patients, and submitted a total of 800 Relative Value Units of Service. During the last year there were 1,000 unduplicated patients treated in the entire specialty network requiring 10,000 RVUs of service. The health plan has 75,000 participants, and the practice has agreed to a capitation rate of $0.50 PMPM. The Market Share and Monthly Capitation Payment calculations are as follows:

Market Share =
$1/2 \times [(100/1000) + (800/10,000)] = 9\%$
Monthly Capitation Payment =
$75,000 \times \$0.50 \times 9\% = \$3,375.00$

HISTORIC MARKET SHARE ANALYSIS

Based on our historic data for Gastroenterology of Four Corners, your current share of our GI specialty network that will be placed under capitation is 15.33 percent. This means that you have treated this percentage of the total number of GI patients who received treatment during 1995. This number does not reflect the number of procedures that you conducted on these patients, nor does it reflect the severity of their conditions.

GASTROENTEROLOGY OF FOUR CORNERS, P.C.

Situation Description

In 1995 Gastroenterology of Four Corners, P.C. (GFC) treated 200 Paragon patients. 1995 net revenue from Paragon patients was $116,295. This constituted 8.3 percent, of GFC's 1995 annual net revenue of $1,401,145.

There were 1,305 Total Unduplicated Specialty Network Patients in 1995. GFC's ratio of Number of Practice RVUs to Total Number of Network RVUs was 13.5 percent.

GFC performed 160 procedures on Paragon patients. Of these 75 were EGDs, 65 were colonoscopies, and 20 were flexible sigmoidoscopies. All of these procedures were performed in the hospital, because Paragon had a policy of not paying tray fees for procedures performed in physicians' offices. The practice, however, has an operating suite, and routinely conducts these procedures in the office for the patients of insurance carriers who do pay tray fees.

Paragon currently pays $85 to physicians for a flexible sigmoidoscopy.

Paragon currently pays hospitals $850 for a colonoscopy and $750 for EGD.

GASTROENTEROLOGY OF FOUR CORNERS, P.C.

RFP

Proposal Points:

- Cap rate of $0.80 PMPM.

- Eliminate RVU elements in the Market Share Formula.
- Carve out flexible sigmoidoscopies. We will accept $50 fee for service, which is $35 less than Paragon's current payment. (Flexible sigmoidoscopy is exclusively a practice-based procedure. Paragon will not pay for conducting this procedure in the hospital.)
- We will accept a tray fee of $300 for performing colonoscopies and EGDs in our office. This will lower the cost to Paragon by $450 to $550 per procedure.
- We will offer a teaching program to primary care physicians that will assist in lowering the cost of H_2 antagonist drugs and other prescription medication to Paragon. Our goal will be to lower this cost by $0.50 PMPM. We propose that all selected GI groups participate in this effort, and that we share in proportion to our market share in a bonus of 25 percent of the cost saving in year one.

Projected Practice Effects:

- Market share = 18%
- Capitation Fee = $133,056
- Prescription Drug Bonus = $3,465
- Tray Fee = $46,980
- Flex. Sig. = $1,762
- Co-payments = $3,992
- Total Paragon Net Revenue = $189,254

DISCUSSION QUESTIONS—A

1. Based on Paragon's proposal, what are Paragon's:
   A. Positions
   B. Interests
2. What sources of internal practice data could you examine to help you respond to this RFP?
3. To what extent are the mix of procedures and the degree to which this may change in the future important for assessing your costs and the risks involved in making a PMPM bid?

Exhibit 13–B1 GIFC Proposal Worksheet

Practice Characteristics

Practice Unique Paragon Patients—1995	200
Procedures on Paragon Patients—1995	160
1995 Paragon Net Revenue—GIFC	$116,295
Total Network Unique GI Patients	1305
Practice % of Unique Patients—GIFC	15.33%
Ratio of Practice RVUs to Network RVUs	13.5%

Breakeven Calculations

At PMPM	$0.874
Market Share Formula	0.144
Total Number Members	77,000
Payment PMPM	$9,691
Annual Net Revenue	$116,295
Net Revenue Impact	$0.00

	PMPM Proposal Outcomes		
PMPM	$0.80	$0.70	$0.60
Total Number Members	77,000	77,000	77,000
Est. Market Share	18%	18%	18%
Net Monthly Capitation Revenue	$11,088	$9,702	$8,316
Annual Capitation Revenue	$133,056	$116,424	$99,792
Tray Fee	$300	$300	$300
Est. Tray Fee Cost	$50	$50	$50
Est. Tray Fee Net Revenue	$250	$250	$250
Est. Number of Tray Fees	188	188	188
Est. Tray Fee Net Revenue	$46,980	$46,980	$46,980
First Year Prescription Savings Goal 50 cents PMPM	$38,500	$38,500	$38,500
GI Providers' Share	$19,250	$19,250	$19,250
Practice Share	$3,465	$3,465	$3,465
Current Flex. Sigs.	30	30	30
Projected Flex. Sigs.	35	35	35
Proposed Fee	$50	$50	$50
Net Revenue	$1,762	$1,762	$1,762
Estimated Annual Co-Pays based on estimated 3% of PMPM	$3,992	$3,493	$2,994
Total Paragon Net Revenue	$189,254	$172,123	$154,993

Source: Copyright © Robert J. Solomon, Ph.D., Irving M. Pike, M.D., and Sentara Health System, used with permission.

4. After examining the cost data in Table 13–B1, what questions do you have about the validity of these data?

5. Examine the market share formula. What questions do you have about the incentives created by this formula? Do you see any perverse incentives created by the formula?

DISCUSSION QUESTIONS—B

1. Do you feel that your responsibilities are defined in the proposal in enough detail?

For example, would you consider carving out any groups of patients for whom you would not be responsible? What kinds of risks would you be trying to control? What sources of data could you examine to help you consider this question? Are there any other counterproposals that you could make to Paragon to control these risks?

2. How would you analyze the net effect on your practice of *not being selected* for the capitation program? What practice changes could you consider making?

DISCUSSION QUESTIONS—C

Consider GIFC's proposal as a devil's advocate position, and develop a response to the Paragon RFP. In your response:

1. quote a PMPM price
2. identify any bonuses and incentives that you think would help your proposal
3. identify any guarantees, minimums, carve outs, or other risk control measures that you would propose

As you develop your proposal, remember to think about *interests versus positions* and *integrative negotiating concepts*, such as:

1. identifying the relevant negotiation issues for both parties
2. opportunities for expanding the pie
3. decomposing compound issues into their component parts
4. log rolling
5. cost cutting (reducing the other's costs)

CHAPTER 14

Business Law

Chapter Objectives

This chapter will provide you with an understanding of fundamental business law concepts. As a result, you will be able to

1. prevent disputes
2. avoid lawsuits
3. anticipate the legal consequences of your actions

The chapter is organized around the following potential sources of liability or conflict:

1. torts
2. contracts
3. employment issues, including equal employment opportunity, employee contracts, contractor agreements, and the Fair Labor Standards Act
4. malpractice, which is a particular type of tort

After reading this chapter, you will understand how the legal system approaches these potential sources of litigation. As a result, you will be able to conduct your daily affairs with due consideration to possible legal consequences.

We are living in an increasingly litigious society. Many explanations have been offered for this, including a declining respect for authority, an ever-increasing number of lawyers, a rise in consumerism, and an evolving interpretation of what constitutes negligence. As a physician, your relationships with your patients expose you to the risk of malpractice litigation. As a physician manager, your organization's arrangements and dealings with insurance companies, landlords, suppliers, employees, contractors, partners, and so on all have potential legal ramifications.

Legal considerations are best handled in anticipation of events. If you are aware of the potential legal consequences of an action, then you can often avoid a legal confrontation or, at a minimum, place yourself in a more favorable legal position. This strategy is called preventive law, and it is analogous to preventive medicine. By eliminating or minimizing problems before they occur, you may avoid the courtroom and all the expense and personal disruption that are associated with this ultimate form of decision making. This chapter will help you recognize when you are entering territory with legal implications. In addition, by understanding the legal aspects of your actions, you will be able to communicate more effectively with your attorney. You should, of course, consult your attorney regarding situations with obvious legal implications, such as a contract, lease, or employment dispute. There will be many unanticipated situations, however, in which understanding the principles of law will allow you to make good operational decisions as well as help you determine when you should involve your attorney.

Legal problems can arise from a number of different sources. In this chapter, these sources are classified as general torts, general contracts, employment issues, and malpractice. When a wrong has been committed that harms a person, that person can seek to recover money damages from the wrongdoer. If the harm was committed through the breach of a contract, then the process is governed by contract law. For example, if you have a contract with a cleaning service and you feel that its performance is inadequate, then your recourse will be governed by the content of the contract and how contracts are interpreted under contract law. When there is no contract, then the wronged party may seek recovery under tort law. For example, if a patient or member of the general public happens to fall in your parking lot, he or she may seek to recover damages under tort law because there is no contract between the two of you. Employment and malpractice cases are, respectively, specific types of contract and tort cases. For example, firing an employee who has an employment contract will be governed by contract law. Malpractice cases are generally governed by tort law, although some cases are filed as a breach of contract between the patient and the physician.

Figure 14–1 outlines the general structure of U.S. law. Statutory law is the result of statutes enacted by state legislatures, ordinances enacted by municipalities, and laws passed by Congress. Common law derives from the decisions of judges:

> Common law . . . makes itself up as it goes along; it sets precedents but they are never unalterable, because they are derived ultimately, not from a book of rules, but from a judge's intuitive feeling for equity and fair play. . . . Common law assumes a freely developing pattern which is nevertheless consistent with itself, like the development of a living language.[1(p.5)]

Criminal law protects society's interest in order, safety, and the integrity of its institutions by defining and prohibiting unacceptable behavior. By definition, criminal law is statutory because it derives from the actions of legislatures and Congress. Civil law also protects society's interests, but it does so by defining the rights and obligations of one person or business vis-à-vis another. Civil law can be constitutional, statutory, or common (case or case based).

GENERAL TORTS

Definition

A tort is a civil wrong that has been committed against another party or another party's property but is not due to a breach of contract. A tort is distinct from a crime, which is an intentionally harmful act that is committed against society. As a result, tort actions are brought by individuals, whereas crimes are prosecuted by the state. Those responsible for a tort are referred to as tortfeasors; those responsible for a crime are referred to as criminals. An act can result in both a tort and a crime, as recently exemplified by the O.J. Simpson cases. Simpson was prosecuted by the state under criminal law and by the injured parties under tort law. It is also possible for there to be a crime with no tort, such as the case of a physician who misrepresents his or her personal property assets to the local tax collector in an attempt to reduce tax liability. Because no individual has been harmed, there is no tort. Finally, there can be a tort with no crime. For example, if a patient inadvertently takes the wrong coat from a waiting room, this is the tort of conversion. This is not a crime, however, because the motivation necessary for theft is absent.

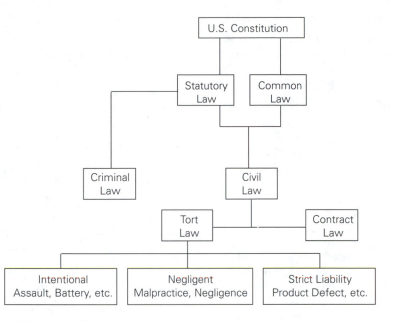

Figure 14–1 The U.S. system of laws.

Liability

The simple fact that a person is harmed or injured does not in itself mean that a tort has occurred. For a tort to occur, there has to be a basis for liability. The following considerations can be used to establish a basis for liability.

Voluntary Action

The tortfeasor's voluntary actions or voluntary failure to act must have contributed to the harm. Actions resulting from immediate peril or fear are generally considered involuntary acts. For example, if you jump back at the sight of a snake and inadvertently strike another person, the action would probably be considered involuntary.

Intent

Some torts require the demonstration of intent, whereas other torts do not. In tort law, the issue of intent relates to whether the tortfeasor intended to commit the act, not whether harm was intended to the other party. To prove intent, it is necessary to demonstrate that the actor either knew or believed that certain results were likely to follow his or her actions. This knowledge is determined on an objective basis: what a reasonable person would be expected to know or would expect to occur under the circumstances.

The following example illustrates the role of intent:

> As a practical joke, Jack pulls a chair out from under Jill as she begins to sit, causing her to fall and sustain a hip fracture. Although Jack actually meant Jill no harm, a court could reasonably find that he knew with substantial certainty that Jill would attempt to sit down where the chair had been, and could fall and be injured. Hence, Jack had the knowledge required to support a finding of intent for tort liability. His intent was to do an act that he could have reasonably foreseen would cause injury to another.[2(p.74)]

Causation

For a tort to be sustained, it must be demonstrated that there was a causal relationship between the wrongful act and the harm. State laws vary regarding how directly the act must be related to the harm for causation to be demonstrated.

The following example illustrates how the causal chain can become extended:

> George Nesselrode was a passenger in an airplane made by Beechcraft Aircraft Corporation. A few minutes after taking off, the plane crashed and all occupants were killed. Action was brought by George's widow against Beechcraft on the theory that it was at fault in failing to prevent the improper installation of certain parts in its airplanes, in consequence of which the parts could be installed in reverse or backwards, and this improper installation had caused the fatal crash. . . .
>
> Judgment [was] against Beechcraft Aircraft Corp. Although no harm would have occurred if third persons had not made an improper installation, the fact remained that the prior failure of Beechcraft to give proper warning was a substantial factor in bringing about the harm. It therefore could not claim that the installation was an act that broke the causal chain. As a substantial contributing factor, the manufacturer was liable even though the wrong installation was the proximate cause and was the act of a third person.[3(p.163)]

Notice that motivation is largely irrelevant to the above four considerations, other than perhaps as a way of demonstrating intent.

Classification

Torts can be classified into three basic groups:

1. Intentional torts result from intended acts, such as assault, battery, malicious prosecution, and defamation.
2. Negligence torts result from unintended acts, such as negligence and malpractice.
3. Strict liability torts result from a liability without fault. Examples include product liability cases in which the manufacturer is held strictly responsible for defective

goods. For example, if a piece of glass was found in a can of soup, the manufacturer would be held strictly liable for any personal injuries suffered.

The following discussion elaborates on some of the torts that a physician might reasonably encounter, as either the victim or the tortfeasor.

Intentional Torts

Assault. Assault is an act (more than words) that creates the apprehension of an immediate harmful contact. The important elements for demonstrating assault are the tortfeasor's action, his or her intent, the perception of fear or apprehension on the part of the assaulted person, and the causal relationship between the assaulted person's fear and the tortfeasor's actions. For example, Mr. Smith is dissatisfied with Dr. Jones's services. He confronts Dr. Jones and points an unloaded pistol at her while threatening to shoot. Assault has occurred because Smith committed an act that a reasonable person would assume would create fear or apprehension whether or not the gun was actually loaded. Dr. Jones had those fears, and they were the proximate result of Smith's actions.

Battery. Battery is intentional, unjustified touching of another person's body. The contact does not have to cause actual physical harm. Battery has occurred even if the action is only offensive or insulting. For example, Dr. Brown intentionally and without consent unjustifiably kisses and fondles Ms. Arnold. Even though no physical harm is done to Ms. Arnold, a battery has taken place.

Defenses against assault and battery suits include consent and privilege. Consent exists if the allegedly wronged party implied or expressly stated that the actions were permissible. Privilege might exist if the alleged tortfeasor acted in self-defense or in the defense of others or of property. The level of force must be reasonable given the circumstances and cannot be retaliatory.

Intentional infliction of emotional distress. This involves disturbing someone's peace of mind through outrageous behavior. The words or actions must be exceedingly severe; otherwise, torts could be claimed based on fictitious psychological damage. Physicians could be exposed to a suit through overly aggressive bill collection procedures that might include abusive or insulting language and threats of violence. Sexual harassment can also result in this tort.

Invasion of privacy. This is an infringement of the right to be left alone. Invasions of privacy fall into four categories. The first is intrusion into another person's private affairs or solitude. The second is disclosure of private, embarrassing facts. The third is publication of information about someone that places the person in a false light. The fourth is the unauthorized use of someone's name or likeness for commercial purposes. A physician can become exposed to an invasion of privacy suit by revealing confidential information about a patient to a third party (e.g., a social acquaintance at a party or even a professional colleague if a proper release has not been obtained from the patient).

Abusive discharge. This tort occurs when an employee who does not have a written contract is discharged for a reason that violates public policy. For example, Dr. Wilson discharges Ms. Blakely because she has become pregnant and he fears that her attendance and job performance will deteriorate. This violation of public policy regarding sexual discrimination could be prosecuted under the equal employment laws and as a tort by Ms. Blakely.

Disparagement or trade libel. This occurs when there are false, injurious statements made about a competitor's reputation. This tort injures the business reputation of the victim and often disparages the conduct of a competing commercial enterprise over time. For example, Dr. Wilson makes condescending and untruthful remarks about Benevolent Daughters Hospital.

Interference with contract. This tort requires that a contract exists between two parties, a third party knows about the contract, and the third party induces one of the other two parties to breach the contract or prevents one of the other parties from fulfilling the contract. For example, Fred Kane is a physical therapist with six months remaining on his employment contract with Dr. Jones. Dr. White is aware of this contract but mentions to Fred that he would be able to give him a higher salary if he would join his practice now. Fred leaves and goes to work for Dr. White. Dr. Jones can sue Dr. White for interference and Fred for breach of contract. It is important to note that it is not necessary for Dr. Jones to prove that Dr. White maliciously intended to harm her. What is important is that Dr. White knew that there was a contract and that his actions interfered with the completion of that contract.

Malicious institution of civil proceedings or malicious prosecution. This occurs when an individual initiates legal proceedings that are both unwarranted and unsuccessful. The plaintiff must show that the tortfeasor lacked probable cause to institute the legal proceedings. In essence, someone cannot instigate a frivolous legal action in an attempt to "even things out."

Defamation. This occurs when a reputation is injured as a result of false statements. If the statement is in writing, then this is called libel. If the defamation occurs verbally or by acts or gestures, then it is called slander. In most cases, the truth is a successful defense, even if the motivation was less than benevolent and even if the accused believed the statements to be false at the time they were made.

Defamation can be a particular concern when one is providing a reference for a former employee.[4] Stick to the facts regarding an employee's job performance. In that regard, your performance appraisal records could be critical to a successful defense (see Chapter 3). It is generally permissible to provide information about a former employee that might on its face appear to be defamatory if the information will help you protect an important interest. Important interests have been defined to include a legal or moral duty to speak, defend your own reputation, warn others of a prospective employee's misconduct or mismanagement, and protect the interests of a third party.

Conveying negative information is a privileged right that may be lost under some circumstances, including the following:

- You did not believe the reference you gave to be true.
- You had no reasonable grounds for your beliefs about the employee, even though you did hold your beliefs in good faith.
- The information you gave was not an appropriate response to the third party's inquiry.
- You gave information to a person who had no need for it.
- You gave information out of malice, which in a legal sense means recklessly, with an improper motive, with an absence of good faith, and with an intention to do harm.

Here are some guidelines to follow when providing references:

- If the employee is being dismissed, explain why, and let the employee review his or her personnel file.
- Tell the employee that, if he or she chooses to use the practice as a reference, you will respond truthfully.
- Have the employee sign a form prepared by your attorney consenting to the release of information (have your attorney prepare a standard release form, and keep copies in your office so that they can be used as needed). Do not release information if the employee refuses to sign the form. If the employee refuses to sign the form and subsequently uses you as a reference, tell the inquirer that you cannot supply information until the former employee signs a release.
- Do not use a release supplied by the other employer. It might not provide you with the appropriate legal safeguards, as would a form drafted by your attorney.
- State that your evaluation of the former employee is your opinion, and provide a full and accurate discussion of the facts supporting your opinion.

- If you forward a written recommendation, be certain to mark the outside envelope *confidential* or *personal*.
- Do not volunteer information that has not been asked for.
- Some employers will give employees who are discharged for inadequate job performance a generic written reference stating that the employee had been a "good employee." Never do this because it could be used against you as evidence of wrongful discharge.

Negligence Torts

Negligence is the most common kind of tort. Negligence occurs when a person or company fails to act with reasonable care under the circumstances. For an injured person to be able to recover for negligence, the following five elements must be demonstrated:

1. *The defendant had a duty to exercise reasonable care.* What constitutes reasonable care is often a subject of debate in the litigation. Generally, the standard that is applied is what an imaginary reasonable person might do under the circumstances. Obviously, this type of standard is going to vary from one occasion to another, and ultimately the issue of reasonableness is only determined after the lawsuit has been resolved.
2. *The defendant breached the duty to behave reasonably.* The standard of performance is not perfection. Rather, the standard is reasonable performance by the defendant under the circumstances. Generally, the more serious the hazard, the more care the defendant must exercise.
3. *Cause in fact.* The plaintiff must demonstrate that the injury would not have happened but for the defendant's acts or omissions.
4. *Proximate cause.* This concept deals with the foreseeability of the consequences of the defendant's act. (The term *proximate* is a lamentable choice of words because the issue has nothing at all to do with

closeness in time or place. The issue relates to how far courts will extend culpability in a chain of events.) Proximate cause exists when there is no intervening cause or chain of causes between the defendant's actions and the harm that occurred to the plaintiff. For example, Andrews is injured in an accident while a passenger in Hill's car. Hill removes Andrews from the car and lays him by the side of the road. Roberts, a passerby, moves Andrews into the roadway, where he is struck by Thompson's car. Hill's alleged negligence is not the proximate cause of the injuries suffered by Andrews as a result of being struck by Thompson's car, although his actions are the proximate cause for the injuries suffered in the original accident.

5. *Injury, damage, or loss.* The plaintiff must demonstrate that personal injury, property damage, or economic loss actually occurred as a result of the act.

The following example illustrates how the elements listed above can combine to form a tort. As a result of a snowstorm, the entrance to Dr. Framingham's office has become slippery. Dr. Framingham has a contract with a cleaning service to provide snow removal. Dr. Framingham learns that the entrance was slippery when he arrives at his office. Before the cleaning service comes to clean the entrance, Mr. Newman slips on the icy entrance and breaks his leg.

Under these circumstances, it is likely that Dr. Framingham was negligent. Courts have generally held that it is a business's duty to provide a safe entrance. The fact that the cleaning service may or may not have responded does not relieve Dr. Framingham of this duty to the public to provide a safe entrance. Therefore, Dr. Framingham breached this duty. The snow at the entrance was the cause in fact of the accident, and the consequences of leaving the entrance covered with snow were foreseeable and known by Dr. Framingham. Finally, Mr. Newman did suffer an injury. As a separate issue, Dr. Framingham may

be able to bring an action against the cleaning service based on the wording of the cleaning contract. For example, if the contract stated that snow would be removed before the office opened in the morning, then the cleaning service may have breached the contract with Dr. Framingham and be liable to him.

Aside from negligent malpractice, which is discussed separately below, a physician manager's greatest exposure to negligence torts lies in the physical state of his or her office. People are very creative in their ability to misuse items and act without forethought. It is essential to examine how patients physically flow through your office and your physical facilities and then rectify any potential hazards. The object is to prevent injuries, not simply provide a reasonable care defense. The following suggestions might be helpful:

- Have all trash removed from your premises (not just your office) as quickly as possible.
- Hallways and entrances should be routinely cleaned and maintained.
- All office furniture should be routinely inspected for loose legs, loose backs, exposed wires, and so on.
- Consider eliminating toys from your waiting room. Playing correlates with activity, and activity correlates with injury. If you must have toys, examine them for sharp edges, points, ingestibility, breakability, or any other potential danger. Instead of toys, stock your waiting room with children's books, and encourage parents to read to their children or let them read.
- Be certain that the receptionist understands that he or she has a responsibility to keep order in the waiting room.
- Be certain that all appropriate safety equipment is properly located and maintained. For example, have an adequate supply of properly placed fire extinguishers, be certain that exit signs are visible, and routinely check safety equipment such as ground fault interrupters, pressure relief valves, and locks.

Malpractice

Malpractice is the tort of negligence as it applies to a professional. For a patient to demonstrate malpractice, he or she must prove by a preponderance of the evidence that the five elements necessary for any tort are present:

1. *Duty*. There was a bona fide physician–patient relationship, and the physician owed the patient a duty to provide a certain standard of care.
2. *Breach of duty or standard of care*. The patient must demonstrate that the physician did not provide a reasonable standard of care.
3. *Causation in fact*. The injury would not have happened but for the actions of the physician.
4. *Proximate cause*. The consequences of the physician's actions would be foreseeable by a reasonable, prudent person.
5. *Injury, damage, or loss*. The injuries caused by the physician resulted in a physical, financial, or emotional loss.

These points are elaborated below.

Duty and breach of duty. Unless there is a physician–patient relationship, there can be no malpractice liability. Once a physician–patient relationship has been formed, however, the physician has an obligation to care for the patient until treatment is completed or the relationship is terminated in a professionally appropriate manner. Failure to terminate a physician–patient relationship properly can result in a charge of abandonment. Proper termination includes providing the patient with reasonable notice, assisting the patient in finding another physician (when requested or when appropriate), and providing medical records when a signed patient record release has been presented by the new physician.

Obviously, the physician must be particularly concerned about the abandonment issue if the patient is in an emergency or crisis situation. Special caution is called for if the patient has been diagnosed with a mental illness because an abrupt termination of the case may exacerbate feelings of loss and abandonment and may precipitate suicidal or other irrational behaviors.

Once it has been established that there was a physician–patient relationship, the standard of care then becomes an issue. The physician owes the patient a certain quality of care, but at the same time the physician is not required to guarantee a favorable outcome. Historically, the standard of care applied in a given malpractice case has usually been related to the standards of the local community and to the specialty and school of medicine practiced by the physician. This standard, however, is usually established through the use of expert testimony. Historically, local experts testified to the standard of care provided in the community. Over the years, the locality rule has eroded, so that experts from outside the defendant's practice area can be used as expert witnesses. As a result, the standard of care is now often regional or even national.

The demise of the locality rule has been due to a number of circumstances, including the hesitancy of local physicians to testify against one another; the adoption of national uniform standards for certification, residency, and training; and requirements for continuing education.[5] The latter two considerations have tended to homogenize and thereby raise the standard of care. Within a specialty, a physician is held to the standard of care of other specialists in the specialty. A general practitioner, for example, is not required to provide the quality of care that would be provided by a specialist. The standard of care for a general practitioner, however, might well require a referral to or consultation with a specialist in a given set of circumstances. The standard of care is also related to the school of medical thought in which the physician was trained. An osteopathic gynecologist is not held to the same standard as an allopathic gynecologist, and vice versa. There is a presumption that patients understand that different schools of medicine may practice differently and that they will take this into account when selecting providers.

Finally, the physician has a duty to provide the patient with the opportunity to consent. If the patient did not consent to a treatment, the physician could be liable for an intentional tort, such as assault or battery. Obviously, it is best always to obtain written consent from the patient, the spouse, or a legal guardian. Consent, however, may be implied in several circumstances, such as these:

- There are extensive discussions between the physician and the patient, as demonstrated by the subsequent actions of both parties.
- An emergency arises, and the physician cannot obtain consent.
- Adjunct treatment is required because of a procedure to which the patient has consented.

If the physician obtains the consent of the patient but the patient has not been properly informed of the potential consequences of the treatment, then the physician has not obtained *informed* consent. Informed consent becomes an issue when the patient alleges that he or she was not provided with sufficient information to make a knowledgeable decision. Some courts have found that the degree of disclosure is determined by the standard of care generally applied by other physicians in similar circumstances. Some states, however, have adopted legislation requiring discussion of risks if a reasonable person in the patient's position would attach significance to the information. Finally, consent only becomes an issue if a reasonable person would have made a different decision as a result of the withheld information. Discuss the content of your state's consent laws with your attorney.

Consent can also be a question when the patient is a minor. Generally, it is best to obtain written consent from the parent of any patient who is younger than 18. Minors can provide consent under certain circumstances, including emergency treatment (when the life of the patient is at risk) and when the minor is emancipated, which can occur as a result of marriage, a court decree, or a failure of the parents to be legally responsible for the child.

Causation in fact and proximate cause. The burden of causation requires that the plaintiff demonstrate by a preponderance of the evidence that the physician's care was the cause in fact and the proximate cause of the damage done to the patient. The courts have tended to take two approaches to determining the question of cause in fact.[6] Using the "but for" standard, the question is whether the harm would not have occurred but for the actions of the physician. If the harm would not otherwise have occurred, cause in fact is taken to be demonstrated. A second standard that courts have applied concerns whether the physician's actions were a substantial factor contributing to the patient's damage. If, for example, there were two causes of the patient's harm, then the substantial factor test would associate liability with the source of each cause. Generally, the burden of proof to demonstrate cause will be on the plaintiff. It can shift to a defendant, however, if one physician is seeking to limit his or her liability with respect to a codefendant.

The issue of proximate cause is related to the foreseeability of the consequences of the physician's actions. Negligence can only be found if the consequences were foreseeable by a reasonable, prudent person. If the consequences were not foreseeable, then the physician did not have a duty to protect the patient from them, even though the physician may have caused them to occur in fact. The old parable "For want of a nail, a shoe was lost; for want of a shoe, a soldier was lost; for want of a soldier, a battle was lost; for loss of a battle, a war was lost" demonstrates the need for the concept of proximate cause. Still, a physician can be negligent because he or she sets a chain of events into motion. The proximate cause standard, however, requires that the physician be an instrumental cause of the injury in the chain of events, as opposed to simply creating conditions in which the harm was possible.

Another way in which cause can be demonstrated is through the doctrine of *res ipsa loquitur*, which is a Latin phrase meaning "the thing speaks for itself." *Res ipsa loquitur* allows a jury to reach a conclusion based on circumstantial evidence without the plaintiff having to demonstrate that the defendant actually caused the harm. This doctrine is often applied, for ex-

406 THE PHYSICIAN MANAGER'S HANDBOOK

ample, when a foreign object has been left inside a patient. The fact that the object is there is sufficient to demonstrate causation. *Res ipsa loquitur* has also been used to demonstrate cause for injuries outside the area of treatment. For example, a patient receives burns during a procedure on a part of the body even though it is distant from the operated site, or a patient develops paralysis after receiving anesthesia. "It speaks for itself" that the harm was done while under the physician's care.

Courts have also applied this doctrine when many people have had control over a patient's unconscious body, such as during the preparation for, conduct of, and recovery from surgery. In this type of situation, it would be difficult if not impossible for the patient to identify the *specific* person responsible for the harm. *Res ipsa loquitur* shifts the burden of proof to the defendant, who must then demonstrate by a preponderance of the evidence that he or she did *not* cause the harm.

For *res ipsa loquitur* to be applied by a court, the plaintiff must demonstrate that:

- the injury is of a type that ordinarily doesn't occur unless there is negligence
- the injury was caused by something that was within the control of the defendant
- the plaintiff did not contribute to the cause of the injury

Damages. For malpractice to be proven, the plaintiff must demonstrate that harm has occurred. The harm can be in the form of financial, emotional, or physical injuries. Compensation can be required for past and future medical costs, loss of income, funeral expenses, pain, mental suffering, and so on. The legal objective is to provide an award of money damages in recompense for the harm done to the plaintiff. In addition, courts occasionally assign punitive and exemplary awards over and above the plaintiff's actual losses, although these awards are usually limited to outrageous, malicious, or intentional acts.

Defenses against Malpractice

There are several defenses to a charge of malpractice. One strategy is to challenge the basis of the tort by claiming that the plaintiff failed to demonstrate that a duty existed, that the standard of care was not breached, that the physician's actions were not causally related to the harm, or that the patient suffered no harm. In addition, the physician can raise substantive defenses, which relate to the facts of the case, and procedural defenses, which relate to the legal basis of the complaint.

Substantive defenses include the contributory negligence and the comparative negligence defenses. Contributory negligence occurs when a patient contributes to the harm that occurred. For example, a patient who fails to follow the physician's directions or provides false or incomplete information may be found to be contributorily negligent. Contributory negligence is a complete defense, which means that if it prevails it will preclude any recovery by the plaintiff. Attorneys may hesitate to use this defense even if it is available because a jury may resent an attempt to equate a minor indiscretion on the part of the patient with a major dereliction on the part of the physician.

Comparative negligence defenses try to apportion the negligence between the plaintiff and the physician. It is not a complete monetary defense, and the award of damages would be in proportion to the harm found to be done by the physician. For example, if it was determined that the physician was responsible for 80 percent of the damage, which was assessed at $100,000, then the physician would be liable for $80,000.

Historically, case law has recognized the doctrine of contributory negligence, but state legislatures have been replacing this doctrine with comparative negligence statutes. The two doctrines are mutually exclusive, and only one will be in force in any given jurisdiction.

A third substantive defense is called assumption of risk. This occurs when the plaintiff knows and appreciates the risk and voluntarily assumes the risk. Obviously, demonstrating that the patient gave informed consent is essential to this defense. Except where informed consent is present, this defense is usually not successful. Generally it is recognized that the physician has superior knowledge of the risks involved and is better able to weigh information in making medical decisions.

A procedural defense relies on a failure to comply with legal procedures. One procedural defense is to claim that the statute of limitations has expired and that the physician has thus been released from liability. A person who alleges injury must initiate legal action before the expiration of the time period referred to in that state's statute of limitations. Some states start the clock on the date when the alleged malpractice occurred. Because some injuries may not be observable for years, it is possible for patients to lose the right to sue before becoming aware of the problem. As a result, many states have adopted statutes that start the clock when the patient discovers or should have discovered the injury.

Some physicians have attempted to limit their liability by having patients sign forms releasing them from liability. These forms are generally worthless because, as a matter of public policy, a person cannot contract away liability for negligence. A release can be valid, however, in the case of experimental or inherently dangerous treatment. Under these circumstances, the release must be signed before the beginning of treatment, and it must pertain to the consequences of properly performed treatment. It will not constitute a defense for improperly or negligently performed experimental or inherently dangerous treatment.

In addition to legal malpractice defenses, you can implement financial defenses. One such defense is called insolvency planning.[7] The object is to make your assets as judgment proof as possible. Because some aspects of insolvency planning may be inconsistent with prudent estate and financial planning, it is essential to consult your attorney and appropriate tax and financial planning consultants so that you can balance these competing interests.

Another financial defense is to maintain sufficient malpractice insurance and periodically reevaluate your level of coverage. Joint ownership of assets can also hamper creditors, especially in states that recognize the concept of tenancy by entirety. This requires that the asset be transferred to both a wife and a husband so that one party's interest cannot be transferred to a third party. Creditors of both the husband and the wife, however, can execute a judgment against this type of ownership. Some states have homestead laws that protect a portion of an owner's equity from a judgment. Retirement plans are also protected from creditors, although distributions from a plan can be subject to a judgment.

Finally, you can give away your assets. You may give up to $600,000 tax free to a spouse over your lifetime, or you may give assets to a reversionary trust (which is irrevocable for a period of time) or to an irrevocable trust. Life insurance that is placed in an irrevocable trust is also not subject to a judgment.

CONTRACTS

The objective of this section is to provide a basic understanding of how contracts are formed and interpreted by the courts. Whenever you are in doubt regarding the meaning of a contract, or whenever a contract includes a substantial commitment of time, money, personnel, or other resources, you should have it reviewed by your attorney.

A contract is a legally binding agreement between two or more parties. Examples of contracts include agreements with your employees, your partners, your suppliers, the telephone company, and your bank. Contracts can be in written or verbal form. As a general rule, you should not enter into any significant contract without first having it reviewed by your attorney. You will probably have to enter into many contracts, however, and it would be time consuming, expensive, and cumbersome to have your attorney review all of them. For example, you engage a security service to install an alarm, a water company to supply bottled water, an employment agency to provide a temporary secretary for this afternoon, a store to supply a wingback chair, and a painter to repaint a chipped file cabinet. All these transactions are contractual, yet probably none of them is of sufficient magnitude that it would warrant the inconvenience and cost of routinely forwarding it to your attorney for review. It is important, therefore, to appreciate how contracts are formed, interpreted, and enforced so that you can identify dubious or potentially disadvantageous situations and selectively use your attorney.

For a contract to exist, the following must occur:

- The parties must be competent.
- They must reach a mutual agreement.
- Consideration must be provided.
- What has been contracted for must be legal.

Competence means that all parties are legally capable of entering into the agreement. Minors, the insane, and individuals who are intoxicated may be considered incompetent to enter into contracts. Entering into a contract with a minor is particularly dangerous because the adult party may be held to the terms of the contract whereas the minor may withdraw at any time. For example, if you treat a minor without the consent of a legal guardian, you may not be able to hold the minor financially accountable, although the minor will be able to hold you to an acceptable standard of care. Although state law may hold the parent financially responsible, you then would have the problem of locating and collecting from the parent.

Mutual agreement means that there was both an offer and an acceptance. An offer means that you intend to be legally bound if the offer is accepted. Because offers may be preceded by preliminary negotiations, it is important to indicate clearly whether you are making an offer or merely expressing an intention to make an offer at some future time. For example, Dr. Kurth may state to Dr. Jackson "I'm interested in selling my practice for $100,000. Would you be interested in buying it?" This is merely an inquiry, not an offer to sell. Dr. Jackson cannot force the sale by producing a check for $100,000. If, however, Dr. Jackson responds by stating "I will buy your practice for $100,000," that would constitute an offer. If Dr. Kurth accepts the offer, a contract would then exist. Phrases such as "Would you be interested in," "I understand that you are looking for," and "How would you feel about" do not constitute offers. Because communications can become complex and the price of misunderstanding can be so great, it is always best to label an inquiry as such.

An offer can be terminated in several ways. The offerer can revoke it at any time before it is accepted by the other party. For example, if Dr. Jackson offers Dr. Kurth $100,000 for the practice, Dr. Jackson can revoke the offer at any point before Dr. Kurth accepts it. The revocation must be received before the offer is accepted for it to be valid.

An offer can be terminated by a lapse of time. For example, an offer can state when it will expire. If the offer contains no stated expiration time, a court will consider the offer valid for a reasonable length of time. What constitutes a reasonable length of time will depend on the facts and circumstances of the case.

An offer will terminate upon rejection or counteroffer. Once an offer is rejected, the person who rejected it cannot change his or her mind and then accept it. If an acceptance is conditional (e.g., "I will accept the offer if . . . "), or if the person to whom the offer is made changes some of the terms, the result is considered a counteroffer, not an acceptance. The original offerer, now the offeree, is free to accept the counteroffer, thereby binding the other party to a valid contract, or to reject it.

Once the person to whom the offer is made accepts the terms of the offer and conveys this acceptance to the offerer, the contract is binding. Communication of acceptance can take place in several ways. If the offer dictates the method of communication, such as by certified mail, then the acceptance must be communicated in that form. If the offer states that the acceptance must be made within a certain time, then once again the acceptance must occur within that time. Generally, an acceptance is considered valid when it is placed in the mail prior to or on the date specified in the offer. To avoid problems with any offers that you make, you should always specify the manner of acceptance and when the offer expires.

Consideration is the exchange that takes place as a result of the agreement. For a contract to be valid, something must be given and something received. For example, consideration exists if you agree to purchase bottled water at $7.50 per jug. Generally, courts are not concerned with the adequacy of consideration; if you strike a bad deal, you will be stuck with it. Consideration does not exist if one party is not truly committed to provide something. For example, an agreement that states "If Dr. Sipos determines that he needs bottled water, he will purchase it for $7.50 per jug from the Gulch Water Company" would be considered an illusory promise. It would not demonstrate consideration because Dr. Sipos is not promising to purchase water. In contrast, an agreement that states "I promise to buy all the bottled water that I need from the Gulch Water Company at $7.50 per jug" would constitute consideration if it was accompanied by the Gulch Water Company's promise to sell all the water needed for $7.50 per jug.

Finally, for a contract to exist, the subject matter must be legal. If a contract is in violation of any statutes or public policy, it is not enforceable. For example, Dr. Smith contracts with Johnson Construction Company to enlarge his office. As part of the contract, he requires that Johnson Construction Company remove the fire doors after the project is completed, so that the building will no longer be in compliance with the building code. This is a violation of local ordinance and cannot be enforced under contract law.

Similarly, contractual terms requiring the violation of public policy will also be unenforceable. The term *public policy* is a loose one, but it generally means "protecting from that which tends to be injurious to the public or contrary to the public good, . . . or any established interest of society."[8] Contracts that obstruct justice, corrupt public officials, are immoral, are offensive to public decency, restrain trade, or discriminate on the basis of race, religion, sex, age, disability, or national origin may violate public policy. For example, if the only two urologists in town contract to fix the price of urological services, this may be construed as a restraint of trade. If one of the urologists then violates the agreement, he or she could claim that there was no contractual relationship because the content of the agreement violated public policy. In addition, both urologists might be prosecuted under federal or state antitrust legislation.

As you can see, the four requirements of a valid contract do not include the necessity of a written document. With certain notable exceptions, verbal contracts are generally enforceable if they are agreed to by competent parties and reflect mutual agreement, consideration, and legal content. Obviously, verbal contracts can be troublesome because memories can become selective. To protect your own interests, you should insist on a written contract whenever the worst possible outcome from a business arrangement is more burdensome than arranging for your attorney to prepare a contract.

Certain types of contracts must be in writing to be enforceable:

- contracts for the sale of land or an interest in land (in some states, a verbal lease of less than one year is enforceable)
- contracts for the sale of goods in excess of $500
- contracts that by their terms cannot be fulfilled within one year
- suretyship contracts (promises to pay for the debts of others)

When a written contract is drafted, it is critical that you or your attorney anticipate all possible consequences of the arrangement and ensure that the contract provides for adequate resolution. If a dispute should arise, a court will apply the "four corners rule" to resolve it. This means that the court will look first to exactly what is contained within the four corners of the contract. Irrespective of what you intended, the contract will be interpreted literally. (There can be exceptions to the four corners rule. For example, if the contract is ambiguous or contradictory, the court may look to parole evidence, which is evidence outside the contract, to determine the intent of the parties.)

Consider the following example. Dr. Jones was working for Dr. Smith. Dr. Jones left Dr. Smith's practice, opened her own practice, and incorporated as Darla Jones, M.D., P.C. Dr. Jones's contract with Dr. Smith had stated that she, Jones, would pay Smith 15 percent of all fees received by her for any patients transferred from the practice for a period of six months. This was in consideration for Smith having provided referrals to Jones and otherwise assisting in building Jones's practice. Jones's practice, Darla Jones, M.D., P.C., paid Jones a salary of 60 percent of collected fees. Jones then paid Smith 15 percent of her salary from transferred patients, or 15 percent of 60 percent of transferred patient collections for six months. Smith objected on the basis that this was simply a subterfuge. Smith maintained that, because Jones "was the corporation," the arrangement was simply a sham to avoid paying 15 percent on all fees collected from transferred patients. Jones refused to comply, and Smith sued Jones.

Judgment was for Jones. The contract clearly stated that the 15 percent payments were payable by Jones on fees collected by Jones. The fact that she interposed a corporation between herself and Smith did not change the clear language of the contract. The court reminded Smith that, if his intention was to have Jones pay a fee on all collections for transferred patients, whether by her or by a corporation employing her, then this should have been so stated in the contract.

Attorneys are skilled at anticipating what can go wrong, drafting language to clarify what the resolution will be if something should go wrong, and positioning their client so that, if a dispute does occur, the client will be in a strong position. Nevertheless, it is important, in any business arrangement, that your attorney fully understand your objectives, your exposure if the other party fails to fulfill the terms of the contract, and protections that you feel you need if the arrangement does not prove to be satisfactory.

You are the ultimate consumer of your legal services, just as you are the consumer of services of an accountant or any other professional consultant. If an attorney does not fully appreciate your needs or drafts a document that does not fully meet your needs, you are the one who will ultimately have to live with the consequences.

EMPLOYMENT ISSUES

Many aspects of the employer–employee relationship have legal implications. The most basic legal consideration in the employer–employee relationship is the employment contract. Other legal considerations include employment discrimination, worker's compensation laws, discrimination law, and the Fair Labor Standards Act. Once again, it is important for you or your business manager to appreciate the legal issues involved so that you will know when to involve an attorney and be able to make daily decisions that are not legally risky.

Employment Contracts

As is the case for other contracts, an employment contract can be written or verbal. Both written and verbal employment contracts can be for a set term or at will. A set term means that the contract is in force for a stated length of time. At will means that the contract can be terminated by either party at its will, which in the extreme can be for good reason, bad reason, or no reason at all.

There are four major reasons why you might want to have a written employment contract with an employee. First, a written contract will decrease the chance that either party will misunderstand the mutual commitments. The process of negotiating the employment contract will require both parties to think about most aspects of the employment relationship, including compensation, vacation time, sick leave policy, work schedules, and termination. If disagreements are discovered in the contracting process, then they can be resolved before they lead to an employer–employee dispute.

Second, if you want a long-term commitment from an employee, it generally should be put in writing. To be enforceable, the contract must be put in writing if it is for one year or longer than one year. For example, if you have a skilled radiology technician and you want to be certain that the employee doesn't leave on the spur of the moment, you could negotiate an employment contract stating that the employment would last for an agreed period of time, such as one year.

Third, you can include in the contract a noncompetition clause that will restrict the ability of the employee to compete with you after leaving your employment. Obviously, the issue of competition is only relevant for physicians or other skilled professionals. Generally, courts have found these clauses to be valid as long as they are limited to a reasonable time period and a reasonable geographical area.

The standards of reasonableness vary with state law and local tradition. In the example above, the 15 percent fee on transferred patients that Dr. Jones was to pay Dr. Smith for six months might well be considered reasonable in many jurisdictions. A contract precluding practice in the same city for five years would generally be considered unreasonable. It is important to remember that the employee has a right to earn a living and that noncompetition clauses contradict the spirit of antitrust laws, which are based on the notion that open, robust competition is beneficial for society. As a result, courts will not enforce a noncompetition clause that unduly restricts this right. Some courts have struck down overbroad noncompetition clauses, whereas others have determined and then applied appropriate geographical and time restrictions. A local attorney's advice is essential in determining what might be a reasonable noncompetition restriction.

Fourth, an employment contract can increase a practice's financial security by committing revenue-generating employees to long-term employment. Practices that employ several physicians can coordinate the lengths of their contracts so that the expiration dates are staggered. This makes it more difficult for the employee physicians to conspire and decimate a group practice by leaving en masse. Other revenue-generating employees, such as nutritionists, physical therapists, and nurse practitioners, should also be considered for employment contracts.

The wording of the termination clause in an employment contract is important. An improperly worded termination clause will restrict your ability to fire an employee. For example, the following termination clause was contained in a nurse's employment contract:

> This Agreement will be in effect for one year from the date upon which it was made and entered into. This Agreement can be terminated before the end of one year:
> 1. at any time by the Employee with 30 days written notice;
> 2. at any time by the Company for inadequate job performance.

During the term of the contract, Nurse Roberts developed strong antiabortion attitudes. He did not allow them to interfere with his job performance, but his participation in public demonstrations and the extremeness of his attitudes caused Dr. Smith, his employer, to feel uncomfortable with Nurse Roberts. Dr. Smith no longer wished to employ him, but because his job performance had been adequate Dr. Smith was committed to retaining him for the remainder of the contract.

From your perspective as an employer, the most favorable termination clause is one that states that the employee serves at your will and that you may terminate the employee for any reason or for no reason and at any time. Although this provision sounds harsh, it can be both legal and highly desirable from your perspective. There are few things as frustrating as not being able to fire an employee immediately when you feel that it is necessary and justified. There are also few things that are as destructive to the morale and effectiveness of an office as a dissatisfied and malevolent employee. Clever employees can be malevolent in passive-aggressive ways that are difficult to document, which can make it hard to show cause for terminating them. It is best to avoid having to show cause by retaining the prerogative to terminate an employee at your will whenever you want.

Because employees, generally, are interested in job security, they will naturally hesitate to sign contracts with strong at-will provisions. They will often seek to limit your ability to terminate them, or at a minimum they will seek severance benefits. Kahn and colleagues propose some provisions that attempt to balance the legitimate needs of physicians to terminate employees with the desires of employees for security[9]:

- There should be a fixed length for the term of the agreement, such as one year, two years, and so on.
- The employer should retain the right to terminate the employee in case of an employee's disability that prevents the employee from carrying out his or her duties, or a failure of the employee to obey orders.
- The employer should retain the right to terminate the employee immediately for misconduct, with no severance benefits. Misconduct is to be defined at the sole and unrestricted discretion of the employer.
- The employer should retain the right to terminate the employee for any reason, with notice (e.g., two weeks).
- The employee should retain the right to resign at any time, with notice to the employer (e.g., two weeks).
- In the case of physician employees, they should agree not to work for a competing practice for a fixed period of time in a stated geographical area.

These termination provisions still give the physician wide latitude to terminate the employee for inadequate job performance or any other reason, yet they provide some measure of job security and financial security for the employee. They also limit the ability of the employee to work for a competitor or to be stolen by a competitor for a higher salary during the term of the agreement.

Exhibit 14–1 contains a checklist of items that should be considered for inclusion in any employment contract. You can use this checklist to help ensure that you explore all relevant issues with the employee or applicant and with your attorney.

In general, you should only enter into written employment contracts with valued employees and only after carefully considering the consequences and having the contracts drafted by an attorney. A written contract will be more restrictive than an unwritten agreement simply because the employee will ask for restrictions that would not occur to him or her with an unwritten agreement. The difficulties and frustrations associated with any restrictions on your ability to terminate hourly employees, for example, should not be underestimated.

Often, the security offered by a long-term contract is illusory. Even if you are able to convince an employee to stay contrary to his or her own true wishes, your victory is almost always merely Pyrrhic. Employees serving against their wishes will take their dissatisfaction out on you, your practice, and your patients, and a written contract will provide you with no effective defense against this form of retribution. It is better to replace employees who simply provide services, such as secretaries, business managers, and nurses, than try to keep them against their will.

Decisions regarding revenue-generating employees are more difficult. Following are three strategies for dealing with revenue-generating employees who are serving against their will:

1. Release them, and consider the lost revenue the price for your own well-being and that of your employees and patients.
2. Negotiate a price for the employee to buy himself or herself out of the contract.
3. Enforce the contract, grit your teeth, and bear it. If you pursue this alternative and the employee leaves, you may seek an injunction barring the employee from working for or becoming a competitor. Courts, however, generally recognize that slavery has been illegal for quite some time, so they are unlikely to force the employee to go back to work for you. Under these circumstances, you may seek mon-

Exhibit 14–1 Employment Contract Checklist

*1. Offer and acceptance of employment.
2. Description of duties, responsibilities, etc.
3. Provision that the employee shall devote full time and attention to the employer's business.
4. Provision that the employee shall not engage in any other employment of any kind without disclosure and written permission.
*5. Duration of the contract.
6. Subsequent renewals (automatic or upon notice).
*7. Compensation.
8. Discipline procedures.
9. Other benefits, such as bonuses, insurance, mileage, etc.
10. Severance benefits (allowed or not, earned or discretionary, accrued or forfeited).
*11. Termination of employment (at will; for cause; whether employee is entitled to any compensation at termination and, if so, under what circumstances).
12. Noncompetition covenants.
13. Nondisclosure of confidential information, such as business plans, patient information, etc.
14. Provision for the employee in the event of sale, merger, etc.
15. "Zipper clause" ("This is the whole of the agreement").
16. Procedure for amending the contract.
17. Definition of what constitutes breach of the contract.
18. Procedure for providing notice to the other party (by certified mail, etc.).
19. Governing law clause ("This contract shall be interpreted according to the laws of the state of . . . ").

*These items must be included in some form.

Source: Adapted with permission from S. Kahn, B. Brown, and B. Zepke, *Personnel Director's Legal Guide, 1988 Cumulative Supplement*, pp. S2-53–S2-54, © 1988, Warren, Gorham, and Lamont.

etary damages. You would have an obligation, however, to mitigate the damages by attempting to replace the employee. The damages that you may be able to recover would be the lost income less the damages that were mitigated, plus your costs for replacing the employee.

For example, Dr. Temple leaves Dr. Johnson's practice in violation of her employment agreement. Dr. Temple generated $200,000 in gross receipts and continues at this rate after leaving. Dr. Johnson hires a replacement, who generates $150,000 during the same time period. Dr. Johnson could seek damages of $50,000. If Dr. Johnson does not attempt to mitigate the damages, the court may decide that there would have been none and may choose to assign no damages. On the other hand, if Dr. Johnson made a good faith effort to find a re-

placement but none was available, Dr. Johnson may be awarded $200,000.

Your choice of strategy will depend on a number of issues, including the precedent that you want to set for other employees, the value of the employee's revenue to the financial health of the practice, and your own peace of mind.

Employment At Will

Employees with no written or stated verbal contract that specifies a term of employment are employed at will. An at-will arrangement, however, implies a contract. When a legally competent employee agrees to provide labor in exchange for compensation, there is consideration, mutual assent, and legal content, and therefore a contract exists. Traditionally, at-will arrangements allowed employers to terminate employees for good cause, bad cause, or no cause at all.

Over the years, however, courts and legislatures have placed limits on the employer's ability to dismiss employees.

Most states currently have laws that restrict the employer's ability to terminate at-will employees unless there is good cause. One type of restriction relates to abusive or retaliatory discharge. This occurs when the discharge is in retaliation for an employee's refusal to violate public policy. For example, many states do not allow dismissal for "whistleblowing" or for failure to perform an illegal activity, such as refusing to commit perjury to protect the employer, refusing to commit bribery, failure to submit false insurance claims, and refusing to falsify records. Many states have made it illegal to dismiss an employee for filing a worker's compensation claim, for refusing to take a polygraph test, or for meeting military or jury duty obligations. In addition, federal and state antidiscrimination laws also limit the employer's ability to dismiss at-will employees without just cause.

An ex-employee's allegation that dismissal was in violation of public policy certainly doesn't mean that a court will uphold this allegation and assign damages. It does mean, however, that the employer may have to provide some evidence for dismissal that refutes the claimed violation of public policy. Documentation of inadequate job performance or insubordination, for example, would be a cornerstone for a successful defense under these circumstances. The need to provide a defense in the first place exemplifies the erosion of the employer's traditional at-will prerogative to terminate an employee for bad cause or no cause at all.

Another challenge to the employer's at-will termination prerogative arises from the concept of implied terms in the employment agreement. Courts have found that oral statements made to the employee, as well as written documents other than the employment contract, can become part of the employment agreement. This, then, makes dismissal conditional upon good cause. For example, some courts have held that an employee handbook can become part of the employee contract. In *Toussaint v. Blue Cross and Blue Shield of Michigan*, the court found that statements in the company's personnel manual indicating that employees would only be terminated for cause became part of the employment contract.[10] Other implied terms have been found in oral statements made at the time of hiring, such as "You'll always have a job here as long as you do as I say" and "I won't fire an employee until I give him or her three chances to improve."

Another attack on at-will employment is application of the doctrine that good faith and fair dealing are implied in any contract. Some courts have interpreted good faith and fair dealing to mean that the employer has an obligation to provide employees with due process and to base terminations on just cause. If the employer has to justify the dismissal or provide an appeal process or a forum for the employee to contest the dismissal, then the at-will option is obviously compromised. This doctrine has been used, for example, to invalidate terminations whose purpose was to avoid paying wages and terminations in which an employee is forced to write a resignation letter.

It should be noted, however, that there is wide variation in how far courts will go to find implied contract provisions. For example, a California court held that "merely exchanging pleasantries about the company during an interview did not imply a promise by the employer of job security."[11(p.S5–25)] Similarly, many courts have held that company handbooks and other written documents are simply unilateral statements. Because there is no "meeting of the minds," there is no contract.

There are several things that you, as an employer, can do to preserve your at-will option to terminate employees insofar as your jurisdiction permits:

- Make no statements in the employment process that could be construed as making an exception to at-will employment. For example, don't say "You'll have a job here as long as you perform well" or "If your work isn't satisfactory, I'll give you a chance to improve."

- Never give an applicant a policy manual or handbook during the employment process. If you do, it may be argued later that its contents were part of the reason that the applicant accepted the job, which will make it part of the employment contract.
- Tell the job applicant that the terms of employment are at will, and explain what that means. Some companies have new employees sign a document at the time of employment in which they acknowledge and accept their at-will status.
- Always document reasons for discharge. Inadequate job performance, absenteeism, and insubordination are among the legitimate reasons for termination, and they can be used to refute allegations of abusive discharge or of an implied contract.
- Have your attorney check state laws and court interpretations and inform you of illegal grounds for termination in your state.
- Always review the facts of a termination with your attorney before you terminate the employee. Do this even if you feel that the facts are clear and your behavior is fully justified. Your attorney may have suggestions regarding how to document the facts and orchestrate the termination to provide you with maximum defensibility.
- Review personnel manuals, employment applications, training materials, and so on for any language that could be construed as limiting your at-will termination authority. These documents should contain a clear statement that employment is at will. In addition, each manual or handbook should contain a disclaimer stating that nothing in it is intended to create or modify a contract with an employee.
- If you create any documents specifying a code of conduct, always include a disclaimer in which you state that the document is illustrative. This will give you latitude because it is impossible to anticipate all the creative ways in which employees can violate the spirit of a policy without clearly breaching its specific content.

- Review the performance appraisal suggestions in Chapter 3. Using these ideas will strengthen your legal defensibility.
- Apply your discipline and termination procedures with consistency.
- Be honest with yourself regarding the real reasons why you are terminating an employee. Sometimes, feelings of anger or betrayal may result in your doing something that isn't legally defensible. If you are honest with yourself, you will be able to avoid a questionable termination.

Equal Employment Opportunity

Federal and state legislation precludes employers from discriminating against employees on the basis of race, religion, sex, national origin, age, and disability. This legislation encompasses all aspects of employment, including hiring, promotion, compensation, access to training, discipline, and termination. Employers covered by this legislation cannot use a person's race, religion, sex, national origin, age (if over 40 years), or disability status to influence an employment decision.

The primary federal equal employment opportunity (EEO) laws are the 1964 Civil Rights Act (in particular, Title VII), the Age Discrimination in Employment Act of 1967 (ADEA), the Age Discrimination Act of 1975, and the Americans with Disabilities Act (ADA). Other relevant pieces of federal legislation include the First, Fifth, Thirteenth, and Fourteenth Amendments to the U.S. Constitution, various executive orders issued by the president, and the Equal Pay Act of 1963.

The Equal Employment Opportunity Commission (EEOC) was created as a result of the Civil Rights Act of 1964. Its mission is to administer Title VII of that act as well as federal age discrimination legislation. The EEOC interprets the meaning of civil rights legislation, provides guidance to employers, and enforces the legislation through prosecution in federal court. As a result of its central position in drafting, interpreting, and enforcing EEO legislation, the

EEOC's interpretations, published in its guidelines to employers, are important.

Many medical practices will not be subject to federal EEO regulation because of their relatively small size. The Civil Rights Act of 1964 and the ADA only cover employers that have 15 employees or more for each working day for 20 calendar weeks or more in the current or preceding year. The ADEA and Age Discrimination Act of 1975 only apply to companies employing 20 employees or more for 20 calendar weeks or more in the current or preceding year. In addition, these two acts only provide protection to employees who are 40 years old or older. Because most federal discrimination enforcement emanates from these acts, many medical practices are effectively exempt from federal EEO regulation. Many of these same practices, however, will be subject to state EEO laws. Because these laws vary considerably from state to state, it is essential that you contact your attorney to understand the compliance requirements in your particular state. In addition, some cities, such as New York and San Francisco, have developed their own civil rights legislation, and once again you should seek guidance from your attorney.

Although the following discussion of federal civil rights legislation only applies directly to those health care organizations that are covered by the various civil rights laws noted above, smaller medical practices nevertheless may want to be familiar with federal guidelines. First, many state laws are based on the EEOC's interpretations of federal legislation. Understanding the EEOC's perspective may help physician managers comply with state legislation. Second, the EEOC's perspective strikes a good balance between society's need for fair and equal treatment of applicants and employees and the employer's need for competent, qualified personnel. Finally, the EEOC's thinking, as embodied in its recommendations to employers, is generally consistent with good personnel management and employment methods. Thus understanding the EEOC's position may help physician managers utilize better personnel management and employment methods.

The primary source of federal EEO enforcement is Title VII of the Civil Rights Act of 1964. Various EEOC publications provide the employer with specific guidance regarding how to hire, compensate, terminate, and otherwise deal with employees without discriminating. The following sections are designed to provide you with an overview of how to comply with the EEOC's recommendations.

Employment Methods

It is important to understand the technical definition of the word *discrimination* as it relates to employment. One form of discrimination is called disparate treatment, which occurs when the employer bases an employment decision on race, color, religion, sex, age, or national origin. In effect, disparate treatment occurs when the employer willfully discriminates. For example, not hiring men or women for certain positions, such as nurse or secretary, constitutes disparate treatment, and it is unlawful.

Another condition that may constitute discrimination is called disparate impact. This occurs when the employer's actions, even though apparently neutral, have the effect of disproportionately excluding one group. For example, during the interviewing process, although you do not consciously screen out women and your interview questions have no obvious gender bias, nevertheless you hire a substantially smaller proportion of women than men. This would constitute disparate impact, but it is not yet discrimination.[12] At this point, the burden shifts to the employer to justify the disparity. A legal defense for disparate impact is business necessity. If the employment method (interviewing) assesses skills that are important and required by the job, then no discrimination has taken place. Persons in the affected groups simply did not possess the necessary skills in as high a proportion as members of other groups. In effect, business necessity is a legal justification for disparate impact.

An employer's ability to demonstrate business necessity will depend on the employment methods that are utilized. For example, suppose that you use an unstructured interview to fill a position. A female applicant who is denied the position claims that the real reason for the rejection was her gender. Your practice has previously rejected a number of female applicants. This fact would be documented by the completion of EEO Form 1, which is required of all employers covered by the 1964 Civil Rights Act. At this point, there is strong evidence for disparate impact. Once this occurs, the burden shifts. It is now up to you to demonstrate that you did in fact use a job-relevant selection method. You cannot show the job relatedness of the unstructured interview questions, however, because you don't have a record of them or of the applicant's responses. It is likely that the EEOC would determine that your employment procedures are discriminatory because there is disparate impact with no documentation of business necessity. More fundamentally, it should be obvious that relying on unstructured interviews is simply bad policy irrespective of its legality. Table 14–1 contains guidelines on preemployment inquiries. These will help you think about the relevance of various interview questions that you might ask and how these questions might be viewed by the applicant.

If, on the other hand, you use a structured interview, you might be able to demonstrate that the content of the interview is closely related to job content and that this particular applicant's performance was inferior to that of the applicant who was hired. By establishing these two points, you would demonstrate business necessity and would probably be able to rebut the charge of discrimination.

Similarly, the nature of the questions that you ask could raise a question of disparate treatment. Table 14–1 provides guidance on preemployment inquiries that have generally been found to be lawful or unlawful.

The same argument holds true for employment tests. If you can illustrate, through the use of a job description, that the tests measure important elements of the job and that the applicant who was hired had higher scores than those who were rejected, you have a strong defense.

Some racial groups and the two genders do, in fact, perform differently on certain types of employment methods. For example, women have lower average scores than men on strength tests. Whites tend to have higher average scores than African Americans on some standardized achievement tests.[13] Undoubtedly, many group differences are due to the effects of socialization, education, and previous discrimination, but rectifying past wrongs is not the employer's legal responsibility. The employer is fully justified in seeking the most qualified applicant irrespective of race, sex, and so on. On the other hand, differences in group averages are not a justification for automatically rejecting any applicants from any group. Each applicant must be evaluated as an individual. If an employment method does have a disparate impact and the method is related to important job performance issues, then the employment method is justified and legally defensible.

The employer can demonstrate the job relatedness of an employment method with disparate impact either quantitatively or qualitatively.[14] In a quantitative demonstration, the employer establishes that groups of employees who performed higher on the employment method also had better job performance than groups with lower employment method evaluations. Some health care organizations covered by Title VII will be too small to demonstrate the job relatedness of their employment methods using statistical methods. When this occurs, most demonstrations will be based on qualitative evidence.

A qualitative validation demonstrates that the content of the employment method is similar to the content of the job. For example, job analysis of a clerical position might show that the job requires word processing skills that are similar in nature to the content of the word processing test that is used to screen applicants. It is important, therefore, to maintain accurate job descriptions and to use employment methods that can be shown to assess the job content. The methods for doing this are described in Chapter 3.

Another qualitative strategy is to use the results of studies conducted by employment test

Table 14–1 Preemployment Inquiries

Subject	Unlawful Inquiry	Lawful Inquiry, but Only if Job Related
Name	If your name has been legally changed, what was your former name?	Have you ever worked in this country under another name? (May be asked of married female applicants to check educational or employment records.)
Age	(Any question that tends to identify applicants age 40 or older.)	Are you over 18 years of age? If hired, can you furnish proof of your age?
Citizenship	Are you a citizen of the United States? Are your parents or spouse U.S. citizens? Are you a naturalized citizen?	If you are not a U.S. citizen, do you have the legal right to remain permanently in the United States? What is your visa status? Do you intend to remain permanently in the United States? (Statement that employment is contingent on identity and eligibility according to U.S. law.)
National origin/ ancestry	What is your national origin/ancestry, parentage, etc.? How did you acquire the ability to speak, read, and write a foreign language? What language is spoken in your home?	What language do you speak, read, or write fluently? Do you have special familiarity with a foreign country?
Race or color	(Any question that directly or indirectly relates to race or color.)	(None.)
Religion	Do you attend religious services or a house of worship? What is your religious denomination, affiliation, parish, pastor? What religious holidays do you observe?	(None.)
Sex	What is your marital status? Do you wish to be addressed as Mr., Mrs., Ms.? What are your plans regarding having children? Do you have the capacity to reproduce?	(None.)
Relatives/marital status	What is your marital status? With whom do you reside? Do you live with your parents? What are the ages of your children?	What are the names of relatives already employed by the company?

continues

Table 14–1 continued

Subject	Unlawful Inquiry	Lawful Inquiry, but Only if Job Related
Physical condition	Do you have any physical disabilities? What is your disability? What caused your disability? What is the prognosis of your disability? Have you had any recent serious illness?	Do you understand the requirements of the job, and can you perform the job? Do you need any special accommodations to perform the job applied for? Explain how you would go about doing the job applied for. (Preemployment offer medical examinations are prohibited, but employment can be made contingent on passing a medical examination.)
Education	(Any question asking specifically the national, racial, or religious affiliation of a school.)	(Questions related to applicant's academic, vocational, or professional education, including schools attended, degrees, dates of graduation, courses of study.)
Experience	(Questions related to military experience in general.)	(Questions related to applicant's work history. Questions related to specific experience in the armed forces.)
Organizations	To what organizations, clubs, societies, and lodges do you belong?	To what organizations, clubs, societies, and lodges do you belong? Exclude those whose name or character indicates the race, religious creed, color, national origin, or ancestry of its members.
Character	Have you ever been arrested?	Have you ever been convicted of a crime? If so, when and where? What was the disposition of the case? (*State laws vary on this issue. Contact your attorney.*)
Work schedule/ training	(Any question related to child care, ages of children, or other subject that is likely to be perceived by a covered group, especially women, as discriminatory.)	Do you have any family, business, health, or social obligations that would prevent you from working consistently/working overtime/traveling? Are there any reasons why you would not consistently arrive for work on time and work according to the company's work schedule?

continues

Table 14–1 continued

Subject	Unlawful Inquiry	Lawful Inquiry, but Only if Job Related
Relocation	(Any question related to spouse's attitudes or other subject that is likely to be perceived by a covered group, especially women, as discriminatory.)	Do you have any family, business, health, or social obligations that would prevent you from relocating? Would you be willing to relocate?
Miscellaneous	(Any inquiry that is not job related or necessary for determining an applicant's potential for employment.)	(Statement or notice to applicant that any misstatements or omissions of significant facts in written application forms or in an interview may be cause for dismissal.)

Source: Adapted with permission from S. Kahn, B. Brown, and M. Lanzarone, *Legal Guide to Human Resources*, pp. 2-51–2-53, © 1996, Warren, Gorham, and Lamont.

publishers and published research studies. Employment tests published by reputable publishers have been validated for various jobs. This research evidence, which is usually reported in the test manual, can also be used to argue that the test is job relevant. To use this strategy, the employer must demonstrate that the job content is similar to jobs reported in the validation study. Once again, having an accurate job description is important for demonstrating this relationship.

Finally, the best and least expensive legal defense is always prevention. Even if an employment method is job related, you always want to consider how it will appear to the applicant. An employment method that doesn't look job related will raise questions in the applicant's mind. A litigious applicant may suspect that the test or interview is merely a subterfuge or an excuse to reject. It is a good idea, therefore, to precede the use of any employment method that is not clearly job relevant with a brief statement concerning why you are asking the applicant to perform this task. You might say, for example, "This questionnaire measures some job-related tendencies, such as your ability to get along with others and your desire to work."

Promotion

The same general issues that arise in the selection of employees also arise in the making of promotion decisions. For example, it is illegal to make a promotion decision based on an employee's race, religion, sex, national origin, or age. Documentation of disparate impact can arise from a number of sources, including a pattern of promotions for a particular race or sex, age category, and so forth, and use of inconsistent promotion standards. Once the adverse impact has been demonstrated, the employer's task is to document the validity of the promotion decision. This can be done by producing performance appraisals and other evidence demonstrating that the promotion decision was based on job performance. Obviously, defenses based on a well-constructed and consistently applied performance appraisal process are more likely to be successful.

Sexual Discrimination

There are several additional points that need to be discussed regarding sexual discrimination. Obviously, there are some jobs in which a person's gender *is* relevant to job performance, such as the preference for an actress for a female role in a play. In this instance, being female is a bona fide occupational qualification. Because of the potential for abuse, bona fide occupational qualifications have been interpreted narrowly by both the EEOC and the courts. For example, a bona fide occupational qualification would not be held to exist in either of the following circumstances:

1. An employer refuses to hire an applicant based on the preferences of coworkers, clients, or patients. It is not permissible to reject a man for a nurse or receptionist position, for example, simply because staff or patients might object or perhaps feel uncomfortable.

2. An employer refuses to hire an applicant based on assumptions about a certain gender, such as "Women are more likely to be sick or to have higher turnover rates."

Discrimination on the basis of pregnancy is also prohibited under Title VII. You cannot terminate or refuse to hire or promote a woman solely because she is pregnant. In addition, it is illegal to set a mandatory pregnancy leave requirement. Pregnancy must be treated as any other short-term disability. Women who take a pregnancy leave have a right to reinstatement once they are able to perform the work if other employees who have been absent because of temporary disability have been allowed to return to work. Correspondingly, if you would terminate injured employees after they had used all their sick leave, then you could treat the pregnancy "disability" in a similar manner. In effect, employers must treat pregnancy in the same way that they treat any other short-term disability in regard to fringe benefits, seniority, and so on. Health care organizations not covered by Title VII may still have to comply with state regulations regarding pregnancy, so it is important to consult with your attorney on this matter.

Sexual Harassment

Sexual harassment has increasingly been a source of litigation over the past decade. In addition to back pay and injunctive relief, plaintiffs often file tort claims in state court for assault, battery, wrongful discharge, invasion of privacy, false imprisonment, and emotional distress. These tort claims create the possibility for both compensatory and punitive damages, and ex-tremely offensive cases have resulted in jury awards exceeding $1 million.

The EEOC has defined sexual harassment as unwelcome sexual advances, requests for sexual favors, and other verbal or physical conduct of a sexual nature when:

- submission to such conduct is made either explicitly or implicitly a term or condition of an individual's employment
- submission to or rejection of such conduct by an individual is used as the basis for employment decisions
- such conduct has the purpose or effect of unreasonably interfering with an individual's work performance or creating an intimidating, hostile, or offensive working environment[15]

Quid pro quo sexual harassment occurs when the employer provides, withholds, or offers job-related benefits based on compliance with sexual requests. "If you don't sleep with me, you won't get a pay raise" or "If you won't go out with me tonight, then I'll give you extra work to do" are two blatant examples. Sexual harassment also occurs if an employer acts in this way, even if it is not overtly stated.

More common, and more difficult to define and address, is sexual harassment arising from a hostile working environment. This occurs when unwelcome sexual conduct interferes with the employee's job performance or creates an intimidating, hostile, or abusive work setting, even though there is no threatened loss of benefits. Examples can include fondling, abusive language, requests for sexual favors, and sexual jokes *if*, according to the U.S. Supreme Court, these are "sufficiently severe to alter the conditions of . . . employment and create an abusive working environment."[16] Generally, an isolated comment, obscenity, request for a date, or invitation to dine does not constitute a hostile environment. There are instances, however, where a single incident, because of its nature, has constituted sexual harassment.

A danger is that two sincere individuals can see the same situation differently, especially if they differ greatly in power, such as a physician and an employee or an administrator and a subordinate. What Dr. Smith views as voluntary and uncoerced, Ms. Wellington may perceive as unwelcome. In the eyes of the law, an event can be both voluntary and unwelcome at the same time. People also vary in their sensibilities. Repeated sexual jokes and gestures can create an atmosphere of discrimination that may be offensive to an employee, although this may not be perceived by the harassing individual. Finally, although men have historically been the harassers, sexual harassment is just as illegal and offensive when it is conducted by a woman.

To reduce the chance that sexual harassment will occur in your organization, and to provide the strongest possible defense should it be alleged, implement the following policies. First, distribute a written policy to all employees that defines and prohibits *quid pro quo* and working environment harassment. Specifically, prohibit sexual advances, requests for sexual favors, intimate relationships between supervisory and subordinate employees unless they are married to each other, and verbal or physical behavior that may be offensive. Emphasize that this is extremely important, and set a personal example by your own behavior. Provide a clear procedure for an employee to complain directly to the "top," such as the managing physician or, in a health care system, a senior executive. State that all incidents will be quickly resolved and documented. Put this policy in any employee manual, conduct training with all employees when it is first implemented, and be certain that it is reviewed with all new employees.

If an event occurs, it is essential to investigate and act upon it immediately. Take *every* complaint seriously, irrespective of who is involved. Harassment can be subtle and encompass a wide range of activities. It is not just young attractive women who are harassed. Some cases may turn into a "he said–she said" confrontation, and it becomes difficult to identify what really happened. Sometimes communication and mutual conciliation between the parties will resolve the matter, but in many cases this will fail. Gener-

ally, courts hold that you as the employer are not responsible for sexual harassment if, once notified, you follow your procedures and take appropriate action. This can include firing the offender, but a strong written reprimand with a threat of future dismissal can be sufficient.

Be certain that you thoroughly and accurately document each employee's job performance on a regular basis and base pay raises, promotions, discipline, and termination on performance appraisals. This can provide the basis for a legal defense in a frivolous harassment claim. Finally, have your attorney review your harassment grievance procedure, and seek legal guidance whenever an employee alleges harassment.

Age Discrimination

The general standards that have been discussed above also apply to age discrimination. Employers who are covered by the ADEA cannot discriminate against an employee who is 40 years old or older on the basis of age. The standard defense to a charge of age discrimination is to document that the job action was based on job performance. If the charge relates to giving preference to a younger employee, then the defense is to document the superior performance of the younger employee in the employment selection process or on the job.

The ADEA also recognizes the concept of bona fide occupational qualifications. As with sexual discrimination, relatively few bona fide occupational qualifications are accepted as legitimate. Generally, these are related to public safety and to instances in which youth is essential to authenticity, such as a youthful part in an advertisement intended to promote the sale of a product to youthful consumers. Age-related bona fide occupational qualifications are largely irrelevant to medical practices.

A medical practice typically encounters the issue of age discrimination when an older person applies for a clerical or technical position. In these instances, utilization of the employment methods and strategies discussed in Chapter 3 will provide the basis for a sound defense based on business necessity if an age discrimination suit is brought. More important, using these methods will ensure that you will hire the best available applicant, who may well be older.

The ADA

The ADA makes it illegal for employers to discriminate against a disabled person who is otherwise qualified for a job in job application procedures, hiring, firing, promotion, compensation, training, or any other conditions or terms of employment. The ADA protects people from employment decisions based on their disability who are otherwise fully qualified to perform a job. The ADA covers individuals who:

- have physical or mental impairments that substantially limit a major life activity, such as standing, talking, walking, seeing, or speaking.
- have a record of such impairment, including those who have recovered from problems such as cancer and drug addiction or who are asymptomatic but test positive for a condition, such as an HIV carrier.
- are regarded as having an impairment, such as obesity or disfigurement, when the employer cannot state a job-related reason for an action. (The inference is that the employer would then be acting on the basis of a stereotype or fear. This provision would also preclude, for example, rejecting an applicant with a chronically ill child on the assumption that this would affect the applicant's attendance record.)

Generally, people with contagious diseases, including AIDS, are covered by the ADA, if their condition does not impose a significant health or safety risk to employees or patients. Former drug addicts and alcoholics also are considered disabled. The employer, however, may set attendance, performance, and behavior standards for all employees. An alcoholic who violates these policies cannot use this condition to avoid or mitigate discipline or termination.

Perhaps the ADA's most controversial provision is the requirement for employers to make reasonable accommodations to employ otherwise qualified disabled applicants. Reasonable accommodation can include making facilities accessible; restructuring jobs; modifying employment methods; adjusting work schedules; acquiring or modifying equipment, procedures, or training materials; and providing qualified readers or interpreters. The employer, however, is not required to make accommodations that would create an undue hardship. Undue hardship occurs when the accommodation would require significant expense or difficulty, taking into account the organization's size and financial resources. If this sounds vague, it is. Defining undue hardship will undoubtedly be the subject of much litigation and regulation writing. It is safe to say, however, that a large hospital system will be held to a standard different from that of a much smaller private practice.

For example, Alister, who is otherwise qualified to be a practice's business manager, uses a wheelchair. He cannot reach all the vertical files, the chair can't enter some of the business areas because of the positioning of furniture and equipment, and the computer desk is too low for him to use with the chair. Reasonable accommodation may mean purchasing lateral files, moving furniture, and putting blocks under the computer desk. These accommodations would probably not constitute an undue hardship, nor would it be permissible to let these accommodations influence the evaluation of Alister's qualifications for the job.

Mary is also otherwise qualified for the position. She lost her sight in an auto accident, however, and she would need a full-time reader, which would cost about $40,000 per year. This almost certainly would constitute an undue hardship for many practices, but what about a health care system generating several hundred million dollars annually? Once again, the litigators and the regulation writers are going to be busy.

Research indicates that the costs of accommodation may not be excessive. One study, based on similar accommodation requirements for the Rehabilitation Act of 1973, found that 81 percent of the accommodations cost less than $1,000 and that 31 percent cost nothing; another reported that 51 percent cost nothing, 30 percent cost less than $500, and 8 percent cost more than $2,000.

The ADA specifically excludes coverage for homosexuality, bisexuality, transvestitism, transsexuality, pedophilia, exhibitionism, voyeurism, gender identity disorders, compulsive gambling, kleptomania, pyromania, sexual behavior disorders, and disorders resulting from using illegal drugs.

To ensure that your organization does not violate the ADA, be certain that all employees with personnel management responsibilities are trained in ADA requirements. In a practice setting, have one managing physician responsible for reviewing all personnel decisions that affect the disabled. This physician's responsibility is to understand enough about the ADA to recognize when the practice is entering dangerous territory and to contact your attorney to avoid or minimize the exposure.

Conduct a thorough job analysis before filling any position, and be certain that the job description clearly defines the tasks that are essential. Review all selection procedures for their job relatedness. Don't use employment tests or other selection criteria that adversely affect the disabled, unless the methods are job related and there are no other choices.

As a physician, you may be called upon to provide physical examinations for other employers. Always ask the employer for a job description. Don't make blanket statements about an individual's general suitability for a job. Don't make any final employment decisions for an employer. Instead, specify the tasks that an individual can't perform or perform safely. The employer should make all final employment decisions.

The Fair Labor Standards Act

This act, also known as the wage and hour law, was enacted by Congress in 1938. Provisions of this act have been copied in so many state laws that the application of its provisions is nearly universal. Among other things, the act sets a national minimum wage, and it also requires the payment of time and a half for overtime in excess of 40 hours per week.

Not all employees are covered by the overtime provision of the act. Employees who are not covered by the overtime provision are referred to as exempt employees. Exempt employees are those who are employed in a bona fide executive, administrative, or professional capacity. Definitions of executive, administrative, and professional employees are found in Exhibit 14–2. Classification of a position as exempt can be difficult, and, given that there may be significant financial implications, you should consult your attorney for the latest interpretations of exempt status. There are many positions in a health care organization that could be classified as exempt, including business manager, office manager, and various nursing and technical positions.

It is important to document all time worked by nonexempt employees. Nonexempt employees can claim to have worked overtime, and if you do not have adequate documentation of their actual work hours, you may have to pay time and a half. The employer has a duty under the Fair Labor Standards Act to keep accurate work records. Exhibit 14–3 lists the data that should be kept for three years for each nonexempt employee. Although the Department of Labor only requires that these records be kept for two years, an employee can bring an action for willful violation of the Fair Labor Standards Act for three years. It is safest, therefore, to retain these records for three years after employment ends. To maintain accurate records on the hours each employee works, time sheets should be completed by every nonexempt employee for each payroll period. Exhibit 9–6 is a sample time sheet for documenting data required by the Fair Labor Standards Act.

Nonexempt employees who work unauthorized overtime must be compensated for this time. To prevent unnecessary overtime, you should do the following:

- Establish and distribute a policy stating that all work beyond normal work hours must be authorized.
- Don't suggest, pressure, or condone coming in early, working late, or taking work home unless you intend to pay for it.

Exhibit 14–2 Fair Labor Standards Act Definitions of Executive, Administrative, and Professional Employees

Executive Employees

- Normally supervises two or more employees.
- Has authority to hire and fire, or whose recommendations in that regard are given serious consideration.
- Primary duty involves managing the practice.
- Regularly exercises discretionary powers.
- Compensation is at least $155 per week.

Also, any employee who receives $345 per week and who manages a department or who supervises two or more employees is considered an executive.

Administrative Employees

- Primary duties consist of office or nonmanual work directly related to management policies or the general operation of the business.
- Exercises discretion and independent judgment on a regular basis.

- Regularly and directly assists executives, performs specialized work, or possesses specialized knowledge and exercises these skills under general supervision only.
- Receives a salary of at least $155 per week.

Professional Employees

- Requires advanced knowledge acquired through a course of specialized intellectual instruction.
- Performs work that is original and is dependent upon the employee's imagination and talent.
- Teaches for an educational institution.
- Performs work that requires the exercise of consistent discretion.
- Performs work that is predominantly intellectual and varied in character.
- Receives compensation of at least $280 per week.

Source: Adapted with permission from S. Kahn, B. Brown, and M. Lanzarone, *Legal Guide To Human Resources*, pp. 16-13–16-17, © 1996, Warren, Gorham, and Lamont.

- Notice when employees arrive and leave. If they are coming in early or staying late, find out why.
- Audit time sheets, and be certain that they are being kept accurately.
- Remember, it is ultimately management's responsibility to make certain that time sheets are accurate and that employees only work the hours that you intend.

Independent Contractor Agreements

An independent contractor is one who contracts to render personal services as well as provides the means to perform those services. Consulting physicians, psychologists, social workers, physical therapists, nurses, and a number of other types of workers are sometimes engaged as independent contractors by health care organizations. The distinction between an independent contractor and an employee has important financial and tax considerations for the em-

ployer. For example, independent contractors are not covered under the Fair Labor Standards Act or worker's compensation laws. Employers also do not have to withhold federal and state taxes on wages, pay the employer's share of FICA, or pay federal and state unemployment taxes for independent contractors. Because of these financial considerations, federal agencies, including the Internal Revenue Service (IRS), may closely examine independent contractor agreements.

Often, the distinction between an employee and an independent contractor is hard to ascertain. Federal agencies, such as the Department of Labor and the IRS, have an interest in classifying workers as employees because that generates more taxes and creates more federal control. The costs associated with treating workers as independent contractors, if the IRS or the Department of Labor subsequently determines them to be employees, can be substantial. The IRS, for

Exhibit 14–3 Fair Labor Standards Act Recordkeeping Requirement for Nonexempt Employees

Full name	Total daily or weekly straight-time earnings
Social Security number	Total overtime compensation for the work week
Home address, including ZIP code	Total additions to or deductions from each pay
Date of birth	period
Sex	Total wages paid each pay period
Job title/occupation	Date of payment and pay period covered by the
Time of day and day of the beginning of the	payment
employee's work week	Amount and nature of each payment excluded
Regular hourly rate	from the regular rate
Basis on which wages are paid ($ per hour, $ per	Total overtime excess compensation for any work
week, $ per month, etc.)	week
Hours worked each day and total hours worked	
per week	

Source: Reprinted from 29 U.S.C. §211(c) (1982).

example, often seeks to collect FICA taxes not withheld plus interest and penalties. As a result, whenever you are considering treating someone as an independent contractor, it is important to discuss this with your attorney. All written independent contractor agreements should be prepared by your attorney.

The overriding issue when determining whether a worker is a contractor or an employee is the degree of control exercised by the employer. There are a number of tests that have been established to determine contractor or employee status. Exhibit 14–4 contains some tests used by the IRS. Imagine that passing a test results in one check mark on the employee or the contractor side of a ledger. The preponderance of the checks may determine the worker's status. The word *may* needs to be stressed because of the predisposition of federal agencies to decide in favor of employee status. Ultimately, both the courts and federal agencies look to the reality of the relationship as opposed to simply counting the number of characteristics associated with contractorship or employee status. The IRS will issue a declaratory ruling for tax purposes. It also may view your inquiry as a red flag, however, and target you for an investigation. If pos-

sible, have your tax attorney or accountant submit the factual information without revealing your identity.

The use of independent contractor arrangements can also create some insulation from liability. Because an independent contractor operates outside the control of the employer, this can provide a defense for the employer in tort cases, such as malpractice. To assert this defense, however, the employer cannot lead a third party, such as a patient, to believe that the contractor is an employee. To ensure that the provider is perceived as an independent contractor, all letterheads, pamphlets, and publications should clearly indicate the provider's contractor status. In addition, request for treatment or financial forms signed by patients should clearly state that the provider is an independent contractor and not under the supervision or control of your organization.

SELECTING AN ATTORNEY

Because the law permeates all aspects of business, it is essential to have an attorney who is readily available. The time to develop a relationship with an attorney is before you find yourself

Exhibit 14–4 IRS Tests To Determine Contractor or Employee Status

Factors Contributing to Employee Status	Factors Contributing to Contractor Status
• The employer has the right to direct and control the individual's performance, including the means, methods, and details of achieving the results. This control does not have to be actually exercised; it simply has to be available to the employer. • The employer can discharge the individual. • The employer furnishes tools and other equipment for performing the work. • The employer furnishes a place to work, and the individual regularly works there.	• The employer only determines the end to be accomplished, not the means to reach the end. • The individual furnishes his or her own tools and normal workplace. • The individual represents himself or herself to the public as available to perform similar duties for others, including being a contractor for others in the same type of business. • The individual does not in fact spend most of his or her time working for one employer.

Source: Adapted with permission from S. Kahn, B. Brown, and B. Zepke, *Personnel Director's Legal Guide, 1988 Cumulative Supplement*, pp. S3-16–S3-17, © 1988, Warren, Gorham, and Lamont.

in a crisis. Consult your attorney whenever you are considering any action with legal implications or receive any document with legal implications. The following documents and actions, among others, require a consultation:

- written employment contracts or verbal employment agreements
- contracts with vendors, suppliers, or independent contractors
- participating agreements with insurance companies
- notification that a lawsuit has been or will be filed against you or your practice
- termination of an employee
- apparent violation of any employment contract or vendor, supplier, or contractor agreement
- injury to any patient, employee, contractor, or member of the general public on your premises
- all leases and other contracts relating to real property

Recommendations from other physicians or health care professionals can be helpful in the screening process when you are choosing an attorney. In addition, you should interview attorneys before making a decision. Many attorneys

will not charge a fee for this type of consultation. Finally, once you select an attorney, you should continue to evaluate the quality and timeliness of his or her work. If you become dissatisfied, discuss this with the attorney; if there is no change, select another attorney.

It is not essential, for your general legal needs, to retain a lawyer or firm that specializes in medical practices. Larger firms have the advantage of being able to offer attorneys who specialize in various parts of the law, such as tax law and employment law. This can also work to your disadvantage, however. For example, if you call with a question that is about a contract but that also may have tax implications, the firm's contract lawyer may consult with the firm's tax lawyer, and you will be billed for both attorneys. Is this kind of intrafirm consultation really required? In some instances it may be, but at other times it may be a strategy for "running the billing clock." In addition, you may find it more difficult to establish a personal relationship with an attorney in a larger firm. If you like to play golf or socialize with your attorney, then you may be more satisfied with a smaller firm that gives you personalized attention.

Keep in mind that you may be a medium or large account to a small firm, whereas you may be a small account to a large firm. A small firm or an attorney with a general business practice will generally possess adequate knowledge to handle most business law questions, and the firm or attorney can always refer you to a legal specialist when necessary. A potential disadvantage to using a solo attorney is that administrative tasks may consume enough time that he or she cannot be as responsive to your needs as an attorney in a large firm.

Fees should be discussed in your initial meeting with the attorney. Generally, the attorney will be your legal representative, file annual corporate papers, and do specified other tasks for a flat fee, which will vary with your geographical location. Additional tasks, such as providing an opinion on a contract, representing you in litigation, or giving advice on how to terminate an employee are generally handled on an hourly basis. Hourly fees will vary with geography and with the experience of the attorney.

CONCLUSION

By reading this chapter, you should have gained an understanding of the legal responsibilities and implications associated with the business side of a health care organization. You should have a basic understanding of contracts and torts that you can use to identify potentially threatening or litigious situations. You should understand the theory of malpractice. You should be able to deal with employment and personnel matters in such a way that you do not implicitly forego your employer prerogatives, while at the same time complying with federal legislation, such as the Fair Labor Standards Act and the Civil Rights Act of 1964. You should understand the role of an attorney and be able to recognize situations in which you should seek legal counsel. Finally, you should have developed an awareness of how to avoid legal conflicts in the daily operation of your health care organization.

REFERENCES AND NOTES

1. V. Maurer, *Business Law: Text and Cases* (New York, N.Y.: Harcourt Brace Jovanovich, 1987).

2. Maurer, *Business Law.*

3. R.A. Anderson, et al., *Business Law* (Cincinnati, Ohio: South-Western Publishing, 1987). See also *Nesselrode v. Executive Beechcraft, Inc.* and *Beechcraft Aircraft Corp.* (MO) 707 S.W. 2d 371 (1986).

4. S. Kahn, et al., *Personnel Director's Legal Guide*, 1988 Cumulative Supplement (Boston, Mass.: Warren, Gorham & Lamont, 1988), S2-27–S2-28.

5. K. Fineberg, et al., *Obstetrics/Gynecology and the Law* (Ann Arbor, Mich.: Health Administration Press, 1984), 21–22.

6. Fineberg et al., *Obstetrics/Gynecology and the Law*, 43–47.

7. Malpractice: Can You Really Protect Your Assets?, *Medical Economics* 30 (October 1989): 129–132.

8. Anderson, et al., *Business Law,* 271.

9. Kahn, et al., *Personnel Director's Legal Guide*, S2-42–S2-43.

10. *Toussaint v. Blue Cross and Blue Shield of Michigan*, 408 Mich. 579, 292 N.W. 2d 880 (1980). See also *Hetes v. Schefman & Miller Law Office*, 393 N.W. 2d 577 (1986).

11. Kahn et al., *Personnel Director's Legal Guide.*

12. The EEOC often applies the four fifths rule to determine disparate impact. This means that if any protected group has a selection rate that is four fifths of the rate of the group with the highest selection rate, then there is disparate impact. For example, if 30 of 100 men are hired (30 percent) but only 10 of 50 women are hired (20 percent), then there is disparate impact because $30\% \times 4/5 = 24\%$.

13. Wonderlic and Associates, *Wonderlic Personnel Test Manual* (Boston, Mass.: Wonderlic and Associates, 1983), 17.

14. Specific technical requirements for demonstrating statistical adverse impact and job relatedness can be found in Uniform Guidelines on Employee Selection Procedures, Federal Register 43 (1979): 38290–38315. These guidelines are also available from the EEOC, which has offices in most large cities.

15. Equal Employment Opportunity Commission, Guidelines on Sexual Harassment in the Workplace, 29 C.F.R., Sec. 1604.11, *Federal Register* 43 (1978): 74676–74677.

16. *Meritor Savings Bank v. Vinson*, 477 U.S.57 (1986).

CHAPTER 15

Managing Information Technology

Chapter Objectives

The goal of this chapter is to familiarize the physician manager with how information technology can be used to support management and clinical decisions. Information technology, such as electronic medical records, resource management and decision support software, telemedicine, and the Internet provide an opportunity to better understand the business aspects of medical decisions, and to operate a more effective medical organization from both clinical and business perspectives. Information technology also creates an opportunity to improve organizational integration by linking diverse parts of the health care system, and by providing new information that help the parts of complex health care organizations work more closely together. Many, however, may resist the changes generated by information technology. This chapter will help the physician manager think about the process of introducing information technology in ways to reduce this resistance.

Information systems provide the physician manager with the data needed to make informed medical and management decisions. We have already discussed the use of several information systems in reference to receivables collection. A clinic's medical office management system (MOMS), for example, is an information system designed for billing and collection functions. Other information systems discussed in Chapter 8 include an aging history database and a collection database. Both these databases are driven by data exported from MOMS. These are all simple information systems that assist management decision making.

Current and near future information systems provide physician managers with potentials that go well beyond the realm of collection and ac-

count management and cross the boundaries of single departments to span organizations. They provide the potential for managing most aspects of medical care, including both clinical and financial functions. They also will help physician managers manage relationships among health care organizations and provide the basis for evaluating both the financial and the clinical performance of organizations and physicians.

Information systems, because they affect every aspect of health care, will in themselves provide a competitive advantage. In Chapter 10 (Figure 10–1), the pentagon and triangle were used to illustrate how the marketing mix or pentagon issues (product/service, place, communication, value, and people) are affected by the underlying triangle infrastructure of systems, logistics, and suppliers. Information technology (IT) increasingly will be an important component of health care management systems, logistics, and supplier management. Effective information systems will allow health care organizations to address the following marketing mix considerations:

- *Design products and services to better meet customer needs.* Most health care organizations have complex customer definitions that include patients, employers, government, insurers, and others. Information systems will help health care organizations determine the product/service attributes that are really desired and then assess the degree to which the provider is meeting this objective.
- *Transcend place distinctions.* Electronic medical records (EMRs) and telemedicine offer the possibility of breaking the link between medical services and specific locations.
- *Offer value.* By identifying care decisions that really affect the quality of outcomes, it will be increasingly possible to reduce costs in areas that don't lead to outcomes that the customer does not value.
- *Communicate in objective ways the quality and value of care.* For example, clinical outcome data that are adjusted for severity, sometimes referred to as case mix data, will provide physicians and health care systems with a way of communicating clinical outcomes to customers. Similarly, these data can be used by specialists to describe the quality and cost of their outcomes to primary care physicians, thereby affecting the referral process.

An outcome from these IT pentagon applications is that the "people" point on the pentagon will change. Physician managers will have to be centrally involved in the emerging information systems, so that the medical perspective will receive proper weight. In addition, health care systems will have to acquire specialized IT skills, which often will mean that positions will have to be allocated to the design and support of clinically useful information systems.

Effective information systems of the future must encompass the complete medical product. In the past, medical information systems generally were specific to either a medical or a financial purpose. Historically, financial information systems evolved first, so that physicians and hospitals could be paid for their work. As the need evolved for clinical systems, they often were cobbled to financial systems because these systems contained some clinical information that was already present for payment purposes. As a result, early clinical applications were usually problematic because the clinical data they accessed were often distorted by the need to generate payments. For example, alcoholism is rarely coded because it is generally not a billable service. Depression, however, is billable, so it is often listed as the primary diagnosis in a financially driven information system. As a result of this problem and others, standalone clinical information systems evolved to fill the void. Their inability, however, to integrate the financial effects of clinical decisions is a major limitation in an era of managed care and capitated contracts. Managed care and capitated contracts affect both medical and financial considerations. As a result, the information systems that health care organizations will need to meet this evolving business and clinical environment will have to capture both the clinical and the business aspects of each case.

The elimination of this artificial and counterproductive distinction between financial and clinical systems is at the heart of the physician manager's role. Physician managers are unique in their ability to integrate financial and medical perspectives to reach a management decision. Physician managers, therefore, will be greatly assisted by information systems that speak to both financial and clinical issues. To achieve this objective, physician managers need to be cognizant of an additional issue.

Information systems are creatures in and of themselves. They represent a new way of thinking about, categorizing, and delivering information. Successful development of health care information systems relies on contributions from physicians, nurses, other users, managers, IT professionals, and quality specialists. Information technologists contribute designs that are functional and productive. Engineering in quality assessment features from the beginning ensures that total quality management thinking and tools, such as "the seven old tools" (see Chapter 12), are intrinsic to the information system, so that appropriate quality data can be easily extracted. Including users, such as physicians, nurses, and managers, in system design increases the probability that systems will provide the data that are necessary in a form that is not unduly intrusive. Successful health care information systems are the result of the work of a design team that includes all these disciplines and perspectives.

THE NATURE OF INFORMATION SYSTEMS

Medical information systems have many specific purposes. Physician managers and their organizations will use several types of information system applications. Ideally, each application will draw on common data sources, so that information is internally consistent. The types of applications fall into the following broad categories: electronic medical record, care automation and resource management, clinical repository, enterprisewide scheduling, and comparative analysis. In many instances, a given software application will cut across several of these categories.

Electronic Medical Record

An electronic medical record (EMR) will be the cornerstone of future clinical information systems. The EMR is essentially a patient chart that is electronic as opposed to paper. EMRs can overcome many problems of paper-based systems and at the same time create many new opportunities. Typical estimates are that paper charts are unavailable about 30 percent of the

time, documentation is deficient about 27 percent of the time, and pulling and filing a chart costs between $4 and $9.[1] In contrast, EMRs can reduce medication errors, and in one study they saved $596 per patient.[2] EMRs also offer the potential to facilitate communication between referring physicians and specialists, improve record legibility, improve timeliness of record-keeping, reduce record access problems, and increase organization integration. EMRs also can provide the basis for evaluating clinical outcomes because input and outcome data are both systematically recorded in a quantitative database.

An example of an EMR screen is shown in Figure 15–1. This particular screen is from an EMR called *Logician*. The screen illustrates a summary view. Other views are selected by choosing from the tabs (Problems, Medications, Warnings, Flowsheet, and Documents) along the top of the screen, with each screen providing additional detail.

In addition to storing basic clinical information, an EMR also should save the physician time, highlight important clinical issues, and provide decision support. For example, the EMR in Figure 15–1 provides a single screen summary of active problems, so that they can be identified quickly. Laboratory results and clinical notes can be searched by date, key word, or level. In addition, EMR clinical information often is arranged in a hierarchy, so that a physician can dive deeper into one line of inquiry, such as recalling all data related to a specific asthma episode.

Some EMRs provide decision support tools. These are capabilities that help the physician make a clinical decision or facilitate the decision once it has been made. Examples of decision support capabilities include the following:

- built-in and easily modified formularies that offer prescription alternatives that are diagnosis sensitive. (Some EMRs provide cost data for prescription alternatives. All should flag potential prescription interactions.)

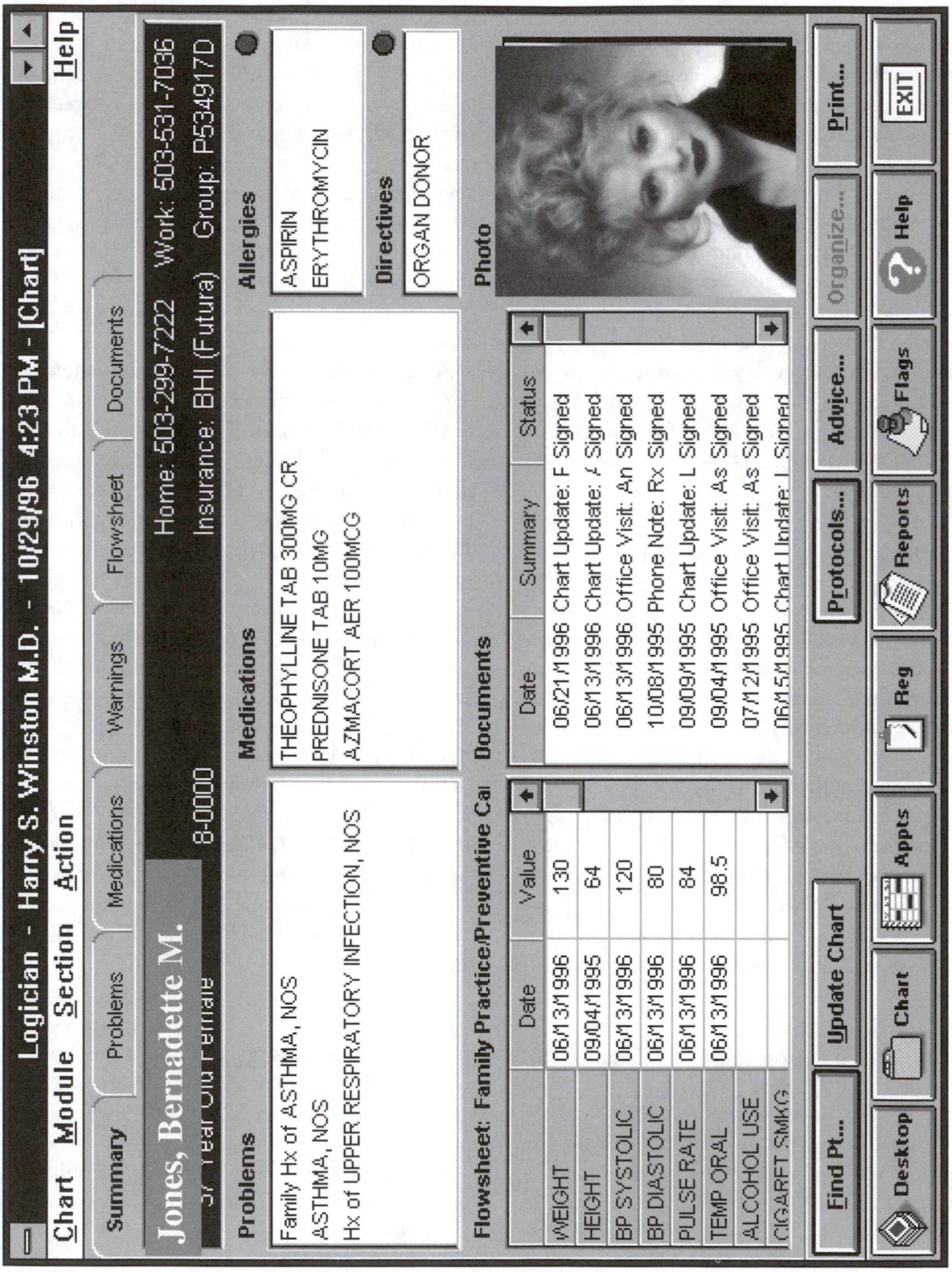

Figure 15–1 Sample EMR screen. Courtesy of Medicalogic, Portland, Oregon.

- identification of tests that are generally useful and not useful before a consultation or referral (Figure 15–2)
- specialist referral guidelines that are sensitive to treatment protocols
- patient education materials that are specific to the patient's needs, diagnosis, or prescription (the material can then be printed at the time of treatment, so that the patient leaves with appropriate reading material)
- suggested treatment protocols based on physician diagnosis
- assessment of patient qualification for a critical pathway and tracking of patient progress on critical paths
- diagnosis assistance

In a true EMR environment, patient charts are electronically updated by all providers. Laboratory results, for example, are "autoflowed" by the laboratory directly into the patient's EMR instead of being keystroked into the chart after a paper report has been sent from the laboratory to the clinic or hospital. Similarly, the laboratory order is generated directly by the physician from the EMR screen, with no paper script.

In some EMR applications, patients can directly enter clinical interview information. For example, Wald and colleagues describe the use of a health history interview with 300 patients at a hospital's primary care practice.[3] Computer-based interviews offer potential advantages of time savings, more structured clinical data collection, greater reliability, and better collection of sensitive or embarrassing information. In this particular study, patients sat at a terminal in the waiting room and completed the computer-based questionnaire before seeing the clinician. Providers felt that the computer system added the most value in the areas of psychiatric information, alternative care, and medical review of symptoms.

For an EMR to function effectively, it must be largely transparent to the clinician. Intrusiveness into the physician's normal routine can be an important issue. In a study conducted at Kaiser Permanente, 46 primary care clinicians and 95

supporting personnel used an EMR on a daily basis between February and December 1994.[4] After four to six months of experience with the system, 85 percent of clinicians disagreed with the statement "If given a choice, I would return to the old system." At two months into the study, time studies indicated that clinicians were averaging 2 minutes 10 seconds longer to complete patient charting. This was due primarily to the tasks necessary to make an order. In addition, it took approximately 30 days before their EMR learning curves matured, during which time physicians lost an average of 38.5 hours of productivity at one site and 24.9 hours at a second location. In addition, training took 16 hours.

Some research does indicate that the use of EMRs can change the nature of the clinical encounter. For example, Urkin and colleagues found that clinicians changed from a conversational pattern, in which they alternated between talking with the patient and recording data, to "block" pattern, in which they first massed patient conversation and data collection and then massed data recording.[5] Aydin and associates addressed the question of patient reaction to computers in the examining room at Kaiser Permanente in the San Diego Preventive Medicine Department.[6] Satisfaction was assessed among 233 patients whose examiners used a computer for medical history and physical examination and 195 patients whose examiners did not use the computer-based system. They found no significant difference in any satisfaction measures. Scales included cognitive (examiner's explanations, information, and patient's understanding of and confidence in the findings of the examination), behavioral (thoroughness and confidence in the examiner), and acceptance (willingness to accept the examiner's advice). The investigators concluded that computer use did not depersonalize the encounter for the patient, but it also didn't enhance patient satisfaction.

Ease of EMR use is facilitated by screens specific to medical applications. For example, Gorman and colleagues describe an EMR that is specific to a diabetes clinic.[7] In this application,

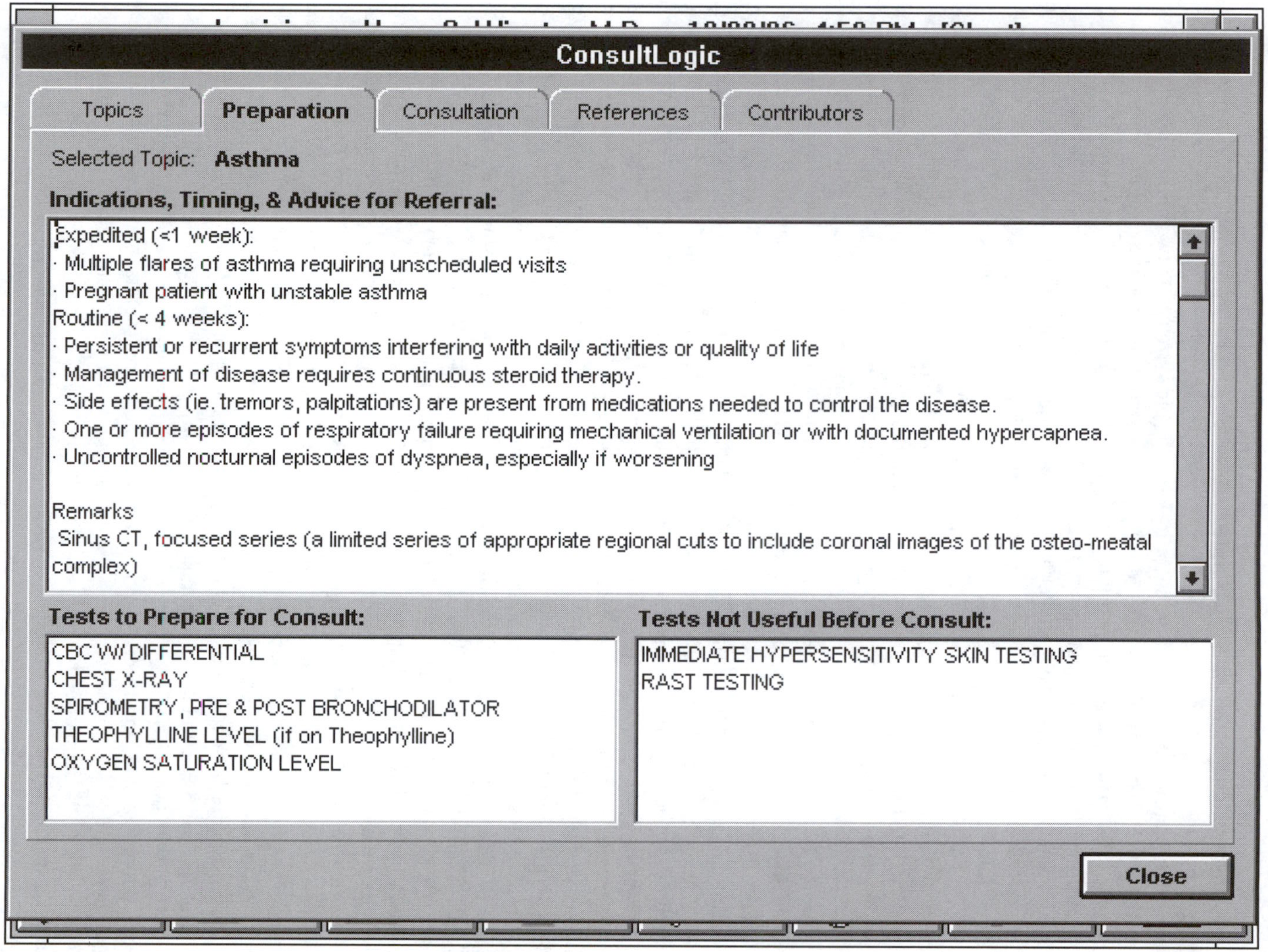

Figure 15–2 EMR suggested test screen. Courtesy of MedicaLogic, Portland, Oregon.

data and presentation screens are optimized to support diabetes-specific encounters, such as initial visits, insulin adjustment visits, dietitian encounters, and the like. DeFriece noted that variability in the entire process of clinical data collection and documentation makes it difficult to design user-friendly EMRs.[8] He proposed designing programs that can learn clinician response patterns to different situations. The program would learn a clinician's most frequently used data elements and actions for a particular problem and then make them quickly accessible.

Most EMRs make extensive use of pull-down menus and touch-screen entry. This results in clinical data coding that is quantifiable and searchable, two qualities that are critical evaluating outcomes. Many physicians, however, rely on dictation. Electronically transcribed dictation can be stored in an EMR as text, but its utility as data for subsequent analysis is limited, such as to searches on key words. Pictures can also be stored as part of the EMR. Patient faces can be helpful for identification, so that staff can provide a more personal greeting. Pictures can also contain clinical data. For example, Fujino and coworkers describe how endoscopic images can be transformed into a video signal, which provides the opportunity for image enhancement and processing as well as storage in an EMR.[9] More widespread is the digitizing of radiographs, which once again can be stored as part of the patient's EMR.

To be as easily used as a paper chart, EMRs must be available instantaneously and simultaneously at all potential treatment sites. In most systems, two locations cannot simultaneously modify the same field, such as primary diagnosis. Multiple locations, however, should be able to work simultaneously with different parts of the same patient record. Touch-screen tablets carried by health care providers that are linked to a server by infrared or wireless transmission represent one approach to providing easy access for data entry. Another alternative is to have data entry terminals in all treatment rooms and physician offices. Some systems use hand-held computers called personal digital assistants. These devices can be loaded with various types of software, such as EMR data entry, prescription, protocol, critical path, spreadsheet, and word processing applications. Generally, personal digital assistants are not on line. They are used to collect data and then download the data to the server at a later point in time, such as at the end of the day or between consultations.

Once an entry to an EMR is posted and signed, it cannot be deleted or changed. Errors are corrected by making additional entries. In addition, only appropriate individuals should be authorized to enter data in specific areas of an EMR. Laboratory personnel, for example, should not be able to make changes to clinical screens, such as symptoms or diagnosis. The EMR is the official legal patient record, and all entries are signed with an electronic signature.

We have previously talked about the importance of integration to the success of large health care systems. An EMR can be a major contributor to system integration. It removes many of the impediments to clinical integration because all authorized providers have access to appropriate parts of the clinical chart in a timely manner. Also, it provides a means of integrating clinical and financial information. The EMR should be the "back end" of the financial information system. Many EMRs electronically transfer clinical information to the billing system, where coding, electronic claims, paper claims, payment, and collection activities take place.

RESOURCE MANAGEMENT AND DECISION SUPPORT

Automating parts of the care delivery process can provide better management of resources and personnel. Automating care can also include providing support for clinical decisions. Resource management and decision support are achieved with an assemblage of discrete capabilities that cut across organization functions and software programs.

One implementation of care automation is computerized order entry. Orders can include discrete events at a point in time for a patient, such as prescribing a medication or a test.[10] Orders also can include transfers across departments or services, such as preadmission, postoperative, and discharge orders. These orders result in many actions in different parts of the health care system. Order systems that automatically notify appropriate locations and prompt for appropriate signatures, authorizations, and cosignatures use automation to better manage time, commodities (e.g., pharmaceuticals), and resources (e.g., hospital beds). They also can help integrate activities across organizational boundaries.

This can, however, intensify previously existing organizational frictions. Massaro described how introducing a physician order system at the University of Virginia Medical Center created strife between different factions.[11] He concluded that introducing IT accentuated existing organizational problems, such as communication and governance. Finally, he concluded that health care systems need to orchestrate the introduction of information systems as part of a conscious change process (see Chapter 11) that is designed to address potential resistance to change. This would include broad participant involvement in the design of systems before implementation.

Another decision support tool is an alert or reminder system. Reminder systems provide feedback by electronic means, flags, letters, and even telephone calls. Research indicates that reminder systems improve clinician compliance with previously accepted protocols by reducing errors that are due to information overload.[12] Rind and colleagues conducted a study of computer-based alerts in a teaching hospital for patients with rising creatinine levels.[13] In a time series experiment involving 14,130 patients, these investigators identified 845 creatinine events among 483 control patients and 728 events among 439 experimental alert system admissions. The mean interval between the occurrence of an event and discontinuation of medication or a dosage change was 97.5 hours for the control group and 75.9 hours for the computer alert group (p<.0001). Of 562 patients admitted who had events involving nephrotoxic medica-

tions, the control group rate for patients who subsequently had serious renal impairment was 7.5 percent; the rate was 3.4 percent for the computer alert group. The investigators concluded that when computer-based alerts were sent to physicians for patients with rising creatinine levels during treatment with nephrotoxic or renally excreted medications, the physicians made more rapid, medically appropriate adjustments.

Decision support can also apply simultaneously to clinical and cost decisions. Evans and associates described a decision-support tool for antibiotic therapy.[14] *Antibiotic Assistant* was linked to the hospital's EMR. Based on clinical data and physician classification of the need for an antibiotic as therapeutic, empiric, or prophylactic, the program suggested an antibiotic and dosage. Mean cost for antibiotics was reduced by $87 per patient during the study. Adverse drug events declined from 2.4 percent to 0.9 percent, although this reduction was not statistically significant.

Linking clinical pathways, clinical documentation, orders, and cost information through the EMR is another example of care automation with resource management implications. In this case, the EMR documents where the patient is on the pathway and identifies the ensuing steps and timing if the patient is to remain on the pathway. With physician concurrence, the care automation system places orders with other departments, such as radiology or pharmacy, to ensure that the patient stays on the pathway.

Figure 15–3 shows a screen from a resource management program called *Resource Case Management System* that displays a patient's status on a pathway. This particular pathway is for a normal delivery. The data in the upper right of the screen indicate that the pathway length of stay is 2 days, with a cost of $2,358 that will generate $4,195 in gross charges with a predicted reimbursement of $3,517, for a margin of $1,159. The current projection is for a one-day stay with a margin of $1,305. The projected variance of –$146 indicates that the one-day length of stay should generate a greater margin than the two-day pathway.

OGG, STACY RENEE   Pathway NormDel – Thu 8/3 10:11P

File   Pathway   Payor   Notes   Codes   View   Options   Help

Name	OGG, STACY RENEE
Age	30
Case No.	05918966
Admit Date	5/31/95
Payor Valid	Yes
Est. Dsc Dt	6/1/95
Path Assigned	Yes
Bed	OB 30601

	LOS	Cost	Charge	Reimb	Margin
Pathway	2	$2,358	$4,195	$3,517	$1,159
Case Est	1	$1,820	$3,494	$3,125	$1,305
Variance	1	$538	$701	$392	($146)

Expand

Popup:
Charges $1,265
Costs
Fixed $196
Variable $194
Total $390

Category	Unit Cost	Path Pre-Admit	Act Pre-Admit	Var Pre-Admit	Path Wed 5/31/95	Act Wed 5/31/95	Var Wed 5/31/95	Var Thu 6/1/95	Path Post Dschg	Act Post Dschg	D
OUTCOMES											
VITALS NORMAL					Y	M					
OBSTETRICS					$1,447	$1,335	$112	$653			
FETAL MONITORING ADD 1/2 HR	$1l				1	6	-5				
BIRTHING ROOM	$39				2		2				
OB,GYN-SEMI PRIVATE	$65				1	1		1			
FATHER'S SCRUB SUIT	$				1	1					
+Other						$611	($611)				
+OPERATING ROOM					$192	$435	($243)				
+LABORATORY					$39	$14	$25				
+CENTRAL DISTRIBUTION					$14	$36	($22)	$14			
+Other											
Total					$1,691	$1,820	($129)	$667			

Figure 15–3 Resource case management system screen critical pathway status with financial data. Courtesy of Medicus Systems, San Diego, California.

The bottom of the chart shows major activity categories. The chart indicates that the path calls for one unit of fetal monitoring, but six units have been used for a –5 variance. Two of the categories, Outcomes and Obstetrics, have been expanded to show more detail. Birthing Room has a unit cost of $390, of which $196 is due to fixed costs and $194 is due to variable costs (see Chapter 6). The data on fixed and variable costs are external to this particular program. Ideally, the data would be generated from a cost accounting system (see Chapter 6). Some health care systems, however, will use a ratio of cost to charges, which at best is speculative and probably invalid. The data entry for this particular system is driven by the billing or admission/discharge/transfer system. This illustrates how management information systems can be integrated. Changes in the EMR drive the billing system, which, through care automation, drives this particular critical path resource management program.

Once pathways are managed in an information system, it becomes possible to see clearly and at any time where the patient is on the pathway. In addition, it also becomes possible to conduct research on the pathway because the aggregation of the patient's EMRs constitutes a database. A research capability is essential to developing effective critical pathways. Figure 15–4 shows a pie chart indicating reasons why an initial antibiotic was not administered within three hours as called for by the pathway. Figure 15–5 shows a scattergram clearly illustrating that compliance with the protocol antibiotic standard was associated with reduced cost variance and reduced average cost. Appropriate statistics, as well as graphics, can be generated by the software.

Having the capability to analyze data easily can form the basis for total quality management analysis (see Chapter 12) of critical pathways. Health care systems that use resource management software have a competitive advantage over those that don't because they will understand better how their resources are being used, where improvement is possible, and which improvements will provide the greatest return. It

should also be noted that these valuable research and system outcomes are a direct result of a more effectively managed clinical process at the patient level.

The ability to analyze data, such as the effects of various medications or changes in the pathway, by using graphing tools built into the resource management software is a minimum characteristic. It is not reasonable, however, to expect this type of software to be as capable at data analysis or as flexible at charting as products developed specifically for these purposes. Care automation and resource management software, therefore, should be capable of exporting data to more powerful statistical software, such as *SPSS* or *SAS*, and higher end spreadsheets, such as *EXCEL*.

CLINICAL REPOSITORY

A clinical repository is a central storage for EMR data. As health care networks expand horizontally to cover larger geographical areas and vertically to cover all types of medical services, a patient's EMR could become fragmented across various locations.[15] For example, the primary care physician, hospital, and specialist might all have an EMR for the same patient. Part of the value of system integration is getting all the information together, so that each clinician can see the complete picture. A clinical repository avoids this fragmentation by basing the EMR in a central location that is accessed by each provider.

A clinical repository also provides an excellent basis for systemwide research. Because all a health care system's clinical data are contained in one accessible location, it is possible to ask systemwide questions. This would not be possible, for example, if each hospital, practice, and outpatient location maintained its own EMRs.

Extending the clinical repository concept a step further could result in each person having a truly transportable medical record that could be accessed nationwide. It is not necessary for all clinical repositories to have the same format, only that they have some common variables and that they use a standard communication format.

Pneumonia Cases

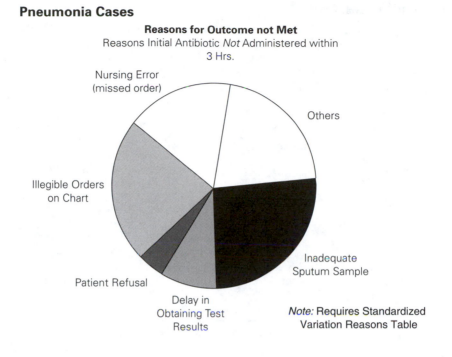

Reasons for Outcome not Met

Reasons Initial Antibiotic *Not* Administered within 3 Hrs.

Nursing Error (missed order)

Others

Illegible Orders on Chart

Patient Refusal

Delay in Obtaining Test Results

Inadequate Sputum Sample

Note: Requires Standardized Variation Reasons Table

Figure 15–4 Resource case management system screen—analysis of unmet outcome. Courtesy of Medicus Systems, San Diego, California.

ENTERPRISEWIDE SCHEDULING

In a health care system striving for integration, patient care will be distributed across several offices, laboratories, and locations. Enterprisewide scheduling helps achieve coordination of schedules, optimum use of health care system resources, and efficient patient processing. The goal of enterprisewide scheduling is to schedule any event at any time by appropriate personnel. One obvious point of scheduling integration should be at the EMR, since data entry into the EMR will generally trigger a referral, script, or follow-up visit.

COMPARATIVE ANALYSIS

Comparative analysis is the process of evaluating physician and health care system outcomes. This is a controversial subject because it touches on the sensitive issue of performance appraisal. Performance appraisal (Chapter 2) is the process of evaluating how well individuals perform their jobs. Management information systems create the opportunity to focus more objectively on clinical and cost outcomes at all levels of health care aggregation, including health care systems, hospitals, practices, and physicians. The difficulty in doing this is that physicians and health care systems have different mixes of patients. In effect, some physicians and systems have sicker patients. If this is not taken into account, then the resulting statistics can be misleading.

One approach to adjusting for this case mix issue was developed at the Johns Hopkins University.[16] It is typical of a number of case mix systems. The Johns Hopkins system adjusts for the fact that patients with certain diagnoses or combinations of diagnoses require more treatment. It is based on diagnosis-related groups (DRGs) that have been compressed into a

Pneumonia Cases: Cost

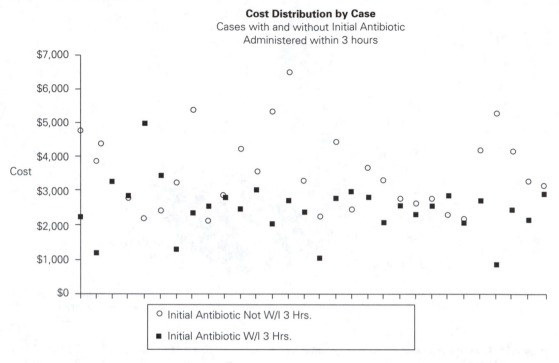

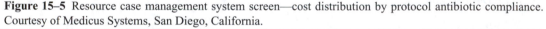

Figure 15–5 Resource case management system screen—cost distribution by protocol antibiotic compliance. Courtesy of Medicus Systems, San Diego, California.

smaller number of ambulatory care groups (ACGs). The distinction is that DRGs classify patients based on the nature of individual encounters or episodes, whereas ACGs classify patients based on age, gender, and illness burden for a 12-month period. A patient's ACG category does not change for 12 months, whereas a DRG might change with each encounter.

The ACG system reduces approximately 6,000 potential diagnoses into 52 mutually exclusive illness burden categories. As a result of this aggregation, cell sizes become large enough to be stable, so that conclusions can be reached about the data. Exhibit 15–1 contains a partial listing of ACG categories. Patients are classified into an ACG category based on an intermediary classification of diagnoses, which are called activity diagnostic groups (ADGs). Notice that ACG–43 is a combination of several ADGs.

Exhibit 15–2 shows an analysis across three locations for five ACG categories. Location A averaged 5.78 visits per patient. Exhibit 15–3 uses the planwide averages for each ACG category to calculate an expected number of visits for each ACG category. The total expected visits for location A is 26,023, for an average of 5.31 visits per patient. Similar statistics could be calculated for locations B and C. Finally, Exhibit 15–4 uses actual, average, and expected numbers to describe location A's activity. The actual/average ratio gives an indication of the unadjusted efficiency with which location A used resources compared with other locations. In this case, location A is using 11 percent more resources than all locations. The expected/average ratio assesses the illness burden, which in this case means that location A is expected to use 2 percent more resources than average. The actual/expected ratio is a measure of efficiency. In this

Exhibit 15–1 Selected ACG Categories

01 Acute Minor, Age < 2	14 Psychosocial, With Psych–Major, Without Psych–Minor
02 Acute Minor, Age 2–5	
03 Acute Minor, Age 6+	15 Psychosocial, With Psych–Major, With Psych–Minor
04 Acute Major	
05 Likely To Recur Condition Without Allergies	16 Preventive/Administrative
	17 Pregnancy
06 Likely To Recur Condition With Allergies	18 Acute Minor and Acute Major
	19 Acute Minor and Likely To Recur Discrete, Age < 2
07 Asthma	
08 Chronic Medical, Unstable	20 Acute Minor and Likely To Recur Discrete, Age 2–5
09 Chronic Medical, Stable	
10 Chronic Specialty, Stable	43 Four or Five Different ADGs, ages 17–44
11 Ophthalmological/Dental	52 No Services Provided
12 Chronic Specialty, Unstable	
13 Psychosocial Only, Without Major Psychiatric Diagnosis	

case, location A is using 109 percent of the resources (visits) expected, given the illness burden of its patients.

Similar analyses can be performed by health care unit or by physician. In addition, the data analyzed can be anything that is measurable and assignable to a unit, such as visits, supplies, medical fees, total cost, or the like. Exhibit 15–5 contains a cost analysis for a specific physician, Dr. Good. The analysis indicates that, given the illness burden of Dr. Good's patients, her total costs are 68 percent of what would be expected. Her costs are above expectations for ambulatory (1.19) and significantly below expectations for hospital (0.41), emergency (0.16), radiology (0.49), and pharmacy (0.49). These data, however, do not tell us whether Dr. Good is providing appropriate medical care. Her 0.68 cost factor may mean that she is treating her patients efficiently, or it may be an indication of undertreatment. What the ACG system does do is to identify Dr. Good as an outlier. Evaluation of what the data mean is a management responsibility that should involve additional data, such as chart audits and discussion with Dr. Good.

Case mix systems, therefore, can be used as screens for quality assurance to identify both overtreatment and undertreatment situations. It is important to point out that the information system is only describing *what* the physician is doing. Judgments regarding the appropriateness or inappropriateness of care should always be the responsibility of a management that includes physicians.

The importance of using case mix adjustments was illustrated by Salem-Schatz and coworkers, who used ADGs to examine retrospectively 37,830 referrals made by 52 primary care physicians to specialists at the Harvard Community Health Plan.[17] Using a regression methodology, the investigators found that, when no case mix adjustment was made, the following variables were significant predictors of specialist referral rate: physician age, years since medical school, years with clinic, health center, laboratory tests per visit, and an inverse relationship with number of hours worked (fewer hours worked resulted in a higher referral rate). When case mix data were entered into the regression, all these variables became nonsignificant and dropped out of the equation. One variable, practice intensity (visits per week/full-time equivalent hours), became significant. This illustrates that the use of unadjusted practice profiles to

Exhibit 15–2 ACG Location Analysis

	Location A		Location B		Location C		Total	Total	Planwide
ACG	Number of Patients	Number of Visits	Number of Patients	Number of Visits	Number of Patients	Number of Visits	Number of Patients	Number of Visits	Average Visits
2	1,000	8,400	500	2,750	800	5,000	2,300	16,150	7.02
5	2,000	11,300	800	3,800	1,200	6,000	4,000	21,100	5.28
14	100	1,000	75	900	125	1,188	300	3,088	10.29
16	1,500	4,500	1,000	2,750	1,250	3,875	3,750	11,125	2.97
17	300	3,100	80	800	150	1,350	530	5,250	9.91
Total	4,900	28,300	2,455	11,000	3,525	17,413	10,880	56,713	

Location	Actual Average Visits per Patient
A	5.78
B	4.48
C	4.94
Total	5.21

Exhibit 15–3 ACG Calculation of Location A Expected Number of Visits

ACG Category	Number of Patients	Planwide Average	Expected Visits
2	1,000	7.02	7,022
5	2,000	5.28	10,550
14	100	10.29	1,029
16	1,500	2.97	4,450
17	300	9.91	2,972
	4,900		26,023
			Expected Average Visits/Patient 5.31

make performance appraisal decisions, such as compensation, sanctions, and employment, is highly questionable.

Management information systems that can supply case mix data can be the basis for a more rational approach to dealing with capitation and assuming the risk for treating a population of patients. In a capitated payment system that is not risk adjusted, an incentive is created for undertreating patients. With risk adjustment, this incentive vanishes because undertreatment can result in lower allocation of resources. In addition, patients and physicians with greater illness burdens are no longer penalized.

Exhibit 15–6 illustrates another risk adjustment system that is used on a federally supplied Medicare database. This system, developed by MEDSTAT Group/Inforum, provides 95 percent confidence intervals around expected val-

Exhibit 15–4 ACG Location A Illness Burden Analysis

	Location A
Actual	5.78
Expected	5.31
Plan Average	5.21
Actual/Average	1.11
Expected/Average	1.02
Actual/Expected	1.09

ues. Actual values that fall outside the expected range can then be identified as outliers. For example, the upper confidence level around the expected mortality level of 11.39 for hospital B is 17.52. Because the observed mortality level of 21 exceeds this limit, further examination is warranted because illness burden has been held constant.

A common response by those who have pointed out the simplifications used by case mix systems, such as those described above, is that they can be gamed through coding inflation and other means. Because any system can be gamed including paper based and subjectively based systems, this is not a reason to reject all information system applications for managed care, risk management, and physician evaluation. This is simply a reason to think more critically about what the data mean, to use them in an intelligent manner, and to develop better comparative data systems.

A legitimate question to ask at this point is whether there is any evidence to indicate that clinical data systems actually improve patient outcomes. In general, studies indicate that information systems are associated with some improved clinical outcomes. Johnson and colleagues, in a review article, found that three of four studies of computer-assisted dosage determination systems reported statistically significant improvement in achieving therapeutic lev-

Exhibit 15–5 Physician Summary Utilization Report

Subject	Actual ($)	Expected ($)	Average ($)	Actual/Average	Expected/Average	Actual/Expected
Dr. Good						
Total cost	638,492	927,956	326,724	1.95	2.84	0.68
Hospital	176,000	427,824	144,724	1.21	2.95	0.41
Ambulatory	342,179	287,342	132,638	2.58	2.16	1.19
Radiology	32,047	64,429	37,244	0.86	1.73	0.49
Laboratory	122,463	179,264	64,322	1.90	2.78	0.68
Emergency	11,427	68,961	29,325	0.39	2.35	0.16
Pharmacy	52,374	104,968	33,107	1.58	3.17	0.49
Preventive	101,324	98,324	42,336	2.39	2.32	1.03
Mental health	80,822	107,772	33,624	2.40	3.20	0.75

Source: Reprinted from N.S. Smith and J.P. Weiner, Applying Population-Based Case Mix Adjustment in Managed Care: The Johns Hopkins Ambulatory Care Group System, *Managed Care Quarterly*, Vol. 2, No. 3, p. 30, © 1994 Aspen Publishers, Inc.

Exhibit 15-6 MEDSTAT Group/Inforum Hospital Outcomes Data

Complication: All Complications
Confidence Level: 95%
DRG:
089   Pneumonia & Pleurisy Age >69 & or CC
090   Pneumonia & Pleurisy Age 18-69 w/o C

	Total Patients	Patients w/Comp	Expected Patients w/Comp	Patients w/Comp Ratio	Comp Lower Conf Int.	Comp Upper Conf Int	Actual Mortality	Expected Mortality	Mortality Ratio	Mortality Lower Conf Int.	Mortality Upper Conf Int.
Hospital B ⟶	193	11	17.76	0.62	9.99	25.54	20	21.13	0.95	13.28	28.99
	>148	7	12.48	0.56	5.91	19.05	21	11.39	1.84	5.25	17.52
	173	7	17.68	0.40	10.01	25.36	18	16.11	1.12	9.11	23.10
	100	8	8.29	0.97	2.94	13.63	6	8.65	0.69	3.49	13.81
	101	11	8.56	1.29	3.17	13.94	8	11.86	0.67	6.30	17.42
	102	6	7.39	0.81	2.32	12.46	7	7.58	0.92	2.82	12.34
	90	1	7.40	0.14	2.35	12.45	4	7.81	0.51	2.82	12.81
	137	10	10.69	0.94	4.61	16.77	8	13.33	0.60	6.90	19.76
	199	12	15.89	0.76	8.48	23.30	16	15.13	1.06	8.33	21.92
	201	9	15.61	0.58	8.24	22.97	12	16.45	0.73	9.16	23.74
	223	13	17.59	0.74	9.79	25.40	19	13.44	1.41	6.66	20.22
	46	3	2.92	1.03	0.00	6.14	2	2.27	0.88	0.00	5.05
	206	11	16.30	0.68	8.78	23.82	25	27.42	0.91	18.96	35.88
	294	16	28.93	0.55	18.98	38.87	20	15.83	1.26	8.59	23.08
	165	20	16.75	1.19	9.32	24.17	15	17.21	0.87	10.07	24.36
	176	9	13.88	0.65	6.95	20.81	8	12.03	0.67	5.89	18.16
	279	18	23.33	0.77	14.38	32.29	19	25.85	0.74	17.31	34.38
	314	32	26.24	1.22	16.73	35.74	31	29.29	1.06	19.60	38.97
	75	9	5.33	1.69	1.00	9.65	1	7.67	0.13	2.82	12.51
	116	7	9.36	0.75	3.66	15.06	17	11.22	1.52	5.58	16.86
	3,338	**220**	**282.38**	**0.78**	**251.25**	**251.25**	**277**	**291.67**	**0.95**	**261.97**	**321.37**

Source: Exhibits are supplied courtesy of The MEDSTAT Group/*Inforum*, a Thompson Healthcare Information company.

*Conf. Int. based on expected values

els.[18] Johnson found no studies, however, that indicated superior patient outcomes. Only one of five studies showed a significant advantage for computer-aided diagnosis. Four of six studies found that computers enhanced the quality of preventive care, such as reminders to provide influenza or tetanus vaccinations. Finally, seven of nine studies indicated that computers improved clinical performance for the treatment of active medical problems.

In a study that was not cited by Johnson's group, Berner and associates had 10 experts create a set of 105 diagnostically challenging clinical case summaries.[19] The cases were designed to be sufficiently complex so that a physician would be likely to seek a diagnostic consultation. Data were then entered into four computer-based diagnostic systems. The proportion of correct diagnoses ranged from 52 percent to 71 percent. On average, less than half the diagnoses that the experts viewed as reasonable were proposed by any of the programs. On the other hand, the programs averaged about two diagnoses that the experts considered feasible but had not originally considered. The investigators concluded that diagnostic support systems appear most effective when they are used to generate hypotheses, to remind physicians of diagnoses that they might not have considered, and to stimulate thinking about related diagnoses.

In an observational study, Pestotnik and colleagues analyzed changes in antibiotic usage and costs that occurred with the use of a computer-assisted decision support system across 162,196 patients discharged from a hospital.[20] They concluded that computer-assisted decision support programs supporting locally derived practice guidelines can improve antibiotic use, reduce costs, and stabilize the emergence of antibiotic-resistant pathogens.

TELEMEDICINE

"What do you call a place the size of New York State with almost no medical, surgical, or pediatric subspecialists? Western Kansas."[21(p.322)]

Herein lies one value of telemedicine. Telemedicine is the process of delivering medical services from one location to another through IT. Patients can receive services more quickly, they can receive services that they otherwise could not receive near home, patients and families don't need to travel long distances to receive specialist services, and their primary care physician can remain involved in the diagnosis and development of a treatment plan.[22] Exhibit 15–7 describes various telemedicine applications.

Telemedicine is not a new idea. Examples can be traced back to the 1960s. Early examples, however, were limited by the capabilities of technology at the time. Recent innovations, such as fiberoptics, compressed video, the Internet, on-line services, and the low cost and high power of desktop computers, have resulted in improved quality, greater accessibility, and lower cost.

Telemedicine can appear in a number of forms, including remote professional consultation, remote patient consultation, and robotics. Remote professional consultation occurs when health care providers consult with other health care providers through IT. This can be face to face (e.g., with two-way interactive video), e-mail, or data transmission. A typical application would be for a rural primary care physician to consult with a specialist regarding a diagnosis or treatment plan. The primary care physician transmits patient clinical data, perhaps the whole EMR, radiographs, and so forth to the specialist, who then communicates back by telephone, video, e-mail, or some other technology process. A variation on this theme is the integrated health care network in which both the primary care physician and the specialist are part of the same organization. Using a common EMR, the specialist simply accesses the patient's clinical history without any need for the primary care physician to undertake any special record assembly or transmission.

One of the most rapidly growing areas of telemedicine is teleradiology. This is a result of advances in imaging technology and database design and management. Applications include

Exhibit 15–7 Telemedicine Application Categories

- Initial urgent evaluation of patients, triage decisions, and pretransfer arrangements.
- Medical and surgical follow-up and medication checks.
- Supervision and consultation for primary care encounters at sites where a physician is not available.
- Routine consultations and second opinions based on history, physical examination findings, and available test data.

- Interpretation of diagnostic images.
- Extended diagnostic work-ups or short-term management of self-limited conditions.
- Management of chronic diseases and conditions requiring a specialist not locally available.
- Transmission of medical data.
- Public health, preventive medicine, and patient education.

computed tomography, magnetic resonance imaging, and ultrasonography as well as traditional radiographs. In this application, the radiographs or other media are digitized and then transmitted to the remote location, where they are interpreted by the radiologist. This can be particularly advantageous if it is desirable to have the radiograph read before the patient is discharged.[23]

Teleradiology also illustrates some of the shortcomings that can be imposed by current technology. Telemammography, for example, is still emerging because of limitations in digital imaging systems and the large volume of information required by this type of radiograph. Scott and colleagues also illustrated some of the current technology limitations.[24] In an experimental design, these investigators had seven senior radiology residents and one radiology fellow evaluate 60 film radiographs and 60 digitized images displayed on a video monitor. All images were of difficult orthopaedic trauma cases. The overall accuracy was 80.6 percent for the film readings and 59.6 percent for the teleradiology readings.

Remote patient consultation is another form of telemedicine. In this application, the physician consults directly with the patient. A number of remote patient consultation systems have been created. The Medical College of Georgia Telemedicine System provides two-way interactive audio and video communications with sev-

eral remote sites in Georgia. The system can also be moved by van to remote locations or emergency settings. In addition to primary care and specialty services, the system is capable of assisting in some surgical procedures, such as endoscopy and laparoscopy. The set-up cost for a remote site is between $95,000 and $115,000. Other patient consultation telemedicine systems have been run by the state of Texas, Kansas University Medical Center, East Carolina University School of Medicine, and the Mayo Clinic. The Mayo Clinic has operated a center at the Pine Ridge Indian Reservation in cooperation with the National Aeronautics and Space Administration. An analysis of the project through postparticipation questionnaires and surveys indicated that two thirds of respondents felt that the telemedicine consultations contributed to their health and that 90 percent felt that the project should continue.[25] Allina Health System in Minneapolis has linked the emergency department of its hospital in Buffalo, Minnesota, with three small hospitals between 50 and 150 miles away through two-way video hookups. Each of the remote hospitals pays $50,000 per year for the service and saves money when compared to staffing an emergency department. Correspondingly, the Buffalo hospital's emergency department has seen a substantial increase in net revenue as a result. Buffalo now handles almost all of the emergencies at the satellite hospitals using specially trained nurses at the remote locations under the direction of Buffalo physicians. Between May 1, 1995, and March 31, 1996, the network handled 243 emergency medical consults.[26]

Another instance of directly delivering medical services to the patient through technology is e-mail between physician and patient. One bottleneck in many clinic settings is communicating messages between patients and physicians. E-mail circumvents this bottleneck. When integrated with an EMR, an e-mail can flag a patient's chart on the physician's activity schedule. In effect, the chart is electronically "pulled" by the e-mail message. Appropriate uses may include providing test results, answering patient questions, and providing follow-up. One physician who has used e-mail to communicate with patients stated:

> It can go on for days [referring to telephone tag]. E-mail puts an immediate end to that problem. . . . A significant population of the university employees here seem to love it . . . and some have recommended me to their friends because it's so easy to use. . . . I'd take only e-mail and not phone messages at all if I could.[27(p.19)]

A variation on the theme of delivering health services from one health facility to another is to deliver them directly into the home. Electronic house calls in a sense take us back to a previous age. Nevertheless, for patients with limited mobility, travel to a clinic or hospital is a real burden. In addition, transportation may be a major component of the total cost of some services, such as renal dialysis and follow-up visits. Remote monitoring, interactive video, e-mail, and even the lowly telephone can make home health care feasible for some patients.

Home-based telemedicine may be particularly effective for follow-up and for monitoring chronic illnesses, such as asthma and diabetes.[28] East Carolina State University has begun remote cardiac rehabilitation using telephone, cable television, and telemetry. The Harvard Community Health Plan placed computer terminals in 150 homes on an experimental basis to help patients manage common illnesses and monitor chronic conditions.

Another emerging telemedicine application is robotics. This technology is based on remote handling systems that were originally developed for use with nuclear materials located in rooms that were inaccessible. Applications in endoscopic surgery, laparoscopy, and battlefield surgery are in the developmental stage. For example, AESOP (Automated Endoscopic System for Optimal Positioning) replaces the technician or physician who holds and maneuvers the endoscopic camera during an operation. AESOP provides a more stable image than a handheld camera; it can remember and return to previous positions, much as an automobile car seat with memory, and it provides substantial cost savings over human operators.

A major obstacle to the growth of telemedicine is reimbursement. Historically, insurers, including the government, only reimbursed for face-to-face delivery of care. There are some exceptions. Teleradiology, telepathology, and electrocardiographic testing are currently reimbursed by the Health Care Financing Administration (Medicare/Medicaid). Probably the greatest obstacle, however, to reimbursement is the lack of evidence demonstrating safety and effectiveness. This is not to imply that telemedicine is unsafe or ineffective. The problem is that the research has not been performed regarding most telemedicine applications. Outcomes have been hard to demonstrate. Many evaluations have been superficial or not controlled enough to conclude clearly that telemedicine was a source of improvement.[29] More thorough evaluations have not shown some expensive applications to offer advantages over low-technology less expensive alternatives, such as the telephone. One inherent problem in conducting research on telemedicine is that the evidence needed to demonstrate safety and efficacy generally requires large clinical trials, but most telemedicine programs are rurally based with small populations. One approach to this problem is to conduct collaborative research across multiple locations to assemble the needed sample sizes.[30]

INTERNET APPLICATIONS

Currently, there is a deluge of interest in the Internet. Unfortunately, a book is the wrong format to discuss Internet medical applications. The Internet, by its nature, is built on change, whereas the book format is more appropriate for less mutable topics. Internet locations change often, new resources become available each minute, and old ones mutate with use. The goal in this section, therefore, is to describe the nature of the Internet for those physicians who are not familiar with it and for those who have had limited Internet experience. For those physicians who currently are Internet users, the discussion that follows will be superfluous.

The Internet is a computer-based network of networks. In theory, any of the computers in any of the networks can talk with any other computer. For example, the School of Business at The College of William and Mary has a computer network that links all the business school faculty, graduate students, and staff through e-mail on a server computer that is called Dogwood. The Dogwood network is also linked to the university's network and to the Internet. Any computer that is on the Dogwood server can access any other Dogwood-, university-, or Internet-connected computer. The type of computer and its operating system are largely irrelevant to its capacity to access the Internet. Windows machines, Macintoshes, UNIX-based computers and mainframes can all communicate with each other using the Internet as an intermediary. The Internet in effect has become a universal translator. This has the potential to solve a major problem that many health care systems face. They possess myriad standalone information systems that cannot talk to each other. Replacing these systems, which continue to do their original functions well, with a new common one would be very expensive and disruptive. By modifying these standalone systems, however, to communicate through the Internet, it becomes possible to link formerly isolated computers and information systems into a large network. Problems of speed and security assurance still need to be resolved. The Internet, however, may provide an inexpensive and quick way to integrate information technology across a health care system.

The major Internet capabilities that are used by health care providers are e-mail, the World Wide Web (WWW), file transfer protocol (FTP), Usenet, and Gopher. E-mail is exactly what its name implies: electronic mail. E-mail messages can be sent from one computer to any other computer on the Internet. Communication with patients and communication with colleagues are two obvious ones. E-mail also can contain attachments of larger documents. For example, while writing this book, I received copies of computer screens as attachments to e-mail messages. These screens contained a lot of data, so they were compressed to a smaller size (stuffed) and then expanded in my Macintosh computer by a program called *Stuffit Expander*. The effect is like freeze drying a large amount of information to package it for easy transportation and then adding water at the other end.

E-mail can be an effective learning device when you communicate with others who have similar interests and concerns, such as family medicine, clinical ophthalmology, managed health care, and so forth. Listserves are an example of e-mail lists of subscribers with a common interest. You subscribe to a listserve by sending a message asking to subscribe to it. Messages from any member to the listserve are automatically sent to all other subscribers. Exhibit 15–8 lists some groups. To subscribe, you send an e-mail to the discussion group address. For example, if I wanted to subscribe to the managed health care quality group in Exhibit 15–8, I would send the following message:

listserv@missoul.missouri.edu
subscribe Mhcare-L (my address)

The WWW is a graphic interface to the Internet that is accessed through a browser program. Examples of browsers are Netscape, Mosaic, and Webcrawler. The most powerful feature of the WWW is that embedded in each image are links to other WWW locations. For example, Figure

Exhibit 15–8 Example of User Group Mail Lists (Listserves)

Group Name	Purpose	Address
Fam-med	Computers in family medicine	listserv@gac.edu
Gasnet	Anesthesiology practitioners	listproc@gasnet.med.yale.edu
CPRI-L	Computerized patient records	listserv@kumchttp.mc.ukans.edu
TDR-scientists	Tropical disease research	listserv@who.ch
Mhcare-L	Managed health care quality	listserv@missoul.missouri.edu

Source: Data from N. Sandlin, "The Internet: What's On It For You?", *American Medical News*, 10 June, 1995, p. 20.

15–6 is a partial screen of the *Journal of the American Medical Association*'s (*JAMA*'s) home page. Each of the 15 boxes in the lower left corner (JAMA, American Medical News, Press Releases, and so on) is linked to those locations. If I click once with my mouse on JAMA, for example, it will take me there. At this screen, I will then have access to a number of other hyperlinks, so that, for example, I can see the table of contents for the current issue of *JAMA*, access abstracts of articles in current and past issues, and in some cases open the actual articles.

"Surfing the Web" means going from hyperlink to hyperlink through a never-ending wave of home pages, documents, pictures, sounds, and even short motion pictures. Home page leads to home page, information leads to information. It literally never ends.

Another useful Internet function is FTP. This is used for downloading information, programs, pictures, and text from another computer to your computer and also for uploading information from your computer to other computers. Often, for example, you can obtain upgrades to software as well as freeware and shareware through downloads. You can FTP from your WWW browser or from services such as America Online (AOL) and CompuServe.

When downloading files, be certain that you have antivirus software installed on your computer and that it is turned on. Some on-line services screen their downloads for viruses, but there are no assurances that your downloads are virus free other than your own safeguards.

Usenet newsgroups are sources of subject-oriented articles that you receive by connecting to a specific newsgroup. In this case, the word

article is used loosely to mean anything ranging from a glorified e-mail to a tome. Remember, anyone can publish anything on the Internet, so the quality begins at junk and ranges upward. About 50,000 articles across 20,000 topics are "published" each day. Examples of newsgroups include telemedicine (sci.med.telemedicine), immunology (sci.med.immunology), and radiology (sci.med.radiology). Articles are grouped into "threads" of similar subject matter. You can examine an article's header to see whether it is of interest before opening it.

Gopher servers are computers that make information available to others. Gopher derives from its source, the University of Minnesota, whose mascot is the Gopher. Gopher also refers to one who gets things for others (go fer this, go fer that), which describes the function of Gopher: to bring to a screen diverse information in an easily accessed hierarchical format. Gopher sites are navigated through plain English hierarchical menus. Gopher menus can link you to other Gopher servers, FTP sites, Usenet archives, and other parts of the Internet including the WWW. For example, a Gopher folder might be entitled Breast Cancer Research and Programs. Opening this folder might reveal documents on early stage breast cancer detection, facts on breast cancer, questions to ask your doctor, and so on. Gopher sites generally contain text although there are some that contain images and sounds.

Examples of Gopher sites include:

- Oncolink—cancer-oriented information including information on clinical trials (gopher cancer.med.upenn.edu)

 File Edit Services Windows AOL FaxMenu   10:33 AM

JAMA Homepage

Home | Back | Forward | Reload | Stop | Load Images | Load Original

Current URL : http://www.ama-assn.org/public/journals/jama/jamahome.html

Link URL :

Page complete   Image complete

the guidance of leading HIV/AIDS authorities and community representatives, this special Web site is made possible by an unrestricted educational grant from *GlaxoWellcome*.

JAMA Subscription Rates

Personal
USA $130, Americas $170, Outside Americas 113 pounds sterling

Regular Rate
USA $175, Americas $220, Outside Americas 152 pounds sterling

AMA Publication Subscription Order Form   NEW

JAMA	NEWS	PRESS RELEASES	Physician Recruitment	What's New!
ARCHIVES				
DERMATOLOGY	FAMILY MEDICINE	OPHTHALMOLOGY	INTERNAL MEDICINE	PEDIATRICS
NEUROLOGY	PSYCHIATRY	OTOLARYNGOLOGY	WOMEN'S HEALTH	SURGERY

Figure 15–6 WWW page (partial) with hyperlinks. *Source:* Reprinted with permission from American Medical Association, © 1996.

- NIAID—a National Institutes of Health gopher on infectious diseases and AIDS (gopher odie.niaid.nih.gov)
- CNET—National Cancer Institute gopher that provides current information to patients and physicians, including research on new treatments (gopher://gan 1.ncc.go.jp:70/0/CNET/All_files/201176).

To access the Internet and all the components described above, you first must be able to connect to it. The first place to look for a connection is on your employer's computer system. Virtually all universities and many larger health care providers have Internet access. If your employer does not, then you have two choices. One choice is to subscribe to a commercial on-line service. On-line services are accessed through a modem and a regular telephone line. Examples include AOL, CompuServe, Prodigy, and Microsoft Network. The advantage of these commercial providers is that they tend to fill the potholes on the information highway. They provide an extra degree of organization that is especially helpful to the novice.

Commercial on-line services also provide built-in Internet search tools. For example, AOL provides Webcrawler. It also provides services that otherwise would have additional subscription fees. For example, as of this date AOL provides access to Medline at no additional cost. Medline is an extensive database of medical publications that provides citations and abstracts that can be located by title or subject matter content. Commercial providers also provide chat groups, which are interactive text conversations among subscribers that are organized around topics. They also have preprogrammed many generally useful Internet locations, so that all you have to do is point to an icon instead of doing a search or typing the WWW address into a search engine.

If your objective is to access the Internet and you do not need an on-line service's proprietary products, you may want to consider a public Internet service provider (ISP). ISPs simply provide access to the Internet along with a search engine, such as Netscape, and e-mail, such as Eudora. Major ISPs include AT&T Worldnet, Sprint, and MCI. The advantage of using an ISP is that their rates are usually lower than those of on-line services. Be aware, however, that some low-priced ISPs have gained a reputation for poor service, such as an insufficient number of access lines, which makes it difficult to gain access during peak hours. ISP users often view on-line services as analogous to being in a box with one slow narrow tunnel out that leads to the Internet. They ask "Why should I get in the box to begin with?"

SECURITY

Physician managers need to be concerned with two types of security. The first relates to the concepts of privacy and confidentiality. Clinical and financial information must be restricted to those with a legitimate need for the information. One security issue, therefore, with regard to EMRs is that only appropriate users can have access, and even then only to appropriate parts of the EMR. For example, coding and billing employees should not have access to clinical data beyond what they need access to in order to do their jobs. Unauthorized use by authorized personnel is a difficult problem because the security process may interfere with appropriate utilization. For example, suppose that a hospital restricts access to a patient's EMR to the attending physician and the assigned nurse out of a concern for privacy and confidentiality. This might slow or prevent the delivery of care by substitute nurses, emergency personnel, or consulting physicians.[31]

When data are being transmitted over public media, such as by satellite, on the Internet, or over telephone lines, the data need to be protected from being read by unauthorized personnel. This requires encryption of the data. Encryption really works. The Workshop on Electronic Data Interchange reported that there have been no known cases of company-to-company encrypted data being compromised.[32] Health care information systems also need to be secure against entry by unauthorized personnel.

Authentication methods, such as passwords, can be used to verify who is gaining access.

Finally, these systems need to be protected from sabotage, such as the entry of viruses, and from physical damage or theft. Viruses can be protected against by controlling access to the system, by retaining logs of users, and by routinely using antivirus software. Data loss as a result of sabotage and theft can be prevented by a well-designed system of data back-ups that store multiple copies of the data at multiple, remote locations.

Physician managers need to be aware that privacy issues are an area of evolving law. Compliance with the federal Privacy Act and relevant state laws requires consultation with knowledgeable legal counsel.

OVERCOMING RESISTANCE

IT will create major changes in how physicians practice medicine. We saw in Chapter 11 that many resist change. Fear is often at the root of this resistance: fear of being unable to adjust, of learning new ways, of losing influence, or of being in less than full control of one's professional life. It was suggested in Chapter 11 that one of the keys to implementing change is to anticipate this resistance and prevent its occurrence or overcome it by using premeditated strategies. All the strategies that were discussed in Chapter 11 are relevant to address the IT resistance issue. As was discussed in that chapter, the "bottom of the list" strategies of manipulation and coercion should generally be avoided unless absolutely necessary (e.g., in the case of an immediate threat to organization survival). Three strategies that are particularly relevant to addressing the resistance that IT may generate are education and communication, participation, and facilitation and support.

One major source of resistance is lack of understanding about the real impact of IT. Physicians who do not understand how IT will help them provide better care or why IT is necessary for organizational competitiveness if not survival cannot justify their own cost in terms of changing how they are used to practicing medi-

cine. To overcome this type of resistance, physician managers must provide an understanding of the nature of the problems that IT will help address. Historically, physicians have defined their job as providing direct clinical care. As we have seen, however, the physician is really at the center of a health care delivery *system*.

This system perspective was illustrated with the pentagon and triangle concepts in Chapter 10. The triangle illustrates how systems are essential to providing a marketing mix (product/service, location, value, communication, and people) that is patient focused. IT is at the core of the systems, logistics, and suppliers and results in customer-focused pentagon points. At the millenium, these triangle issues can best be managed by thoroughly pervasive information systems. If you don't use IT to manage these systems to provide the best level of customer-focused service, your competitors will, and as a result they will do it better and at lower cost. Physicians who do not appreciate the significance of this marketing perspective and how their role as physicians fits into the overall product that the system provides cannot appreciate why their jobs must change. *Education, therefore, is an essential element to introducing IT successfully.*

In a similar manner, physicians who do not understand the financial considerations of medical decisions (see Chapter 6) cannot fully understand why IT changes are necessary. Providing fundamental education on the nature of costs and the importance of and difficulties associated with determining costs will help justify the construction of complex and, on occasion, intrusive IT systems.

Education and communication are strategies to lower resistance by providing perspective on the nature of the challenges faced by health care providers. They reduce resistance by demonstrating that IT can help find solutions to managed care problems. It is important in true education and communication, however, to avoid messages that state that management has the specific solution. To do so is to distort education to the point that it becomes propaganda. Avoid stating, for example, "The XYZ EMR is the answer to all our problems!" True education provides a justification for change, it provides background, and it provides context. It is not a tool that management should use to try to sell a specific solution to an otherwise skeptical audience.

Participation is one of the most powerful tools to overcome IT resistance. Effective IT systems can only be developed when physicians are part of the design process. Because physicians will be the primary users of many health care IT systems and will be affected by others, they possess valuable knowledge that should be included in the design of systems or the evaluation of competing systems. When physicians are included in the design process, they develop a sense of ownership. Generally, owners have a strong incentive to make their ideas work.

The danger of using participation is that physicians with a predisposition to resist IT changes may use their opportunity for input to delay or minimize change. Preceding participation with a thorough education program that stresses the need for change may reduce the chance that participation will be used as an opportunity to obstruct.

Finally, facilitation and support will provide physicians with the skills that they will need to operate in an IT environment. Facilitation and support should begin at the time of initial education about the need for IT systems. At this point, management should make statements, reassurances, and, to the degree possible, commitments that it will provide thorough training in IT system use. When the product development or selection phase is undertaken with physician participation, one of the charges that those designing or selecting the system should undertake is development of a training process. Designers must also consider ease of use as a major development goal or selection criterion. Finally, as system implementation approaches, physicians should receive training in a hands-on environment. Ideally, physician leaders should be trained before system roll-out to test the system before general implementation. This is often referred to as the beta test phase. These physicians,

to the extent possible, should be involved in subsequent physician training to take advantage of their medical perspective, system experience, and medical collegiality.

A general strategy, therefore, to reduce or overcome resistance to IT change is to use these three change methods in a complementary fashion. Education and communication provide perspective. Participation results in systems that meet physician and organization needs less obtrusively and creates ownership and thereby commitment. Facilitation and support reduce fear by providing a clear path from the present to the future.

INTEGRATION

Improving organization integration is one of the great potential benefits of IT. In Chapter 11, two of the four general factors that were identified as inhibiting integration—complexity and physical size and distance—are directly addressed by IT. Two of the three integration barriers that are specific to health care—embryonic development of most clinical information systems and separate unintegrated financial and clinical information systems—are also directly addressed by IT. IT therefore offers major opportunities to increase organization integration dramatically.

Integration, however, is not fundamentally an IT problem so much as it is a human and management problem. Unfortunately, IT by itself will not improve integration. Computers did not create the nonalignment of incentives among various parts of health care systems; people did. Computers also did not create differentiation, the systematic differences in values, attitudes, and behaviors that often characterize health system subunits. Computer systems by themselves will solve none of these problems.

Achieving integration is fundamentally a management problem. Physicians and physician managers, because of their central role in the delivery of health care, must be important players in the design of information systems that align with personal and organizational goals. Once incentives are created so that, for example, medical, nursing, and laboratory services have a common incentive to work together to get a DRG through the hospital on average four hours sooner than the competition across town, IT will help them achieve this objective. In the absence of a self-interested commitment to work toward this goal, IT will simply provide more data for each faction to justify why it is right and the others are wrong. Introducing ever more powerful IT systems into health care organizations in which the parts are acting like medieval dukedoms, each competing and intriguing to obtain advantage, will only contribute to the problem.

Managed care companies, payers, and consumers are increasingly asking for demonstrated outcomes.[33] This requires more than simply communicating information across intrasystem boundaries. It requires a commitment on the part of all players to use IT data in creative ways to improve the quality of services and demonstrate important outcomes. Once the easier intradepartment improvements are achieved, this will leave the more difficult interdepartment/organization challenges as the only remaining improvement frontier. Improvements of this type cannot occur in health care systems that are still managed as an assemblage of competing interests.

Currently, the real IT integration challenge is masked in many health care systems by the babble of standalone information systems that were designed for singular purposes and do not communicate with each other. These are easy targets, and they obscure the more difficult and important IT integration challenge. Typical of the easy targets are the billing and clinical systems that are coincidentally acquired by health care systems when they purchase independent medical practices and hospitals. Other examples are legacy systems that were designed for specific standalone purposes years ago, such as billing, scheduling, and ordering. Without an integrated management plan and a shared vision by all important players (physicians, nursing, laboratories, pharmacy, finance, top management,

etc.), large health care systems will continue to automate with incompatible management and control systems that will optimize for each user and will suboptimize for the whole organization and, more important, its customers.

CONCLUSION

The physician manager's role in IT management has been alluded to throughout this chapter. First, physician managers need to be certain that they are included in the design and development of all IT projects. Physicians are at the core of the health care delivery system. They possess valuable and unique information about how information systems must function if they are to provide the most valuable contributions to patient care and organization effectiveness. This can only be achieved when physicians are instrumental in information system design.

The physician manager's role in the change process is to keep it focused on outcomes that make a difference. All too often, information systems are developed because they are "developable," not because they make a difference in terms of demonstrated clinical and financial outcomes. As a result of their training, physician managers have a natural predisposition to look first toward outcomes. That is a healthy screen to use when you are evaluating IT projects.

Second, physician managers need to be cognizant of the potential for physicians and others to resist the introduction of IT solutions. Use of resistance reduction strategies should be an integral part of any IT system development or selection process. Physician managers need to take the lead in providing education, participating in system design, and ensuring that appropriate training will be provided for all physicians, including those who are not currently computer literate. This means that one training program may not be suitable for all physicians.

Third, the research on information system outcomes is in its infancy. Initial results in some areas are promising (reminders), but in other areas (diagnosis) the research indicates that significant development is necessary before effective systems can be put in place. This picture may change rapidly, and physician managers need to stay abreast of the research literature so that they can make informed decisions about the introduction of new IT solutions. Some IT solutions, however, may never work, and a healthy skepticism and a "show me" attitude represent a healthy approach for physician managers to take when considering IT solutions.

In an area of such rapid technological change, designers will be constantly stretching technology to its limits. Physician managers must be keenly aware of whether they are implementing IT solutions that can deliver what is promised or whether the products offered are just system engineers' toys. Considerations such as real clinical and cost effectiveness, low-cost and low-technology alternatives, unobtrusive use, and patient acceptance cannot be sacrificed to create an impression of progress. Physician managers, because of their unique education and experience, are in an excellent position to weigh all these considerations. As in most organizational situations, vacuums will be fleeting. If physician managers don't step in and assert their power or influence, others will, and the medical perspective will not be properly represented.

REFERENCES AND NOTES

1. Wall Street Journal (6 April 1992).

2. E. Drazen, *Patient Care Information Systems* (Boston, MA: Arthur D. Little, 1995).

3. J.S. Wald, et al., Patient Entries in the Electronic Medical Record: An Interactive Interview Used in Primary Care, *Proceedings of the Annual Symposium of Computer Applications in Medical Care* (1995):147–151.

4. M.A. Krall, Acceptance and Performance by Clinicians Using an Ambulatory Electronic Medical Record in an HMO, *Proceedings of the Annual Symposium of Computer Applications in Medical Care* (1995):708–711.

5. J. Urkin, et al., How Does a Computerized Medical Record Affect Physicians' Work Style?, *Proceedings of the American Medical Informatics Association's 1993 Spring Congress* (1993):89.

6. C.E. Aydin, et al., Computers in the Examining Room: The Patient's Perspective, *Proceedings of the Annual Symposium of Computer Applications in Medical Care* (1995):824–828.

7. C. Gorman, et al., A Clinically Useful Diabetes Electronic Medical Record: Lessons from the Past; Pointers toward the Future, *European Journal of Endocrinology* 134 (1996):31–42.

8. R.J. DeFriece, Design Considerations for Intelligent Data Entry: Development of MedIO, *Proceedings of the Annual Symposium of Computer Applications in Medical Care* (1995):91–95.

9. M. Fujino, et al., Electronic Endoscopy in Perspective, *Journal of Gastroenterology* 29 (1994):85–90.

10. J.M. Teich, et al., Enhancement of Clinician Workflow with Computer Order Entry, *Proceedings of the Annual Symposium of Computer Applications in Medical Care* (1995):459–463.

11. T.A. Massaro, Introducing Physician Order Entry at a Major Academic Medical Center: I. Impact on Organizational Culture and Behavior, *Academic Medicine* 68 (1993):20–25.

12. K.B. Johnson, et al., Medical Informatics and Pediatrics, *Archives of Pediatric and Adolescent Medicine* 149 (1995):1371–1380.

13. D.M. Rind, et al., Effect on Computer-Based Alerts on the Treatment and Outcomes of Hospitalized Patients, *Archives of Internal Medicine* 154 (1994):1511–1517.

14. R.S. Evans, et al., A Decision Support Tool for Antibiotic Therapy, *Proceedings of the Annual Symposium of Computer Applications in Medical Care* (1995):651–655.

15. As hospitals, practices, and other care organizations merge, an emerging challenge is to combine these organizations' EMRs or existing clinical repositories into a centralized repository. For a discussion of one system's approach to this problem, see K.A. Marrs and M.G. Kahn, Extending a Clinical Repository To Include Multiple Sites, *Proceedings of the Annual Symposium of Computer Applications in Medical Care* (1995):387–391.

16. N.S. Smith and J.P. Weiner, Applying Population-Based Case Mix Adjustment in Managed Care: The Johns Hopkins Ambulatory Care Group System, *Managed Care Quarterly* 2 (1994):21–34.

17. S. Salem-Schatz, et al., The Case for Case-Mix Adjustment in Practice Profiling, *Journal of the American Medical Association* 272 (1994):871–874.

18. M.E. Johnson, et al., Effects of Computer-Based Clinical Decision Support Systems on Clinician Performance and Patient Outcome: A Critical Appraisal of Research, *Annals of Internal Medicine* 120 (1994):135–142.

19. E.S. Berner, et al., Performance of Four Computer-Based Diagnostic Systems, *New England Journal of Medicine* 330 (1994):1792–1796.

20. S.L. Pestotnik, et al., Implementing Antibiotic Practice Guidelines through Computer-Assisted Decision Support: Clinical and Financial Outcomes, *Annals of Internal Medicine* 124 (1996):884–890.

21. A. Allen, Telemedicine in Kansas: Introduction, *Kansas Medicine* 93 (1992):322.

22. B.J. Vaughan, et al., A Client/Server Approach to Telemedicine, *Proceedings of the Annual Symposium of Computer Applications in Medical Care* (1995):776–780.

23. D.V. Beard, et al., Real-Time Radiologist Review of Remote Ultrasound Using Low-Cost Video and Voice, *Investigative Radiology* 28 (1993):732–734.

24. W.W. Scott, et al., Subtle Orthopedic Fractures: Teleradiology Workstation versus Film Interpretation, *Radiology* 187 (1993):811–815.

25. T.E. Kottke, et al., The Pine Ridge–Mayo–National Aeronautics and Space Administration Project: Program Activities and Participant Reactions, *Mayo Clinic Proceedings* 71 (1996):329–337.

26. G. Borzo, Telemedicine Program Demonstrates Market Value, *American Medical News* (29 July 1996): 12.

27. Talk with Patients, *American Medical News* (12 June 1995): 19.

28. U.S. Congress, Office of Technology Assessment, *Bringing Health Care Online: The Role of Information Technologies.* OTA-ITC-624 (Washington, D.C.: U.S. Government Printing Office, September 1995), 166.

29. P. McLaren and C.J. Ball, Telemedicine: Lessons Remain Unheeded, *British Medical Journal* 310 (1995): 1390–1391.

30. D.A. Perednia, Telemedicine System Evaluation and a Collaborative Model for Multi-Centered Research, *Journal of Medical Systems* 19 (1995):287–294.

31. Office of Technology Assessment, *Bringing Health Care Online,* 116.

32. Office of Technology Assessment, *Bringing Healthcare Online: The Role of Information Technologies* (Washington, D.C.: GPO, 1995), 116.

33. G. Borzo, Integrated Networks Depend on Integrated Information Systems, *American Medical News* (14 October 1996):49–50

CHAPTER 16

Some Final Thoughts

INTEGRATING THE PHYSICIAN MANAGER'S MANAGEMENT SKILLS

We have discussed the issue of integration as the challenge of getting the parts of a health care organization or system to work in a synergistic, coordinated manner. Similarly, physician managers need to use their management skills in an integrated fashion. One of the difficulties of presenting a survey of business issues is that, to organize the process so that the content would be most understandable, the book had to be divided into homogeneous chapters. As a result, the chapters are organized around specific content, such as finance, performance appraisal, marketing, and so forth. The physician manager's job, however, is more than the sum of each of the chapters in this book.

In reality, the lines between the knowledge areas discussed in this book either do not exist or are at best indistinct. Leadership blends into negotiation. Motivation blends into leadership. Financial information blends into performance appraisal. Marketing becomes strategy. Total quality management becomes organization structure, performance appraisal, motivation, and leadership. Information systems are an organization's neural network that extends everywhere. Part of the skill of being an effective physician leader is developing the intuition to look beyond the immediate situation to envision additional implications of your actions.

THE PHYSICIAN MANAGER'S PERSONAL CHALLENGE

In life, what usually creates the most pain, hurt, disappointment, and difficulty for us are our own expectations or, better stated, our own unrealistic expectations of ourselves and others. What happens when expectations are unrealistic? They play havoc with our emotions, thereby interfering with our interpersonal relationships, with our feelings about ourselves, and with our ability to act in a rational, problem-centered manner. Fear, anger, anxiety, and a need for retribution begin to control us, and we act in ways that are ineffective and self-defeating.

Many physicians initially have unrealistic expectations concerning the demands of running a business or working in a large health care organization. For some, reality causes them to adjust their expectations to more realistic levels. Other physicians, however, begin with unrealistic expectations and never give them up. They continue to assume that their expectations are realistic and that the world simply isn't cooperating!

Understanding and mastering the personal and emotional aspects of managing and working with others are essential for the physician manager to succeed. This is important for three reasons:

1. You may be able to react more quickly to and work more effectively with personal

and emotional issues if you are aware that they are real and that they can affect your decision making.

2. If you believe that your difficulties are unique, you may begin to feel helpless and hopeless. By understanding that they are not unique and that others have undergone similar ordeals, you may be less frightened or troubled during times of great stress.

3. Understanding what underlies your personal reactions to a situation may give you a more positive mind set. This may help you deal more effectively with employees, patients, partners, and colleagues and obtain more enjoyment from your job.

What, then, are typical expectations that physician managers have that may affect their ability to act effectively? They basically fit into two categories. The first category is expectations of others, including employees and associates as well as yourself. The second category is expectations regarding how the business world operates.

EXPECTATIONS OF OTHERS AND SELF

For practice-based physician managers, owning and running a practice is an exciting, motivating process. Similarly, physician managers in management positions in larger health care organizations generally have challenging, responsible positions with considerable organizational visibility. In both types of settings, physician managers are frequently involved in important decisions at the highest levels of their organization. It is easy for physicians managers in these positions to become caught up in the excitement of their jobs. It is also easy for them to fall into the trap of expecting others, especially employees, to have similar feelings and degrees of commitment.

Others may initially be equally enthusiastic, but their enthusiasm often fades. No one will care as much about "your baby" or your project as you do, and no one will be as willing as you to sacrifice and struggle when times are difficult. For practice-based physicians, this can also be a problem with other partners, who perhaps don't have as large a financial stake or who simply don't have the same degree of psychological investment as you do.

Others' lack of caring may manifest itself in a number of ways. For example, your receptionist might walk through the waiting room and fail to pick up a candy wrapper that is lying on the floor. On a more serious plane, one of your partners might promise to review the practice's aging analysis on Saturday but instead spends the entire weekend on a camping trip. Perhaps you have a report for the hospital chief executive officer (CEO) on the status of the new electronic medical record project. Your word processing clerk leaves at 5:00 P.M. and never informs you that it won't be finished for your meeting with the CEO tomorrow morning at 8:00 A.M.

These incidents have two levels of significance. First, you should be concerned because someone did not perform a task that you felt should have been performed. In this regard, providing immediate feedback along with a clear statement of your future expectations can address the performance issue. At another level, however, you may be exasperated, perhaps even exhausted, if these are the latest in a series of events that are symbolic of an uncaring, irresponsible attitude. When this happens, you may have an emotional reaction, such as disappointment, anger, or perhaps even hopelessness.

Managers often find themselves in this circumstance. Expecting others to have the same degree of investment or insight into how their actions affect others is simply setting yourself up for disappointment. Although you probably accept that it is unrealistic to expect that employees who have no ownership or who don't share in the rewards of top management should have the same degree of commitment that you have, it is always disappointing when they don't.

Employees work for the goals that are important to them. Expectancy theory, discussed in Chapter 5, suggests that you should not expect employees to work as though they were owners or top level executives when they will not in fact enjoy the rewards or benefits of these positions. Many nonexempt employees, especially, will perceive demands beyond the ordinary perhaps minimal duties of their jobs as inequitable. Generally, employees who perceive inequity will regain equity indirectly, for example by being cold or uncaring toward a patient or leaving for the day with a project incomplete. Unrealistic expectations of others will result in disappointment, doubts about your own management ability ("If I was a good manager, he never would have . . . "), and employee turnover.

When a partner or other executive behaves in ways that you perceive as unfair or irresponsible, then feelings of disappointment, anger, and even betrayal are common. What should you do about the situation? You don't have many choices. Either you can look the other way, knowing that this may perpetuate if not reinforce the behavior, or you can immediately discuss the matter with the other individual. If you choose to discuss the problem, consider undertaking this discussion at both the factual and the emotional level. Tell the partner or peer about your expectations and how his or her actions made you feel. If you were disappointed or angry, let him or her know this. This will be helpful to you because you will reduce your frustration by "getting it off your chest." It also tells the partner or peer that the behavior has affected you, and the discussion process may help clarify any misperceptions regarding mutual expectations.

Usually, directly addressing the circumstances will result in both parties adjusting their behaviors and expectations. Suppose, however, that the other individual is a partner who continues to behave in ways that you perceive as inequitable. Assuming that you have tried to clarify your expectations, you may then conclude that the transgressions were the result of conscious decisions. Your partner simply doesn't care about your feelings or what you need. In effect, your partner is not functioning as a partner and is probably focusing more on his or her personal needs. When circumstances reach this

point, you may need to consider getting a "divorce," such as the situation that we saw at Oregon Sports Medicine with Drs. Able, Baker, and Cane.

This is the time to protect your own interests and to weigh the financial and personal value of continuing the relationship against the frustration, inconvenience, and financial costs, as well as benefits, associated with dissolving the business relationship. Once again, the underlying theme is that people work for themselves. If a group practice is such that one party will tolerate a disproportionate share of the burden, then another party will invariably take advantage of this situation. Conducting civil war to regain equity will almost certainly lead to an organization that is dysfunctional. If you and your partners cannot work together without feelings of unfairness, then it may be best to recognize this reality and end the relationship.

You should, however, place your dissatisfaction into perspective. As practices have become larger and physicians find themselves working in larger health care organizations, work life simply has become much more complex. Simply having more people around, all of whom carry their own perspectives, agendas, and personal and organizational self-interests, ensures that the level of potential discord in organizations in which physicians are now finding themselves will be larger than in the past. Physicians as a profession are beginning to experience more of the frustrations of organizational life that much of the rest of society has been living with for most of the 20th century. Holding out for a standard of perfection and perfect agreement and allowing relatively minor levels of disagreement transgression or inequity to destroy a generally beneficial relationship, group practice, or your future in a large organization is self-defeating. Before you enter into civil war or organization or professional suicide, think long and hard about the cost–benefit relationship.

Personally, over the years I have had to work with a number of other professors, partners, and practice employees whose views of their organizational responsibilities were not similar to mine. On occasion, discussions got heated, sometimes even abusive. My goal, however, which I have achieved with varying degrees of success, always has been to evaluate these occurrences in the larger context, to refrain from making an emotional response, and to evaluate as best as I possibly could my long-term self-interest. Sometimes this has meant swallowing my pride, on other occasions it has meant acting swiftly and decisively, and on others it has meant biding my time and acting when the circumstances were to my advantage.

The expectation that you will be truly in control and that you can force events to occur the way that you wish is a fantasy. You can influence events to varying degrees, but you cannot control your practice, employees, or health care organization as if it were an extension of yourself. The larger the organization of which you are a part, the more it takes on a life of its own that to some extent meets the competing needs of employees, partners, departments, shareholders, patients, the community, and to some degree yourself. You cannot be everywhere all the time, and when and where you are absent these other constituencies may make decisions based on their needs; decisions that are not always in your best interest.

Someone once said that running a business is like being in a war. You are going to have casualties, and the casualties may be your needs and desires. The goal is to take acceptable casualties in relation to the objectives you achieve. No secretary will be perfect. Some fees will not be collected, and some telephone messages will be lost. Occasionally, charts will be misfiled. Others whom you counted on for political support will defect. Employees, partners, and patients will not live up to their promises. The list of daily failures can appear endless, if you choose to count them. If you are of a mind to, you can create an inexhaustible list of events over which to become upset. What you must keep in mind, however, is whether, in spite of these failures, you are achieving the objectives that are really critical to you and to your organization. This is not to say that you should be unconcerned about

setting high performance standards because, if you don't set them, no one will. Instead, this is a call for balance and realism. Effective managers know when to push. They push when it makes a real difference, and they back off when it doesn't. Effective managers also know when it's important to care and when to shrug their shoulders and recognize that tomorrow is another day.

It also is vitally important for you to examine your own need for perfection. A perfectionistic attitude can result in pushing for perfection at the wrong times or in the wrong places. Virtually every element of a physician's development and training encourages perfectionism. Perfectionism is adaptive in the practice of clinical medicine because inattention to detail can significantly affect the well-being of patients. Medicine attracts people who are intellectually oriented toward facts and details and enjoy pursuing cause-and-effect relationships. The demands of medical education tend to eliminate those who are not concerned with nuances. Finally, the physician–patient relationship is an unequal one. The patient is in a dependent position, which tends to reinforce the physician's expectation that his or her requests will be followed unquestioningly.

Unbridled perfectionism can result in striving for that last 10 percent when it really doesn't matter. If you don't choose when to be demanding, you will waste a lot of energy fighting battles of no great consequence, and you will create a tense, confrontational work environment for no good reason.

BUSINESS EXPECTATIONS

It is important to have a realistic understanding of the relationship between your practice, hospital, or health care system and others in your market. In many ways, business relationships are like the criminal justice system. In the criminal justice system, each side advocates its strongest possible position. The competition of ideas and facts, as filtered by the law, reveals the truth, which is determined by a judge or jury. In the business world, each business seeks to maximize its own gain by offering its most competitive products or services. Business law, business ethics, standards of practice, and community standards serve as the law in this competition, and the marketplace, which is both jury and judge, will determine the value of the competing services. Cooperation between adversaries, such as we see when suppliers work with hospitals to achieve mutual gain, always occurs because it is to both parties' advantage.

In the current health care market, your gain is generally a competitor's loss, and vice versa. In addition, everyone in your business environment is trying to survive, and someone else's survival might be at your expense. Every time you turn around, someone will be trying to take money out of your pocket. Employees expect pay raises, cities increase taxes on revenues and personal property, suppliers raise their prices, insurance companies increase their premiums while simultaneously tightening their claims payment criteria, some patients will not pay for services, equipment will break, new forms of providing and organizing health care services will evolve,

competitors will move into the market, others will consolidate . . . the list is endless.

This sounds like the Law of the Jungle, and it is. For many physicians, however, these business realities have been masked by a forgiving jungle in which there has been a plentiful supply of patients at fees that were tolerant of business inefficiency. Tigers can become fat and complacent when the food supply is abundant. Many health care organizations expect that revenues will always flow irrespective of the competition and changing market conditions. "It will never happen here" is still a common refrain in many regions and in many health care organizations.

For some physicians in some specialties or in well-positioned health care organizations, this may continue to be the case, for a time. Others, however, are finding a market in which increasing competition or declining patient demand requires them to run a leaner, more effective medical business now. This book provides the skills that you will need to manage that leaner, more effective medical business, whether it is in a practice, hospital, or other health care delivery system.

Index

Page numbers in italics indicate figures and exhibits
Page numbers followed by "t" indicate tables.